Lecture Notes in Computer Science 7058

Commenced Publication in 1973
Founding and Former Series Editors:
Gerhard Goos, Juris Hartmanis, and Jan van Leeuwen

Andreas Holzinger   Klaus-Martin Simonic (Eds.)

Information Quality in e-Health

7th Conference of the Workgroup
Human-Computer Interaction and Usability Engineering
of the Austrian Computer Society, USAB 2011
Graz, Austria, November 25-26, 2011
Proceedings

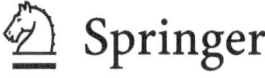 Springer

Volume Editors

Andreas Holzinger
Klaus-Martin Simonic

Medical University of Graz (MUG)
Institute of Medical Informatics, Statistics and Documentation (IMI)
Research Unit Human–Computer Interaction
Auenbruggerplatz 2/V, 8036 Graz, Austria
E-mail: {andreas.holzinger, klaus.simonic}@medunigraz.at

ISSN 0302-9743   e-ISSN 1611-3349
ISBN 978-3-642-25363-8   e-ISBN 978-3-642-25364-5
DOI 10.1007/978-3-642-25364-5
Springer Heidelberg Dordrecht London New York

Library of Congress Control Number: 2011941083

CR Subject Classification (1998): H.4-5, D.2, C.2, I.2, J.3, K.4.2

LNCS Sublibrary: SL 2 – Programming and Software Engineering

Typesetting: Camera-ready by author, data conversion by Scientific Publishing Services, Chennai, India

Printed on acid-free paper

Springer is part of Springer Science+Business Media (www.springer.com)

Preface

The topic of the USAB 2011 conference is of tremendous importance: information quality in healthcare. We envision this as the means to bridge the hiatus theoreticus, and as a means to bring technology and medicine closer together. While some aspects of human factors of technology have already been incorporated into medical informatics, information quality combines aspects understood by both fields.

Medical information systems are already highly sophisticated; however, while computer performance has increased exponentially, human cognitive evolution cannot advance at the same speed. Consequently, the focus on interaction and communication between humans and computers is of increasing importance in medicine and healthcare. The daily actions of medical professionals must be the central concern of any innovation. Simply surrounding and supporting them with new and emerging technologies is not sufficient if these increase rather than decrease the workload. Information systems are a central component of modern knowledge-based medicine and health services; therefore, it is necessary for knowledge management to continually be adapted to the needs and demands of medical professionals within this environment of steadily increasing high-tech medicine. Information processing, in particular its potential effectiveness in modern health services and the optimization of processes and operational sequences, is also of increasing interest.

It is particularly important for medical information systems (e.g., hospital information systems and decision support systems) to be designed with the daily schedules, responsibilities and exigencies of the medical professionals in mind. Within the context of this symposium our end users are medical professionals and justifiably expect the software technology to provide a clear benefit: to support them efficiently and effectively in their daily activities.

In biomedicine, healthcare, clinical medicine and the life sciences, professional end users are confronted with an increased mass of data. Research in human-computer interaction (HCI) and information retrieval (IR) or knowledge discovery in databases and data mining (KDD) has long been working to develop methods that help users to identify, extract, visualize and understand useful information from these masses of high-dimensional and mostly weakly structured data. HCI and IR/KDD, however, take very different perspectives in tackling this challenge; and historically, they have had little collaboration. Our goal is to combine these efforts to support professionals in interactively analyzing information properties and visualizing the relevant information without becoming overwhelmed. The challenge is to bring HCI and IR/KDD researchers to work together and hence reap the benefits that computer science/informatics can provide to the areas of medicine, healthcare and the life sciences.

Working in an interdisciplinary area requires the ability to communicate with professionals in other disciplines and the willingness to accept and incorporate their points of view.

USAB 2011 was organized in order to promote a close collaboration between software engineers, biomedical engineers, psychology researchers and medical professionals.

USAB 2011 received a total of 103 submissions. We followed a careful and rigorous two-level, double-blind review, assigning each paper to a minimum of three and maximum of six reviewers from our international scientific board. On the basis of the reviewers' results only 18 full papers were accepted (an acceptance rate of approx. 18%). Additionally, 29 short papers and 2 posters were accepted; resulting in a total of 49 regular papers plus 2 keynote papers (51 contributions) from 21 different countries: USA, UK, Japan, India, Iran, Korea, Finland, Italy, Cyprus, Germany, Austria, Portugal, Switzerland, Poland, The Netherlands, Belgium, Slovenia, Croatia, Greece, Turkey, and Slovakia.

The organizers saw USAB 2011 as a bridge within the scientific community, between technology and medicine. The people who gathered together to work for this conference showed great enthusiasm and dedication.

We cordially thank each and every person who contributed towards making USAB 2011 a success, for their participation and commitment: the authors, reviewers, partners, organizations, supporters, the team of the Research Unit Human–Computer Interaction for Medicine and Health Care (HCI4MED) of the Institute of Medical Informatics, Statistics and Documentation of the Medical University Graz and all the volunteers. Without their help, this bridge would never have been built.

November 2011   Andreas Holzinger
                                                      Klaus-Martin Simonic

Organization

Program Chairs

Andreas Holzinger   Medical University of Graz, Austria
Klaus-Martin Simonic   Medical University of Graz, Austria

Program Committee

Patricia A. Abbot   Johns Hopkins University, USA
Ray Adams   Middlesex University London, UK
Sheikh Iqbal Ahamed   Marquette University, USA
Henning Andersen   Technical University Denmark, Denmark
Patrick Baudisch   University of Potsdam, Germany
Russel Beale   Birmingham University, UK
Marilyn Sue Bogner   Institute for the Study of Human Error,
                             LLC Bethesda, USA
John M. Carroll   Pennsylvania State University, USA
Tiziana Catarci   Università di Roma la Sapienza, Italy
Luca Chittaro   University of Udine, Italy
Andy Cockburn   University of Canterbury, New Zealand
Matjaz Debevc   University of Maribor, Slovenia
Alan Dix   Lancaster University, UK
Judy Edworthy   University of Plymouth, UK
Jan Engelen   Katholieke Universiteit Leuven, Belgium
Pier Luigi Emiliani   National Research Council, Italy
Geraldine Fitzpatrick   Vienna University of Technology, Austria
Matjaz Gams   University of Ljubljana, Slovenia
Vlado Glavinic   University of Zagreb, Croatia
Sabine Graf   Athabasca University, Canada
Andrina Granic   University of Split, Croatia
Eduard Groeller   Vienna University of Technology, Austria
Lisa Gualtieri   Tufts University School of Medicine Boston,
                             USA
Sissel Guttormsen   University of Bern, Switzerland
Martin Hitz   Klagenfurt University, Austria
Timo Honkela   Helsinki University of Technology, Finland
Ebba P. Hvannberg   University of Iceland, Reykjavik, Iceland
Bin Hu   Birmingham City University, UK
Bo Hu   SAP Research Belfast, UK
Homa Javahery   IBM Centers for Solution Innovation, Canada
Chris Johnson   University of Glasgow, UK

Anirudha N. Joshi   Indian Institute of Technology, Bombay, India
Kinshuk   Athabasca University, Canada
Georgios Kouroupetroglou   University of Athens, Greece
Effie Lai-Chong Law   University of Leicester, UK
Denise Leahy   Trinity College Dublin, Ireland
Zhengjie Liu   Dalian Maritime University, China
ZongKai Lin   Chinese Academy of Science Peking, China
Gitte Lindgaard   Carleton University, China
Julie Maitland   Georgia Institute of Technology, USA
Flora Malamateniou   University of Pireaus, Greece
Silvia Miksch   Donau University Krems, Austria
Shogo Nishida   Osaka University, Japan
Hiromu Nishitani   University of Tokushima, Japan
Nuno J Nunes   University of Madeira, Portugal
Anne-Sophie Nyssen   Université de Liege, Belgium
Erika Orrick   GE Healthcare, Carrollton, USA
Anna-Lisa Osvalder   Chalmers University of Technology, Sweden
Philipe Palanque   Université Toulouse, France
Vimla Patel   Arizona State University, USA
Helen Petrie   University of York, UK
Margit Pohl   Vienna University of Technology, Austria
Robert W. Proctor   Purdue University, USA
Harald Reiterer   University of Konstanz, Germany
Carsten Roecker   RWTH Aachen University, Germany
Yvonne Rogers   University College London (UCL), UK
Demetrios Sampson   University of Piraeus, Greece
Anthony Savidis   ICS FORTH, Heraklion, Greece
Albrecht Schmidt   Fraunhofer IAIS/B-IT, University of Bonn,
                             Germany
Andrew Sears   UMBC, Baltimore, USA
Ahmed Seffah   EHL Lausanne, Switzerland
Cecilia Sik Lanyi   University of Pannonia, Hungary
Daniel Simons   University of Illinois at Urbana Champaign,
                             USA
Christian Stary   University of Linz, Austria
Constantine Stephanidis   ICS FORTH, Heraklion, Greece
Harold Thimbleby   University of Swansea, UK
Hironomu Takagi   Tokyo Research Laboratory, IBM, Japan
A Min Tjoa   Vienna University of Technology, Austria
Jean Underwood   Nottingham Trent University, UK
Geoff Underwood   Nottingham University, UK
Gerhard Weber   Technische Universität Dresden, Germany
Karl-Heinz Weidmann   FHV Dornbirn, Austria
William Wong   Middlesex University, London, UK
Panayiotis Zaphiris   University of Cyprus, Cyprus

Ping Zhang   Syracuse University, USA
Jiajie Zhang   University of Texas Health Science Center, USA
Martina Ziefle   RWTH Aachen University, Germany

International Scientific Workshop Committee

Mounir Ben Ayed   École Nationale d'Ingénieurs de Sfax (ENIS) and
                            Université de Sfax, Tunisia
Matt-Mouley Bouamrane   University of Glasgow, UK
Remy Choquet   Université Paris, France
Kapetanios Epaminondas   University of Westminster, London, UK
Alexandru Floares   Oncological Institute Cluj-Napoca, Romania
Adinda Freudenthal   Technical University Delft, The Netherlands
Wolfgang Gaissmaier   Max Planck Institute of Human Development,
                            Berlin, Germany
Jun Luke Huan   University of Kansas, Lawrence, USA
Anthony Hunter   UCL University College London, UK
Kalervo Järvelin   University of Tampere, Finland
Igor Jurisica   IBM Life Sciences Discovery Centre and
                            University of Toronto, Canada
Jiří Klema   Czech Technical University, Prague,
                            Czech Republic
Lubos Klucar   Slovak Academy of Sciences, Bratislava,
                            Slovakia
Patti Kostkova   City University London, UK
Damjan Krstajic   Research Centre for Cheminformatics,
                            Belgrade, Serbia
Natsuhiko Kumasaka   Center for Genomic Medicine (CGM), Tokyo,
                            Japan
Nada Lavrac   Jožef Stefan Institute, Ljubljana, Slovenia
Luca Longo   Trinity College Dublin, Ireland
András Lukacs   Hungarian Academy of Sciences and
                            Eötvös University, Budapest, Hungary
Avi Ma' ayan   The Mount Sinai Medical Center, New York,
                            USA
Ljiljana Majnaric-Trtica   Josip Juraj Strossmayer University, Osijek,
                            Croatia
Martin Middendorf   University of Leipzig, Germany
Silvia Miksch   Vienna University of Technology, Vienna,
                            Austria
Antonio Moreno-Ribas   Universitat Rovira i Virgili, Tarragona, Spain
Ant Ozok   UMBC, Baltimore, USA
Jan Paralic   Technical University of Kosice, Slovakia
Gabriella Pasi   Università di Milano Bicocca, Milan, Italy
Armando J. Pinho   Universidade the Aveiro, Portugal

Margit Pohl	Vienna University of Technology, Vienna, Austria
Paul Rabadan	Columbia University College of Physicians/Surgeons, New York, USA
Heri Ramampiaro	Norwegian University of Science and Technology, Norway
Dietrich Rebholz	European Bioinformatics Institute, Cambridge, UK
Giuseppe Santucci	La Sapienza, University of Rome, Italy
Paola Sebastiani	Boston University, USA
Andrzej Skowron	University of Warszaw, Poland
Neil R. Smalheiser	University of Illinois at Chicago, USA
Olof Torgersson	Chalmers University of Technology, Sweden
Patricia Ordonez-Rozo	University of Maryland, Baltimore County, Baltimore, USA
Jianhua Ruan	University of Texas at San Antonio, USA
Pinar Yildirim	Okan University, Istanbul, Turkey
Minlu Zhang	University of Cincinnati, USA
Xuezhong Zhou	Beijing Jiaotong University, China

Organizing Committee

Marcus Bloice	Medical University Graz
Markus Fassold	Medical University Graz
Michael Geier	Medical University Graz
Manuela Haid	Medical University Graz
Andreas Holzinger	Medical University Graz and Austrian Computer Society (Chair)
Gabriele Kröll	Medical University Graz
Gig Searle	Medical University Graz
Klaus-Martin Simonic	Medical University Graz (Co-chair)

Partners

We are grateful to all our partners, companies and institutions for their support in our aims to bridge science and business and industry and research. Their logos are displayed on our conference webpage: http://www.medunigraz.at/imi/usab2011/supporters.php

Table of Contents

Information Usability and Clinical Workflows (Session S1)

Education and Patient Empowerment (Session S4)

Patient Empowerment and Health Services (Session S 7)

Information Visualization, Knowledge and Analytics (Session S 10)

Information Usability and Accessibility (Session S 2)

Governmental Health Services and Clinical Routine (Session S 5)

Information Retrieval and Knowledge Discovery (Session S 8)

Decision Making Support and Technology Acceptance (Session S 11)

Information Retrieval, Privacy and Clinical Routine (Session S 12)

Usability and Accessibility Methodologies (Session S 9)

Information Usability and Knowledge Discovery (Session S 6)

Human-Centred Computing (Session S 3)

Poster Presentations (within Session C 4)

Biomedical Informatics in Health Professional Education (Plenary Session P 2)

Cognitive Approaches to Clinical Data Management for Decision Support: Is It Old Wine in New Bottle?

Vimla L. Patel[1] and Thomas G. Kannampallil[2]

[1] Center for Cognitive Studies in Medicine and Public Health
New York Academy of Medicine
1216 Fifth Avenue
New York, New York 10029
[2] Center for Cognitive Informatics and Decision Making
School of Biomedical Informatics
University of Texas Health Science Center
1941 East Road, Houston, TX 77054
Vimla.Patel@shortliffe.net, Thomas.Kannampallil@uth.tmc.edu

Abstract. Most current health information technology (HIT) is not designed to support the cognitive aspects of clinicians decision-making task. We propose a case for cognitive support systems (CSS), a class of support systems whose design rationale is based on aligning the decision making process closely with the empirical results on clinicians organization of knowledge structures. Using examples drawn from our current and past studies, we explain an epistemological framework of medical knowledge and how experts' representations could be better visualized within CSS for efficient and safe decision making. We discuss the state of the current research as well as the challenges for the development of patient-centered decision support, and the cognitive support for other members of the healthcare team, all within the constraints of clinical workflow.

Keywords: cognitive support systems, clinical decision making, intermediate constructs, knowledge elicitation, knowledge representation, cognitive science.

1 Introduction

Current Health Information Technology (HIT), such as Electronic Health Record systems is not designed to support the cognitive aspects of healthcare providers' decision-making tasks. EHRs often serve as a medium for information storage and are often not aligned with the mental processes underlying clinical decisions. Theory of comprehension suggests that the way information is stored at the time of input dictates the success one has at the time of retrieval [1].

In the clinical environment relevant patient-related information has to be retrieved just in time in the right context for it to be useful in providing support for healthcare providers in making clinical decisions. Thus, comprehensive understanding of the mental processes that underlie clinical tasks for making decisions are critical for decision support [2].

A. Holzinger and K.-M. Simonic (Eds.): USAB 2011, LNCS 7058, pp. 1–13, 2011.

Unlike the traditional decision support systems (DSS), cognitively based decision support, integrates cognitive aspects of the decision making including memory (help in reduction of information overload), perception (management of multiple data streams through current channels), comprehension (filtering out of irrelevant information), problem solving (use of relevant strategies for problem solutions) [3].

Clinicians' attention is a precious resource, which in the current health care practice is consumed by the cognitive demands of information overload, time pressure, multi-tasking and the need to aggregate and synthesize information from disparate sources.

The use of information processing theories from cognitive science provides a holistic framework for considering cognitive support. Comprehension of information is driven by what is perceived from the environment (e.g., reading a patient note). Comprehension also involves a complex process of perceiving the representations, matching it to existing knowledge schemas and interpreting these within the context of perceived information. The traditional mechanism of decision support is to provide support at the point of making decisions (e.g., after reading a narrative, the clinician decides to write some orders). In contrast, we propose a cognitively driven approach of supporting the comprehension of the user. In other words, cognitive support is aimed at better problem comprehension, eventually leading to better decisions and actions (see Figure 1).

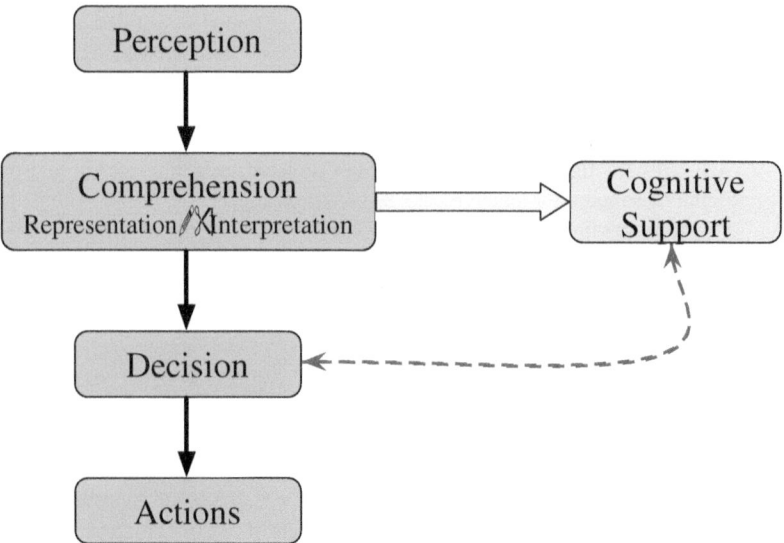

Fig. 1. Theoretical framework showing the relationship between comprehension, decision-making and the role of cognitive support. Arrows depict directionality of information flow.

2   Memory, Comprehension and Expertise

Studies on cognitive aspects of decision making has shown that as one develops expertise in a domain (e.g., chess, sports, dance, music, physics), the   knowledge of the task domain is organized in such a way that facilitates the decision making process [4].

Similarly, studies of clinical decision-making using theories and methods from cognitive science have shown that expert healthcare providers mentally organize information in task-specific ways for efficient, effective and safe diagnostic or therapeutic decisions [3].

We also know that novice clinicians frequently organize information haphazardly, according to the order in which information in entered, rather than performing any restructuring of information (like the experts).

A series of studies from late 1980s to early 1990 showed the relationship between comprehension of medical information and problem solving [3, 5-7]. Ability to separate relevant and critical information from irrelevant information was one of the major factors that identified an expert in medical domains. Development of an adequate schema was found to be necessary for this, since comprehension of information involves the development of schemata, which serve to filter relevant information selectively, thereby circumventing limitations of memory [1].

Prior research has also shown that comprehension or understanding of a clinical situation is a necessary prerequisite for accurate problem solving and decision making, and that expert clinicians are distinguished by their ability to organize information in ways (i.e., problem-specific mental representations) that facilitate rapid generation of effective and accurate solutions. A well-developed knowledge structure, as seen in the case of experts, facilitates development of better problem solving and decision making strategies [5, 6, 8].

3   Organization of Medical Knowledge

Medical knowledge can be organized as a hierarchy of concepts formed by observations at the lowest level, followed by findings, facets, and, diagnoses, as illustrated in Figure 2 [9]. This structure provides the medical domain epistemology based on the INTERNIST model [10]. Observations are units of information that are recognized as potentially relevant in the problem-solving context.

However, they do not constitute clinically useful facts. For example, a patient reporting dry skin, knee joint pain as well concentrated urine constitute as observations.

Findings include only the observations that have potential clinical significance, since not all observations are relevant to the patient problem under investigation. Establishing a finding reflects a decision made by a doctor that an array of data contains a significant cue or cues that need to be taken into account. In the above problem, only the dry skin and concentrated urine may be relevant. Facets consist of clusters of findings that indicate an underlying medical problem or class of problems, such as concept of dehydration (the above case). They reflect general descriptions of pathologic conditions, and these concepts can be generated for different clusters of findings.

For example, children with Malaria also show signs of dehydration. Facets resemble constructs used by researchers in medical artificial intelligence to describe the partitioning of a problem space [7].

Diagnosis is the level of classification that subsumes and explains all levels beneath it. Finally, the systems level consists of information that serves to contextualize a particular problem, such as the cardiovascular or endocrinology problem. An empirically tested epistemological framework such as this allows us to characterize differential organization of information in a range of tasks, from writing clinical case summaries to reasoning for diagnostic or therapeutic decisions [11].

We illustrate the various levels of the framework with an example. Consider a patient presenting to the emergency department with chest pain, shortness of breath, leg swelling, excessive sweating and a weak pulse. As described earlier, chest pain, leg swelling and excessive sweating would be considered as observations in the framework.

The presence of a deep vein thrombosis (DVT) through a Doppler scan is finding that is evolved from the preliminary observation regarding a leg swelling. These deductions (along with other evidence) can lead the physician to reach an intermediary conclusion regarding the presence of embolic phenomena in the patient. The embolic phenomena can be considered as facets, narrowing the problem space of the clinicians' possible diagnoses. They are interim hypotheses that serve to divide the information in the problem into sets of manageable sub-problems and to suggest possible solutions. Facets also vary in terms of their levels of abstraction. The conclusion in this case could be a diagnosis of pulmonary embolism (a condition where one or more arteries in the lungs become blocked).

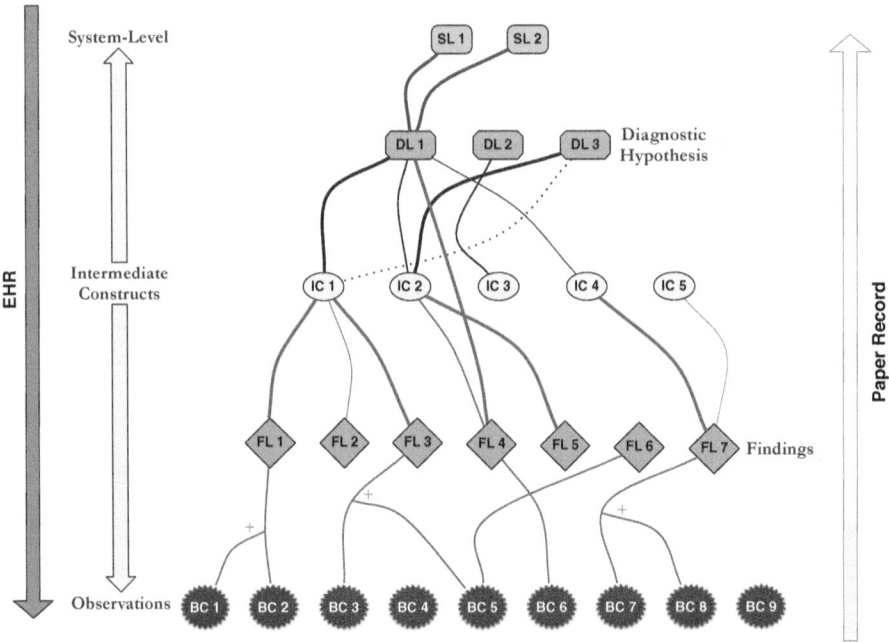

Fig. 2. Epistemological framework representing the structure of medical knowledge for clinical problem solving. The lowest or the basic concept level [10] represents the observations; FL represents the findings level; IC represents the intermediate constructs; DL represents the diagnostic hypothesis level and SL represents the systems level. Arrows represent the direction of information processing.

The framework also represents two other important characteristics: first, paper-based records support a bottom-up (i.e., from the observations to diagnosis) model of clinical diagnosis leading to a tedious, and lengthy process. Such a process is inefficient and can often affect the effectiveness of the clinicians. Second, in contrast, electronic records cater to a top-down processing of information, where clinicians first encounter system-level information. This is due to nature of organization of information in electronic health record systems, such as a clinical support filter (e.g., from the drop down menus). In effect, this leads to a few observations that narrow the search options for the clinicians.

This framework has been used as a basis for building reference models for medical knowledge [5], for coding inferences in studies of medical text comprehension [1-3, 12, 13] for characterizing clinical reasoning [5, 6] and doctor–patient interactions [8]. These reference models, which are idealizations or benchmarks of accurate reasoning, can then be mapped to clinicians' representations of clinical information.

Research results have shown that physicians understand and reason about clinical information at different levels, depending on their level of expertise. Knowledge of these differences can be useful for the design of decision-support or training systems in which information (e.g., reminders, help) could be presented at multiple levels of the aggregation. In this way, information can be matched to the level of medical knowledge a user is more likely to understand.

4   Intermediate Constructs for Cognitive Support

Characterizing the knowledge structures that underlie specific decisions can be an effective component for supporting the decision making process. To this end, utilizing the specific configurations of knowledge structures that are utilized by experts across various domains would be important. Intermediate constructs (IC's in Figure 2) facilitate effective and accurate representations of the intermediate solutions that can potentially lead to a final solution (or diagnosis). For example, in the medical domain, experts often develop such intermediate findings that are not in themselves diagnosis but help the physicians in narrowing the diagnostic search space.

Examples of the utilization of intermediate constructs can be found across several domains of problem solving. For example, expert chess players recognize higher-level patterns and perceive them as units (e.g., a queen side castle is recognized as a unit consisting of a number of chess pieces as opposed to the individual pieces) [14]. Similar constructs have been reported in the domains of sports, music as well as art [4].

Numerous similar examples are also encountered in the medical domain. Below we provide a detailed example (using a common condition, development of Sepsis, in the critical care context), on the identification of intermediate constructs through a knowledge elicitation process with clinicians. Sepsis is a bacterial infection that can affect one or more body systems and is accompanied by multiple symptoms including altered mental status, fever, hyperventilation, increased heart rate and decreased urine output. Diagnosis of sepsis involves identification of the infection and its source (e.g., kidneys). Multiple tests including blood gases, kidney functions, white blood cell (WBC) and platelet counts are used to identify the infection and its source.

In order to capture the structure of the clinical knowledge of experts regarding sepsis, we conducted interviews with pairs of clinicians where they discussed the diagnostic and/or therapeutic conditions. One key element of developing appropriate knowledge models is the use of appropriate empirical methods. We used the technique of knowledge acquisition (KA) --the process of identifying and eliciting knowledge from domain experts-- and subsequently encoding that knowledge for use. We used knowledge acquisition from two experts, through a consensus-development process. The field of cognitive science offers several methods for understanding the reasoning processes and knowledge used by experts when they solve problems.

The entire effort to capture and utilize knowledge in building a knowledge representation model in computerized form is predicated on the recognition that knowledge has a central role to play in providing tailored guidance through decision support systems [15]. In order to gain insight into their mental processes, the experts are asked to talk aloud about what they are doing and thinking while they are performing the task. In the world of cognitive science, such responses generated during problem solving are known as think-aloud protocols [16].

Participants were encouraged to discuss the condition and generate a visual representation of the organization of their knowledge on a white-board, which was captured for further analysis. The clinicians were also steered toward discussing meaningful clusters of information that they would utilize for their decisions. These sessions were audio-recorded and transcribed, and key sets of concepts were captured as Concept Maps [17, 18] using the CMapTools software [19].

From our knowledge elicitation sessions, we found that physicians organize their knowledge regarding the diagnosis and treatment of sepsis in specific ways. We present one of the examples from our knowledge elicitation sessions on how physicians utilized SIRS (Systemic Inflammatory Response Syndrome) as an intermediary step during the diagnosis and management of sepsis.

One of the initial stages in the diagnosis (and treatment) of sepsis is the identification of the inflammatory condition, SIRS. In other words, SIRS is a

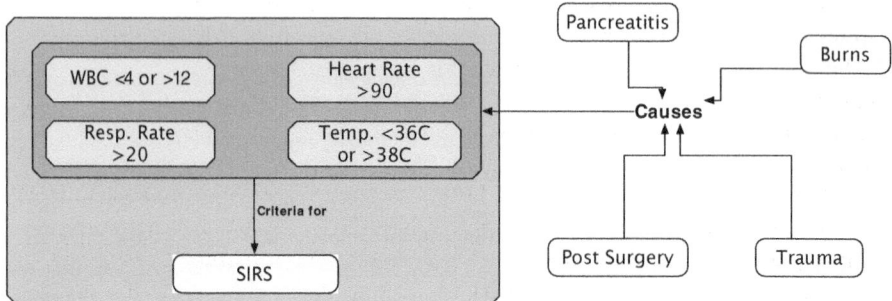

Fig. 3. An extract of the concept map showing the SIRS criteria. When two of the four relevant criteria match, the patient is considered to have SIRS.

preliminary finding of potential infection and the physician has to further explore to find the source and cause of such infection. Conditions for the manifestation of SIRS include (but not limited to) body temperature less than 36 degrees or greater than 38 degrees, heart rate greater than 90 beats per minute, tachypnea (or respiratory rate greater than 20 per minute) and white blood cell count less than 4000 cells/mm^3 or greater than 12,000 cells/mm^3 (Society of Critical Care Medicine). SIRS is diagnosed when two or more of these symptoms are present. An excerpt from a concept map that captures concepts relevant to decision making in SIRS is shown in Figure 3 (within the box the four criteria are depicted). Encapsulated in the figure are the diagnostic criteria for SIRS, which include a set of reference ranges for WBC, Heart Rate, Respiratory Rate and Temperature.

It was evident from our knowledge elicitation sessions that the physicians utilized SIRS as an intermediate stage, where they explicitly aggregated information from multiple sources, towards the diagnosis of the sources of infection and sepsis. The decision as to whether a patient exhibits SIRS as a sub-component of a larger decision process, which includes an assessment of the probability of underlying infection, and an exploratory search for likely causes of this infection. However, we focus on the physicians' ability to identify "is this SIRS?" as an illustrative example of how experts organize their knowledge during the diagnosis and management of complex medical conditions.

In the above-mentioned example of intermediate constructs of SIRS, there are several purposes that are served: first, the intermediate constructs act as a starting point for further investigation and diagnosis. By abstracting the problem space and narrowing the available choices to a limited number of options, the expert clinician is able to quickly reduce an open-ended, ill-structured [20, 21] diagnostic problem in to manageable proportions. Second, the intermediate constructs allow for the flexible investigation of a diagnostic case. For example, by quickly identifying the intermediate constructs (SIRS), the clinician can further investigate key aspects of the parameters that led to SIRS (e.g., temp, heart rate or respiratory rate) or go on to the specific case diagnosis. This flexibility early on in the diagnostic process provides clinicians ability to better comprehend the problem at a granular level (e.g., from observational values) or from a global level (disease or hypothesis level).

Additionally, the nature and properties of the intermediate constructs also make it amenable for its incorporation into clinical decision support systems. Next, we discuss how intermediate constructs can be incorporated into clinical systems for providing better real-time cognitive support.

5   Utilizing Intermediate Constructs for Clinical Decision Support

Utilizing theories and concepts from human reasoning and decision-making can provide a foundation for the design of better systems to support healthcare practice. Knowledge elicitation techniques, methods and theories from cognitive science can be used to effectively characterize the processes that underlie human interaction with information technology.

Such characterization and understanding provides a basis for the development of support tools that can aid physicians for making clinical decisions. These support tools, which we refer to as cognitive support systems, aim to *support* human behavior by closely aligning the decision-making process with the cognitive processes of human decision making.

The need for cognitive support systems is also driven by the fact that physicians attention is consumed by cognitive demands from information overload, time pressure, distributed information and complex patient conditions [11]. In order to make efficient and appropriate clinical decisions, the physician must be supported with tools that align with and aid their medical reasoning and decision-making [7].

Our approach towards the design of cognitive support systems is derived from over two decades of research on medical cognition and decision-making. Prior research has shown that experts develop significant abilities to organize information in a manner that facilitates quick and efficient diagnostic solutions. We proposed a case for cognitive support systems bridging the cognitive theories of medical cognition, medical knowledge organization and reasoning, based on *intermediate constructs* that play a significant role in expert decision making [6]. As suggested in the previous section, intermediate constructs afford several potential advantages for clinical decision-making.

One of the aspects of an effective decision support system is to support the analytical reasoning process of decision-maker. Complex patient conditions present significantly challenging, ill-structured problems for the physician. The problem is compounded by the multitude of information about the patient that is available in multiple formats (e.g., images, graphs, text). The different sources of information include lab results, flow sheets, medications, prior medical history and x-rays. Prior research [6] has shown that expert physicians selectively attend to the available information based on their prior knowledge and the context of the problem.

Use of intermediate constructs gives the physicians the added ability to flexibly move between the levels of knowledge (see Figure 2) depending on their understanding of the patient condition. For example, in the case of the SIRS example, the physician can choose to examine the specific components of the SIRS hypothesis (e.g., temperature, HR) or proceed to investigate the inherent sources and causes of the infection by looking into further test results. Additionally, such a process allows designers of cognitive support systems to provide mechanisms for supporting such flexible investigation through appropriate visualization techniques.

One of the insights that we gained from our knowledge elicitation session was that physicians utilized certain operators to describe the nature of information that they would need to further explore their available data.

We call these, conceptual operators [22], which allow for the categorical evaluation of the parameters that are involved in making decisions regarding an intermediate construct. In other words, these conceptual operators were the analytical mechanism by which physicians evaluated various criteria when arriving at atomic decisions (e.g., an intermediate decision regarding the presence of SIRS in a patient). A detailed description and coding of conceptual operators can be found elsewhere (See [23]), but for the purposes of clarity and explanation we provide a summary with a few examples (See Table 1).

Table 1. Example of the various operators that were derived from our analysis (adapted from [23])

Operator	Example
Compare to norm	Physician 1: "And white count is greater than 12 but less than 4" Physician 2: "right" Physician 1: "and fever is greater than 38 or less than 36"
Compare to expected	Physician 2: " it would, so there's variations where obviously if you have heart condition, you may not get to a heart rate of 90, um, if you are on sedative drugs"
Compare over time	Physician 2: " over the course of 2-3 days if it goes up you start worrying about it"

We describe three conceptual operators: (a) compare-to-norm involves the comparison of an observed parameter to a specific known reference ranges (e.g., a WBC count of less than 4 or greater than 12), (b) compare-to-expected is the comparison under mitigating circumstances to the reference ranges (e.g., when the patient is sedated, the reference values for heart rate can be different) and (c) compare-over-time involves a time-variant evaluation of the changes in a considered variable (e.g., how temperature changed over the last 24 hours). The use of conceptual operators to investigate variables provides an opportunity to embed visualization tools for that support specific cognitive requirements of the physicians. For example, one can consider conceptual operators as a basis for designing the visual elements that can provide analytical evaluation mechanisms for the clinicians. While further research, especially on empirical evaluation of such operators, still needs to be done, our current data provides potential avenues for improving the state of the art of decision support.

Another related potential benefit in integrating intermediate constructs into clinical decision support systems is its ability to provide contextual focus for the clinician. In other words, experts' utilization of intermediate constructs during their diagnostic decision making process helps in situating a problem within a specific focus (e.g., SIRS within the larger context of sepsis) while allowing for a higher-level perspectives. Such focus + context approaches [24] are utilized in information visualization to allow users to get a clear idea of the primary interest presented in full detail along with the perspective of the larger problem as a whole. Such visualization approaches (e.g., see the hyperbolic browser) allow the user to focus on the specific data point of interest and easily within the larger context of the whole data set. Navigating to new data points put that point in focus within the context of the entire data set. Similarly, the utilization of intermediate constructs allows for focusing on specific atomic decision points within the context of the overall diagnostic problem.

The utilization of intermediate constructs also helps in breaking down a complex diagnostic problem into simpler categories and related concepts that can be more easily understood and resolved. As argued elsewhere (e.g., [6]), breaking down complex problems into more manageable proportions helps in quicker, and more appropriate solutions.

A cognitive support system that has intermediate constructs included will allow for such problem decomposition and is more likely to make diagnostic problem solving more efficient.

Theoretically, the role of intermediate constructs for clinical decision-making makes a great deal of common sense, However, there is limited empirical evidence on the utility and efficacy of these constructs as mechanism for cognitive support in clinical settings. Currently, we are running simulated laboratory-based experiments to test the use of intermediate constructs. We also have planned evaluations of a cognitive support system in clinical settings that use intermediate constructs as the underlying mechanism for cognitive support.

Based on this expert knowledge, new technological support can be created to help clinicians to make better decisions. In addition, this support system, properly implemented, must include the concepts, principles, and procedures of the work domain, together with cognitive nature of the task performed by the clinicians in their natural clinical environment. So, our next natural step was to collect field data from the critical care environment. We investigated physicians' information needs during clinical rounds in the medical intensive care unit [25] and found significant sub-optimal patterns in the manner and mode of information seeking and organization. Most of the current decision support is provided through EHRs and the current use of the electronic and paper records together adds another set of complicating factor in real time decision making. These results on clinical workflow together with how experts elicit and use knowledge in their natural setting and will help us understand the nature of their information needs, which will provide reality check on our cognitive support design for EHR.

6   Future Directions and Challenges

We presented a case for using intermediate constructs as a basis for the development of cognitive support systems for medical decision-making. Drawing from over two decades of research in cognitive science and medicine, we have argued for incorporation of these intermediate level constructs into cognitively driven clinical decision support systems and how the new representation can potentially improve the efficiency and effectiveness of clinical decisions for patient care. In spite of its several suggestive advantages, further research is necessary before we can truly utilize intermediate constructs into real world applications. Below we describe some of the challenges (and opportunities) for incorporating intermediate constructs into cognitive support systems.

We have addressed the issues surrounding expert cognitive decision support, but the task becomes more complex once we start discussing cognitive approaches to patient data management for *patient-centered* decision making and cognitive support. *Patient centered decision-making* is relevant to patients as well as to the clinicians during their interaction. Patient-centered decision support (PCDS), although not a new phenomenon, has recently attracted renewed attention [26]. In the health care environments, clinicians work as teams, and so knowledge representations of the clinical team that support team decisions need to be considered.

For example, how can intermediate constructs be used to provide a unified perspective regarding a patient case in a team setting where there are clinicians of different expertise (e.g., attending physicians, nurses, residents, and fellows)? In addition, various clinical personnel who are not clinical experts also use decision support systems. Embellishing the decision model for these less-than-experts will also be necessary.

It is clear from the empirical studies of support system that implementation and recommendations for their design that integration with workflow is key to success [26]. How to integrate the new representations into patient centered decision support and then introduce within clinicians' workflow, remains a challenge, in part because there are no current standards for clinical workflow [27]. In addition to integration with the workflow, the success of such implementation or intervention is determined by the policies, norms, constraints, and tasks of the organization in which they are being used [27, 28]. Although many of the challenges and barriers experienced during the design stage of any HIT can be overcome, additional ones (intended and unintended) may arise during the implementation phase [28, 29].

In this paper, we argued that decision models based on the underlying human decision-making process could form the basis for a cognitive support system. Our notion differs radically from the conventional notions of a decision support system, partly in that we attempt to support human cognition at the level of perception, synthesis and comprehension of information rather than unilaterally make diagnostic or therapeutic decisions, although we consider the latter to be important.

Clinicians have appropriately been unwilling to entrust their diagnostic and therapeutic decision-making to machinery. To do so would deprive the patient of a set of expertise that is uniquely human. However, at the proximal point of these decisions, where information must be selected, organized and synthesized, opportunity exists for a computerized system to play a pivotal, collaborative role in the decision-making process.

Acknowledgments. Part of the work reported in this paper was supported by an award from James S McDonnell Foundation (220020152) and from the US Office of the National Coordinator for Health Information (10510592). We thank the members of our research team, Trevor Cohen, Eric Li, Ram Vedam, Dinesh Gottipati, Naveen Kommera, Bela Patel and Khalid Almoosa.

References

1. Kintsch, W.: The role of knowledge in discourse comprehension construction-integration model. Psychological Review 95, 163–182 (1988)
2. Groen, G.J., Patel, V.L.: Relationship Between Comprehension and Reasoning in Medical Expertise. Lawrence Erlbaum (1988)

3. Patel, V.L., Arocha, J.F., Kaufman, D.R.: Diagnostic Reasoning and Expertise. The Psychology of Learning and Motivation: Advances in Research and Theory 31, 137–252 (1994)
4. Ericsson, K.A.: The road to excellence: the acquisition of expert performance in the arts and sciences, sports and games. Lawrence Erlbaum (1996)
5. Patel, V.L., Groen, G.J.: Knowledge-based solution strategies in medical reasoning. Cognitive Science 10, 91–116 (1986)
6. Patel, V.L., Groen, G.J.: The General and Specific Nature of Medical Expertise: A Critical Look. In: Ericsson, A., Smith, J. (eds.) Towards a General Theory of Expertise: Prospects and Limits, pp. 93–125. Cambridge University Press, Cambridge (1991)
7. Patel, V.L., Kaufman, D.R.: Cognitive science and biomedical informatics. In: Shortliffe, E.H., Cimino, J.J. (eds.) Biomedical Informatics: Computer Applications in Health Care and Biomedicine, 3rd edn., pp. 133–185. Springer, Heidelberg (2006)
8. Patel, V.L., Evans, D.A., Kaufman, D.R.: Cognitive framework for doctor-patient interaction. In: Evans, D.A., Patel, V.L. (eds.) Cognitive Science in Medicine: Biomedical Modeling, pp. 253–308. MIT Press, Cambridge (1989)
9. Patel, V.L., Kaufman, D.R.: Clinical Reasoning and Biomedical Knowledge. In: Higgs, J., Jones, M. (eds.) Clinical Reasoning in the Health Professions, pp. 117–128. Butterworth Heinemann, Oxford (1995)
10. Miller, R.A., Pople, H.E., Myers, J.D.: INTERNIST-1: An Experimental Computer-Based Diagnostic Consultant for General Internal Medicine. New England Journal of Medicine 19, 307 (1982)
11. Patel, V.L., Kaufman, D.R., Arocha, J.F.: Emerging Paradigms of Cognition and Medical Decision Making. Journal of Biomedical Informatics 35, 52–75 (2002)
12. Norman, G.R., Coblentz, C.L., Brooks, L.R., Babcook, C.J.: Expertise in visual diagnosis: a review of the literature. Academic Medicine 67, 78–83 (1992)
13. Sharda, P., Das, A., Cohen, T., Patel, V.L.: Customizing clinical narratives for the electronic medical record interface using cognitive methods. International Journal of Medical Informatics 75, 346–368 (2006)
14. Chase, H., Simon, H.A.: Perception in Chess. Cognitive Psychology 4, 55–81 (1973)
15. Shortliffe, E.H., Patel, V.L.: Generation and Formulation of Knowledge: Human-Intensive Techniques. In: Greenes, R.A. (ed.) Clinical Decision Support - The Road Ahead, pp. 207–226. Elsevier (2007)
16. Ericsson, K.A., Simon, H.A.: Protocol Analysis: Verbal Reports as Data. MIT Press (1993)
17. Cañas, A.J., Novak, J.D.: A concept map-centered learning environment. In: Proceedings of the 11th Biennial Conference of the European Association for Research in Learning and Instruction, EARLI (2005)
18. Patel, V.L., Arocha, J.F.: Cognitive models of clinical reasoning and conceptual representation. Methods of Information in Medicine 34(1), 1–10 (1995)
19. Cañas, A.J., Hill, G., Carff, R., Suri, N., Lott, J., Eskridge, T.: CmapTools: A knowledge modeling and sharing environment (2004)
20. Simon, H.A.: Structure of ill-structured problems. Artificial Intelligence 4(3-4), 181–201 (1973)
21. Simon, H.A.: The Sciences of the Artificial. MIT Press (1996)
22. Hassebrock, F., Prietula, M.J.: A Protocol-Based Coding Scheme for the Analysis of Medical Reasoning. International Journal of Man-Machine Studies 37(5), 613–652 (1992)
23. Cohen, T., Kannampallil, T.G., Patel, V.L.: Perils of Thoughtless Design: A Case for Cognitive Support Systems Under Review (2011)

24. Lamping, J., Rao, R., Pirolli, P.: A Focus+Context Technique Based on Hyperbolic Geometry for Visualizing Large Hierarchies. In: Proceedings of the Proc. ACM Conf. Human Factors in Computing Systems, CHI (1995)
25. Gottipati, D., Nguyen, V., Myneni, S., Almoosa, K.L., Kannampallil, T.G., Patel, V.L.: Information Integration Model in Critical Care Setting: Role of Electronic Health Records. In: Proceedings of the AMIA Annual Symposium (2011)
26. Stead, W., Lin, H.: Computational Technology for Effective Health Care: Immediate Steps and Strategic Directions. National Research Council (2009)
27. Agency for Healthcare Research and Quality U.S. Department of Health and Human Services, C. N. Challenges and Barriers to Clinical Decision Support (CDS) Design and Implementation Experienced in the Agency for Healthcare Research and Quality CDS Demonstrations (2010)
28. Ash, J.S., Sittig, D.F., Poon, E.G., Guappone, K., Campbell, E., Dykstra, R.H.: The extent and importance of unintended consequences related to computerized provider order entry. Journal of American Medical Informatics Association 14, 415–423 (2007)
29. Bloomrosen, M., Starren, J., Lorenzi, N.M., Ash, J.S., Patel, V.L., Shortliffe, E.H.: Anticipating and addressing the unintended consequences of health IT and policy: a report from the AMIA 2009 Health Policy Meeting. Journal of American Medical Informatics Association 18(1), 82–90 (2011)

Visualization of Patient Samples by Dimensionality Reduction of Genome-Wide Measurements

Huilei Xu and Avi Ma'ayan[*]

Department of Pharmacology and Systems Therapeutics, Systems Biology Center New York
(SBCNY), Mount Sinai School of Medicine, New York, NY 10029
avi.maayan@mssm.edu

Abstract. As the cost of genome-wide profiling is decreasing, the possibility for using such technologies for routine diagnostics as well as for classification and stratification of patients in clinical settings is increasing. However, the high dimensionality of such data makes it challenging to interpret and visualize for comparing and contrasting patient samples. Here we propose two visualization methods that display unsupervised clustering of genome-wide profiling of mRNA from breast cancer tumors from patients as images that can quickly show clusters of patients based on their expression profiles with perspective of their clinical outcome. The first visualization method converts expression profiles into a sparse network, whereas the second method visualizes patient samples on a hexagonal grid. Both visualization methods use the first three coordinates from principle component analysis (PCA) applied to reduce the dimensionality of the data. Colors of nodes in the network or hexagons are based on clinical outcome or tumor estrogen receptor (ER) status. Such visualization methods could be useful for grouping patients in an unsupervised manner to predict outcome and tailor personalized therapeutics.

Keywords: Microarrays, Graph Theory, Hexagonal Grid, Principle Component Analysis, Dimensionality Reduction, Data Visualization.

1 Introduction

Efforts are abound to reduce the dimensionality of high-dimensional objects for the purpose of visualizing the similarity between these objects in two-dimensional space. The most popular method for achieving such visualization is Principle Component Analysis (PCA) scatter plot, but there are other alternative approaches. For example, some relevant prior work developed the methods Locally Linear Embedding (LLE) [1], Isometric Feature Mapping (IFM) [2], and Mapper [3] to visualize multivariate non-linear objects into low-dimensional space. LLE attempts to find non-linear functions that can be mapped onto the Euclidean space of the objects with neighborhood-preserving embedding of the high-dimensionality of the objects. IFM combines classical Multidimensional Scaling (MDS) with estimation of geodesic

---

[*] Corresponding author.

A. Holzinger and K.-M. Simonic (Eds.): USAB 2011, LNCS 7058, pp. 15–22, 2011.

distances between pairs of objects of high-dimensional space by computing pair-wise shortest paths between objects. The basic idea behind Mapper is to preserve the nearness distances between high-dimensional objects while distorting the larger distances through various distance functions. Later, Nicolau et al. [4] applied Mapper to analyze gene expression samples from breast cancer patients. Indeed, there is a growing need to develop computational methods for visualizing high-dimensional genome-wide expression datasets collected from patients for stratifying patients for disease sub-classification and personalized medicine. Existing methods are complicated and produce displays that are not showing clearly and directly the relationships between patient samples. Here we introduce two dimensionality reduction unsupervised clustering visualization methods that combine Principle Component Analysis (PCA) with graph-based or self-organizing-map-based visualizations of genome-wide expression data from breast cancer tumors combined with clinical outcome data.

2   Methods

The patients samples used are from a genome-wide mRNA expression microarray dataset collected from 310 patients (GEO accession GSE25055) with newly diagnosed HER2-negative breast cancer, treated with taxane-anthracycline chemotherapy pre-operatively and endocrine therapy if ER-positive, as reported in reference [5]. In [5] the response of patients was assessed at the end of neoadjuvant treatment and distant-relapse-free survival was followed for at least three years post-surgery. Probesets from the microarray dataset were mapped to genes. For genes with multiple probesets average expression was calculated.

Principle Component Analysis (PCA) and construction of patient-patient similarity matrix was then performed as follows: Coefficient of variation C_V was used to measure the variability of gene expression across all samples. For each gene, C_V was calculated as follows:

$$C_V(g_i) = \frac{stddev(g_i)}{mean(g_i)} . \tag{1}$$

Genes were then sorted based on C_V and PCA was performed on the top 1000 genes. Distance between pairwise patients was then calculated as the Euclidean distance between two patients in the principal component space in respect to their loading scores of the first three principal components. Specifically, for two patients $X = (x_1, x_2, x_3)$ and $Y = (y_1, y_2, y_3)$, where x_k and y_k was the score of X and Y to the kth principal component, respectively, the distance between patient X and Y is:

$$d(X,Y) = \sqrt{\sum_{k=1}^{3} (x_k - y_k)^2} \ . \tag{2}$$

All analyses were performed using the statistic toolbox of MATLAB (Natick, MA). The patient-patient similarity network was then constructed based on this distance matrix where nodes represent patients and edges represent patient-patient similarities. To minimize connectivity for clear visualization, each node was connected to its two closest neighbors based on the Euclidean distance matrix. Network layout was automatically determined by the yEd software using the organic layout settings.

The hexagonal visualization of patient samples was done as follows: The data described above was reorganized into a $N \times M$ data matrix D where rows represent tumor samples and columns are the top three loading scores from the principal component analysis. Using simulated annealing, the patient samples were rearranged on the hexagonal grid based on correlations between sample loading scores using the same technique implemented to develop the software GATE [6]. Specifically, the data matrix D was rearranged on the hexagonal array H by a mapping function $f(D) \to H$. In order to find the mapping $f(D)$ that captures a high quality clustering result, we assigned the fitness function $\mathrm{Fit}[f(D)]$ to each mapping:

$$-1 \leq \mathrm{Fit}[f(D)] = \frac{\sum_{i=1}^{N} \sum_{j \in N_i} C_{ij}}{6N} \leq 1 \ . \tag{3}$$

where C_{ij} is the Pearson correlation coefficient between two variables and N_i are the six neighbors of hexagon h_i. This way we identify a mapping $f_*(D)$ with near-optimal fitness using a standard simulated annealing algorithm.

Finally, we replace nodes and hexagons with silhouettes of a person colored based on the clinical outcome or ER status.

3   Results and Conclusions

Our goal is to summarize and compare in a neat display individual patients based on their molecular profiles and clinical outcomes. As an example, here we applied our methods to published invasive breast cancer genome-wide mRNA expression data where clinical outcome was available [5]. Currently the molecular stratifying of breast cancer patients is mainly achieved through their estrogen-receptor (ER) status. If the ER gene is over-expressed the tumor is deemed ER positive. ER positive patients are more likely to have a better outcome, mostly because current drugs can target the ER pathway by antagonizing it with drugs that inhibit ER activity. However, the ER status only shows a

(A)

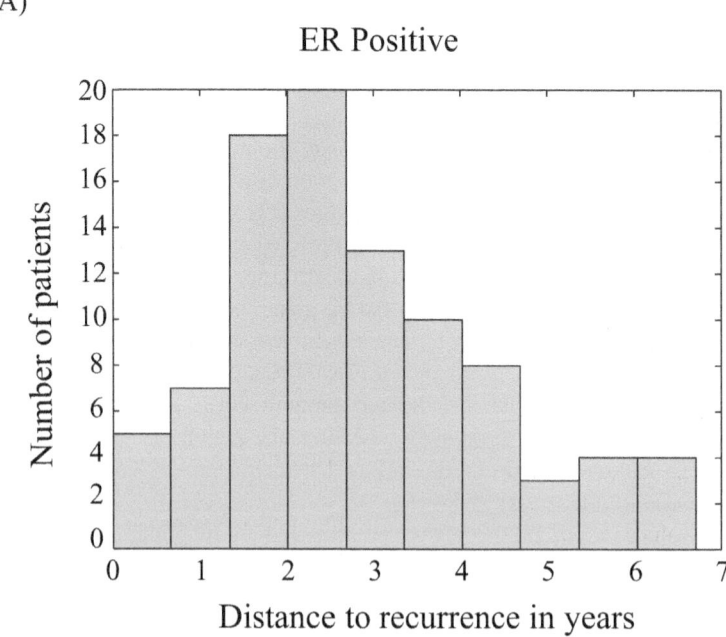

(B)

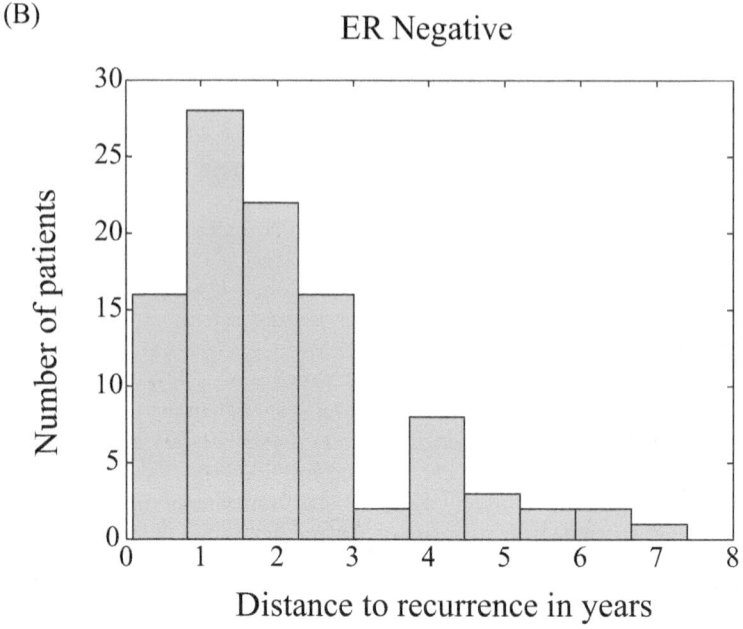

Fig. 1. Histograms of distance to recurrence for ER positive and negative patients. Distribution of the distance to recurrence in years for (A) ER-positive and (B) ER-negative patients.

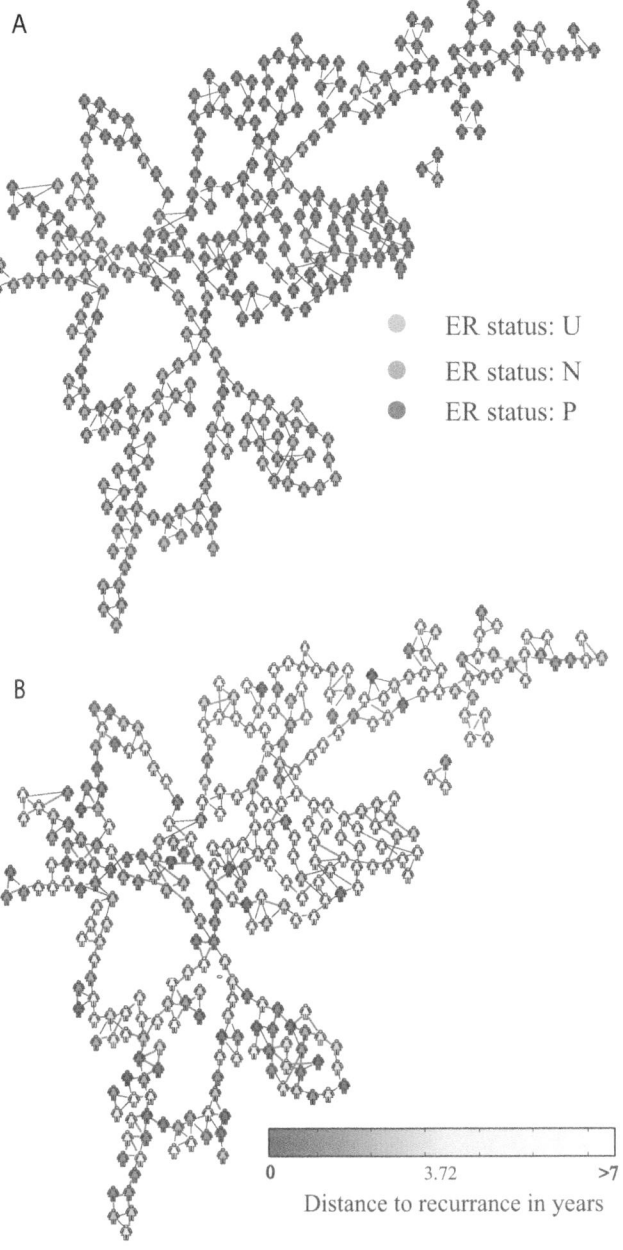

A

ER status: U

ER status: N

ER status: P

B

0   3.72   >7
Distance to recurrence in years

Fig. 2. Unsupervised network visualization of gene expression microarrays of breast cancer patients. In the network, nodes represent profiled tumors from patients, (A) color-coded based on ER status, or (B) distance to recurrence in years. Each patient sample is connected to the two closest neighbors based on pairwise Euclidean distance extracted from the first three principal components. ER status: P-positive; N-negative; and U-undetermined.

(A)

(B)

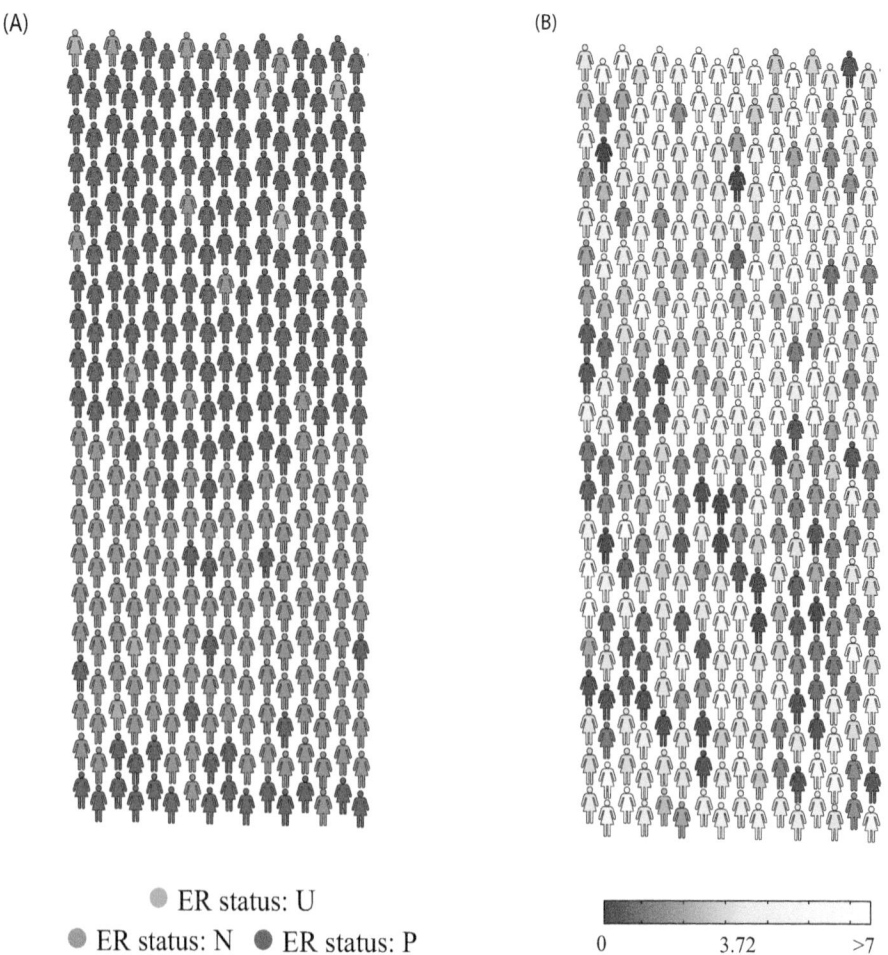

⬤ ER status: U

⬤ ER status: N   ⬤ ER status: P

0   3.72   >7

Fig. 3. Hexagonal grid visualization of patients. Each human icon represents a profiled tumor biopsy from individual patients and is color-coded based on (A) ER status or (B) distance to recurrence in years. The hexagonal grid folds on itself to form a torus such that hexagons at the edges are close to hexagon from the opposite side. Patients are arranged based on correlation of their first three principal component loading scores.

trend in recurrence outcome, making stratification of patients by this one variable alone very fuzzy, as seen when plotting a histogram of the recurrence distribution of the ER positive and negative patients from reference [5] (Fig. 1). To better visually explore the relationship between ER status and recurrence outcome, we visualized patient-patient similarity based on the mRNA expression profiling data collected from the 310 breast cancer patients [5]. To visualize this data we first identified the most variable genes, then applied PCA on the matrix of variable genes and patient samples, then applied Euclidian geometry using the top three principle components from the principal component space for each sample to construct a network (Fig. 2), or to display the data on a hexagonal grid (Fig. 3). In each of the visualization displays, nodes in the networks or hexagons on the grid are drawn as human-shaped silhouette icons colors based on the ER status or distance to recurrence outcome. The resultant networks (Fig. 2) and hexagonal grids (Fig. 3) are highly consistent with the ER status of the patients. This means that the global expression profiles of the patients can be mostly divided into two groups based on ER status. In other words, ER status has a strong effect on the entire global expression state of the tumors. However, as seen from the histogram in Fig. 1, distance to recurrence is only trending with ER status, suggesting that there are other confounding factors that affect distance to recurrence that could be unrelated to the initial gene expression profiling. The visualization of the network or hexagonal grid color-coded with the distance to recurrence outcome, right next to the same plot showing the ER status identifies, to some extent, subgroups of patients in the ER positive and negative groupings that have either favorable or unfavorable outcomes. Such refined clustering intuitively helps in understanding the dataset better. Therefore, our visualization methods may be helpful for placing newly profiled patients within their respective clusters for outcome prediction and potentially can help physicians to make appropriate and better decisions about treatment options in clinical settings. These visualization methods can be applied to other diseases profiled with other types of genome-wide profiling technologies in other clinical settings.

Acknowledgements. This work was supported by NIH grants P50GM071558-03, R01DK088541-01A1, RC2LM010994-01, P01DK056492-10, RC4DK090860-01, and KL2RR029885-0109.

References

1. Roweis, S.T., Saul, L.K.: Nonlinear dimensionality reduction by locally linear embedding. Science 290(5500), 2323–2326 (2000)
2. Tenenbaum, J.B., de Silva, V., Langford, J.C.: A global geometric framework for nonlinear dimensionality reduction. Science 290(5500), 2319–2323 (2000)
3. Singh, G., Mémoli, F., Carlsson, G.: Topological Methods for the Analysis of High Dimensional Data Sets and 3D Object Recognition. In: Eurographics Symposium on Point-Based Graphics (2007)

4. Nicolau, M., Levine, A.J., Carlsson, G.: Topology based data analysis identifies a subgroup of breast cancers with a unique mutational profile and excellent survival. Proc. Natl. Acad. Sci. U.S.A 108(17), 7265–7270 (2011)
5. Hatzis, C., Pusztai, L., Valero, V., Booser, D.J., Esserman, L., Lluch, A., Vidaurre, T., Holmes, F., Souchon, E., Wang, H., et al.: A genomic predictor of response and survival following taxane-anthracycline chemotherapy for invasive breast cancer. JAMA 305(18), 1873–1881 (2011)
6. MacArthur, B.D., Lachmann, A., Lemischka, I.R., Ma'ayan, A.: GATE: software for the analysis and visualization of high-dimensional time series expression data. Bioinformatics 26(1), 143–144 (2010)

Contextual Search: Issues and Challenges

Gabriella Pasi

Università degli Studi di Milano Bicocca, Viale Sarca 336, 20131 Milano, Italy
pasi@disco.unimib.it

Abstract. To overcome the "one size fits all" behavior of most search engines, in recent years a great deal of research has addressed the problem of defining techniques aimed at tailoring the search outcome to the user context to the aim of improving the quality of search. The main idea is to produce context-dependent and user-tailored search results. Search tasks are subjective, and often complex; the user-system interaction based on keyword-based querying and on the presentation of search results as a list of web pages ordered according to their estimated relevance is often unsatisfactory. In this paper a short overview of the main issues related to contextual search are outlined.

Keywords: Information Retrieval, Context modeling, User Modelling, Search Personalisation.

1   Introduction

The advent of the Internet and the birth of the World Wide Web have caused a strong resurgence of interest in Information Retrieval [1]. With the diffusion of the World Wide Web the amount of information available on-line has increased to a point to generate great demand for effective systems that allow easy and flexible access to information relevant to some specific needs. By flexibility it is meant the capability of the system to both manage imperfect (vague and/or uncertain) information, and to adapt its behaviour to the search and user context [1,2]. Moreover, more recently, the increasing interest in defining the so called Semantic Web requires the definition of a more powerful and flexible basic infrastructure than the existing one to organise, link, and give meaning to the huge amount of available data/information, and to allow for better (more natural) communication between humans and machines.

Search engines constitute the tip of the iceberg of Information Retrieval. However, despite the above mentioned needs most search engines apply the "one size fits all" search paradigm, by which distinct users formulating the same query obtain the same retrieval results in spite of the fact that their preferences could be defined by different criteria and with different aims. In textual information retrieval (i.e. the automatic process of retrieving texts relevant to specific users' needs) the terms extracted from or associated with the texts (called the index terms) constitute the information granules on which the IR systems work.

The central, but ill-defined, concept in IR is the concept of relevance; the main objective of Search Engines is to estimate the relevance of Web pages to the

A. Holzinger and K.-M. Simonic (Eds.): USAB 2011, LNCS 7058, pp. 23–30, 2011.

information needs expressed in the user's query. However, only the user can determine the true relevance of a document, i.e., the usefulness, pertinence, appropriateness, or utility of that document with respect to the user search intents formally sketched in a query. Relevance is time, situation, and user specific. Moreover, in assessing the utility of a document, users are influenced by many factors that go beyond topical relevance, i.e. whether or not a given document is about the topics covered in the users' queries. Relevance is in fact a multi-dimensional notion that depends on many complex factors related to the user, to her/his context, and to the document and search context too. An effective automatic estimate of the relevance of documents to a query should attempt, in some way, to take into account a context model, and to asses document relevance based on several dimensions, related to document usefulness and quality.

An important objective in contextualizing search is not to burden the user-system interaction with the need of explicitly specifying contextual information; on the contrary, a good context aware system should be able to identify the useful context information by making the user unaware of this. Moreover a good system should be able to detect the often complex and dynamic characteristics of users search tasks. Users often employ a search engine to the aim of undertaking a complex search, or, on the contrary, an exploratory search [3]. In a complex search what the user is looking for is clear, but it is the result of a complex task she/he has in mind, while in exploratory search the user does not have a precise idea of what she/is is looking for [3]. An effective system should be reactive in the case of a complex search; it should understand that a search mission is ongoing, and offer a user a high level interaction, by giving her/him suggestions and help, by also keeping track of the user's actions and the collected information (context) and using it. On the contrary, in the case of exploratory search, the system should avoid to interfere with the user's search. The identification of the kind of search the user is willing to undertake is a difficult task, which deserves research efforts [2].

This paper addresses the problem of modeling and using context to improve search; it shortly presents and reviews a few main issues and problems related to contextualizing search, by trying to outline both the research challenges and the user role and involvement in the various identified tasks.

2   Contextualizing Search

In recent years there has been increasing research interest in the problem of contextualizing search in order to overcome the limitations of the "one size fits all" search paradigm, which is generally applied by Search Engines. By this paradigm the keyword-based query is considered as the only carrier of the users' information needs. As a consequence, the document relevance estimate is system-centered, as the user context is not taken into account. Instead, a contextual Search Engine relies on a user-centered approach since it involves processes, techniques and algorithms that exploit as much contextual factors as possible in order to tailor the search results to users [4],[5],[6],[7],[8],[9],[10].

A context aware search system should be able to produce answers to a specific query, by also taking into account the contextual knowledge formally expressed in a context model. The key notion of context has multiple interpretations in Information Retrieval [11]; it may be related to the characteristics and topical preferences of a specific user or group of users (in this case contextualization is referred to as personalization), or it may be related to spatio-temporal coordinates, it may refer to the information that qualifies the content of a given document/web page (for example its author, its creation date, its format etc.), or it may refer to a social or socio-economic context.

The development and increasing use of tools which either help users to express or to automatically learn their preferences, along with the availability of devices and technologies that can detect users' location (such as GPSs) and monitor users' actions, allow to capture the user's context. Moreover, the Internet of Things and the Web of Things will increasingly offer means and opportunities to model context as well as to exploit context for improving and tailoring several applications to specific user needs [12],[13],[14].

To model new paradigms for contextualized search, a significant amount of research has addressed two main problems:

1) How to learn and model context, and
2) How to exploit it in the retrieval process in order to provide context-aware results.

In recent years several research works have offered possible solutions to the above problems related to the considered interpretation of context, leading to the creation of specific IR sectors such as personalized IR, mobile IR, social IR. Although the contextual models proposed within these branches of research vary (due to the different aspects of context that need to be modelled), their common issue is to improve the quality of search by proposing to the user results tailored to the considered context. The majority of the proposed approaches are related to personalization, i.e. enhancing the search outcome based on knowledge and consideration, in the retrieval process, of a user model (also called user profile) that explicitly represent the information characterizing a person or group of persons (personal information) and his-her/their preferences.

An important and difficult problem that should be addressed by the research aimed at search personalization is that users often switch from a search interest to another, and they alternate search related to long term interests with search related to temporary interests. In the case of a query that is unrelated to the user's topical interest, the consideration of the user topical preferences not useful, and could be even noisy and unproductive to enhance search. Therefore a big research challenge is to make systems able to capture user's interest shifts (especially temporary ones).

In the following sub-sections some main issues related to contextualizing search are shortly addressed.

2.1   The Context Modeling Issue

In a context dependent IR strategy, the definition of the context model encompasses three main activities: identification/extraction of the basic knowledge which characterizes the context, choice of a formal language in which to represent this knowledge, and a strategy to update this knowledge (to adapt the representation to context variations). A large amount of research has addressed the first problem, i.e. identifying information useful to characterize the context; in order to capture contextual information related to the user, two main techniques are currently employed: explicit and implicit [15],[16],[17],[18],[19]. The former requires an explicit user-system interaction, while the latter does not force the user to play an active role for communicating to the system his/her contextual information. By the explicit approach in fact the user is asked to be proactive and to directly communicate his/her personal data and preferences to the system. By the implicit approach several techniques have been proposed to automatically capture the user's interests, by monitoring the user's actions, and by implicitly inferring from them the user's preferences [20]. The proposed techniques range from click-through data analysis, query log analysis, desktop information analysis, etc.

As a subsequent step, the process of organization and representation of the information obtained by the context acquisition phase implies the selection of an appropriate formal language to define the user context model. In the literature several representations for the user model have been proposed, ranging from bag of words and vector representations, to graph-based representations [21], and, more recently, to ontology based representations [22],[23],[24],[25]. The more structured and expressive the formal language is, the more accurate the user model can be.

The approaches more widely employed to define user profiles are based on words or concept features; with the objective of also representing the relations between words/concepts, usually an external knowledge resource, such as the ODP (Open Directory Project [26]), Wordnet [27], and more recently Wikipedia is required.

As previously outlined, a problem that can raise by making use of user profiles in search sessions is that they are representative of long term topical interests. In the case of random session (i.e. sessions unrelated with usual interests) it is not meaningful to make an association of the query with the topical user interests. An important research issue is then related to making the system able to identify positive and negative associations of the user context with the queries formulated by the users so as to define correct contextual processes.

2.2   Definition of Methods and Models for Search in Context

The second key point of contextual search is related to the problem of effectively exploiting the context knowledge to improve the outcome of the search. This is usually done by defining specific algorithms, which make explicit use of the information in the context representation to produce the search results related to a specific query.

The main approaches proposed in the literature can be categorized in three main classes [9]:

- Approaches that concur to relevance assessment
- Approaches that modify/reformulate the user query to enrich it with the context information

- Approaches for result re-ranking; these approaches are aimed at modifying the relevance assessments computed by a traditional search engine, based on the information represented in the context model.

Among the approaches belonging to the first category we cite the PageRank based methods, based on modifications of the PageRank algorithm that include user modelling into rank computation, to create personal views of the Web [28],[29].

The more numerous approaches are re-ranking techniques that may differ both in the adopted context   model and in the re-ranking strategy [17],[23],[30]. Query modification techniques are aimed at exploiting the user profile as a knowledge support to select information that is useful for defining more accurate queries via a query expansion or modification technique [19],[31],[32].

A challenging research direction to implement contextual search is related to exploiting the user social context. As outlined in [2], using collective behavior is particularly important when the user undertakes a complex search activity. A first way to do this is to gather data about the actions undertaken by a large group of individuals (especially related to Web usage) to the aim of assisting the user; this is one of the fundamental ideas behind the so-called wisdom of crowds [33]. The limits behind this idea are related to the fact that the information collected may be biased due to the presence of spam and low quality data. Some measure of trust or reliability of users may alleviate this problem; but in general this is only worth if the user shares the crowd's values [2]. A second way to use social information is related to the so-called collaborative search approach, where like-minded people actions are considered to leverage the search undertaken by an individual of the considered community [34].

2.3   Aggregation in Context

An interesting aspect which emerges when addressing the problem of contextual search is that the availability of a multi-dimensional model of context makes it possible to consider several new dimensions in the relevance assessment process. The birth of Web Search Engines as well as the evolution of IR techniques have implied a shift from topical relevance assessment (which was the only dimension to assess relevance in the first IRSs) to a multi-dimensional relevance assessment, where the considered relevance dimensions encompass topical relevance, page popularity (based on link analysis in web search engines), geographic and temporal dimensions, etc. The availability of a user model (and more generally the availability of more structured context models), make the dimensions which are available to concur in the process of relevance assessment still more numerous. As a consequence, there is the need for combining the relevance assessments related to the considered dimensions. The consideration and representation of a context model makes the multi-dimensionality of the information available to assess relevance still more evident.

This problem has been generally faced so far by adopting simple linear combination schemes applied independently of the user's preferences over the relevance dimensions. An interesting research direction that has been recently addressed is to explicitly consider the user preferences in determining such an aggregation scheme: this can be simply done by making the aggregation dependent on the user's preferences over the single relevance dimensions. In this way, for a same query and a same context-model, different document rankings can be obtained based on the user's preference over the relevance dimensions. To this aim priority based aggregation operators have been defined and applied in the IR context [35],[36]. With the proposed approach user-dependent aggregation schemes are defined as linear combinations where weights of relevance dimensions are automatically computed by a user preference-based priority order over the dimensions.

2.4   The User-System Interaction Issue

An important issue related to the use of search engines concerns the user-system interaction paradigm; with the increasing need for complex and exploratory search paradigms the question which arises is if search engines will offer more expressive interactions that go beyond keyword-based search. As outlined in [2], an important issue is to maintain the interaction simple; query suggestion is a form of improvement of the user-system interaction, which does not require any explicit user action. However, as discussed in [2] the position of search companies seems to be conservative.

Another important aspect of the user-system interaction is related to the visualization of search results: one of the main problems when using search engines is that, although the information relevant to the user's needs expressed in a query could be probably found in the long ordered list of results, it is quite difficult to locate them. It is in fact well know that users seldom go beyond an analysis of the first two/three pages of search results. So the definition of alternative visualization paradigms is an important research direction (cluster based organization of search results is an example of alternative organization and presentation of the search outcome). To enhance results visualization through the knowledge of the user's context and preferences is an interesting topic; recently, an approach aimed to help users to visually identify bad and good results through two or three-dimensional presentations of search results, by also taking into account the user's preferences [37].

An important issue of context-aware systems is privacy. To apply personalization search engines need data from the user as well as explicit consent. Google personalized search offers an example of centralized solution to the "one size fits all" approach. To avoid the privacy concern client-side applications can be developed. In [38] an interesting analysis of the privacy issue is presented.

3   Conclusions

To overcome the "one size fits all" behavior of most search engines and Information Retrieval Systems, in recent years a great deal of research has addressed the problem of defining techniques aimed at tailoring the search outcome to the user context. This paper has briefly outlined a few main issues related to the two basic problems beyond these approaches: context representation and definition of processes which exploit the context knowledge to improve the quality of the search outcome.

References

1. Manning, C.D., Raghavan, P., Schütze, H.: Introduction to information retrieval. Cambridge University Press (2008)
2. Baeza-Yates, R., Boldi, P., Bozzon, A., Brambilla, M., Ceri, S., Pasi, G.: Trends in Search Interaction. In: Ceri, S., Brambilla, M. (eds.) Search Computing II. LNCS, vol. 6585, pp. 26–32. Springer, Heidelberg (2011)
3. White, R.W., Kules, B., Drucker, S.M., Schraefel, M.C.: Supporting Exploratory Search, Introduction. Communications of the ACM 49(4), 36–39 (2006)
4. Brusilovsky, P., Kobsa, A., Nejdl, W. (eds.): The adaptive web: methods and strategies of web personalization. LNCS, vol. 4321. Springer, Heidelberg (2007)
5. Ingwersen, P., Järvelin, K.: The Turn: Integration of Information Seeking and Retrieval in Context. Springer, Heidelberg (2005)
6. Pasi, G.: Issues in Personalizing Information Retrieval. IEEE Intelligent Informatics Bulletin (IIB), 3–6 (December 2010)
7. Pasi, G.: Modelling Users' Preferences in Systems for Information Access. International Journal of Intelligent Systems 18(7), 793–808 (2003)
8. Pitkow, J., Schutze, H., Cass, T., Cooley, R., Turnbull, D., Edmonds, A., Adar, E., Breuel, T.: Personalized search. Communications of the ACM 45(9), 50–55 (2002)
9. Micarelli, A., Gasparetti, F., Sciarrone, F., Gauch, S.: Personalized Search on the World Wide Web. In: Brusilovsky, P., Kobsa, A., Nejdl, W. (eds.) Adaptive Web 2007. LNCS, vol. 4321, pp. 195–230. Springer, Heidelberg (2007)
10. Bloice, M., Kreuzthaler, M., Simonic, K.M., Holzinger, A.: On the Paradigm Shift of Search on Mobile Devices: Some Remarks on User Habits. In: Leitner, G., Hitz, M., Holzinger, A. (eds.) USAB 2010. LNCS, vol. 6389, pp. 493–496. Springer, Heidelberg (2010)
11. Tamine-Lechani, L., Boughanem, M., Daoud, M.: Evaluation of contextual Information Retrieval effectiveness: overview of issues and research. Knowledge Information Systems 24, 1–34 (2010)
12. Berners-Lee, T.: The Web of Things. ERCIM News 72 (January 2008)
13. Guinard, D., Trifa, V., Mattern, F., Wilde, E.: From the Internet of Things to the Web of Things: Resource Oriented Architecture and Best Practices. In: Uckelmann, D., Harrison, M., Michahelles, F. (eds.) Architecting the Internet of Things, pp. 97–129. Springer, Heidelberg (2011)
14. Zhong, N., Ma, J.H., Huang, R.H., Liu, J.M., Yao, Y.Y., Zhang, Y.X., Chen, J.H.: Research Challenges and Perspectives on Wisdom Web of Things (W2T). Journal of Supercomputing, 1–21 (2010)
15. Agichtein, E., Brill, Dumais, S., Ragno, R.: Learning user interaction models for predicting Web search preferences. In: ACM SIGIR Conference on Research and Development in Information Retrieval 2006, pp. 3–10 (2006)
16. Claypool, M., Brown, D., Le, P., Waseda, M.: Inferring user interest. IEEE Intern. Comput., 32–39 (2001)
17. Shen, X., Tan, B., Zhai, C.X.: Implicit user modeling for personalized search. In: International Conference on Information and Knowledge Management, CIKM 2005, pp. 824–831 (2005)

18. Speretta, M., Gauch, S.: Personalized Search Based on User Search Histories. In: IEEE/WIC/ACM International Conference on Web Intelligence 2005, pp. 622–628 (2005)
19. Teevan, J., Dumais, S., Horvitz, E.: Personalizing search via automated analysis of interests and activities. In: International ACM SIGIR Conference on Research and Development in Information Retrieval 2005, pp. 449–456 (2005)
20. Kelly, D., Teevan, J.: Implicit feedback for inferring user preference: A bibliography. SIGIR Forum 37(2), 18–28 (2003)
21. Daoud, M., Tamine-Lechani, L., Boughanem, M.: Towards a graph-based user profile modeling for a session-based personalized search. Knowl. Inf. Syst. 21(3), 365–398 (2009)
22. Calegari, S., Pasi, G.: Ontology-Based Information Behaviour to Improve Web Search. Future Internet 4, 533–558 (2010)
23. Sieg, A., Mobasher, B., Burke, R.: Web search personalization with ontological user profiles. In: International Conference on Information and Knowledge Management, CIKM 2007, pp. 525–534 (2007)
24. Speretta, M., Gauch, S.: Miology: a Web Application for Organizing Personal Domain Ontologies. In: International Conference on Information, Process and Knowledge Management, EKNOW 2009, pp. 159–161 (2009)
25. Trajkova, J., Gauch, S.: Improving Ontology-Based User Profiles. In: RIAO 2004 Conference, pp. 380–390 (2004)
26. The Open Directory Project, http://dmoz.org/
27. Wordnet, http://wordnet.princeton.edu/
28. Jeh, G., Widom, J.: Scaling Personalized Web Search. In: 12th International World Wide Web Conference (WWW 2003), Budapest, Hungary, pp. 271–279 (2003)
29. Havelivala, T.H.: Topic-sensitive PageRank. In: 11th International World Wide Web Conference (WWW 2002), Honolulu, Hawai, May 7-11 (2002)
30. Ma, Z., Pant, G., Sheng, O.: Interest-based personalized search. ACM Transaction on Information Systems 25(5) (2007)
31. Chirita, P., Firan, C., Nejdl, W.: Personalised Query Expansion for the Web. In: ACM SIGIR Conference on Research and Development in Information Retrieval 2007, pp. 287–296 (2007)
32. Liu, C., Yu, C., Meng, W.: Personalized Web Search For Improving Retrieval Effectiveness. IEEE Transactions on Knowledge and Data Engineering 16(1), 28–40 (2004)
33. Surowiecki, J.: The wisdom of crowds. Knopf Doubleday Publishing Group (2005).
34. Smyth, B.: A Community-Based Approach to Personalizing Web Search. IEEE Computer 40(8), 42–50 (2007)
35. da Costa Pereira, C., Dragoni, M., Pasi, G.: Multidimensional Relevance: A New Aggregation Criterion. In: Boughanem, M., Berrut, C., Mothe, J., Soule-Dupuy, C. (eds.) ECIR 2009. LNCS, vol. 5478, pp. 264–275. Springer, Heidelberg (2009)
36. da Costa Pereira, C., Dragoni, M., Pasi, G.: Multidimensional relevance: Prioritized aggregation in a personalized Information Retrieval setting. Infomation Processing and Management (online version, July 2011)
37. Ahn, J.-W., Brusilovsky, P.: Adaptive Visualization of Search Results: Bringing User Models to Visual Analytics. Information Visualization 8(3), 167–179 (2009)
38. Kobsa, A.: Privacy-Enhanced Web Personalization. In: Brusilovsky, P., Kobsa, A., Nejdl, W. (eds.) Adaptive Web 2007. LNCS, vol. 4321, pp. 628–670. Springer, Heidelberg (2007)

Data Certification Impact
on Health Information Retrieval

Carla Teixeira Lopes[1] and Cristina Ribeiro[1,2]

[1] DEI, Faculdade de Engenharia, Universidade do Porto
[2] INESC-Porto
Rua Dr. Roberto Frias s/n, 4200-465, Portugal
{ctl,mcr}@fe.up.pt

Abstract. The Web is being increasingly used by health consumers to search for health information. In this domain, the quality of the retrieved contents is crucial to avoid healthcare hazards. To address this problem and help the user identify reliable and credible contents, initiatives have appeared that certify the compliance of health websites to quality standards. In this work we explore the impact of medical certification on several aspects of health information retrieval performance. Moreover, we analyze the usefulness of certification categories to the personalization of the search experience. Our findings suggest that medical certification might be incorporated as a ranking criterion. We conclude that the medical accuracy of the resulting knowledge is enhanced by the use of certified information and depends on the users' comprehension of the document. In general, we also conclude that there is space for personalization in search by health consumers.

Keywords: Medical Certification, Health Information Retrieval, Context, Health Consumers, User Study.

1   Introduction

The use of the Web to search for health information is gaining popularity among patients, their family and friends. A Harris Interactive poll reported, in 2010, that 88% of the US online population has searched for health information on the Web, the highest percentage and year-over-year increase since the first study of this type [6]. The characteristics of the Web make it a medium where publishing is easy and accessible to everyone. This, allied with the impact that online health resources have on people's life and well-being, emphasize the importance of mechanisms that help identify the quality of online health information. A 2009's Pew Internet report [4] found that "about one in ten online health inquiries have a major impact on someone's health care or the way they cared for someone else".

The problem of finding quality information exists since the first developments on information retrieval. Health domain specificities have triggered research

A. Holzinger and K.-M. Simonic (Eds.): USAB 2011, LNCS 7058, pp. 31–42, 2011.

initiatives parallel to the general ones. A systematic review of studies that assess the quality of health information for consumers on the Web has been done by Eysenbach et al. [2]. To address the problem of health information quality, initiatives like the Health on the Net Foundation Code of Conduct (HONcode) certification or the URAC's Health Web Site Accreditation Program have emerged. They both intend to help the user identify reliable and credible content through a seal that identifies the sites that satisfy their code of conduct or quality standards. HONcode certification is considered the most successful initiative [1].

Typically, a search session starts in a generalist search engine instead of health-specific websites [3] and Google is commonly the chosen search engine [8]. Studies that compare the performance of generalist and health-specific search engines mostly conclude that the former outperform the latter. Regarding the quality of information, some studies report that health-specific search engines provide higher quality contents while fewer conclude that quality is the same in both types of search engines [5].

With this context in mind, we conducted a user study to analyze the impact of limiting the collection of a search engine to certified health documents, having the HONcode certification as a base. This impact is measured in terms of precision, medical accuracy, documents' comprehension by users, documents' readability and users' motivational relevance. In the end, our findings may indicate how medical certification can help generalist search engines provide a better service to their users in consumer health retrieval. A second goal of our study is to evaluate how useful are the HONcode categories for personalizing the search experience in a generalist engine. For example, we want to know if sites "for patients" are preferred to sites "for professionals" or if sites "for women" are actually more valued by women.

This paper is structured as follows. After briefly explaining health information certification in Section 2, we describe the user study in Section 3. Results are presented in Sections 4 and 5. The studys ndings, along with their implications, are discussed in Section 6 and the conclusions follow in Section 7.

2   Health Information Certification

As previously said, health websites may be certified by external entities that assure that every site that has a certification seal respects a certain code of conduct. There are two widely known certification programs, one promoted by the Health on the Net Foundation (HON) and the other promoted by URAC. They are both non-profit organizations and they differ in scope. URAC intends to promote health quality in a global way, not only through the quality of online information as is the case with HON.

The URAC Health Web Site Accreditation Program evaluates websites against 48 quality standards[1]. A search of URAC accredited companies on their

---

[1] Available at http://www.urac.org/docs/programs/URACHW2.1factsheet.pdf

web site returns only 19 records. This confirms the greater popularity of the HONcode certification program that has 7,200 HONcode certified websites [1].

Details about the HONcode certification system can be found on their website[2]. Briefly, any health site can request the certification, free of charge, whether or not it has a health focus. Requests are then examined by a committee that includes health professionals and verifies if all the HONcode ethical principles are respected. The ethical principles are: authority, complementarity, confidentiality, attribution, justifiability, transparency, financial disclosure and advertising. A certified website is subjected to regular monitoring.

3 Case Study

Our user study involved 40 undergraduate students (25 females, 15 males) of a programme in Information Science. Users are medically lay people and have a mean age of 22.25 years (sd = 6.42). We defined 8 information needs[3] based on questions submitted to the health category of the Yahoo! Answers service. Each information need requires finding a treatment for a particular disease or condition and is associated with 4 different queries formulated by the researchers. We have used Google as a black-box search engine with two collections, Google's entire collection and Google's indexed webpages with HONcode certification. We filtered the collection through Google custom search, a tool provided by Google in which it is possible to create custom search engines that work with specific sets of websites or webpages. Henceforward, we will call WebSys to the system working with the first collection and HONSys to the system working with the HONcode certified collection.

For each query and system, we collected the top-30 results. To reduce the risk of Google learning from the previous submitted queries, we ensured that returned links were never clicked. Further, to prevent changes in the search engine or in the HON collection, we submitted all queries within a very short time span.

A query run on one of the retrieval systems leads to a task that a user can execute. Each user was assigned a set of 8 different tasks in which he had to assess, in a 3-value scale, the relevance and comprehension of the top-30 documents and to answer a post-search questionnaire. A Latin-square like procedure was adopted during task assignment to guarantee that each user assessed the relevance of every information need and was exposed to each retrieval system the same number of times. We have also guaranteed that each system is associated with each information need the same number of times. To prevent possible bias owing to human behavior, we have also permuted the order of tasks and forced users to complete them in the prescribed order. Additionally, to preempt users' fatigue, each task had to be performed in different days, that is, tasks had to be separated by an interval of, at least, 24 hours. Users did not have time limits to perform each task.

---

[2] Available at `http://www.hon.ch/HONcode/Patients/Visitor/visitor.html`
[3] Available at `http://www.carlalopes.com/research/userstudy3.html`

4   Impact Analysis

Our analysis will focus on three aspects: comparison of search systems, comparison of certified and non-certified documents and comparison of shared and non-shared documents. A shared document is a document that is retrieved by both systems.

Henceforward, we will use * and ** to sign significant results at the levels of significance (α) of 0.05 and 0.01, respectively. Additionally the following nomenclature will be used to identify information about hypothesis tests: $\chi^2(df)$ corresponds to the chi-square distribution with df degrees of freedom; W is the statistic calculated for the Wilcoxon rank-sum test, a non-parametric test for assessing whether two independent samples of observations have equally large values; $t(df)$ is the Student's t distribution with df degrees of freedom; $F(df)$ is the F-distribution with df degrees of freedom used in the ANOVA test to compare the means of several distributions; TukeyHSD is presented before the confidence limits of the Tukey's Honestly Significance Difference test, used in multiple comparisons after the ANOVA test; and p is the abbreviation of *p-value*.

4.1   Precision

To analyze precision we use the Graded Average Precision (GAP) and Graded Precision (gP) measures recently proposed by Robertson et al. [7]. These measures are based on a probabilistic model that, assuming the user always has a binary view of relevance, generalizes precision and average precision to the case of multi-graded relevance.

As can be seen in Figure 1, in terms of precision, the HONSys had a worse performance in every measure: GAP, gP@5 and gP@10. As expected, the statistical dispersion is lower with GAP, since this is an average measure that considers the top-30 results. Differences between systems are significant in every measure at $\alpha = 0.01$ which means that users prefer the WebSys even including non-certified documents.

In the WebSys, we computed the correlation between each measure and the proportion of certified documents in each session (for GAP), in each top-5's session (for gP5) and in each top-10's session (for gP10). In GAP and gP10, the correlation is approximately 0.18 and is significantly higher than 0 at $\alpha = 0.05$. The almost null correlation in gP5 and the low correlation values in gP10 and GAP make us believe that the HONCode certification is not a major factor influencing relevance assessments, mainly in the top-ranked results.

Since GAP, gP5 and gP10 are measures that evaluate the performance of a set of documents, we cannot use them to compare certified with non-certified documents. For that reason, we will compare these two sets of documents using documents' individual relevance assessments. In the WebSys, the non-certified documents (column *No* in Figure 2) are almost equally distributed in terms of relevance assessments, having each level of the relevance scale about 33% of the non-certified documents. Since the number of documents in each category

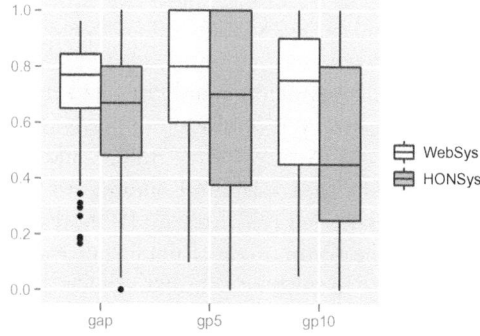

Fig. 1. GAP, gP5 and gP10 boxplots on both systems

presented in the x-axis of Figure 2 is variable, in the y-axis we plotted the proportion of not-relevant, partially relevant and totally relevant documents instead of the documents' counting. On the other hand, in certified documents, the proportion of non-relevant documents is much lower (27%) and significantly lower than partially relevant ($\chi^2(1) = 11.89$, p=0.0003**) and totally relevant documents ($\chi^2(1) = 19.1$, p=6.24e-06**). In WebSys certified documents, the most likely is to find a *totally relevant* document (38%). We also conclude that, in WebSys, certified documents are associated with higher relevance scores than non-certified ones. In fact, the proportion of *not relevant* documents is higher in WebSys non-certified documents ($\chi^2(1) = 13.54$, p=0.0001**) and the proportion of *totally relevant* documents is higher in WebSys certified documents ($\chi^2(1) = 6.47$, p=0.005**).

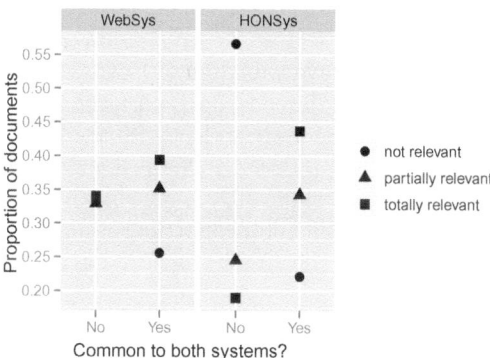

Fig. 2. Proportion of documents by search system, share status and relevance assessment

In the HONSys, all documents are certified but we can distinguish two groups of documents, the ones that are also retrieved by the WebSys and the ones that are not. As can be seen in Figure 2, these two groups of documents have an opposite behavior in terms of relevance. When both groups are compared, shared documents are associated with a significantly higher relevance, expressed by a lower proportion of *not relevant* documents ($\chi^2(1) = 283.37$, p<2.2e-16**) and a higher proportion of *partially relevant* ($\chi^2(1) = 28.77$, p=4.07e-08**) and *totally relevant* ($\chi^2(1) = 203.78$, p<2.2e-16**) documents.

It is also interesting to note that, although having a similar pattern, shared documents are assessed with a higher relevance on HONSys than on WebSys, perhaps influenced by the relative comparison to the other results. Comparing rank positions of shared documents in both systems we notice that, as expected, these documents appear first in HONSys ranks (rank median of 4) than in WebSys' ranks (rank median of 11). This difference is statistically significant (W=304150, p<2.2e-16**). Certified documents appearing in the top-30 in the WebSys have characteristics beyond certification that distinguish them from the other certified documents that do not appear on these top-30 and appear on the HONSys top-30 ranks. These characteristics are intimately related with Google's criteria for ranking. Comparing the results of certified and non-certified documents on WebSys, we can conclude that the certification is a criterion that should be integrated in the set of criteria used by search engines.

4.2   Medical Accuracy

After each task, users were asked to write the treatment(s) they found for the condition mentioned in the information need. Each answer was evaluated by a medical doctor regarding their correct and incorrect contents. The combination of these two measures leads to a variable which we named *medical accuracy* that varies between 0 (lowest accuracy) and 4 (highest accuracy). The median of the medical accuracy on the HONSys is significantly higher than the one on the WebSys ($W = 11326$, p=0.03*). An analysis by answers' correctness and incorrectness shows that, in terms of correct contents, both systems have a similar behavior. Both systems have a median of 1 (*answer with some value*) and have no significant proportion differences in each level of the correctness scale. In terms of incorrect contents, the WebSys leads to more incorrect answers than the HONSys ($W = 10815.5$, p = 0.004**). The proportion of answers classified with *some incorrect content* is significantly higher in the WebSys (39% against 28% - $\chi^2(1) = 3.59$, p=0.03*) and the proportion of answers with *no incorrect content* is significantly higher in the HONSys (57.5% against 42% - $\chi^2(1) = 7.2$, p=0.004**).

Based on the previous finding, we investigated if, on the WebSys, the medical accuracy, correctness and incorrectness of contents increase with the number of certified pages. In terms of medical accuracy and correct contents, we detected no significant differences and no pattern inline with our hypothesis. In terms of incorrect contents, we found significant differences in the mean number of certified pages between levels of the incorrectness scale (F(2)=3.63, p=0.03*). Surprisingly, a pairwise comparison showed that sessions of answers with *no incorrect content* have less certified pages than sessions of answers with *some* *incorrect content* (TukeyHSD: (-2.61; -0.04), p=0.04*). This is the opposite of what we expected and, assuming there are no incorrect contents in certified documents, we conclude there are several non-certified documents that have *no incorrect contents* and suspect that a few documents with incorrect contents have the power to damage the knowledge acquired in the overall search session. This strengthens our previous conclusion that certification must occupy a prominent place in the set of criteria used by search engines.

4.3   Readability

Documents readability was automatically evaluated using the Simple Measure of Gobbledygook (SMOG) metric. A higher SMOG means the document contains more polysyllables and is, therefore, more difficult to read. We found that documents retrieved by HONSys (mean SMOG of 7.55) are more complex (W = 9287206, p=0.001**) than WebSys documents (mean SMOG of 7.38). However, if we make this comparison by certification status, we find that non-certified documents have a higher SMOG mean (7.46 against 7.4). Although this last difference is not significant, these two results show a contradictory trend. We also compared the SMOG mean according to the system and the URL share status (Table 1). In the WebSys, the non-certified documents have a mean SMOG higher than the one in certified documents, a difference that is statistically significant (W=1413680, p=8.88e-16**). In the HONSys, documents that are also retrieved by the WebSys have a lower SMOG when compared to non-shared ones, a significant difference (t(911.76)=6.0029, p=1.4e-09**) that evidences that document's readability may be used by Google to rank documents. Since the median rank of shared documents on the HONSys is significantly lower than the one in the WebSys, we conclude this criterion predominates in smaller collections where other criteria may probably not be met.

Table 1. Mean SMOG by system and share status

URL	WebSys	HONSys
Shared	6.9	6.84
Not shared	7.46	7.59

4.4   Comprehension

The comprehension of the documents was assessed by the users during the search task using a 3-value scale: 0 - *I did not understand*, 1 - *I partially understood* and 2 - *I totally understood*. We found that users understand better the documents retrieved by the WebSys than the HONSys documents. In fact, the former system has a significantly lower proportion of *not understood* URL ($\chi^2(1) = 15.07$, p=5.18e-05**) and a significantly higher proportion of *totally understood* URL ($\chi^2(1) = 10.98$, p=0.0005**). Although the complexity of the text is not the only factor affecting the comprehension of a document, this is in agreement with the readability results reported in the previous section. An analysis by documents' certification status revealed that non-certified documents are better understood by users when compared to certified ones. The former have a significantly lower proportion *not understood* assessments ($\chi^2(1) = 7.16$, p=0.004**) and a significantly higher proportion of *totally understood* assessments ($\chi^2(1) = 4.78$, p=0.01*). Specifically in the WebSys, we detected no significant differences between certified and non-certified documents comprehension. In the HONSys, shared documents have a significantly lower proportion of *not understood* classifications when compared with non-shared documents ($\chi^2(1) = 10.89$, p=0.0005**). This is a sign that shared documents are better understood by users and is inline with the readability results.

4.5   Motivational Relevance

After the search task, users evaluated their degree of satisfaction according to the provided information need in a scale of 1 (*I did not succeed in this task*) to 5 (*The information need is completely satisfied*). We compared both retrieval systems and found that the WebSys is associated with a higher degree of satisfaction (W=14265, p= 0.03*). In the WebSys, we did not find significant differences on the mean number of certified pages between the 5 levels of satisfaction.

5   Contextual Analysis

During the HON certification process, websites are classified according to their purposes. Some of the categories are: "for health professionals", "for patients", "for women" and "for men". In this section we compare users' relevance and comprehension assessments in the four categories mentioned above. In the two last categories, we also consider the users' characteristics. Additionally, in the first two categories, we compare documents' readability.

The categories "for health professionals" and "for patients" are not mutually exclusive, with some documents being classified for both audiences. There are also documents that do not belong to any of these categories. In our sample there are 118 URL for health professionals and 456 directed for consumers. We have applied several proportion tests to verify if these documents differ in terms of comprehension and relevance scores. In Table 2, for each level of comprehension and relevance, we present the proportion difference found ($<$ or $>$) along with its significance and test value. For example, regarding comprehension, in level 0 we found that "nP<P", i.e., documents "for health professionals" (P) have a higher proportion of documents "not understood" (level 0) than documents that are not in the "health professionals" group (nP).

Through the results presented in Table 2, we conclude that documents that are not in the "for health professionals" category are better understood by users than the ones that do. The former category has a smaller proportion of documents that are not or are partially understood and a larger proportion of totally

Table 2. Proportion tests performed by level of comprehension, relevance and HON Categories. n= not, P = Professional, C = Consumer. $\chi^2(1)$ value in parenthesis.

Level	Comprehension	Relevance
0	nP<P** (11.28)	nP>P** (8.92)
	nC>C** (56.6)	nC>C** (22.93)
1	nP<P** (86.46)	nP<P** (21.94)
	nC>C** (34.78)	nC<C* (3.43)
2	nP>P** (115.38)	nP>P (1.74)
	nC<C** (88.89)	nC<C** (12.85)

understood documents. On the other hand, documents that belong in the "for patients" (C) category are better understood than the ones that do not (nC). The behavior of the "for patients" category is similar to the one presented above for the documents that do not belong in the "for health professionals" category.

Regarding readability, we found significant differences between SMOG means that are in accordance with the previous results. We found that documents "for health professionals" are more complex (W=1338060, p=2.55e-07**) than documents that do not belong to this group just like documents that are not "for patients" (t(3116.6)=5.9, p=1.86e-09**) in comparison with documents in the "for patients" group.

In terms of relevance, the "for patients" documents are more relevant than the documents that are not linked to this category. On the "for health professionals" category the behavior is opposite but less clear. The professional documents seem to be more relevant than the documents that do not belong to this category.

In our sample there are 60 assessments of 8 documents "for women" and 50 assessments of 6 documents "for men". In these categories we do an analysis similar to the previous one but we also consider the gender of the user. In terms of comprehension we found that documents "for women" are better understood by the general user and, more specifically, by the women. In fact they have a lower proportion of documents classified with 1 ($\chi^2(1) = 4.54$, p=0.02* in the general user and $\chi^2(1) = 3.71$, p=0.03* in the women) and a higher proportion of documents assessed with 2 ($\chi^2(1) = 7.75$, p=0.003** in the general user and $\chi^2(1) = 5.94$, p=0.007** in the women). In terms of relevance, the only significant result we have found is that men assess documents "for men" as *not relevant* more frequently than they do in documents not classified as "for men" ($\chi^2(1) = 5.56$, p=0.009**).

6   Discussion

In the comparison between retrieval systems, the system that had the Web as a collection, including certified and non-certified documents, has a better performance in all aspects but medical accuracy. Users assess relevance higher in this system, understand better its documents, feel more satisfied after the search sessions and their documents are less difficult to read. However, this system is associated with more incorrect contents than the one that only includes certified documents. In this matter, we found that this difference is not due to the higher number of non-certified pages in this system because the proportion of certified documents in sessions with *some incorrect content* is significantly higher than sessions with *no incorrect contents*. Assuming there are no incorrect contents in certified documents, either the problem is on the comprehension of certain documents or in a few non-certified documents that may have the power to damage the knowledge acquired in the overall search session. We found that non-certified documents are better understood by users than certified ones. Since readability is not significantly different between both types of documents, the comprehension differences may be related with the existence of medical concepts that are not apprehended. We also found that certification does not affect relevance assessments, mainly in the top-rank results. This may be justified by a conclusion of a previous study [3] that found that "three-quarters of health seekers do not consistently check the source and date of the health information they find online".

A more profound analysis was done in three groups of documents: non-certified documents (WebSys non-shared documents), certified documents retrieved by both WebSys and HONSys (shared documents) and certified documents retrieved only by HONSys (HONSys non-shared documents). We found that shared documents are the ones with better performance in terms of relevance and readability. This is not strange since this set of documents meets the general criteria of Google search engine and have all the quality standards defined in the HON-Code. In terms of comprehension, these documents are better understood than HONSys non-shared ones but have no significant differences when compared with WebSys non-shared ones. As expected, these documents rank higher in the HONSys than in the WebSys. After this set of documents, the ones with better performance in relevance, readability and comprehension are the WebSys non-shared documents.

In the contextual analysis we also considered the HONCode categories. We found that documents "for patients" and documents that are not "for health professionals" are easier to read and understand. The readability of a document can be a good evidence of its adjustment to health consumers. In terms of relevance, users find documents "for patients" and "for health professionals" more relevant. Although users understand worse the latter type of documents, we believe these documents convey a professionalism and confidence that makes users rate their relevance higher. In addition, documents "for women" are better understood by the general user and, more specifically, by the women.

7   Conclusion

In this work we analyze the impact of medical certification on several aspects of health information retrieval performance. We conclude that users value the diversity provided by generalist search engines even if this means including non-certified documents. Yet, we found that the medical accuracy of generalist search engines may be in risk if users do not understand documents or if the session has a few documents with unreliable information. As we have seen, to assure the comprehension of the documents, besides their readability, engines must also guarantee that document terminology is adjusted to the users' knowledge. To improve the performance of generalist search engines on health tasks and to assure the credibility of the top results, the ones that receive more attention, it is advisable to incorporate the medical certification in the set of criteria currently in use by the search engine. As we have shown, the documents retrieved by the WebSys with HON certification are the ones with best overall performance. Supported by findings of previous studies and the fact that certification has no impact on users' relevance judgments, we have reasons to believe that health consumers do not consistently check if the health information they find is certified. Since users' unawareness of information reliability may be associated with some dangers, the inclusion of medical certification in the set of search engines' criteria becomes even more important.

We also concluded that the classification of documents as "for patients" and "for health professionals" may be useful to personalize the search experience. In this sense, it would be important to explore as future work which page characteristics may be used to automatically classify documents. On the other hand, there is also the need to predict if the user is a lay person or a professional and his level of expertise on the topic. Since documents' readability is tightly connected with the HONCode categorization and it proved to be discriminating in several comparisons, it may be a good indicator of documents that are valued and understood by users.

Acknowledgments. Thanks to Fundação para a Ciência e a Tecnologia for partially funding this work under the grant SFRH/BD/40982/2007. Thanks to Dagmara Paiva for the medical evaluation of users' answers on each task.

References

1. Baujard, V., Boyer, C., Geissbühler, A.: Evolution of Health Web certification. In: 23rd Annual days of the Swiss Society of Medical Informatic (2010)
2. Eysenbach, G., Powell, J., Kuss, O., Sa, E.R.: Empirical Studies Assessing the Quality of Health Information for Consumers on the World Wide Web: A Systematic Review. JAMA 287(20), 2691–2700 (2002),
http://dx.doi.org/10.1001/jama.287.20.2691
3. Fox, S.: Online Health Search 2006. Tech. rep., Pew Internet & American Life Project (October 2006),
http://www.pewinternet.org/ /media//Files/Reports/2006/
PIP_Online_Health_2006.pdf.pdf
4. Fox, S., Jones, S.: The Social Life of Health Information. Tech. rep., Pew Internet & American Life Project (June 2009),
http://www.pewinternet.org/ /media//Files/Reports/2009/
PIP_Health_2009.pdf
5. Lopes, C.T., Ribeiro, C.: Comparative evaluation of web search engines in health information retrieval. Online Information Review (2011)

6. Petrock, V.: Cyberchondriacs Becoming Empowered Health Information Seekers, http://www.emarketer.com/blog/index.php/cyberchondriacsempowered -health-seekers/ (cited May 11, 2011); archived by WebCite http://www.webcitation.org/5ym7xLoYp (August 2010)
7. Robertson, S.E., Kanoulas, E., Yilmaz, E.: Extending average precision to graded relevance judgments. In: Proceeding of the 33rd International ACM SIGIR Conference on Research and Development in Information Retrieval, SIGIR 2010, pp. 603–610. ACM, New York (2010), http://dx.doi.org/10.1145/1835449.1835550
8. Schembri, G., Schober, P.: The Internet as a diagnostic aid: the patients' perspective. Int. J. STD AIDS 20(4), 231–233 (2009), http://dx.doi.org/10.1258/ijsa.2008.008339

Literature Mining for the Diagnostic Procedures of Osteoporosis

Pınar Yıldırım[1] and Çınar Çeken[2]

[1] Pınar Yıldırım, Department of Computer Engineering, Faculty of Engineering and Architecture, Okan University
pinar.yildirim@okan.edu.tr
[2] Çınar Çeken, Department of Physical Medicine and Rehabilitation
The Ministry of Health of Turkey Antalya Education and Research Hospital
cinar_ceken@hotmail.com

Abstract. In this paper, we highlight the importance of osteoporosis disease in terms of medical research and healthcare and we consider a knowledge discovery approach regarding the diagnostic procedures of osteoporosis from a historical perspective. Osteoporosis is characterized by low bone mass, micro-architectural deterioration of bone tissue, and increased bone fragility and susceptibility to fracture. Osteoporosis affects an estimated 75 million people in Europe, the USA and Japan, with 10 million people suffering from osteoporosis in the United States alone. Osteoporosis may significantly affect life expectancy and quality of life and is a component of the frailty syndrome. We use a freely available biomedical search engine based on text-mining technology to extract the diagnostic procedures used in osteoporosis from MEDLINE articles. We conclude that there are some changes in diagnostic procesures in the last four decades and Dual energy x-ray absorptiometry is the most commonly used technique today.

Keywords: Biomedical Text Mining, Osteoporosis, Information Extraction, Diagnostic Procedure.

1   Introduction

The scientific literature in biomedicine contains rich knowledge resources for biomedical research. MEDLINE is one of the most popular database and its abstracts and full-text documents include a database of over 20 million citations (abstracts) of biomedical articles dating back to the 1960s [1]. The database is currently growing at the rate of 500,000 new citations each year. With such explosive growth, it is extremely challenging to keep up to date with all of the new discoveries and theories even within one's own field of biomedical research. Text mining is one of the major approaches to aid researchers to deal with information overload, which makes it possible to discover patterns and trends from huge collections of unstructured text. It consists of many different techniques such as natural language processing, information retrieval, information extraction and data mining [1].

There are many web-based tools to explore and analyze the biomedical literature. These tools provide many opportunities for the analysis of co-occurrences between

A. Holzinger and K.-M. Simonic (Eds.): USAB 2011, LNCS 7058, pp. 43–51, 2011.
© Springer-Verlag Berlin Heidelberg 2011

biomedical entities such as disease, drugs, genes, proteins and symptoms [2]. Some text mining systems which are mostly used include:

- Textpresso: uses a custom ontology to query a collection of documents for information on specific classes of biological concepts (e.g. gene, cell) and their relations (e.g. association and/or regulation)[1].
- iHOP: visualizes the interactions between genes[2].
- EBIMed: retrieves sentences based on detecting co-occurrences between biological entities[3].
- PolySearch: uses heuristic weighting of different co-occurrence measures and includes a detailed guide to implementation and vocabularies [4].
- NovoSeek: leverages the Web 3.0 and text mining technology to identify biomedical relevant concepts within life sciences text[5].

Osteoporosis is widely recognised as an important public health problem because of the significant morbidity, mortality and costs associated with its complications, namely fractures of the hip, spine, forearm and other skeletal sites [3]. Across the whole of Europe, an estimated 3.1million fragility fractures occur each year in men and women age 50 years or over, including 620,000 cases of hip fracture, 490,000 clinical vertebral fractures and 574,000 forearm fractures. The incidence of fractures is highest amongst elderly white women, with one in every two women suffering an osteoporosis related fracture in their lifetime. Attention is often focussed on hip fractures because they incur the greatest morbidity and medical costs for health services. However, fractures at other sites are also associated with significant morbidity and costs , and both hip and vertebral fractures are associated with an increased risk of death, and increased dependence on nursing homes and private and public care services for the basic activities of daily living. In the European Union the combined annual costs of all osteoporotic fractures exceeds 20 billion. Because of the ageing population the prevention of fractures will assume increasing importance. Although for many years there was awareness of the morbidity and mortality associated with fragility fractures, real progress only came with the ability to diagnose osteoporosis before fractures occur, and with the development of effective treatments. Bone density scanning played an important role in both these developments. Until the mid-1980s measurements of bone mineral density (BMD) were used mainly in research, and it was only with the introduction of dual-energy X-ray absorptiometry (DXA) scanners in 1987 that they entered routine clinical practice. Further significant developments included the first publication showing that bisphosphonate treatment can prevent bone loss [10], the publication of the World Health Organisation (WHO) report defining osteoporosis in postmenopausal white women as a BMD T-score at the spine, hip or forearm of −2.5 or less, and the Fracture Intervention Trial confirming that bisphosphonate treatment can prevent fractures [4,5,6,7].

---

[1] http://www.textpresso.org/
[2] http://www.ihop-net.org/UniPub/HOP/
[3] http://www.ebi.ac.uk/Rebholz-srv/ebimed/index.jsp
[4] http://wishart.biology.ualberta.ca/polysearch/
[5] http://www.novoseek.com

All osteoporosis fractures are associated with significant morbidity and mortality, but hip fractures are particularly traumatic. Twenty percent of women who suffer a hip fracture die within the first year. Because of the ageing population, it is estimated that the number of hip fractures could double or even triple in the U.S.A. by 2020 [6].

In this paper, we present knowledge discovery on the diagnostic procedures of osteoporosis in a historical perspective. We use a web-based biomedical text-mining tool to search and analyze MEDLINE articles in different periods of time. Considering the point of view of physicians, it allows them to get hidden knowledge in medical articles and to interpret them. From the perspective of healthcare initiatives, they can evaluate the diagnostic techniques over the time periods (1970-2010) and develop new effective strategies that provide better diagnostic procedures.

2   Diagnosing of Osteoporosis

An examination to diagnose osteoporosis can involve several steps that predict fractures, diagnose osteoporosis, or both. It might include:

- An initial physical exam
- Various x rays that detect skeletal problems
- Laboratory tests that reveal important information about the metabolic process of bone breakdown and formation
- A bone density test to detect low bone density[8-9].

Measurement of bone mineral density (BMD) is the basis of the diagnosis of osteoporosis. The risk of fracture increases with decreasing bone mineral density, which can be measured using several different techniques. Common bone mineral density (BMD) tests Include:

- DEXA (Dual Energy X-ray Absorptiometry)
- pDXA (Peripheral Dual Energy X-ray Absorptiometry)
- SXA (Single Energy X-ray Absorptiometry)
- pQCT (Peripheral Quantitative Computed Tomography)
- RA (Radiographic Absorptiometry)
- QCT (Quantitative Computed Tomography)
- QUS (Quantitative Ultrasound)

In these techniques, DEXA is is considered the gold standard for the diagnosis of osteoporosis.

Screening
The U.S. Preventive Services Task Force (USPSTF) recommended in 2011 that all women 65 years of age or older should be screened with bone densitometry. They recommend screening women of any age with increased risk factors that puts them at risk equivalent to a 65 year old without additional risk factors. The most significant risk factors is lower body weight (weight < 70 kg), with less evidence for history of smoking or family history. There was insufficient evidence to make recommendations about the optimal intervals for repeated screening and the appropriate age to stop

screening. Clinical prediction rules are available to guide selection of women ages 60–64 for screening. The Osteoporosis Risk Assessment Instrument (ORAI) may be the most sensitive.

The USPSTF concludes that the harm versus benefit of screening for osteoporosis in men of any age is unknown. Others have however claimed that screening may be cost effective in those 80 to 85 years of age [10].

3   Method

The following steps are applied to extract information about the diagnostic procedures for osteoporosis:

STEP 1: Select a Search Engine
Kleio text mining tool is used to diagnostic procedures from the relevant articles. Kleio is an advanced information retrieval (IR) system developed at the UK National Centre for Text Mining (NaCTeM). The system offers textual and metadata searches across MEDLINE and provides enhanced searching functionality by leveraging terminology management Technologies [11].

Kleio draws upon one of the technologies from the NaCTeM text mining tool kit to enhance automated detection and mark-up of biologically important terms appearing in text, such as gene/protein names. One of these tools is AcroMine, which disambiguates acronyms based upon the context in which they appear.   This functionality plays a key role in searching large document collections by allowing users to expand their queries and to include synonymous acronyms without losing the specificity of the original query.

The rich variety of term variants is a stumbling block for information retrieval as these many forms have to be recognised, indexed, linked and mapped from text to existing databases. Typically, most of the currently available information retrieval systems for the biomedical domain fail to deal with the problems of term ambiguity and variability. Kleio addresses this problem for reducing the diversity of term variation.   Another key innovation of Kleio is dealing with the variety of names (terms) for denoting the same concept. To map these forms (e.g. IL2, IL-2 and Interleukin-2) to biological databases we use machine learning based term normalisation techniques which reduce term variation (e.g. il2).   An advantage of applying term normalisation is to permit efficient look-up and to discover ambiguous and variant terms in the resources. The novelty of this work lies in using existing resources to automatically learn term variation patterns [11].

STEP 2: Enter Search Criteria
Kleio offers some search options for users. For example, in order to find and analyze articles published in the period of 1970-1980 and relevant to osteoporosis, a researcher can use the time range option by setting a "1970-1980" date range with the query "osteoporosis". Figure 1 shows the query results for the last date range.

STEP 3: Get Search Results
Diagnostic procedures section in the query results has been expanded and the results have been copied to a spreadsheet table. This query has been modified for other time

periods to collect time specific articles and extract diagnostic procedures. Table 1 shows the total number of articles obtained for osteoporosis during the considered time periods.

Table 1. The number of articles found for the keyword osteoporosis

Time Period	Number of Articles
1970-1980	1345
1980-1990	3441
1990-2000	9808
2000-2010	20486

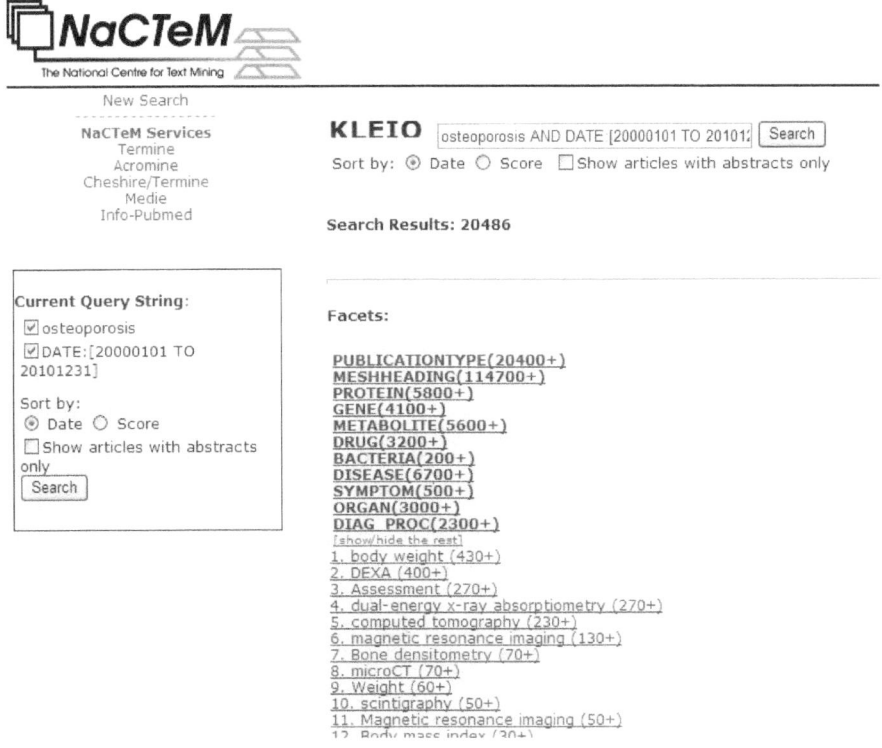

Fig. 1. The query results from Kleio for osteoporosis from 2000 to 2010

STEP 4: Interpret Results

In this step the changes in the diagnostic procedures, changes in time and rank are analyzed. More details about why some diagnostic procedures are emerged or abandoned are investigated using the related articles.

Table 2 shows extracted and ranked list of diagnostic procedures in four consecutive time periods. The Table 2 also provides a time-based comparison for the diagnostic procedures of osteoporosis. In addition, the ranking list can show the popularities of the diagnostic procedures over a certain time period. For example, some procedures can be more preferred in a certain period than others or new techniques emerge in some other time periods.

4   Results and Discussion

According to Table 2, some techniques such as autopsies, xeroradiography, arthrography are only seen in 1970-1980 time period. In addition, other techniques such as breast examination, endometrial biopsy, pap smear, skinfold thickness and angiography which are not specific diagnostic techniques used for osteoporosis are also seen in this period.

Today, bone biopsies are rarely used to diagnose or manage patients with osteoporosis due to the procedure's invasiveness, lack of technical training among clinicians, pain, cost, lack of specialized centers to interpret bone samples, time delays between biopsy and pathology report, and limited understanding of histological results. These real or perceived limitations have prompted an ongoing search to develop noninvasive bone markers to predict bone turnover, mineralization status, bone volume, cellular abnormalities, and potential accumulation of toxic elements, such as aluminum[12].

A large variety of different modalities from conventional X-rays and DEXA to CT and MRI have been developed to assess bone structure at the macro- and microlevels. As it is seen in Table 2, DEXA is the most commonly used technique today. This scan is a simple, quick test similar to having a low-energy x-ray. Since the test is non-invasive, it is painless and produces no known side effects [13]. While only DEXA can be used for diagnostic classification according to criteria established by the World Health Organization, DEXA and some other Technologies may predict fracture risk and be used to monitor skeletal changes over time.[14] These technologies such as Computed Quantitative Computer Tomography (QCT) are capable of measuring the bone's volume, and are, therefore, not susceptible to the confounding effect of bone-size in the way that DEXA results are susceptible.[15]. The ionising radiation dose of spinal QCT is higher than for DEXA, but the dose compares favorably with those of other radiographic procedures (spinal radiographs) performed in patients suspected of having osteoporosis [16]. Compared with other modalities CT-based techniques have also some advantages. In contrast to DEXA, volumetric quantitative CT (vQCT) offers three-dimensional (3D) information and cortical and trabecular bone can be separately analysed. In contrast to MRI, vQCT acquisition is much quicker and technically less demanding. Also standard whole body clinical CT scanners can be used for acquisition. These are more widely available and easier to operate than MRI equipment. Dedicated peripheral CT scanners are available for assessing BMD in the radius and tibia as well as for measuring trabecular structure of the forearm. The imaging of specimen, bone biopsies and small animals for the investigation of bone

Table 2. The extracted and ranked diagnostic procedures in time periods from 1970 to 2010

1970-1980	1980-1990	1990-2000	2000-2010
photon absorptiometry	photon absorptiometry	body weight	body weight
body weight	dual photon absorptiometry	computed tomography	DEXA
microradiography	computed tomography	DEXA	dual-energy x-ray absorptiometry
scintigraphy	body weight	photon absorptiometry	computed tomography
bone biopsy	single photon absorptiometry	dual-energy x-ray absorptiometry	magnetic resonance imaging
tomography	scintigraphy	single photon absorptiometry	bone densitometry
bone scan	dual photon absorptiometry	dual photon absorptiometry	microCT
skinfold thickness	DEXA	magnetic resonance imaging	scintigraphy
xeroradiography	bone biopsy	scintigraphy	body mass index
angiography	bone densitometry	bone densitometry	positron emission tomography
arthrography	bone scan	dual energy x-ray absorptiometry	bone scan
autopsies	microradiography	FEV1	
biopsy	magnetic resonance imaging	dual energy x-ray absorptiometry	
bone densitometry	biopsy	body mass index	
breast examination		differential diagnosis	
endometrial biopsy		ultrasonography	
joint imaging		biopsy	
pap smear		dual photon absorptiometry	

structure currently is almost exclusively done with microCT (μCT) scanners. Over the past decade, several commercial companies have been offering an increasing variety of μCT scanners for different applications. In addition, active research in μCT is going on at several academic institutions [17].

Quantitative ultrasound (QUS) techniques are also capable of assessing fracture risk. QUS cannot be used as the sole measurement for the diagnosis of osteoporosis. The main field of application is in the prediction of future fractures since QUS measurements have been shown to predict fracture risk in the older population. However, QUS has many advantages in assessing osteoporosis. The modality is safe, small, portable and no ionizing radiation is involved, measurements can be made quickly and easily, and the cost of the device is low compared with DEXA and QCT devices. The calcaneus is the most common skeletal site for quantitative ultrasound assessment because it has a high percentage of trabecular bone that is replaced more often than cortical bone, providing early evidence of metabolic change. Also, the calcaneus is fairly flat and parallel, reducing repositioning errors. The method can be applied to children, neonates, and preterm infants, just as well as to adults. Once microimaging tools to examine specific aspects of bone quality are developed, it is expected that quantitative ultrasound will be increasingly used in clinical practice [18, 19].

A further facility of the new bone densitometry technology is the option for vertebral morphometry. There are errors of accuracy in all bone densitometry techniques and also in the interpretation of the data they provide. Biochemistry is widely used in the differential diagnosis of secondary osteoporosis. Suspicions of osteomalacia or invasive processes in the bone marrow are the most common indications for bone biopsy. Finally, although history and physical examination are insufficient in diagnosing primary osteoporosis, they are important in targeting other investigations to exclude secondary forms of osteoporosis [20]. Conventional X-rays are available for the diagnosis of osteoporosis. In the first instance, conventional X-rays serve to document osteoporotic fractures, but alone are not suitable for establishing an early diagnosis of osteoporosis [21].

Magnetic resonance imaging(MRI) is currently used to predict osteoporosis. Significant progress has been made in the development of MR methods for assessing the skeletal status during the last few years. Insufficiency fractures can be detected early with MR imaging. Advances in basic MR hardware may significantly improve the impact of HR-MRI, diffusion MR imaging and MR spectroscopy for the study of trabecular bone [19].

5   Conclusion

Osteoporosis is a major health problem in the world. Given the impact of osteoporosis on individuals, families, and society, there is a great interest in diagnosis and prevention of this disease.

A decision on which technique to use for the assessment of osteoporosis is not easy. The clinicians should select the appropriate technique based on the age of the patient and the clinical context. Dual energy X-ray absorptiometry (DEXA) measurements of bone mineral density (BMD) have an important role in the evaluation of individuals at risk of osteoporosis, and in helping clinicians advise patients about the appropriate use of anti-fracture treatment.

We consider the importance of osteoporosis disease in terms of medical research and healthcare initiatives and carry out a study based on disease-diagnostic procedures relationships in MEDLINE articles. The MEDLINE contains huge number of articles thus biomedical search engines working on text mining techniques make important contributions in extracting useful information within published articles. We use a free biomedical text mining tool to extract diagnostic procedures in the articles and search general issues in the diagnosis of osteoporosis. Our results show that some techniques such as bone biopsy is rarely used today and Dual energy X-ray absorptiometry (DEXA) is the dominating technique in the last two decades.

References

1. Cohen, A.M., Hersh, W.R.: A survey of current work in biomedical text mining. Briefing in Bioinformatics 6(1), 57–71 (2005)
2. Yildirim, P., Çeken, K., Saka, O.: Knowledge discovery for the treatment of bacteria affecting liver. Turkish Journal of Medical Sciences 41(1) (2011)
3. Hoblitzell, A., Mukhopadhyay, S., You, Q., et al.: Text mining for bone biology. In: HPDC 2010 (2010)
4. Honeywell, M., Philips, S., Vo, K., et al.: Teriparatide for Osteoporosis: A Clinical Review. Drug Forecast 28(11) (2003)
5. Cummings, S.R., Melton III, L.J.: Epidemiology and outcomes of osteoporotic fractures. Lancet 359(9319), 1761–1767 (2002)
6. Carmona, R.H.: Bone Health and Osteoporosis: A Report of the U.S. Surgeon General (2004)
7. Blake, G.M., Fogelman, I.: The clinical role of dual energy X-ray absorptiometry. European Journal of Radiology 70, 406–414 (2009)
8. Physician's Guide to prevention and Treatment of Osteoporosis. Copyright ©. National Osteoporosis Foundation, 1232 22nd Street NW, Washington, D.C. 20037–1292 (2003)
9. http://www.niams.nih.gov/Health_Info/Bone/Osteoporosis/diagnosis.asp#b (cited August 28, 2011)
10. http://en.wikipedia.org/wiki/Osteoporosis (cited August 22, 2011)
11. Nobata, C., Cotter, P., Okazaki, N., et al.: Kleio: A Knowledge-enriched Information Retrieval System for Biology. In: Proceedings of the 31st Annual International ACM SIGIR Conference on Research and Development in Information Retrieval, pp. 787–788. ACM (2008)
12. Malluche, H.H., Mawad, H., Monier-Faugere, M.: Bone Biopsy in Patients with Osteoporosis. Current Osteoporosis Reports 5(4), 146–152 (2007), doi:10.1007/s11914-007-0009-x(12)
13. http://www.livestrong.com/article/93681-tests-osteoporosis (cited August 22, 2011)
14. Engelke, K., Adams, J.E., Armbrecht, G., et al.: Clinical Use of Quantitative Computed Tomography and Peripheral Quantitative Computed Tomography in the Management of Osteoporosis in Adults: The 2007 ISCD Official Positions. Journal of Clinical Densitometry: Assessment of Skeletal Health 11(1), 123–162 (2008)
15. http://en.wikipedia.org/wiki/Dual-energy_X-ray_absorptiometry (cited August 20, 2011)
16. Adams, J.E.: Quantitative computed tomography. Eur. J. Radiol. 71(3), 415–424 (2009)
17. Genant, H.K., Engelke, K., Prevrhal, S.: Advanced CT bone imaging in osteoporosis. Oxford Journals Medicine & Rheumatology 47(suppl. 4), iv9–iv16 (2008)
18. http://portableultrasoundmachines.net/ultrasound-and-osteoporosis/74 (cited August 22, 2011)
19. Damilakis, J., Maris, T.G., Karantanas, A.H.: An update on the assessment of osteoporosis using radiologic techniques. Eur. Radiol. 17(6), 1591–1602 (2006)
20. Kröger, H., Reeve, J.: Diagnosis of osteoporosis in clinical practice. Ann. Med. 30(3), 278–287 (1998)
21. Kraenzlin, M.E.: Diagnosis of osteoporosis. How do you manage it?, MMW Fortschr. Med. 144(21), 24–30 (2002)

Challenges Storing and Representing Biomedical Data

Joel P. Arrais, Pedro Lopes, and José Luís Oliveira

DETI/IEETA, University of Aveiro
Campus Universitário de Santiago, 3810 – 193 Aveiro, Portugal
{jpa,pedrolopes,jlo}@ua.pt

Abstract. The scientific achievements coming from molecular biology depend greatly on the capability of computational applications to manage and explore laboratorial results. One component that is commonly underrated is the need for proper user interfaces that allow researchers to visually explore the results and extract biological evidences.

In this paper, we review the main challenges of dealing with complex biomedical datasets, namely regarding data storing, communicating, representing and visualizing biomedical experimental data. We emphasize the need for proper human computer interaction paradigms and underlying data management architectures in order to achieve a correct interpretation of the experimental results.

Keywords: Biomedical Data, Data Integration, Data Mining, Data Representation.

1   Introduction

Advances in biomedical research have created a data deluge whose analysis requires proper methods and computer infrastructures. One major challenge consists in the creation of data structures that store relevant information in a form that is easy for computer programs to manipulate and that is accessible for human interpretation.

The comprehensive analysis of an experiment commonly requires combining and studying the locally obtained results with third-party biological data [1, 2]. This need arises from the inherent complexity of both living organisms and the biological structures that define them; for instance, a single phenotype may be the result of interactions involving genetic elements. Other reason is associated with function conservation, because prior information about the biological function of a gene in one organism can be used to evaluate its function in others. Therefore, in order to fully understand the role of a gene, a scientist usually needs its nucleotide sequence, metabolic pathways and known drug interactions amongst a myriad of other equally important factors and concepts that need to be placed in context in order to facilitate knowledge extraction. Such a need becomes especially important when high throughput techniques, such as microarrays, produce results that only become meaningful after being matched with additional, previously known data residing at public databases [3, 4]. Thus, providing a unified view of multiple kinds and often

A. Holzinger and K.-M. Simonic (Eds.): USAB 2011, LNCS 7058, pp. 53–62, 2011.

large sets of data confers a catalyzing effect on the investigation process and, as such, its importance cannot be stressed enough.

In this paper, we present a review of the main challenges for storing, communicating, representing and visualizing biomedical experimental data. The results and discussion presented outline the main difficulties and envisage the opportunities and directions of a still emerging field where the paradigms for human computer interaction will play a critical role. Furthermore, both the issues found in dealing with biomedical data are detailed, and two representative examples introduced, where the visual representation of biomedical data is crucial for the correct interpretation of the experimental results.

2   Challenges for Biomedical Data Management

Like in many other areas, the growing number of biomedical resources has drastically increased the level of heterogeneity in the biomedical field. As the "omics" revolution unfolds, new software and hardware are created to meet clinicians and researchers' demands. Consequently, end users are overwhelmed with the amount and diversity of available tools and information.

Managing biomedical data has been the subject of various research projects tackling two great challenges in the field: the integration and interoperability from and amongst distributed resources [5-7]. Whereas the former played a key role in bioinformatics evolution over the last couple of decades [8, 9], the latter is a modern topic, allowing for continuous improvements. Whilst these challenges cannot be approached independently, we can benefit from using similar service composition strategies in their resolution.

2.1   Integration

The main goal of integration architectures is to provide support for a unified set of features, working over disparate and heterogeneous applications, and presenting a holistic view to end-users. Along with technical restrictions such as software/hardware platforms, model disparities or content locations, there are also other hindrances to the integration tasks, such as enterprise/academic boundaries or political/ethical issues [10]. Whether we are simply dealing with the integration of a set of files resulting from microarray experiments or with distributed database instances containing reference genomics data, integration relies on service composition and coordination methods to centralize distributed information or to give the idea that data are centralized.

Strategies for data integration revolve around three key structures, differing mostly on the amount and kind of data that are merged in the central system and, respectively, on the it's final performance and efficacy (Fig. 1). Warehouse solutions (Fig. 1 A) consist on the creation of warehouses collecting data gathered from several resources. Integrated datasets are entirely replicated in the warehouses, raising issues regarding data model mappings and data updates, among others [11-13]. In bioinformatics, Bio2RDF [14] is the edge-of-breed solution. Mediator-based solutions require the implementation of

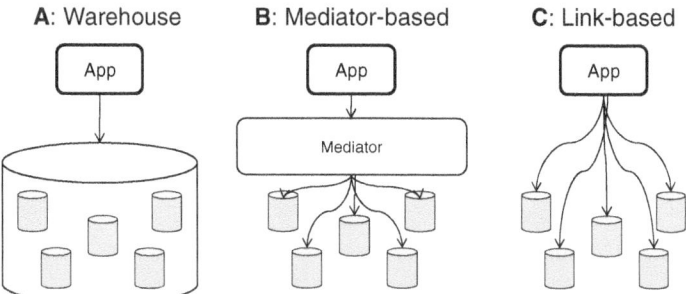

Fig. 1. Data integration models categorized according to their relation with the integration application and the integrated external resources

software wrappers, connecting the central application to the external resources (Fig. 1 B). The result is a virtual warehouse, with a dynamic middleware layer extending the access scope to distributed resources [15, 16]. The third widely used approach is link-based resource integration (Fig 1. C). This strategy consists in the aggregation of pointers to relevant distributed resources, without explicitly importing their data [17]. WAVe uses this strategy for the integration and enrichment of genetics datasets, presenting them using augmented browsing techniques [18].

Despite the fact that these approaches cover almost all possible solutions for data integration, most bioinformatics developers craft ad-hoc hybrid solutions, mixing direct warehousing integration for some resources with wrappers and pointers to others.

2.2   Interoperability

Interoperability is a feature to facilitate integration and collaboration between distinct software. Interoperable systems can access and use parts of other systems, exchange content with other systems and communicate using predefined protocols that are common to both systems. Software interoperability is defined as the level where multiple software components can interact regardless of their implementation programming language or software/hardware platform. Syntactic software interoperability may be achieved with data type and specification level interoperability. Data type interoperability consists in distributed and distinct programs supporting structured content exchanges whether through indirect methods, such as writing in the same file, or direct methods, like Application Programming Interfaces (APIs), invoked inside a computer or through a network. Specification level interoperability encapsulates knowledge representation differences when dealing with abstract data types, thus, enabling programs to communicate at higher levels of abstraction – web service level for instance.

In modern biomedical data management, interoperability plays a key role in scenarios where several hardware/software tools must exchange data. Whether developers are dealing with Picture Archival and Communication Systems (PACS) or Electronic Health Records systems (EHRs), service composition and coordination strategies are implemented for enhanced performance [20, 21]. For example, the underlying challenges for establishing intelligent data connections in breast cancer diagnosis, treatment and monitoring, involve the design of shared data models and interoperable services, which ultimately result in improved patient care. These are required for a coherent data flow from radiology departments to a genetic diagnostics lab and to patient digital records available for clinicians, leveraging the need for highly expertise regarding the software interoperability domain.

2.3   Service Composition

The development of hybrid integration and interoperability approaches has gained momentum in recent years, especially through the introduction of novel web-based data access techniques and workflow enactment applications [22]. This trend consists in making resources, data or tools, available as web services, allowing dynamic and real-time communication and data exchanges.

Web services are the most widely used technology for the development of distributed web applications. The World Wide Web Consortium (W3C) defines web services "as software system designed to support interoperable machine-to-machine interaction over a network". This broad definition allows us to consider a web service as any kind of online-available resource, as long as it enables machine-to-machine integration and interoperability. Despite this all-embracing definition, we can divide existing web services in two main groups: web services following W3C's standards and application-specific REST services.

Standardised web services have the main purpose of providing a unified data access interface and a constant data model of the data sources. Simple Object Access Protocol (SOAP), Universal Description, Discovery and Integration (UDDI) and Web Services Description Language (WSDL) are the currently used standards and they define exchanges at all software interoperability levels, ranging from the data transport protocol to the query languages used [24]. REST web services usage is growing as they are emerging as a viable alternative to standardised web services. REST services consist in simple web applications that respond to HTTP requests. HTML, XML, JSON, CSV or, most simply, free text, are used in replies, leaving the data handling tasks to the original application [25].

As a whole, web service composition [26] defines the collection of protocols, messages and strategies that have to be applied in order to coordinate a heterogeneous set of web services to reach a given goal. Biomedical data integration and interoperability scenarios involve the adoption of service composition strategies, requiring the development of a composition infrastructure that is able to control the workflow's coordinated execution, communicate with the distinct web services and organize the information flow between the web services.

2.4   Beyond Integration and Interoperability

In the healthcare domain, integration and interoperability are directly intertwined. We can only extract the full added value from our software if we use these concepts within the same strategy. We argue in accordance with Slater [27] and colleagues, whose research underlines drawbacks intrinsic to current techniques, recognizing the need for novel approaches based on distinct skills and ideals. For this, Semantic Web methodologies arise as the desired resolution in spite of their projected slow adoption [29].

Tim Berners-Lee, the self-proclaimed inventor of the modern Internet and director of W3C, promoted semantic Web developments in 2001. The W3C Semantic Web Activity group has already launched a series of standards to promote the developments in this area, such as URI, RDF, OWL and SPARQL [30]. A URI is a simple and generic identifier that is built on a sequence of characters and that enables the uniform and unique identification of any resource. RDF was designed as a standard to enable the description of web resources in a simple fashion [31]. The syntax neutral data model is based on the representation of predicates and their values. A resource can be anything that is correctly referenced by an URI. In RDF we can represent concepts, relations and taxonomies of concepts. This triplet characteristic results in a simple and flexible system: relationships are established through subject-predicate-object formalizations. SPARQL is an SQL-like query language that acts as a friendly interface to RDF information. Ontology consists on the collection of consensual and shared models in an executable form of concepts, relations and their constraints tied to a scaffold of taxonomies. In practical terms, we use ontologies to assert facts about resources described in RDF and referenced by an URI.

Combining these technologies will enable integration and interoperability between distributed and heterogeneous resources, resulting in the possibility of data in one source to be transparently and intelligently connected with data in a distinct source [34]. In a long-term perspective, adopting these technologies will result in vast improvements over current systems. By establishing more meaningful relationships amongst data in our repositories, we will be able to obtain deeper insights from the collected knowledge. It is clear that the innate complexity of the life sciences domain, amplified in biomedical data management software, requires large efforts and expertise to be overcome. With the Semantic Web, a truly integrative and interoperable knowledge network will cover the entire life sciences domain.

3 Challenges Representing Biomedical Data

While biomedical data management triggers complex computer science challenges, this area is of crucial importance to the development of improved human interaction methods to analyze clinical and experimental data. Next we explore two scenarios where the combination of resource integration with rich user interfaces is essential to the interpretation of experimental results.

3.1 Microarray Study

Microarray analysis is, currently, a very important technique for the study of gene expression patterns. The principle supporting this technique is the ability of a given nucleic acid sequence binding specifically to, or hybridizing to, another nucleic acid of complementary base composition. Therefore, this technology provides a global, simultaneous view on the transcription levels of many or all genes of an organism under a range of conditions or processes. The information obtained by monitoring gene expression levels in different developmental stages, tissue types, clinical conditions and different organisms can help in understanding gene function and gene networks, assist in the diagnostic of disease conditions and reveal the effects of medical treatments.

A key step in the analysis of gene expression data is the identification of groups of genes that manifest similar expression patterns that is equivalent to the algorithmic problem of clustering genes based on their expression data. The data used for clustering consists of a vector for each gene with the expression values for each individual condition under study. Because we usually have thousands of genes the typical results is a matrix of expression levels. This vector is indeed complemented with the annotations from the external databases resulting in a cube. It is the analysis of this cube that holds the key to the interpretation of the experiment. Is therefore of critical importance the need for intuitive interfaces to explore this data aggregation.

A common approach consists in the use of cluster analysis is usually complemented with related biomedical data, in order to understand the active process under the conditions under study. The goal is to partition the elements into subsets, which are called clusters, so that two criteria are satisfied: homogeneity, elements in the same cluster are highly similar to each other; and separation, elements from different clusters have low similarity to each other.

Fig. 2 outlines the challenges representing the sum of data from a microarray experiment, namely the multiple dimensionalities of the data as the high number of biomedical terms associated with each term.

3.2   Network Representation of Gene-Disease Association Studies

The identification of genes responsible for the cause or prevention of diseases is critical knowledge in the development of new diagnostics and therapies. Over the past few years, several computational methods have been used to obtain candidate genes for a disease and although the results require experimental validation, they provide important clues for selecting the best targets.

A group of computational methods that have been successfully applied are based on biomedical networks. This networks is obtained by integrating data from disparate data sources including Gene Ontology (GO) (http://www.geneontology.org), pathway annotations (KEGG), Online Mendelian Inheritance in Man (OMIM), and multiple literature and ontology databases (Fig. 3).

Regarding the web interface, we envisage an ontology-driven semantic search system, which should provide all the functionalities of the system in a simple to use interface. We will focus mostly in investigating visualization techniques to map the query result structure, so that a user can easily see how concepts relate to each other, allowing the assessment of the explicit relations among the searched terms. The application interface should be intuitive, providing links to the original documents in PubMed, and to the pages describing the concepts identified in each document.

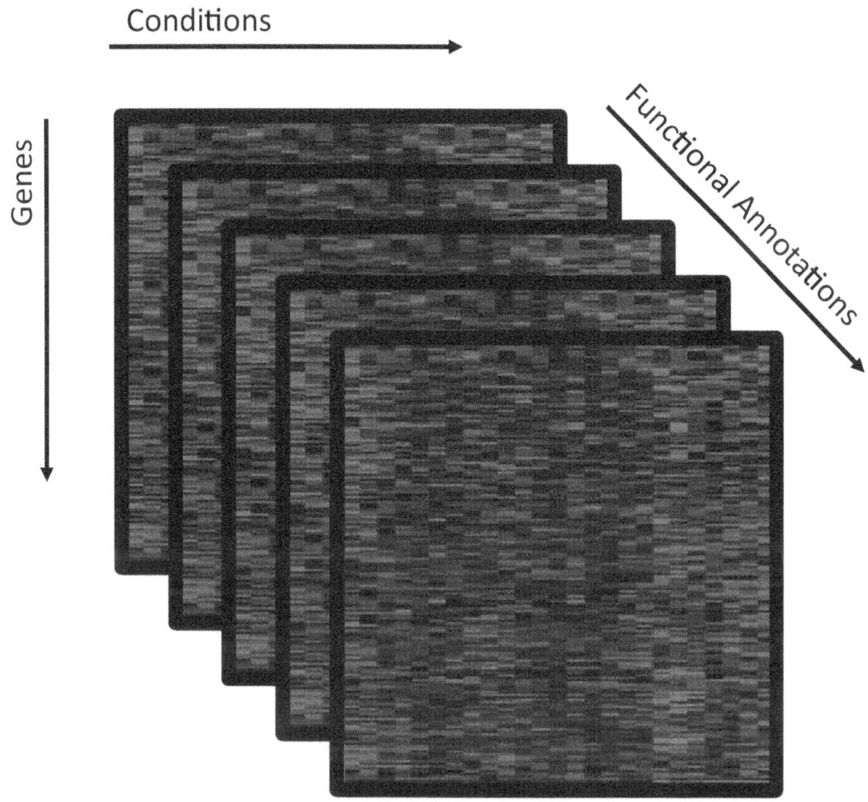

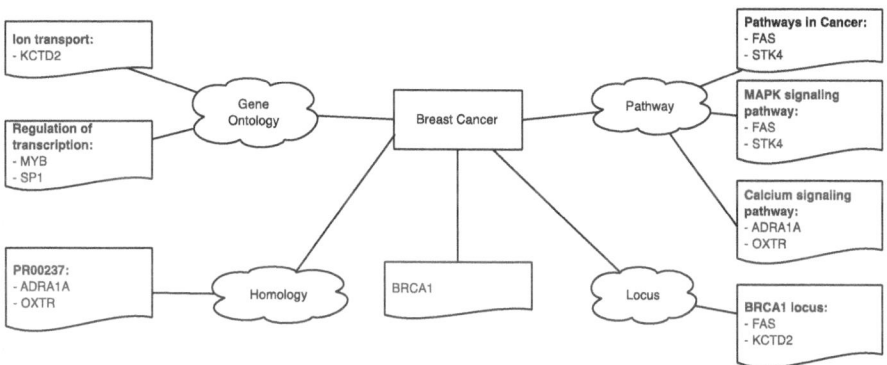

Fig. 2. Data cube representing the functional interpretation of a microarray experiment

Fig. 3. Example that demonstrates the usage of GeNS to obtain the network of concepts related with Breast Cancer disease

Besides exploiting web interfaces for the semantic network representation, the use of innovative interaction paradigms, based on a 2D/3D scanner and gesture tracking, and its impact on user acceptance and productivity. The visual abstractions that we will follow provide another major challenge. Many approaches to network visualization use graphs or trees, representing nodes and links through different sizes, shapes and colors. This approach has the benefit of allowing a wide variety of layout algorithms, contributing to the overall flexibility of the visualization system. However, other approaches can provide more useful results, such as abstract geometrical shapes, city abstractions, landscapes, tree maps, relative neighborhood graphs, correlation plots, heat maps and many others. The user will be able to navigate along the network representation, modify visualization attributes such as the perspective, lighting, camera position and zoom, either in static or animated mode.

4   Conclusion

The integration and interoperability among heterogeneous resources is a classic problem in biomedical software, where the ability to provide a unified view of conceptually different sets of data offers scientists a much broader view of a given subject, thus making it much easier to extract conclusions that may not have been visible otherwise. In this paper we review the main challenges for the storage, interoperability, representation and visualization of biomedical clinical and experimental data.

Furthermore, results and discussion presented in this manuscript are used as a seed for the awareness of the opportunities and directions in a still emerging field, where the paradigms for human computer interaction are sustained by advanced data management strategies to fulfill their critical role.

References

1. Stein, L.: Creating a bioinformatics nation. Nature 417(6885), 119–120 (2002)
2. Goble, C., Stevens, R.: State of the nation in data integration for bioinformatics. J. Biomed. Inform. 41(5), 687–693 (2008)
3. Al-Shahrour, F., et al.: From genes to functional classes in the study of biological systems. BMC Bioinformatics 8, 114 (2007)
4. Fang, Z., et al.: Knowledge guided analysis of microarray data. J. Biomed. Inform. 39(4), 401–411 (2006)
5. Trifiro, G., et al.: EU-ADR Healthcare Database Network vs. Spontaneous Reporting System Database: Preliminary Comparison of Signal Detection. Studies in Health Technology and Informatics 166, 25–30 (2011)
6. Webb, A.J., Thorisson, G.A., Brookes, A.J.: An informatics project and online "Knowledge Centre" supporting modern genotype-to-phenotype research. Human Mutation 32(5), 543–550 (2011)
7. Ring, H.Z., Kwok, P.-Y., Cotton, R.G.: Human Variome Project: an international collaboration to catalogue human genetic variation. Pharmacogenomics 7(7), 969–972 (2006)

8. Goble, C., Stevens, R.: State of the nation in data integration for bioinformatics. Journal of Biomedical Informatics 41(5), 687–693 (2008)

9. Smedley, D., et al.: BioMart - biological queries made easy. BMC Genomics 10(1), 22 (2009)

10. Hohpe, G., Woolf, B.: Enterprise Integration Patterns: Designing, Building, and Deploying Messaging Solutions. The Addison-Wesley Signature Series. Addison-Wesley (2004)

11. Polyzotis, N., et al.: Meshing Streaming Updates with Persistent Data in an Active Data Warehouse. IEEE Transactions on Knowledge and Data Engineering 20(7), 976–991 (2008)

12. Zhu, Y., An, L., Liu, S.: Data Updating and Query in Real-Time Data Warehouse System. In: 2008 International Conference on Computer Science and Software Engineering (2008)

13. Arrais, J., Pereira, J., Oliveira, J.L.: GeNS: A biological data integration platform. In: ICBB 2009, International Conference on Bioinformatics and Biomedicine. WASET, World Academy of Science, Engineering and Technology, Venice (2009)

14. Belleau, F., et al.: Bio2RDF: towards a mashup to build bioinformatics knowledge systems. J. Biomed. Inform. 41(5), 706–716 (2008)

15. Haas, L.M., et al.: DiscoveryLink: A system for integrated access to life sciences data sources. IBM Systems Journal 40(2), 489–511 (2001)

16. Matos, S., et al.: Concept-based query expansion for retrieving gene related publications from MEDLINE. BMC Bioinformatics 11(1), 212 (2010)

17. Lopes, P., Dalgleish, R., Oliveira, J.L.: WAVe: Web Analysis of the Variome. Human Mutation 32 (2011)

18. Lopes, P., Dalgleish, R., Oliveira, J.L.: WAVe: web analysis of the variome. Hum. Mutat. 32(7), 729–734 (2011)

19. Arrais, J., et al.: GeneBrowser: an approach for integration and functional classification of genomic data (2007)

20. Garde, S., et al.: Towards semantic interoperability for electronic health records. Methods Inf. Med. 46(3), 332–343 (2007)

21. Blazona, B., Koncar, M.: HL7 and DICOM based integration of radiology departments with healthcare enterprise information systems. Int. J. Med. Inform. 76(suppl. 3), S425–S432 (2007)

22. Ludascher, B., et al.: Taverna: Scientific Workflow Management and the Kepler System. Research Articles, Concurrency and Computation: Practice & Experience 18(10), 1039–1065 (2006)

23. W3C, W.W.W.C., Web Services. World Wide Web Consortium (2002)

24. Wang, Y.-H., Liao, J.C.: Why or Why Not Service Oriented Architecture. In: International Conference on Services Science, Management and Engineering 2009 (2009)

25. Rosenberg, F., et al.: Composing RESTful Services and Collaborative Workflows: A Lightweight Approach. IEEE Internet Computing 12(5), 24–31 (2008)

26. Milanovic, N., Malek, M.: Current solutions for Web service composition. IEEE Internet Computing 8(6), 51–59 (2004)

27. Slater, T., Bouton, C., Huang, E.S.: Beyond data integration. Drug Discovery Today 13(13/14), 584–589 (2008)

28. Kozhenkov, S., et al.: BiologicalNetworks 2.0 - an integrative view of genome biology data. BMC Bioinformatics 11(1), 610 (2010)

29. Cannata, N., et al.: A Semantic Web for bioinformatics: goals, tools, systems, applications. BMC Bioinformatics 9(suppl. 4), S1 (2008)

30. Berners-Lee, T., Hendler, J., Lassila, O.: The Semantic Web. Sci. Am. 284, 34–43 (2001)
31. Miller, E.J.: An Introduction to the Resource Description Framework. Journal of Library Administration 34(3), 245–255 (2001)
32. Uschold, M., Gruninger, M.: Ontologies: Principles, Methods and Applications. Knowledge Engineering Review 11(2), 93–155 (1996)
33. Stevens, R., Goble, C.A., Bechhofer, S.: Ontology-based knowledge representation for bioinformatics. Brief Bioinform. 1(4), 398–414 (2000)
34. Hepp, M.: Semantic Web and semantic Web services: father and son or indivisible twins? IEEE Internet Computing 10(2), 85–88 (2006)

Semantic Analytics of PubMed Content[*]

Dominik Ślęzak[1,2], Andrzej Janusz[1], Wojciech Świeboda[1],
Hung Son Nguyen[1], Jan G. Bazan[3,1], and Andrzej Skowron[1]

[1] Institute of Mathematics, University of Warsaw
ul. Banacha 2, 02-097 Warsaw, Poland
[2] Infobright Inc.
ul. Krzywickiego 34 lok. 219, 02-078 Warsaw, Poland
[3] Chair of Computer Science, University of Rzeszów
ul. Rejtana 16A, 35-310 Rzeszów, Poland

Abstract. We present an architecture aimed at semantic search and
synthesis of information acquired from the document repositories. The
proposed framework is expected to provide domain knowledge interfaces
enabling the internally implemented algorithms to identify relationships
between documents, researchers, institutions, as well as concepts extracted from various types of knowledge bases. The framework should
be scalable with respect to data volumes, diversity of analytic processes,
and the speed of search. In this paper, we investigate these requirements
for the case of medical publications gathered in PubMed.

Keywords: Semantic Search and Analytics, PubMed, MeSH, RDBMS,
Document Repositories, Decision Support Systems, Behavioral Patterns.

1 Introduction

Rapid development of freely available biomedical databases, such as PubMed
[21], allows users to search for documents containing highly specialized biomedical knowledge. This article outlines the **SONCA** (**S**earch based on **ON**tologies
and **C**ompound **A**nalytics) [6] framework, whose aim is to extend the functionality of such databases not only by more efficient search of relevant documents,
but also by more intelligent extraction and synthesis of information, as well as
more advanced interaction between users and knowledge sources.

[*] This work was supported by the grant N N516 077837 from the Ministry of Science
and Higher Education of the Republic of Poland and by the National Centre for Research and Development (NCBiR) under the grant SP/I/1/77065/10 by the Strategic
scientific research and experimental development program "Interdisciplinary System
for Interactive Scientific and Scientific-Technical Information (SYNAT)". We would
like to acknowledge the whole SYNAT team, in particular: Marek Grzegorowski, Michał Kijowski, Marcin Kowalski, Adam Krasuski, and Krzysztof Stencel (co-creators
of database model; Section 3), Kamil Herba, Grzegorz Jaśkiewicz, Michał Meina,
Sinh Hoa Nguyen, and Marcin Szczuka (co-creators of experimental framework; Section 4), as well as Przemysław Pardel and Sebastian Stawicki (responsible for loading
and parsing PubMed data). Special thanks go to Stanisława Bazan-Socha for her remarks on possible future usage of SONCA by biomedical experts.

A. Holzinger and K.-M. Simonic (Eds.): USAB 2011, LNCS 7058, pp. 63–74, 2011.
© Springer-Verlag Berlin Heidelberg 2011

Although development of SONCA is still at its relatively preliminary stages, our ambition is to construct the engine enabling to formulate decision support types of queries in a simplified, domain-specific language, and assembly the answers basing on a chain of operations on semantic indexes cyclically recomputed over a repository of documents and other information sources, stored in both structural and relational fashion. In this paper, we discuss this vision with respect to potential expectations of biomedical experts, using the contents of PubMed and one of the corresponding domain ontologies as a case study.

The paper is organized as follows. In Section 2, we outline SONCA's architecture. In Section 3, we elaborate on RDBMS model supporting analytic processes. In Section 4, we show some examples of basic functionalities and the corresponding experiments. In Section 5, we discuss future steps.

2   Requirements and Components

SONCA is aimed at the analysis of documents of different origin and format. It should be also able to utilize domain ontologies or specialized databases. Knowledge bases, such as, e.g., MeSH[1] [26], can be employed as the source of domain knowledge, as well as the means for communicating with the users or the basis for discovering meaningful patterns in data. SONCA is characterized by ability to represent various types of entities, such as documents, authors, concepts, results, images, data sets. It also uses available knowledge bases to produce semantic indexes that facilitate search and information synthesis [23].

SONCA needs to be scalable with respect to the volumes of data and a variety of usage patterns. It should be characterized by a modern database architecture, as well as support for various approximate and hierarchical reasoning algorithms [5,19]. There might be no single methodology addressing all scalability expectations. For example, document stores seem to be the best for gathering and managing original files and metadata. On the other hand, analytic-oriented RDBMS engines are a better choice for managing information about documents and other related entities in order to build more useful semantic indexes.

Figure 1 outlines the main SONCA's modules: the repository of documents, the analytic index server, the search index server, and the user interfaces. The repository stores original documents or links to some external sources. The analytic index server computes intermediate tables and final semantic indexes. The search index server provides scalable external access to the results of analytic processes. The interfaces parse and decompose user requests basing on domain-knowledge-driven hierarchical modeling [5,14]. Requests can be usually addressed by the search index server, in combination with links to original documents. However, some parts of more advanced requests may be redirected to intermediate analytic structures or generic tables described in Section 3.

---

[1] MeSH is a medical ontology created by United States National Library of Medicine. It contains over 26 thousands of concept records (also called subject headings), most of which consist of a definition, a list of synonyms, and links to related entries.

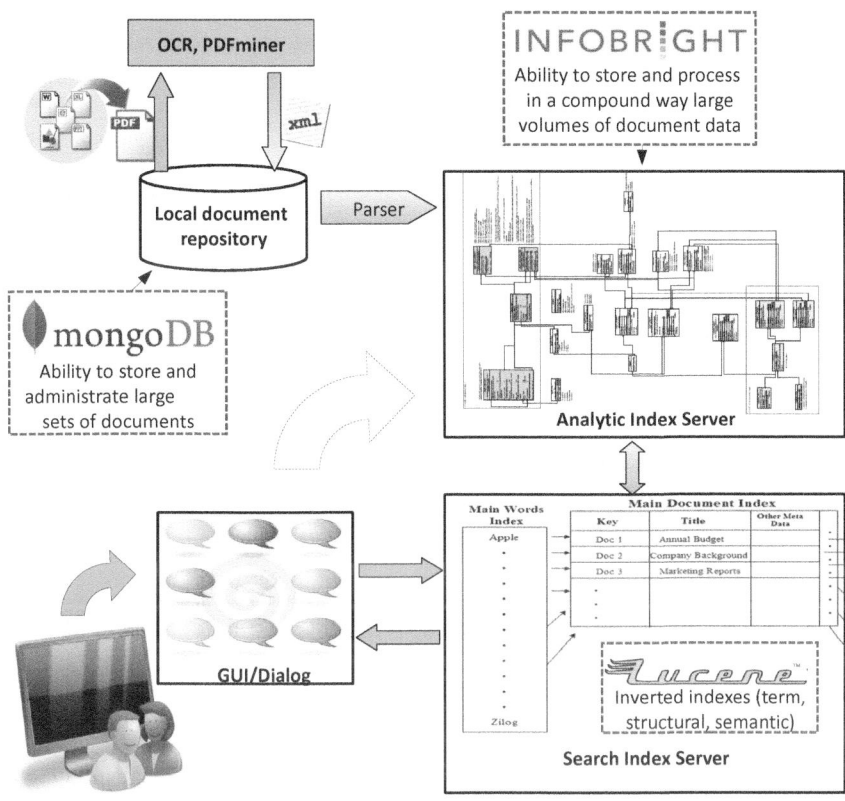

Fig. 1. The architecture of SONCA along with some of software components

Figure 1 also shows software solutions that we applied at the prototype stage in order to meet the outlined requirements. We use MongoDB [8], Infobright [22], and, among the others, Lucene [17] to represent information in three forms: repository-oriented, analytics-oriented, and search-oriented. The choice of tools for building the user interfaces is still under investigation.

3   RDBMS Model

SONCA's analytic index server is based on the relational database schema aimed at efficient storing and querying documents, as well as entities corresponding to researchers, institutions, scientific areas, and others. We adapted some types of relations from the CERIF project [15]. We also store detailed information about parsed documents in order to conduct analytics in combination with domain knowledge about scientific topics, by means of standard SQL and RDBMS management. Of course not all documents are available in their full form. For example, we treat as documents also the items parsed from bibliographies of available

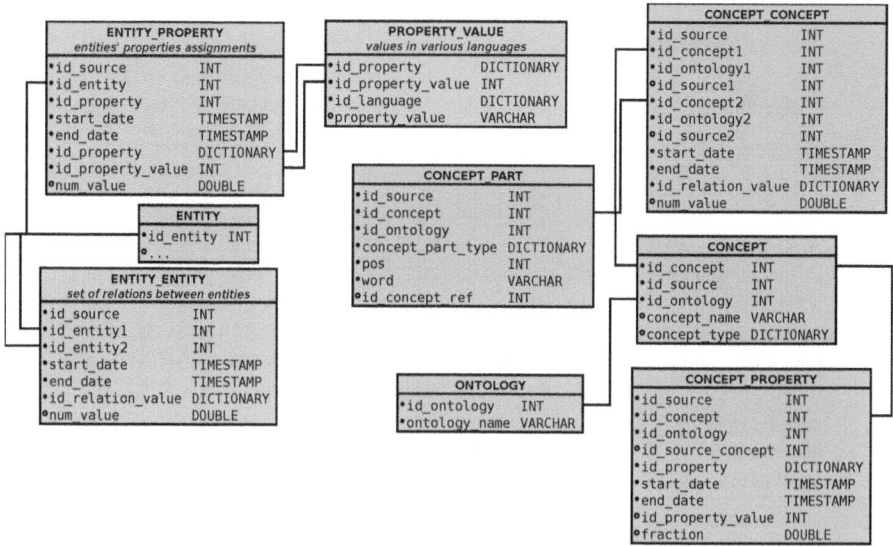

Fig. 2. General schema for assigning properties to entities and relations to entity pairs (left). There are three types of entity semantics: instances, objects, and concepts (right).

publications. This leads to a need of applying analytic and search methods capable to work with incomplete, often uncertain information.

We store information about all properties of entities and all relations between entities in two kinds of tables: ENTITY_ENTITY and ENTITY_PROPERTY (see Figure 2). This way, we avoid an uncontrolled amount of tables. We utilize this universal layout in the three major areas of our model described below.

The first area, referred as generic, contains table INSTANCE, which stores information about instances – entities distinguishable while parsing input files. It follows a general ENTITY layout. It also reflects decomposition of each of documents onto parts, such as abstract, section, or bibliography, with their hierarchy levels encoded by column instance_type (see Figure 3). Each decomposed part is treated as a separate instance. It enables us to operate with the parts of documents when creating semantic indexes and conducting ad-hoc analytics. For example, investigation of current trends in the field of genetic research may be enriched by the analysis of changes in occurrences of related concepts in the concluding sections of articles published in several consecutive years.

All metadata enclosed in input files or gained from other sources are stored in two tables: INSTANCE_PROPERTY and INSTANCE_INSTANCE. The latter one includes connections between persons and organizations, which should be revealed during analyzing publication (e.g.: affiliations), between organizations and publications (e.g.: editors of documents from references), between persons and publications (e.g.: relation of being an author of publication) and so on.

We assume temporality of properties and relations. We address it by adding columns defining validation time windows. This allows us to model various

```
<Document>
  <Abstract>
    Effects of magnesium on...
  <\Abstract>
  <Section>
    High magnesium doses were...
  <\Section>
<\Document>
```

id_instance	id_superinstance	start_pos	end_pos	instance_type	word
1		0	2984	Document	
2	1	0	512	Abstract	
3	2	0	1	word	Effects
4	2	1	2	word	of
5	2	2	3	word	magnesium
6	2	3	4	word	on
⋮	⋮	⋮	⋮	⋮	⋮
513	1	513	1393	Section	
514	951	513	514	word	High
515	951	514	515	word	magnesium
516	951	515	516	word	doses
517	951	516	517	word	were
⋮	⋮	⋮	⋮	⋮	⋮

Fig. 3. A part of a file from PubMed and its corresponding RDBMS representation

situations more realistically. For example, in order to express information about researchers in medicine, we need such temporal properties and relations as, e.g., 'MedicalSpeciality' and 'PlaceOfMedicalPractice'.

In order to verify whether it is realistic to put such a huge volume of data into a relational database schema, we conducted a simple experiment with Infobright's software [22], optimized for data compression and SQL-based analytics. We parsed 235,000 documents from the PubMed Central Open Subset [21]. The size of this text corpus was about 385 GB. We measured compression ratios for data stored in RDBMS. Physical size of table INSTANCE turned out to be almost 40 times smaller than the corresponding tabular data obtained from the parsing algorithm. The sizes of tables INSTANCE_INSTANCE, INSTANCE_PROPERTY, and PROPERTY_VALUE were, respectively, 30, 20, and 5.5 times smaller.

The second area, referred as analytic, is analogous to the generic area of the schema. The difference is that now we work with objects corresponding to classes of instances grouped together by matching algorithms, executed cyclically over the content of generic tables. Relationships between identifiers of instances and objects are stored in table OBJECT_MATCH, which is the bridge between generic and analytic layers. The corresponding attributes in tables describing objects are synthesized by algorithms basing on OBJECT_MATCH and INSTANCE. Such synthesis may significantly increase information completeness. For example, the same article can occur in bibliographies of many documents, with different parts of information provided. After matching multiple article's instances together, we can operate with merged information about the corresponding object. Surely, such matching and synthesizing techniques can work on heuristic basis.

The third area refers to ontologies, which can be regarded as models of knowledge with distinguished entities, their properties and relations between them. We call such ontology-based entities as concepts (see Figure 2, on the right). Precisely, by a concept we treat every entity that can be retrieved from a source provided by an expert (and using algorithms accepted by an expert). A technical challenge in this area is to provide fairly universal framework for storing information about concepts acquired from different sources, such as, e.g., Wikipedia or MeSH [26]. Such information is contained in table `CONCEPT`. We also need representation of concepts as texts. As one can represent a concept by different text descriptions, we introduce column `concept_part_type`. There is, however, a difference between this column and `instance_type` in the table `INSTANCE` as we did not find a reason for introducing a hierarchy for concept descriptions. For example, in MeSH each subject heading, apart from its short definition, may be described by an annotation, a historical note, and a list of synonyms. Table `CONCEPT_PART` allows storing this information in a unified way.

Table `CONCEPT_OBJECT` consists of relations between ontological concepts and analytic objects. An important relation that we can derive, store and use is labeling documents or scientists with topics from ontologies (e.g.: from MeSH). Going further, we can do it not only for the whole documents but also for their particular parts, which can lead to some interesting document structure-aware analytics. One example may be to reason about the most promising areas of science, e.g., by means a query formulated by a student who searches for potential topics of future thesis, where SQL-based heuristics may extract topics occurring frequently in the concluding parts of documents but with no significant representation in bibliographies and major parts of documents. Table `CONCEPT_OBJECT` is built analogously to `ENTITY_ENTITY` in Figure 2, where the first entity becomes analytic object and the second entity becomes ontological concept.

To conclude this section let us discuss how to extend SONCA by adding new types of entities. Consider an example of microarray experiments [3,12]. In this case, we need two new types of objects – an experiment and a gene. Additionally, one may consider a collection of microarray experiments as an entity itself. Information about all experiments may be stored within the previously-described tables or, optionally, in a separate table comprising of columns `experiment_id`, `collection_id`, `gene_id`, and `gene_expression_value`. New entities may have unique properties and unique types of relations with other objects. Genes may be labeled by a symbol, synonyms in various ontologies, a type, a taxon, and a sequence. They can be in relation with, e.g., collections of experiments, in which they were examined. Moreover, all the above-discussed new entities may be related to some documents. For example, a microarray data set can be used in a study described by a document, which draws a conclusion regarding a role of a specific gene. Such relations, if discovered, can be used to enrich analytic results. Further types of entities may origin from log files, upper ontologies, annotated medical images, patent databases, patient histories, and so on.

4   Basic Functionalities

By the support for the methods of semantic indexing and user interaction with data sources, SONCA is intended to become a problem-solving tool. Our ultimate goal is to allow querying the system in a semi-natural language, e.g., with a use of a controlled vocabulary. Such queries would be mapped into our data model using domain knowledge and translated into the corresponding SQL statements. Their intermediate results would be then post-processed by dedicated information synthesis modules and finally presented to the users.

Consider the following query as an example: "Provide a summary of the current state of knowledge about X", where "X" may refer to a condition, a chemical compound, or a patient's history. In this case, the system would have to identify the concept "X", find the most related pieces of information, and construct a summary that could be returned in a variety of formats, including figures, tables, links to original sources, and so on. Other useful queries may look like: "Give me a definition of X"; "What are the most related research problems?"; "When was it first used in the literature?"; "Which academic units work on a given problem?"; "Which workshops and conferences discuss the topic?". Ability to answer such queries would doubtlessly benefit the community.

Let us now briefly describe three examples of basic computational blocks that can eventually lead towards hierarchical execution of the above types of queries in SONCA. It is interesting to look at them as a chain of information transmission that can be scheduled in order to provide user interfaces with the most efficient indexes. In particular, structural and semantic information extracted by the first two of the following modules will be used in the third one.

Source unification. Given the requirement of handling document content from various data sources, it is crucial to unify the underlying documents' structure. While choosing a suitable data format, we were inspired by the NLM Archiving and Interchange DTD used within PubMed [21]. We refer to this data format as NXML, after the filename suffix of the PubMed documents. Actually, Figure 3 contains a fragment of text in the NXML format (on the left).

Converting the source documents to the NXML files is prone to errors. The corresponding modules require appropriate measures of validity. The PubMed documents provide a natural benchmark data, as they are available both in digital PDF and NXML formats. Thus, we could test our algorithms by converting those PDFs to the (simplified) NXML files. For each input document, (partial) comparison was related to the tree structures and the NXML file content. One may take into account multi-column texts, hyphenations, detection of titles, authors and bibliographic entries, as well as such structural entities as tables, figures or footnotes. In theory, such comparisons can be implemented both within the local document repository and the analytic index server. However, it is more intuitive and efficient to run them at the repository level.

Semantic indexing. Medical document databases use external knowledge bases to facilitate the searching process. For example, documents in PubMed are semi-manually tagged with concepts from MeSH. Queries sent to the database are then automatically extended by the corresponding MeSH headings. One of possible usages of SONCA is to extend such tagging process. Indeed, the ontological part of our data model supports storage of information from different external knowledge bases, such as MeSH or DBpedia. Therefore, we may implement some universal methods for detecting associations between documents and concepts. We can automatically tag documents with the notions from their domain of origin and store the outcomes in table CONCEPT_OBJECT, ready to facilitate search and retrieval. The obtained tags can be then utilized in various processes, such as grouping of search results or topical classification (e.g.: automatic classification of documents into MeSH's topical qualifiers).

The extracted semantic information can also serve as a way of extending the commonly used bag-of-words representation of text documents [7]. The key concepts assigned to a document form representation that we call a bag-of-concepts. As a step toward this direction, we implemented within SONCA the Explicit Semantic Analysis (ESA) technique [10], where natural language definitions of concepts from an encyclopedia or an ontology are matched against texts to find the best associations. Let us recall that we keep processed text descriptions of concepts in table CONCEPT_PART. Thus, we can easily construct an inverted semantic index that maps words occurring in such descriptions into related concepts. For each new document, concepts that correspond to its words basing on such inverted index are retrieved and aggregated to form an extended bag-of-concepts. For a larger set of documents it is worth implementing the whole operation in the analytic index server and gather all bag-of-concepts representations within a single intermediate analytic structure ready for further usage.

We applied the above method in combination with MeSH and DBpedia to index PubMed documents. We verified effectiveness of our approach in two ways. First, we clustered small subsets of documents represented by bag-of-words and bag-of-concepts using a simple k-means algorithm and found out that the semantic representation frequently yields better results [23]. We also compared the key MeSH concepts assigned to selected documents with the corresponding tags assigned by the PubMed experts. Preliminary results of this analysis reveal that the ESA method produces quite reasonable tags (see Table 1).

Online document grouping. Online grouping methods utilize content of usually up to several hundreds snippets (contexts for the searched term occurrences) returned by the Web search engines. The output is a list of labeled groups assigned with some objects (typically Web pages). The goal of grouping is then to provide a navigational rather than a summary interface [20]. On the other hand, a document retrieval system can usually access higher quality information about documents, which sets up expectations at a different level. In such a case, the groups based merely on snippets' content may not be informative enough to provide a meaningful overview of documents returned by the query. This suggests that enriching snippets may lead to a higher quality clustering.

We conducted experiments which utilized document representations based on inbound and outbound citations (i.e.: the lists of documents that are referenced by and that reference each given paper), semantic indexes described earlier in this section, as well as snippets extended by document abstracts. MeSH terms assigned by the PubMed domain experts to documents provided natural means of validation for each of clustering methods, as ideally the system would group documents in a similar way that the experts would do it [20,23]. Table 2 shows an

Table 1. Exemplary tags assigned to documents by PubMed experts and SONCA. The "∗" in the "MeSH tags by PubMed" column indicates the primary headings.

Document title	MeSH tags by PubMed	MeSH tags by SONCA
Cockroaches (Ectobius vittientris) in an intensive care unit, Switzerland.	Cockroaches∗, Insect Control∗, Intensive Care Units∗, Cross Infection, Insect Vectors	Cockroaches, Intensive Care Units, Klebsiella Infections, Pest Control, Cross Infection
Serotonin transporter genotype, morning cortisol and subsequent depression in adolescents.	Depressive Disorder∗, Genetic Predisposition to Disease∗, Serotonin Plasma Membrane Transport Proteins∗, Genotype, Multilevel Analysis	Depressive Disorder, Genome-Wide Association Study, Multilevel Analysis, Cohort Studies, Adolescent Psychiatry
Capacity of Thailand to contain an emerging influenza pandemic.	Disaster Planning∗, Health Policy∗, Disease Outbreaks, Health Resources, Influenza Human	Health Care Rationing, Health Resources, Epidemics, Evidence-Based Medicine, Influenza B virus

Table 2. A cluster labeled "Body Weight" discovered after a baseline document representation was extended with citation information. Column "Grouping (abstract)" shows original (baseline) groups assigned to each document (two of them were previously unassigned to any group). The third column lists MeSH terms associated with each document (these terms were unavailable for the fourth document). We emphasized concepts that seem (subjectively) to be similar to the group label.

Title	Grouping (abstracts)	MeSH keywords
Effects of antenatal dexamethasone treatment on glucocorticoid receptor and calcyon gene expression in the prefrontal cortex of neonatal and adult common marmoset monkeys.	Molecular; Dexamethasone	Age Factors; Animals; Animals, Newborn; **Body Size**; **Body Weight**; Callithrix; Dexamethasone; Female; Glucocorticoids; Male; Membrane Proteins; Prefrontal Cortex; Pregnancy; Prenatal Exposure Delayed Effects; Receptors, Glucocorticoid; Receptors, Mineralocorticoid; RNA, Messenger
The body politic: the relationship between stigma and obesity-associated disease		Adiposity; Age Factors; **Body Mass Index**; Electric Impedance; Female; Humans; Male; **Obesity**; Prejudice; Risk Factors; Sex Factors; Stress, Psychological
Prenatal Stress or High-Fat Diet Increases Susceptibility to Diet-Induced Obesity in Rat Offspring.	High-fat Diet	Animals; Child; Diabetes Mellitus, Type 2; **Dietary Fats**; **Energy Intake**; Female; Genetic Predisposition to Disease; Humans; Infant; Male; **Obesity**; Pregnancy; Prenatal Exposure Delayed Effects; Rats; Rats, Sprague-Dawley
The TNF-α System: Functional Aspects in Depression, Narcolepsy and Psychopharmacology.		

example of cluster that was discovered after extending document representations by information about citations. We expect that extraction of more meaningful snippets can further improve our results in the nearest future.

In our experiments (single server setup, documents from PubMed), SONCA performed comparably to other information retrieval engines with respect to execution time of simple queries. Moreover, expressiveness of the relational database model allowed us to construct queries using joins or filters on structural and semantic relations between objects (e.g: "return documents published in the given journal, whose primary MeSH headings match any document written by the given author"). While the user interface modules responsible for query generation are still under investigation, the computational overhead can be minimized by materializing indexes that substitute or approximate implicit joins in queries. For example, in order to facilitate online grouping, we constructed an auxiliary table joining every term from our corpus with snippets. Such a table, containing over 4.6 billion rows, dramatically speeded up the document representation enhancement process. On the other hand, given characteristics of the applied software (see Figure 1), both the size and the speed of cyclic reconstruction of that table are fully acceptable in terms of SONCA requirements.

5   Further Perspectives

Our primary motivation to develop SONCA is to extend functionality of the currently available search engines towards document based decision support and problem solving, via enhanced search and information synthesis capabilities, as well as richer user interfaces. For this purpose, we have been seeking for inspiration in many projects and approaches, related to such fields as, e.g., semantic web [2], social networks [18], or hybrid information networks [13]. Surely, there are plenty of aspects to be further investigated, in particular, in what form the results should be transmitted between modules and eventually reported to users. With this respect, we can refer to some research on, e.g., enriching original contents [1] and linguistic summaries of query results [16].

Another challenge is how to manage a hierarchy of computational tasks in order to assembly the answers to compound queries. Basing on initial observations in Section 4, we can see that the framework for specifying intermediate components of search and reasoning processes is crucial for both performance and extendability of the system [4,27]. The chain of computational specifications may follow a way human beings interact with standard search engines in order to summarize knowledge they are truly interested in. Thus, it is crucial to know how to represent and learn behavioral patterns followed by domain experts while solving problems [28]. Some hints in this area may come out from our previous research related to ontology-based approximations of compound concepts and identifying behavioral patterns in biomedical applications [5,11].

We also need to work on completion of the list of query types that should be supported. Besides examples mentioned in the previous sections, one may be interested in questions such as: "Who specializes in the treatment of a given condition (countries, states, hospitals)?"; "What are the current and past methods of diagnosis and treatment (e.g.: links to patient histories and medical images)?"; "What is their effectiveness (which could be depicted on a timeline)?"; "What are the most typical and least typical cases of a given condition?"; "What are morphological, molecular, genetic, functional or other aspects relevant in a given context?"; "Which pharmaceutical patents are relevant to treatment of the condition?"; "Which drugs are registered or approved in different regions?"; "What are typical interactions or complications after treatment?".

Furthermore, the user-system dialog may go beyond answering to queries (see e.g. [24]). The system may be actually more active by means of proposing solutions, suggesting additional pieces of information that should be completed, or even identifying the existing pieces that might need to be reexamined. For example, let us imagine a SONCA-based diagnostic support system based on a repository of medical documents and clinical data sets, where a medical doctor should be able to enter information about a patient's history and, within a context of specific queries, expect some guidelines with regards to further medical treatment and, if necessary, further data acquisition and verification.

The above use cases additionally illustrate the importance of establishing clear but powerful language of communication. The challenge is actually related not only to a syntax that the users are supposed to follow while formulating their queries (although this is a huge research topic by itself; see e.g. [9]). It is related also to all other layers of SONCA's architecture, wherein interfaces should parse the input queries, identify their components that may be addressed by the existing indexes or computational blocks, and, if possible, dynamically resolve the missing parts of the information flow by analogy to some previously applied strategies. From this perspective, we may refer, e.g., to such fundamental issues of mathematics as understanding of the concepts of proof, similarity of proofs, analogies between theorems, analogies between strategies of proofs used in different domains, and so on [25]. We may also refer to our own experience with evolution of languages applied to constructing and describing information granules [14] that, in the framework of SONCA, correspond to the hierarchy of intermediate tables and structures required to achieve the final goal.

References

1. Agrawal, R., Gollapudi, S., Kannan, A., Kenthapadi, K.: Enriching Education through Data Mining. In: Kuznetsov, S.O., Mandal, D.P., Kundu, M.K., Pal, S.K. (eds.) PReMI 2011. LNCS, vol. 6744, pp. 1–2. Springer, Heidelberg (2011)
2. Badr, Y., Chbeir, R., Abraham, A., Hassanien, A.: Emergent Web Intelligence: Advanced Semantic Technologies. Springer, Heidelberg (2010)
3. Baldi, P., Hatfield, G.W.: DNA Microarrays and Gene Expression: From Experiments to Data Analysis and Modeling. Cambridge University Press (2002)
4. Barwise, J., Seligman, J.: Information Flow: The Logic of Distributed Systems. Cambridge University Press (1997)
5. Bazan, J.G.: Hierarchical Classifiers for Complex Spatio-temporal Concepts. Transactions on Rough Sets 9, 474–750 (2008)
6. Bembenik, R., Skonieczny, Ł., Rybiński, H., Niezgódka, M. (eds.): Intelligent Tools for Building a Scientific Information Platform. Springer, Heidelberg (2011)
7. Butcher, S., Clarke, C.L.A., Cormack, G.: Information Retrieval: Implementing and Evaluating Search Engines. MIT Press (2010)
8. Chodorow, K., Dirolf, M.: MongoDB: The Definitive Guide: Powerful and Scalable Data Storage. O'Reilly Media (2010)
9. Davies, J., Grobelnik, M., Mladenic, D.: Semantic Knowledge Management: Integrating Ontology Management, Knowledge Discovery, and Human Language Technologies. Springer, Heidelberg (2009)
10. Gabrilovich, E., Markovitch, S.: Computing Semantic Relatedness using Wikipedia-based Explicit Semantic Analysis. In: Proc. of the 20th Int. Joint Conf. on Artificial Intelligence (IJCAI), pp. 6–12 (2007)
11. Góra, G., Kruczek, P., Skowron, A., Bazan, J.G., Bazan-Socha, S., Pietrzyk, J.J.: Case-based Planning of Treatment of Infants with Respiratory Failure. Fundamenta Informaticae 85(1-4), 155–172 (2008)

12. Grużdź, A., Ihnatowicz, A., Ślęzak, D.: Interactive Gene Clustering - A Case Study of Breast Cancer Microarray Data. Information Systems Frontiers 8(1), 21–27 (2006)
13. Han, J.: Construction and Analysis of Web-Based Computer Science Information Networks. In: Kuznetsov, S.O., Ślęzak, D., Hepting, D.H., Mirkin, B.G. (eds.) RSFDGrC 2011. LNCS (LNAI), vol. 6743, pp. 1–2. Springer, Heidelberg (2011)
14. Jankowski, A., Skowron, A.: Wisdom Technology: A Rough-Granular Approach. In: Marciniak, M., Mykowiecka, A. (eds.) Bolc Festschrift, vol. 5070, pp. 3–41. Springer, Heidelberg (2009)
15. Jörg, B., Jeffery, K., van Grootel, G., Asserson, A., Dvorak, J., Rasmussen, H.: CERIF 2008 - 1.2 Full Data Model (FDM) Introduction and Specification (2008), http://www.eurocris.org/Index.php?page=CERIF2008\&t=1
16. Kacprzyk, J., Zadrożny, S.: Computing With Words Is an Implementable Paradigm: Fuzzy Queries, Linguistic Data Summaries, and Natural-Language Generation. IEEE Transactions on Fuzzy Systems 18(3), 461–472 (2010)
17. McCandless, M., Hatcher, E., Gospodnetić, O.: Lucene in Action, 2nd edn. Manning Publications (2010)
18. Mika, P.: Social Networks and the Semantic Web. In: Proc. of the 2004 IEEE/WIC/ACM Int. Conf. on Web Intelligence (WI), pp. 285–291 (2004)
19. Nguyen, H.S.: Approximate Boolean Reasoning: Foundations and Applications in Data Mining. Transactions on Rough Sets 5, 334–506 (2006)
20. Nguyen, H.S., Ho, T.B.: Rough Document Clustering and the Internet. In: Pedrycz, W., Skowron, A., Kreinovich, V. (eds.) Handbook of Granular Computing, pp. 987–1003. John Wiley & Sons, Inc., New York (2008)
21. Roberts, R.J.: PubMed Central: The GenBank of the Published Literature. Proc. of the National Academy of Sciences of the United States of America 98(2), 381–382 (2001), http://www.pnas.org/content/98/2/381.abstract
22. Ślęzak, D., Wróblewski, J., Eastwood, V., Synak, P.: Brighthouse: An Analytic Data Warehouse for Ad-hoc Queries. Proc. of the VLDB Endowment (PVLDB) 1(2), 1337–1345 (2008)
23. Szczuka, M., Janusz, A., Herba, K.: Clustering of Rough Set Related Documents with use of Knowledge from DBpedia. In: Yao, J., Ramanna, S., Wang, G., Suraj, Z. (eds.) RSKT 2011. LNCS (LNAI), vol. 6954, pp. 394–403. Springer, Heidelberg (2011)
24. Tenenbaum, J.M., Shrager, J.: Cancer: A Computational Disease that AI Can Cure. AI Magazine 32(2), 14–26 (2011)
25. Ulam, S.: Analogies Between Analogies: The Mathematical Reports of S. M. Ulam and His Los Alamos Collaborators. University of California Press (1990)
26. United States National Library of Medicine: Introduction to MeSH - 2011 (2011), http://www.nlm.nih.gov/mesh/introduction.html
27. Valiant, L.G.: Robust Logics. Artif. Intell. 117(2), 231–253 (2000)
28. Vapnik, V.: Learning Has Just Started (An interview with Vladimir Vapnik by Ran Gilad-Bachrach) (2008), http://seed.ucsd.edu/joomla/index.php/articles/12-interviews/9-qlearning-has-just-startedq-an-interview-with-prof-vladimir-vapnik

Complexity Profiles of DNA Sequences Using Finite-Context Models

Armando J. Pinho*, Diogo Pratas, and Sara P. Garcia

Signal Processing Lab, IEETA / DETI
University of Aveiro, 3810–193 Aveiro, Portugal
{ap,pratas,spgarcia}@ua.pt

Abstract. Every data compression method assumes a certain model of the information source that produces the data. When we improve a data compression method, we are also improving the model of the source. This happens because, when the probability distribution of the assumed source model is closer to the true probability distribution of the source, a smaller relative entropy results and, therefore, fewer redundancy bits are required. This is why the importance of data compression goes beyond the usual goal of reducing the storage space or the transmission time of the information. In fact, in some situations, seeking better models is the main aim. In our view, this is the case for DNA sequence data. In this paper, we give hints on how finite-context (Markov) modeling may be used for DNA sequence analysis, through the construction of complexity profiles of the sequences. These profiles are able to unveil structures of the DNA, some of them with potential biological relevance.

1 Introduction

Modeling plays a key role in data compression. With the invention of the first practical algorithm for arithmetic coding [1], the problem of finding out an efficient representation for a certain information source could be restated as a data modeling problem. For our purposes, a model is a mathematical description of the information source, providing a probability estimate of the next outcome. The entropy of this model sets a lower bound on the compression performance of the arithmetic encoder. This bound is tight, meaning that it is possible to generate a bitstream with average entropy as close as desired to the entropy of the model, suggesting that the effort should be made to find good models of the information sources.

For about the last ten years, we have been addressing the problem of data compression using arithmetic coding. Initially in the context of image coding and, more recently, in the context of DNA coding, we have been relying on

* This work was partially funded by FEDER through the Operational Program Competitiveness Factors - COMPETE and by National Funds through FCT - Foundation for Science and Technology in the context of project FCOMP-01-0124-FEDER-010099 (FCT reference PTDC/EIA-EIA/103099/2008).

A. Holzinger and K.-M. Simonic (Eds.): USAB 2011, LNCS 7058, pp. 75–82, 2011.

finite-context (Markov) models for describing the data in an efficient way. Finite-context models assume that the source has Markovian properties, i.e., that the probability of the next outcome of the information source depends only on some finite number of (recent) past outcomes. This past is normally referred to as the "context", hence the name "finite-context model".

In the context of DNA data compression, these models have been usually associated with the task of providing compression when the main method fails. However, they have also been used as the main method, both for representing protein-coding regions of DNA [2] and for representing unrestricted DNA, i.e., DNA with coding and non-coding regions [3,4,5,6,7]. In this paper, we present and discuss the problem of computing complexity profiles (or information sequences) using finite-context models. Basically, a complexity profile indicates how many bits are required to represent each symbol (DNA base). These complexity profiles are of interest because they reveal structures inside the chromosomes, structures that are often associated with regulatory functions of DNA [8].

2   Finite-Context Models

Consider an information source that generates symbols, s, from an alphabet $\mathcal{A}$, and denote by $x^n = x_1 x_2 \ldots x_n$ the sequence of symbols generated by the source after n outcomes. A finite-context model of an information source (see Fig. 1 for an example where $\mathcal{A} = \{0, 1\}$) assigns probability estimates to the symbols of the alphabet, according to a conditioning context computed over a finite and fixed number, k, of past outcomes (order-k finite-context model) [9,10,11]. At instant n, we represent these conditioning outcomes by $c^n = x_{n-k+1}, \ldots, x_{n-1}, x_n$.

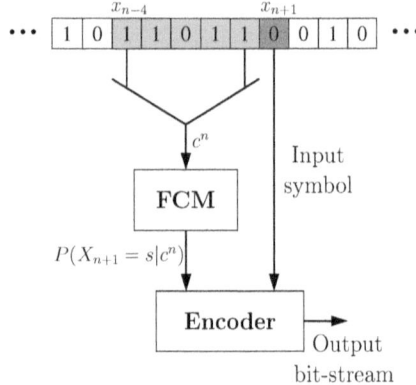

Fig. 1. Example of a finite-context model for the binary alphabet, i.e., for $\mathcal{A} = \{0, 1\}$. The probability of the next outcome, X_{n+1}, is conditioned by the k last outcomes. In this example, $k = 5$.

In practice, the probability that the next outcome, X_{n+1}, is $s \in \mathcal{A}$, is obtained using the estimator

$$P(X_{n+1} = s|c^n) = \frac{N_s^n + \alpha}{\sum\limits_{a \in \mathcal{A}} N_a^n + |\mathcal{A}|\alpha}, \tag{1}$$

where $|\mathcal{A}|$ denotes the size of the alphabet, and N_s^n represents the number of times that, in the past, the information source generated symbol s having c^n as the conditioning context. The parameter α controls how much probability is assigned to unseen (but possible) events, and plays a key role in the case of high-order models. In fact, when k is large, the number of conditioning states, $|\mathcal{A}|^k$, is high, implying that statistics have to be estimated using only a few observations. This estimator reduces to Laplace's estimator for $\alpha = 1$ [12] and to the frequently used Jeffreys/Krichevsky estimator when $\alpha = 1/2$ [13,14].

Initially, when all counters are zero, the symbols have probability $1/|\mathcal{A}|$, i.e., they are assumed equally probable. The counters are updated each time a symbol is encoded. Since the context is causal, the decoder is able to reproduce the same probability estimates without needing additional information.

The block denoted "Encoder" in Fig. 1 is an arithmetic encoder. It is well known that practical arithmetic coding generates output bitstreams with average bitrates almost identical to the entropy of the model [9,10,11]. The number of bits that are required to represent symbol x_{n+1} is given by $-\log_2 P(X_{n+1} = x_{n+1}|c^n)$. Therefore, the average bitrate (entropy) of the finite-context model after encoding N symbols is given by

$$H_N = -\frac{1}{N} \sum_{n=0}^{N-1} \log_2 P(X_{n+1} = x_{n+1}|c^n) \quad \text{bps}, \tag{2}$$

where "bps" stands for "bits per symbol".

3 Applications to DNA Data

DNA sequences are sequences of symbols (bases) from a 4-symbol alphabet: adenine (A), cytosine (C), guanine (G), and thymine (T). Several specific coding methods have been proposed for compressing these sequences (see, for example, [15,16,17,18,19,20,21,2,22,23,3,4,6,7]). Most of these methods are based on searching procedures for finding exact or approximate repeats, both directly and in their reversed complemented versions (A $\leftrightarrow$ T, C $\leftrightarrow$ G). Although this approach has been quite effective in terms of compression rates, it also requires a significant computational effort. Low-order finite-context models are typically used in those methods as a secondary, fall back mechanism. Our goal has been to investigate DNA compression methods based only on finite-context models.

Modeling DNA data using only finite-context models has advantages over the typical DNA compression approaches that mix purely statistical (for example, finite-context models) with substitutional models (such as Lempel-Ziv based algorithms): (1) finite-context models lead to much faster performance, a characteristic of paramount importance for long sequences (for example, some human chromosomes have more than 200 million bases); (2) the overall model may be easier to interpret, because it is made of sub-models of the same type.

Initially, we proposed a three-state finite-context model for DNA protein-coding regions, i.e., for the parts of the DNA that carry information regarding how proteins are synthesized [2]. This three-state model proved to be better than a single-state model, giving additional evidence of a phenomenon that is common in these protein-coding regions, the periodicity of period three.

More recently [3,4,6,7], we investigated the performance of finite-context models for unrestricted DNA, i.e., DNA including coding and non-coding parts. In that work, we have shown that a characteristic usually found in DNA sequences, the occurrence of inverted repeats, which is used by most of the DNA coding methods (see, for example, [18,19,20]), can also be successfully integrated in finite-context models. Inverted repeats are copies of DNA sub-sequences that appear reversed and complemented in some parts of the DNA.

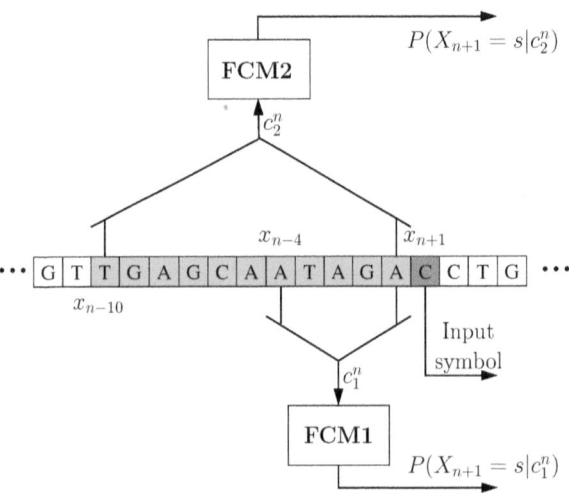

Fig. 2. Example of the use of multiple finite-context models for encoding DNA data. In this case, two models are used, one with a depth-5 context and the other using an order-11 context.

DNA is non-stationary, with regions of low information content (low entropy) alternating with regions with average entropy close to two bits per base. This alternation is modeled by most DNA compression algorithms by using a low-order finite-context model for the high entropy regions and a Lempel-Ziv dictionary-based approach for the repetitive, low entropy regions. We have been studying approaches relying only on finite-context models for representing both regions, leading us to conclude that DNA can be much better represented by Markov models than what it was previously believed.

Moreover, our studies have shown that multiple finite-context models can be more effective in capturing the statistical information along the sequence

[4,6,7]. Figure 2 gives an example of these multiple models, that can operate in a competitive or cooperative way. When in competitive mode, the best of the models is chosen for encoding each DNA block, i.e., the one that requires less bits is used for representing the current block [7]. When in cooperative mode of operation, the probability estimates of the several models are combined using an adaptive mixture model [6].

4   Complexity Profiles of DNA

The work of researchers such as Solomonoff, Kolmogorov, Chaitin and others [24,25,26,27,28,29], related to the problem of defining a complexity measure of a string, has been of paramount importance for several areas of knowledge. However, because it is not computable, the Kolmogorov complexity of a string A, $K(A)$, is usually approximated by some computable measure, such as Lempel-Ziv complexity measures [30], linguistic complexity measures [31] or compression-based complexity measures [32].

One of the important problems that can be formulated using the Kolmogorov theory is the definition of similarity. Following this line, Li et al. [33] proposed a similarity metric based on an information distance [34], defined as the length of the shortest binary program that is needed to transform strings A and B into each other. This distance depends not only on the Kolmogorov complexity of A and B, respectively $K(A)$ and $K(B)$, but also on conditional complexities, for example $K(A|B)$, that indicates how complex string A is when string B is known. Because this distance is based on the Kolmogorov complexity (not computable), they proposed a practical analog based on standard compressors, which they call the normalized compression distance [33].

According to [33], a compression method needs to be "normal" in order to be used in the normalized compression distance. One of the conditions for a compression method to be normal is that compressing string AA (the concatenation of A with A) should generate essentially the same number of bits as compressing A alone [35]. This characteristic holds, for example, in Lempel-Ziv based compressors, making them a frequent choice in this kind of applications.

The construction and analysis of DNA complexity profiles has been an important topic of research, due to its applicability in the study of regulatory functions of DNA, comparative analysis of organisms, genomic evolution and others [36,37]. For example, it has been observed that low complexity regions of DNA are often associated with important regulatory functions [38].

Several measures have also been proposed for evaluating the complexity of DNA sequences. Among those, we find the compression-based approaches the most promising and natural, because compression efficiency is clearly defined (it can be measured by the number of bits generated by the encoder).

One of the key advantages of DNA compression based on finite-context models is that the encoders are fast and have $\mathcal{O}(n)$ time complexity. As we mentioned already, most of the effort spent by previous DNA compressors is in the task of finding exact or approximate repeats of sub-sequences or of their inverted

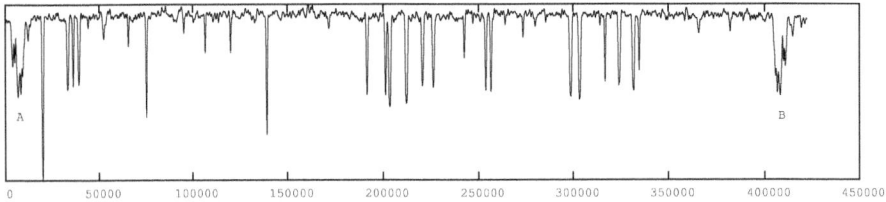

Fig. 3. Complexity profile of chromosome 1 of the *Cyanidioschyzon merolae* organism, obtained with a multiple finite-context modeling approach. We can see several regions where the complexity value goes well below the baseline level that, for an entropy-based complexity profile of DNA, can be set at two bits per DNA nucleotide. The two regions which we have marked with letters A and B correspond to telomeric inverted repeated sequences.

complements. No doubt, this approach has proved to give good returns in terms of compression gains, but normally at the cost of long compression times. Although slow encoders could be tolerated for storage purposes (compression could be ran in batch mode), for interactive applications they are certainly not appropriate. For example, the currently best performing DNA compression techniques, such as NML-1 [22] or XM [23], could take hours for compressing a single human chromosome. Compressing one of the largest human chromosomes with the techniques based on finite-context models takes less than ten minutes in a 1.66 GHz laptop computer. These DNA sequences have about 240 million bases.

Figure 3 shows an example of one of those complexity profiles (corresponding to chromosome 1 of the *Cyanidioschyzon merolae*) as generated by a multiple finite-context model DNA encoder. We can observe several regions where the complexity is very small, meaning that a reduced number of bits was required for compression those regions. Of particular interest are the two regions which we have marked with letters A and B, corresponding to telomeric inverted repeated sequences.

5   Conclusion

It has been shown that finite-context models are a powerful tool for representing DNA sequences, as demonstrated by the good compression results that they are able to provide [6,7]. However, they may also be useful in other tasks, such as in data analysis. The construction of complexity profiles is an obvious case. These information sequences allow a quick analysis of long sequences, unveiling locations of low information content, which are usually associated with DNA regions of potential biological interest. This seems to be a very promising line of research, clearly deserving further investigation.

References

1. Rissanen, J.: Generalized Kraft inequality and arithmetic coding. IBM J. Res. Develop. 20(3), 198–203 (1976)
2. Pinho, A.J., Neves, A.J.R., Afreixo, V., Bastos, C.A.C., Ferreira, P.J.S.G.: A three-state model for DNA protein-coding regions. IEEE Trans. on Biomedical Engineering 53(11), 2148–2155 (2006)
3. Pinho, A.J., Neves, A.J.R., Ferreira, P.J.S.G.: Inverted-repeats-aware finite-context models for DNA coding. In: Proc. of the 16th European Signal Processing Conf., EUSIPCO 2008, Lausanne, Switzerland (August 2008)
4. Pinho, A.J., Neves, A.J.R., Bastos, C.A.C., Ferreira, P.J.S.G.: DNA coding using finite-context models and arithmetic coding. In: Proc. of the IEEE Int. Conf. on Acoustics, Speech, and Signal Processing, ICASSP 2009, Taipei, Taiwan (April 2009)
5. Pratas, D., Pinho, A.J.: Compressing the Human Genome Using Exclusively Markov Models. In: Rocha, M.P., Rodríguez, J.M.C., Fdez-Riverola, F., Valencia, A. (eds.) PACBB 2011. AISC, vol. 93, pp. 213–220. Springer, Heidelberg (2011)
6. Pinho, A.J., Pratas, D., Ferreira, P.J.S.G.: Bacteria DNA sequence compression using a mixture of finite-context models. In: Proc. of the IEEE Workshop on Statistical Signal Processing, Nice, France (June 2011)
7. Pinho, A.J., Ferreira, P.J.S.G., Neves, A.J.R., Bastos, C.A.C.: On the representability of complete genomes by multiple competing finite-context (Markov) models. PLoS ONE 6(6), e21588 (2011)
8. Pinho, A.J., Pratas, D., Ferreira, P.J.S.G., Garcia, S.P.: Symbolic to numerical conversion of DNA sequences using finite-context models. In: Proc. of the 19th European Signal Processing Conf., EUSIPCO 2011, Barcelona, Spain (August 2011)
9. Bell, T.C., Cleary, J.G., Witten, I.H.: Text compression. Prentice-Hall (1990)
10. Salomon, D.: Data compression - The complete reference, 4th edn. Springer, Heidelberg (2007)
11. Sayood, K.: Introduction to data compression, 3rd edn. Morgan Kaufmann (2006)
12. Laplace, P.S.: Essai philosophique sur les probabilités (A philosophical essay on probabilities). John Wiley & Sons, New York (1814); translated from the sixth French edition by Truscott, F.W., Emory, F. L. (1902)
13. Jeffreys, H.: An invariant form for the prior probability in estimation problems. Proc. of the Royal Society (London) A 186, 453–461 (1946)
14. Krichevsky, R.E., Trofimov, V.K.: The performance of universal encoding. IEEE Trans. on Information Theory 27(2), 199–207 (1981)
15. Grumbach, S., Tahi, F.: Compression of DNA sequences. In: Proc. of the Data Compression Conf., DCC 1993, Snowbird, Utah, pp. 340–350 (1993)
16. Rivals, E., Delahaye, J.P., Dauchet, M., Delgrange, O.: A guaranteed compression scheme for repetitive DNA sequences. In: Proc. of the Data Compression Conf., DCC 1996, Snowbird, Utah, p. 453 (1996)
17. Chen, X., Kwong, S., Li, M.: A compression algorithm for DNA sequences. IEEE Engineering in Medicine and Biology Magazine 20, 61–66 (2001)
18. Matsumoto, T., Sadakane, K., Imai, H.: Biological sequence compression algorithms. In: Dunker, A.K., Konagaya, A., Miyano, S., Takagi, T. (eds.) Genome Informatics 2000: Proc. of the 11th Workshop, Tokyo, Japan, pp. 43–52 (2000)
19. Manzini, G., Rastero, M.: A simple and fast DNA compressor. Software—Practice and Experience 34, 1397–1411 (2004)

20. Korodi, G., Tabus, I.: An efficient normalized maximum likelihood algorithm for DNA sequence compression. ACM Trans. on Information Systems 23(1), 3–34 (2005)
21. Behzadi, B., Le Fessant, F.: DNA Compression Challenge Revisited. In: Combinatorial Pattern Matching. In: Apostolico, A., Crochemore, M., Park, K. (eds.) CPM 2005. LNCS, vol. 3537, pp. 190–200. Springer, Heidelberg (2005)
22. Korodi, G., Tabus, I.: Normalized maximum likelihood model of order-1 for the compression of DNA sequences. In: Proc. of the Data Compression Conf., DCC 2007, Snowbird, Utah, pp. 33–42 (March 2007)
23. Cao, M.D., Dix, T.I., Allison, L., Mears, C.: A simple statistical algorithm for biological sequence compression. In: Proc. of the Data Compression Conf., DCC 2007, Snowbird, Utah, pp. 43–52 (March 2007)
24. Solomonoff, R.J.: A formal theory of inductive inference, part I. Information and Control 7(1), 1–22 (1964)
25. Solomonoff, R.J.: A formal theory of inductive inference, part II. Information and Control 7(2), 224–254 (1964)
26. Kolmogorov, A.N.: Three approaches to the quantitative definition of information. Problems of Information Transmission 1(1), 1–7 (1965)
27. Chaitin, G.J.: On the length of programs for computing finite binary sequences. Journal of the ACM 13, 547–569 (1966)
28. Wallace, C.S., Boulton, D.M.: An information measure for classification. The Computer Journal 11(2), 185–194 (1968)
29. Rissanen, J.: Modeling by shortest data description. Automatica 14, 465–471 (1978)
30. Lempel, A., Ziv, J.: On the complexity of finite sequences. IEEE Trans. on Information Theory 22(1), 75–81 (1976)
31. Gordon, G.: Multi-dimensional linguistic complexity. Journal of Biomolecular Structure & Dynamics 20(6), 747–750 (2003)
32. Dix, T.I., Powell, D.R., Allison, L., Bernal, J., Jaeger, S., Stern, L.: Comparative analysis of long DNA sequences by per element information content using different contexts. BMC Bioinformatics 8(suppl. 2), S10 (2007)
33. Li, M., Chen, X., Li, X., Ma, B., Vitányi, P.M.B.: The similarity metric. IEEE Trans. on Information Theory 50(12), 3250–3264 (2004)
34. Bennett, C.H., Gács, P., Vitányi, M.L.P.M.B., Zurek, W.H.: Information distance. IEEE Trans. on Information Theory 44(4), 1407–1423 (1998)
35. Cilibrasi, R., Vitányi, P.M.B.: Clustering by compression. IEEE Trans. on Information Theory 51(4), 1523–1545 (2005)
36. Nan, F., Adjeroh, D.: On the complexity measures for biological sequences. In: Proc. of the IEEE Computational Systems Bioinformatics Conference, CSB 2004, Stanford, CA (August 2004)
37. Pirhaji, L., Kargar, M., Sheari, A., Poormohammadi, H., Sadeghi, M., Pezeshk, H., Eslahchi, C.: The performances of the chi-square test and complexity measures for signal recognition in biological sequences. Journal of Theoretical Biology 251(2), 380–387 (2008)
38. Gusev, V.D., Nemytikova, L.A., Chuzhanova, N.A.: On the complexity measures of genetic sequences. Bioinformatics 15(12), 994–999 (1999)

Representing and Visualizing Mined Artful Processes in MailOfMine*

Claudio Di Ciccio, Massimo Mecella, and Tiziana Catarci

Sapienza – Università di Roma
Dipartimento di Ingegneria Informatica, Automatica e Gestionale Antonio Ruberti
{cdc|mecella|catarci}@dis.uniroma1.it

Abstract. Artful processes are informal processes typically carried out by those people whose work is mental rather than physical (managers, professors, researchers, engineers, etc.), the so called "knowledge workers". MailOfMine is a tool, the aim of which is to automatically build, on top of a collection of e-mail messages, a set of workflow models that represent the artful processes laying behind the knowledge workers activities. This paper presents its innovative graphical syntax proposal and the interface for representing and showing such mined processes to users.

Keywords: process mining, process visualization, artful process.

1 Introduction

For a long time, formal business processes (e.g., the ones of public administrations, of insurance/financial institutions, etc.) have been the main subject of workflow related research. Informal processes, a.k.a. "artful processes", are conversely carried out by those people whose work is mental rather than physical (managers, professors, researchers, engineers, etc.), the so called "knowledge workers" [18]. With their skills, experience and knowledge, they are used to perform difficult tasks, which require complex, rapid decisions among multiple possible strategies, in order to fulfill specific goals. In contrast to business processes that are formal and standardized, often informal processes are not even written down, let alone defined formally, and can vary from person to person even when those involved are pursuing the same objective. Knowledge workers create informal processes "on the fly" to cope with many of the situations that arise in their daily work. Though informal processes are frequently repeated, they are not exactly reproducible even by their originators – since they are not written down – and can not be easily shared either. Their outcomes and their information exchanges are done very often by means of e-mail conversations, which are a fast, reliable, permanent way of keeping track of the activities that they fulfill. Understanding artful processes involving knowledge workers is becoming crucial in many scenarios. Here we mention some of them:

---

* This work has been partly supported by Sapienza – Università di Roma through the grants FARI 2010 and TESTMED, and by the EU Commission through the FP7 project Smart Vortex. The authors would like also to thank Monica Scannapieco and Diego Zardetto for useful insights and discussions.

A. Holzinger and K.-M. Simonic (Eds.): USAB 2011, LNCS 7058, pp. 83–94, 2011.

- *personal information management (PIM)*, i.e., how to organize one's own activities, contacts, etc. through the use of software on laptops and smart devices (iPhones/iPads, smartphones, tablets). Here, inferring artful processes in which a person is involved allows the system to be proactive and thus drive the user through its own tasks (on the basis of the past) [9,18];
- *information warfare*, especially in supporting anti-crime intelligence agencies: let us suppose that a government bureau is able to access the *e*-mail account of a suspected person. People planning a crime or an act out of law are used to speak a language of their own to express duties and next moves, where meanings may not match with the common sense. Though, a system should build the processes that lay behind their communications anyway, exposing the activities and the role of the actors. At that point, translating the sense of misused words becomes an easier task for investigators, and allows inferring the criminal activities of the suspected person(s);
- *enterprise engineering*: in design and engineering, it is important to preserve more than just the actual documents making up the product data. Preserving the "soft knowledge" of the overall process (the so-called product life-cycle) is of critical importance for knowledge-heavy industries. Hence, the idea here is to take to the future not only the designs, but also the knowledge about processes, decision making, and people involved [1,2,14].

The objective of the MAILOFMINE approach, proposed in [12], which this paper is based upon, is to automatically build, on top of a collection of *e*-mail messages, a set of workflow models that represent the artful processes laying behind the knowledge workers activities. Here, we discuss how we addressed the challenge of showing artful processes to users, i.e., knowledge workers, through a graphical interface which is flexible, functional and easy to understand. It is designed to be validated and further improved in collaboration with them. A user-centered methodology is going to be applied, not only to the development of the graphical interface, but also to the specification of the visual notation symbols that describe processes.

The work here presented is related to the so called *process mining*, a.k.a. *workflow mining* [4], that is the set of techniques allowing the extraction of structured process descriptions, stemmed from a set of recorded real executions (stored in the *event logs*). ProM [5] is one of the most used plug-in based software environment for implementing workflow mining techniques.

Most of the mainstream process mining tools model processes as Workflow Nets (WFNs – see [3]), explicitly designed to represent the control-flow dimension of a workflow, and visualizes processes in various graphical notations, all of them basically graph-based. Also, the most of standard graphical notations for processes, such as UML Activity Diagrams and BPMN – Business Process Modeling Notation, basically visualize an entire process as a graph, in order to provide the users with a one-shot view of the process.

The need for flexibility in the definition of processes leads to an alternative to the classical "imperative": the "declarative" approach. Rather than using a procedural language for expressing the allowed sequences of activities, it is based on the description of workflows through the usage of constraints: the idea is that every task can be performed, except what does not respect them. Such constraints, in [15] (Chapter 6) are formulations of Linear Temporal Logic ([11] – Chapter 3). DecSerFlow [6] and ConDec [16] provide graphical representations for processes described through the declarative approach.

Nonetheless, we believe that the declaration of collaborative workflows constraints can be expressed by means of regular expressions, rather than LTL formulae: regular expressions express finite languages (i.e., processes with finite traces, where the number of enacted tasks is limited). LTL formulae are thought to be used for verifying properties over semi-infinite runs instead. On the contrary, human processes have an end, other than a starting point. We envision the process schemes like grammars describing the language spoken by collaborative organisms in terms of activities, thus being more related to formal languages rather than temporal logic. In this paper we propose a novel graphical notation for such languages.

2 The MailOfMine Approach

The MAILOFMINE approach (and the tool we are currently developing) adopts a modular architecture, the components of which allow to incrementally refine the mining process. The architecture is shown in Figure 1; before briefly presenting it, we need to introduce some basic concepts needed in the following. The details of the architecture, as well as the formal definitions of concepts, are presented in [12].

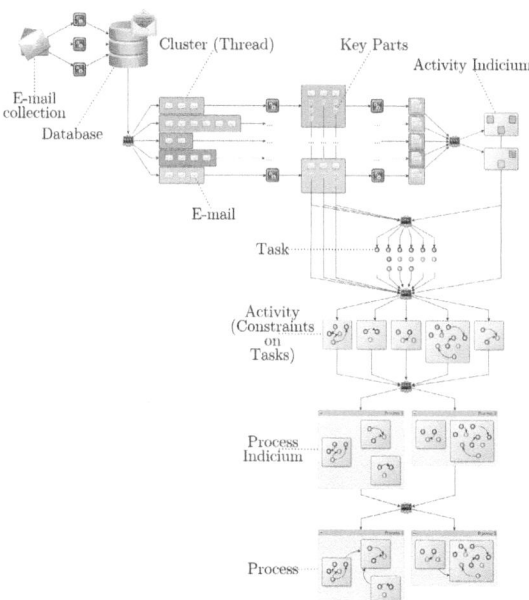

Fig. 1. The MAILOFMINE approach [12]

An *actor* is the subject directly or indirectly taking part in the progress of a work. A *task* is an elementary unit of work. Each task is connected to *(i)* its expected *duration, (ii)* zero or more *outcomes, (iii)* one or more *actors*. An *activity* is a collection of tasks or (recursively) other activities. A *key part* is each *unique* piece of text belonging to the *e*-mail messages exchanged in a communication trace. Thus, given a collection of duplicated pieces of text (coming from the same or different *e*-mail messages in the trace), just a single representative is selected as key part. For instance, HTML signatures used by the sender of the *e*-mail, quotations of previous *e*-mail messages used in replies, etc., are all examples of redundant information that may appear in a communication trace, but is filtered out by means of the *key part* concept. On the other hand, any piece of text not appearing in any other *e*-mail message in the discussion thread is interpreted as a *key part*. An *indicium* is any communication trace, or part of it, attesting the execution of a task, an activity, or a process instance.

A *process scheme* (or *process* for short) is a semi-structured set of activities, where the semi-structuring connective tissue is represented by the set of constraints stating the interleaving rules among activities or tasks. Constraints do not force the process instance to follow a tight sequence, but rather leave it the flexibility to follow different paths, while performing the execution, though respecting a set of rules that avoid illegal or non-consistent states.

In [12], we argued that each constraint is expressible through regular grammars. Regular grammars are recognizable through Finite State Automata (FSA) [10] (either deterministic or non-deterministic [17]). The FSA recognizing the correct traces for processes (i.e., accepting the valid strings) is the intersection of all the FSAs composing the set of constraints. This is the theoretical basis for the reasoning core that internally manages the process scheme to be finally shown to the user.

Initially, we need to extract *e*-mail messages from the given archive(s). The outcome is the population of a database, on the basis of which all the subsequent steps are carried out. The first of them is the clustering of retrieved messages into extended communication threads, i.e., flows of messages which are related to each other. Once the communication threads are recognized, we can assume them all as activity indicia candidates. Afterwards, messages are analyzed in order to identify key parts. Key parts are gathered by combining the technique for the removal of quoted material, presented in [8], with an iterative approach over the *e*-mail messages in the thread. MAILOFMINE can thus build the activity indicia as the concatenation of all the key parts belonging to the messages of a communication thread. Then, the clustering algorithm is used again, this time to identify the matches between activity indicia. By taking into account the activities set and the key parts (task indicia candidates), the clustering algorithm checks for matching key parts: those are considered tasks.

Taking as input all of the preceding outcomes, MAILOFMINE starts searching for execution constraints between tasks within the activities they belong to. To this intent, we exploit and extend the SPIRIT techniques for regular patterns mining ([13]). Specifically, on the basis of all the possible constraints, a selection of those that are valid over most of the activity indicia is made.

Once activities and tasks are recognized, a supervised learning process takes place, in order to cluster activities into processes. Once processes are identified, MAILOFMINE performs the second step for the construction of the process scheme, i.e., the mining of production rules among activities inside the same process, by using the SPIRIT techniques for regular pattern mining again.

3   Process Visualization

The literature dealing with the representation of processes typically aims at visualizing the processes all at once, by means of diagrams that show the complete grid of interconnections among activities. Here we propose a change in the viewpoint. As stated before, we want to model artful processes as a collection of constraints, through the declarative approach. Being highly flexible, this kind of representation does not necessarily impose a pre-defined order on activities, neither explicit nor implicit. For instance, it is not mandatory to specify which the initial activity is, and the following step depends on the previous choices. In other words, the process schema itself can change according to the things that may have happened before. This is why we do not consider as the best suitable solution adopting a static graph-based global representation alone, on one hand: a local view should work better in conjunction with it. On the other hand, no knowledge worker is expected to be able to read and understand the process by reading the list of regular-expression based constraints: a graphical representation, easy to understand at a first glimpse, must be used.

The process schema and the running processes are respectively modeled through *(i)* a set of diagrams, representing constraints on workflows (static view: Section 3.1) and *(ii)* an interactive evolutionary graphical representation for the visualization of running instances (dynamic view: Section 3.2). Furthermore, we propose two complementary views on constraints: *(i)* a local view focusing on one activity at a time and *(ii)* a global view providing a bird-eye sketch of the whole process schema.

As activities are basically collections of tasks (thus, they can be single tasks too), which have to be compliant with the same constraints as tasks, in the following we will consider tasks only, for sake of simplicity. The same statements remain valid for activities, though.

3.1   Process Schema

The local view. It is very hard to show a process schema all at once and keep it easily readable, due to the high flexibility of the declarative representation. Thus, given that the declarative approach is based on constraints, we collect all of those related to every single task, i.e., where the task (e.g., t) is either *(i)* directly implied (e.g., if s is done, then t must be done), or *(ii)* directly implying (e.g., if t is done, no matter when, u was done before or must be done

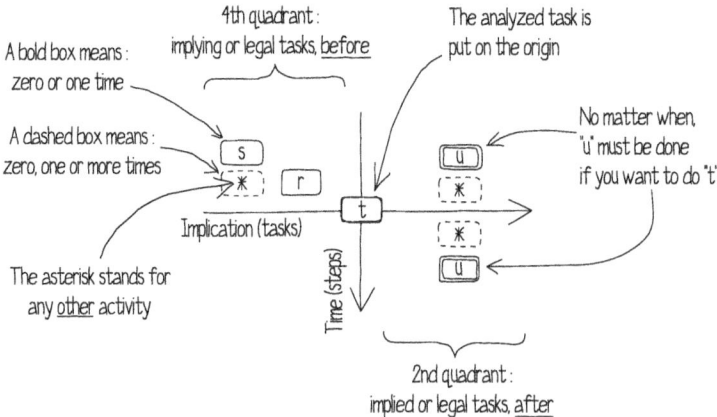

Fig. 2. The tasks static view rationale

in the future). The *directly* adverb is used due to the need not to make things too much complicated and to follow the rationale of having a local view only. For instance, if r was a task implying that s could not be done further (and if s is done, then t must be done), such a chain of constraints is not taken into account, unless we are looking at the constraints regarding t. This avoids the confusion of too many cross-implications to consider at a time (for sake of readability) and respects the principle of declarative approaches: you can not do s if r was done; though, if r was not done, no constraint on s must hold, then we do not care it as a side-effect on t.

The representation of relation constraints is based on three main degrees of freedom, namely *(i)* time, *(ii)* implication, *(iii)* repeatability. The time is considered here as a discrete ordered set of steps the tasks can take place in. We ideally consider each task as spending a single unit in this conception of time. The implication is a binary set (implying, implied). The repeatability is a space of four values, standing for the number of times a task can be consequently fulfilled: *(i)* zero, one or more times; *(ii)* zero or one time; *(iii)* exactly once; *(iv)* zero times.

Our graphical notation represents time and implication as the coordinates of a bidimensional drawing, where time is on the ordinates. This ideal y axis divides the plane space into two separate regions: one for each value of the implication dimension (implying, implied), on the abscissae. The x axis divides the plane space into two regions: upwards, what can (or can not) happen *before* the task is executed, and, downwards, what can (or can not) happen after. Indeed, on the origin of this chart, inspired to the cartesian coordinate system, we put the task under examination. See Figure 2 for a sketch of the rationale.

Differently from the classical orientation, we consider the y axis oriented towards the bottom. This for following the reading directionality. For the same reason, the implication relation order flows from the left to the right. Of course, this detail can change according to the localization of the software running:

e.g., users from Arabic countries might prefer a mirrored version, where the implied tasks are on the left, the implying on the right.

The repeatability is expressed by the thickness of the boundaries round the boxes representing tasks: dashed for tasks that can be done zero, one or more times, bold for zero or one times, double-line for exactly one time. The task box turns into a cross shape when repeatability is zero. The repeatability is referred to the quadrant the box appears in. For instance, u must appear once either before or after t took place. We recall here that the scope of repeatability, as all of the other degrees of freedom, is not extended to the whole process instance existence, but only for what concerns the time surrounding of the single task in analysis.

For sake of readability, we do not explicitly mention every possible task the process can be composed of, on the graph. Instead, we render only such tasks which are interested in focused constraints. Though, visualizing the tasks involved in constraints only, might look like a way to force the actor to execute nothing else than the ones that are shown. On the contrary, declarative models allow to do more: roughly speaking, what is not mentioned, is possible. Thus, we make use of a wildcard ($*$) not intended as "every task" in the usual all-comprehensive form, but in the typical human conception: "any task", where it is understood that the other rules remain valid (e.g., if it is stated that s can not be executed before t, a $*$ before t means "any task, except s). Examples of the diagrams are in Figure 3.

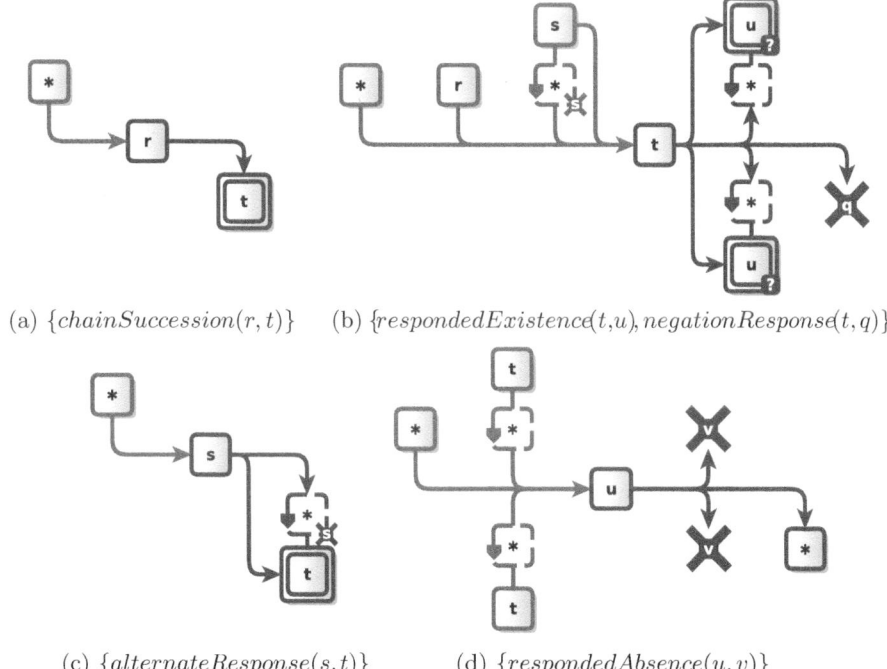

(a) $\{chainSuccession(r,t)\}$ (b) $\{respondedExistence(t,u), negationResponse(t,q)\}$

(c) $\{alternateResponse(s,t)\}$ (d) $\{respondedAbsence(u,v)\}$

Fig. 3. The MailOfMine local static constraint diagrams

The graphical notation is enforced by arrows, easing the user to go across the flow of tasks, from the implying before to the implied afterwards. Colors are used for sake of readability and comprehensibility, as additional arrows making a loop on zero-one-more-repeatable tasks, though the overall rationale is the same: such diagrams must be easy to be sketched by a pen, as well.

The local view can focus on a possible sub-trace of executed tasks, as in Figure 4.

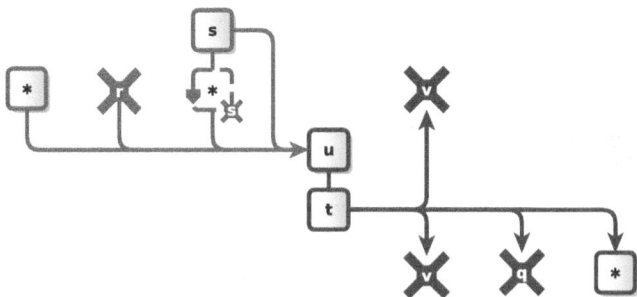

Fig. 4. The $< u, t >$ tasks subtrace constraints diagram

The global view. The aim of the global view (Figure 5) is to show the relations between tasks, namely *(i)* whether the presence of one implies a further constraint (on the graph, a dot on the tail of an arrow, starting from the implying task and ending on the implied), *(ii)* which task must be performed after, between the implying and the implied, if known (on the graph, an arrow, put on the head or the tail), *(iii)* whether the presence of one implies the absence of another (a cross in the middle of the arrow), or not (no cross put upon). All of the previous information bits are independent of each other, hence all the possible combinations are allowed. This is the restricted basic graphical syntax used in Figure 5a. Indeed, it is not explicitly expressed how strong the constraint is (e.g., whether other tasks can be performed between the implying and the implied), in order to tidy the diagram up and provide a fast view of the overall process, without entering in details that are likely better explained through the local views: they can rely, in fact, on dimensions spread on axes the cartesian way, not as in graphs.

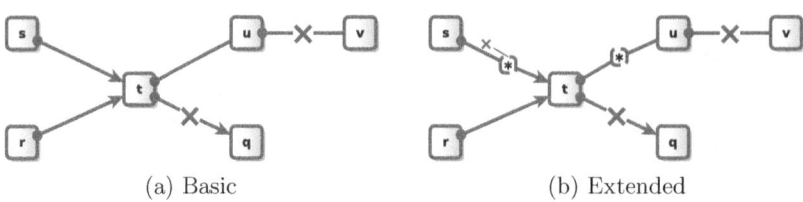

(a) Basic   (b) Extended

Fig. 5. The MAILOFMINE global static constraints diagram

Nonetheless, skilled users might want to have a complete vision of the constraints involved, even though it might result in a reduced readability, due to the unavoidable increase of graphical symbols to draw in the diagram. Thus, a richer graphical syntax is needed. Its design rationale is to extend the basic, though keeping coherence with *(i)* the visual language terms used and *(ii)* the graph structure. This allows the user to be required of a minimal cognitive effort in order to learn its semantics, on one hand, and lets her toggle between the basic and the extended view. Indeed, only arcs are loaded with new symbols, as depicted on Figure 5b: no additional shape nor any change in the graph topology are required.

The global view is inspired to the graphical syntax of [7]; only a minimal subset of the DecSerFlow constraints are represented: this makes it easier for future developers to introduce new constraints, that inherit the basic relations (before/after, implying/implied, existence/absence), without introducing new graphical notations, but only modifying the local view graphical patterns.

Coupling this diagram with the local view is useful for avoiding the misunderstanding that could arise by the usage of oriented graphs. Indeed, Finite State Automata, Petri Nets, State Transition Networks, UML Activity Diagrams, Flowcharts, and so forth, all use the same semantics: roughly speaking, nodes are places to traverse one by one, following a path that respects the direction given by arrows along the arcs. Here, it is not the case: e.g., considering Figure 5, one could intuitively suppose that, done t, the next task is u. It is not true: after t, s or t itself could be performed, even many times, and only after a while, u.

A GUI sketch. Figure 6 draws a prototype of the window showing a local view, on the t task. The additional information regarding the cardinality of the task, the actors involved and so forth is located on the bottom of the window. The global view, put on the right, is used as a navigation tool on the process schema. Conversely, it will be possible at any point in time to activate the local view of a task selected on the global view screen, in order to freely switch from one to another.

3.2   Running Instances

A dynamic view is associated to the static process scheme, for the management of running instances. Such a view is designed to be interactive, i.e., to let the user play with the model, so to control the evolution of the running process. Moreover, she can better learn the constraints mechanism by looking at the process evolving. Indeed, it is based on the same visual notation provided for the traces constraints visualization (see Figure 4), based in turn on local view diagrams. This choice is made in order to remark the user that global views do not explicitly express the evolution of the system over time, whereas local views do. Figure 7 depicts a sample evolution of a process instance.

From a starting task onwards, the user is asked to specify which the next task to perform is. At each step, the following tasks that can be enacted are shown, by means of the same visual language used for static views. After one of them is fired, all the *possible* and *mandatory* following tasks are shown. And so forth.

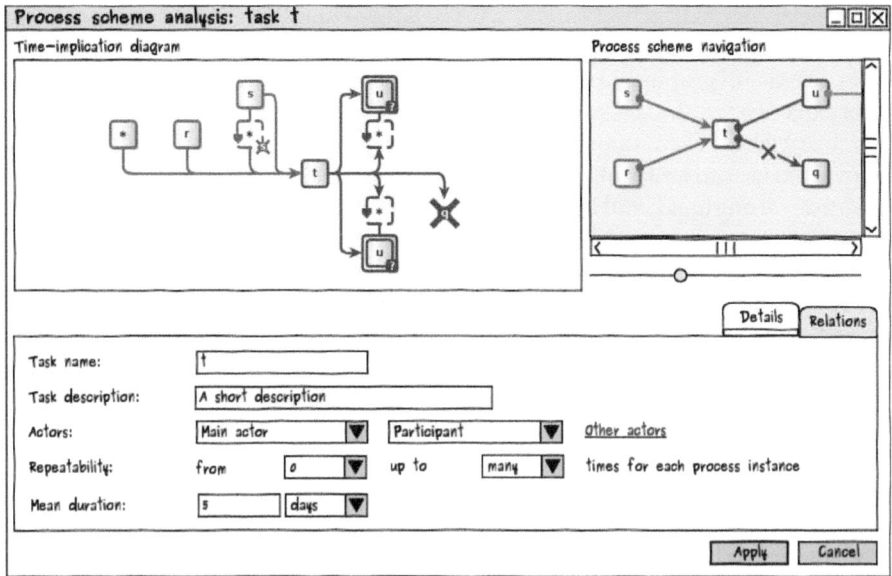

Fig. 6. The task details screen

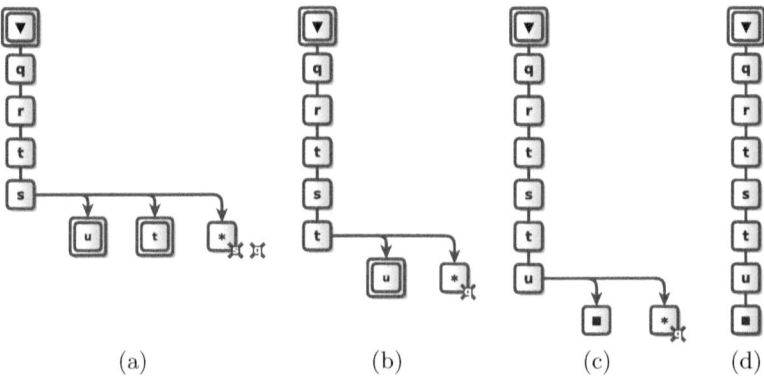

Fig. 7. The MAILOFMINE dynamic process view

We recall here that the recognition of the possible initial tasks, as far as the evolution which follows, is a view on the current state of the FSA obtained as the intersection of all the FSA's expressing the constraints in the process scheme. We are currently implementing such process scheme viewer.

A GUI prototype sketch. Figure 8 is a prototype sketch. It remarks two main features. The first is that users can adapt the timing in two different ways: either *(i)* as if every task lasts a time unit only, ignoring pauses between the preceding and the following, or *(ii)* showing the actual time consumption for both tasks completion and pauses in between. The former is useful for a compact

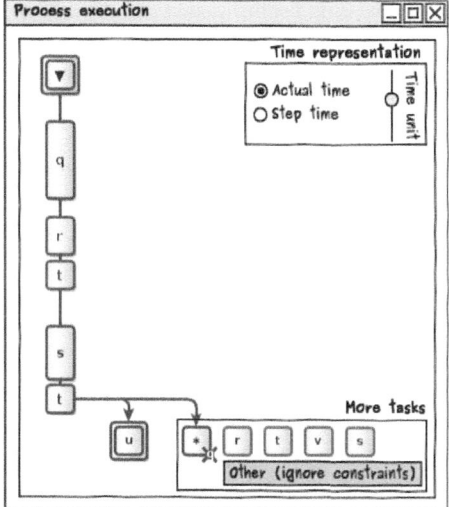

Fig. 8. The process execution management window

representation, the latter for a realistic snapshot of the time the running process is taking, with the evidence of delays. The second remarked feature is that users may even violate constraints: artful processes are subject to frequent changes, thus imposing a strict respect of constraints could be frustrating for the user who would like to do something else. This, on the other hand, can be a useful information for the process miner, since it can in turn refine the evolution of the process scheme itself, if a sufficient quantity of deviations from the expected paths are detected. For the next tasks to take over, the user will be asked to choose whether she wants to *(i)* delete the violated constraint from the overall process scheme, or *(ii)* proceed as if it was a point deviation only, namely keeping the constraints untouched. The former option is manageable thanks to the fact that each constraint is an FSA: this allows to immediately identify the violated constraint, on one hand, and recalculate the updated process scheme, on the other hand. During the execution of the process instance, in fact, not only the validity of the path on the global intersection FSA is considered: every step is monitored by the evolution of the individual constraint FSA components as well. So, when one or more of them are violated, they can be deleted from the set, on top of which the intersection FSA is computed. Once removed, the FSA is recalculated. Finally, the same history, up to the deviation, is enacted back on the new FSA. The next possible tasks to perform are shown accordingly.

4   Conclusions

In this paper we outlined the MailOfMine approach for mining artful processes from e-mail messages collections, focusing on the visualization aspects, i.e., the graphical syntax, the diagrams drawn and its GUI. We are currently in the process of realizing the various techniques into a working prototype. Then, we are going to validate it over a large *e*-mail messages collection. At the same time, we are testing the validity of our user interface with knowledge workers. The idea is to propose a graphical language for expressing artful processes, tailored to the users who will actually interact with it the most. Thus, symbols, connectors and all the other graphical details for modeling processes will be validated with them, rather then decided a priori by a team of experts in the business process management domain. In other words, we will exploit a user centered design for developing not the application only, but its core graphical language too.

References

1. Shaman. FP7 IP Project, http://shaman-ip.eu/shaman/
2. Smart Vortex. FP7 IP Project, http://www.smartvortex.eu/
3. van der Aalst, W.M.P.: Verification of Workflow Nets. In: Azéma, P., Balbo, G. (eds.) ICATPN 1997. LNCS, vol. 1248, pp. 407–426. Springer, Heidelberg (1997)
4. van der Aalst, W.M.P.: The application of petri nets to workflow management. Journal of Circuits, Systems, and Computers 8(1), 21–66 (1998)
5. van der Aalst, W.M.P., van Dongen, B.F., Günther, C.W., Rozinat, A., Verbeek, E., Weijters, T.: ProM: The process mining toolkit. In: BPM 2009 Demos (2009)
6. van der Aalst, W.M.P., Pesic, M.: Decserflow: Towards a Truly Declarative Service Flow Language. In: Bravetti, M., Núñez, M., Tennenholtz, M. (eds.) WS-FM 2006. LNCS, vol. 4184, pp. 1–23. Springer, Heidelberg (2006)
7. van der Aalst, W.M.P., Pesic, M., Schonenberg, H.: Declarative workflows: Balancing between flexibility and support. Computer Science - R&D 23(2) (2009)
8. de Carvalho, V.R., Cohen, W.W.: Learning to extract signature and reply lines from email. In: CEAS (2004)
9. Catarci, T., Dix, A., Katifori, A., Lepouras, G., Poggi, A.: Task-Centred Information Management. In: Thanos, C., Borri, F., Candela, L. (eds.) Digital Libraries: R & Development. LNCS, vol. 4877, pp. 197–206. Springer, Heidelberg (2007)
10. Chomsky, N., Miller, G.A.: Finite state languages. Information and Control 1(2), 91–112 (1958)
11. Clarke, E.M., Grumberg, O., Peled, D.: Model Checking. MIT Press (2001)
12. Di Ciccio, C., Mecella, M., Scannapieco, M., Zardetto, D., Catarci, T.: MailOfMine – Analyzing mail messages for mining artful collaborative processes. In: SIMPDA (2011)
13. Garofalakis, M.N., Rastogi, R., Shim, K.: Spirit: Sequential pattern mining with regular expression constraints. In: VLDB (1999)
14. Heutelbeck, D.: Preservation of enterprise engineering processes by social collaboration software. Personal Communication (2011)
15. ter Hofstede, A.M., van der Aalst, W.M.P., Adams, M., Russell, N.: Modern Business Process Automation: YAWL and its Support Environment. Springer, Heidelberg (2010)
16. Pesic, M., van der Aalst, W.M.P.: A Declarative Approach for Flexible Business Processes Management. In: Eder, J., Dustdar, S. (eds.) BPM Workshops 2006. LNCS, vol. 4103, pp. 169–180. Springer, Heidelberg (2006)
17. Rabin, M.O., Scott, D.: Finite automata and their decision problems. IBM J. Res. Dev. 3, 114–125 (1959)
18. Warren, P., Kings, N., et al.: Improving knowledge worker productivity - The ACTIVE integrated approach. BT Technology Journal 26(2), 165–176 (2009)

Checking User-Centred Design Principles in Distributed Cognition Models: A Case Study in the Healthcare Domain

Paolo Masci and Paul Curzon

School of Electronic Engineering and Computer Science
Queen Mary University of London, United Kingdom
{paolo.masci,paul.curzon}@eecs.qmul.ac.uk

Abstract. We propose a constructive procedure for building a distributed cognition model of a system out of contextual / ethnographic data. We then show how such a model can be conveniently used for studying, in a repeatable and justifiable way, if a system correctly implements selected user-centred design principles. Our approach thus complements user studies in that it enables reasoning about the situated use of a teamwork system even before direct user involvement. We have applied our procedure to a healthcare case study. In particular, we have re-analysed a well-known adverse incident that led to a fatality and for which a comprehensive investigation report is in the public domain. By reasoning about the distributed cognition model, we identified several issues that were not addressed in the incident report nor in other subsequent analyses.

1 Introduction and Motivation

Information technologies are improving healthcare systems by enabling greater control in drug delivery and enhanced patient monitoring. However, there is also evidence that the use of information technologies is causing serious problems to care givers and patients: not only delay and emotional distress [22], but also severe injury or death [19,12,10,17]. In 2010, the Food and Drug Administration (FDA) agency of the United States Department of Health and Human Services logged more than eight hundred thousands reports on incidents where medical devices may have caused death or serious injury to patients — almost a fifty percent increase from 2009 [20]. Although FDA advises that *"the number [of logged adverse events] is not intended to be used either to evaluate rates of adverse events or to compare adverse event occurrence rates across devices"*, such a number provides evidence that we are facing a serious and widespread problem.

An important consideration is that healthcare systems are teamwork systems relying on work-flows and protocols that have been finely tuned over long periods of time. Disrupting any work-flow or protocol is a potential source of unintended consequences [21]. Therefore, it is important to understand how the system works before introducing any modification. Contextual studies such as

A. Holzinger and K.-M. Simonic (Eds.): USAB 2011, LNCS 7058, pp. 95–108, 2011.

ethnographic studies represent a suitable means for understanding how a system works in practice. They involve collecting information from people actually working in the system, including observing activities as they are carried out in the real workplace. This contrasts with studies based on experimental or simulated settings. A common difficulty in ethnographic studies is that ethnographers need to know *what* to look for and *when*. Distributed cognition [14] is a conceptual framework that can help ethnographers address those issues. The idea of distributed cognition is that cognition is not confined to the mind of humans, but it spans across humans and artefacts. As such, cognition is a property of the whole system, and can be described in terms of transformations of the representational state of information.

To date, ethnographic data and distributed cognition models have been used for gaining a better understanding of how a range of systems work, highlighting strengths and weaknesses – see for instance [3]. However, the possibility of using the same data and related models for checking if the system adheres to known user-centred design principles has been largely overlooked in favour of experimental studies. In this paper, we explore the utility of using distributed cognition models for checking user-centred design principles in teamwork systems concerned with situation awareness.

Our contributions are (i) the definition of our constructive procedure for building, out of contextual study data, a distributed cognition model of the system that can be mechanically checked against properties of interest; (ii) a demonstration of how a distributed cognition model can be conveniently used for studying, without direct user involvement and in a repeatable and justifiable way, if a system correctly implements selected user-centred design principles. Our approach thus complements user studies. We consider a case study in the healthcare domain. The case study is based on contextual data collected by others during the investigation of an adverse incident in outpatient care [10].

The paper is organised as follows. In Section 2, we briefly introduce the concept of distributed cognition, and then present a constructive procedure for building a distributed cognition model that can be mechanically checked against properties of interest. In Section 3, we describe a healthcare case study, summarising the contextual data collected by others during an incident investigation. In this case it was primarily based on interview data. We then describe how we mechanically build a distributed cognition model of the system out of such data. In Section 4, we introduce the concept of situation awareness, and then we use the distributed cognition model of the system for checking selected situation awareness design principles. In Section 5, we discuss the utility of the presented approach. In Section 6, we summarise related work and draw the conclusions.

2   Distributed Cognition Models

Distributed cognition [14] is a conceptual framework proposed by Hutchins in the mid 1980s. The framework has gained attention in the research community because of its capacity to capture the key mechanisms that form the basis of complex teamwork systems. The idea behind the framework is that cognition is a property of the whole system rather than something confined to the heads of individuals. In other words, the cognitive activities of an individual are not self-contained in the mind of the individual, and external artifacts and other people constitute part of it. Based on this view, Hutchins argues that it is possible to deduce important information on the cognitive activities of the users of the systems by reasoning about the observable representational states of information. Hutchins, indeed, observes that even if the cognitive activities of users remain hidden, in many cases the representational state of information and the kind of errors made by users impose constraints that are tight enough to enable an accurate identification of the plausible mental models (i.e., the internal representations and processes) that the users must be adopting. An important implication is that the design of artifacts and technologies can be used not only for understanding plausible mental models, but also for *shaping* them to ones that are "syntactically correct", in the sense that they can provide guidance to the person that has to perform a task, thus making the path to the solution apparent. In our work, we aim to study if the overall system design supports such a correct shaping of mental models. To do this, we build a distributed cognition model of the system out of contextual / ethnographic data, and we check if such a model consistently implements user-centred design principles.

2.1   Procedure for Building a Distributed Cognition Model

A distributed cognition model describes the behaviour of the system in terms of transformations of the observable representational states of information [14]. To date, the construction of a distributed cognition model has been a prerogative of analysts holding a deep knowledge of the domain. One of the reasons behind this is that Hutchins' distributed cognition framework [14] provides a set of abstract principles for modelling the system, but it does not actually provide an explicit constructive procedure for building the model. Other works, such as [3], have defined various distributed cognition models for studying the system in a structured way, but they also lack a constructive procedure for building the model. In this work, we aim to fill this gap.

We aim to identify a heuristic procedure that can help any analyst to mechanically build a distributed cognition model that reasonably resembles how the system works. The proposed heuristic procedure is based on the identification of recurrent reasoning strategies deducible from the narrative descriptions of different distributed cognition models built by different authors in various studies, such as [15,14,3,11,1,13,7].

In order to build such a model from ethnographic or other contextual data, we need to answer the following questions: (i) what are the relevant information items for the system? (ii) what level of detail is needed for specifying the representational state? (iii) what are the relevant transformations needed for modelling the behaviour of the system? In the following, we define a three-step constructive procedure for answering the above questions.

Step 1: define the relevant information items. Two good starting points for deriving the relevant information items are the specification of the aim of the system, which gives a bird's eye view on the intended functionalities of the system, and the specification of the system requirements, which provides insights on what parameters matter for the system. Any information item included in such specifications can be considered relevant for describing how the system works. For example, for a healthcare system, a specification of the aim might be that patients receive the correct medication; a requirement can be that a medication can be given to a patient only after his or her blood samples have been tested by the laboratory and checked by a medic. In this case, the information items relevant for the system would be: patients, medics, laboratory, medications, and blood samples.

Step 2: define the observable representations. Given the relevant information items, the second step is to define which media hold their observable representations within the system. Intuitively, we need to answer the following question: *how does the system remember the relevant information items?* To answer this question, we need to "follow" the information items within the work-flows of the system, and identify the elements (humans, artefacts, technologies) whose observable features hold characteristics of the information item. For example, if we follow a medication in a healthcare system, the observable representations can be given by the medication itself, fields of electronic records, paperwork (including labels), data stored in medical devices, and utterances.

Step 3: define the behaviour of the system. The behaviour of the system is specified in terms of transformations of observable representations. In this context, a transformation corresponds to an activity carried out by a system element. Given an information item, the relevant activities for such an item are those modifying the representational state of the item. As with Step 2, activities and relations between activities can be identified by "following" the observable representations of an information item within the work-flows of the system. For example, if we consider a prescription, which is an observable representation of a medication in a healthcare system, an activity can be defined by a physician entering the prescription into an electronic order.

The obtained specification of the behaviour of the system is compatible with Hutchins' view of tasks and work-flows as distributed computations — they create, transform and propagate the representational state of information across a series of heterogeneous "representational media". Note that the specification of the behaviour of the system obtained from the above procedure may include more details than a typical procedural description. Indeed, rather than identifying only the type of activities and the dependency relations among activities, the procedure points out also the role of the different elements in the system and, as such, it provides a description of the cognitive tasks faced by individual members of the team [14].

3   Case study

To illustrate the utility of our approach, we consider contextual data reported in the fluorouracil incident root cause analysis report [10] by the Institute of Safe Medication Practices (ISMP) Canada. The data was collected by a team of five healthcare professionals for the investigation of an adverse incident in outpatient care. A young woman, Denise Melanson, received by mistake an infusion of a chemotherapy drug (fluorouracil) over 4 hours instead of 4 days. Due to the toxicity of the drug, the overdose caused her death.

For the purpose of our study, we consider the data relative to the preparation of the drug doses in the hospital. In the following, we report the integral text of an introductory paragraph of the report, which summarises the contextual data collected, and we summarise some additional information contained in the report about the preparation of the doses. The complete report can be found in [10].

> *"The patient had previously been treated with chemotherapy and radiation from May 10 to June 22 and was to start three cycles of adjuvant chemotherapy with cisplatin and fluorouracil. At this clinic visit [on Friday, July 28], the clinic nurse reviewed the orders, the results of lab work, and the patient's height and weight to ensure all was in order for chemotherapy administration on Monday, July 31. The bay pharmacist also reviewed the order and completed the calculations required for pharmacy staff to enter the drug order into the pharmacy information system and prepare the dose."*

The bay pharmacist used a computerised physician order entry system (page 35, fluorouracil incident root cause analysis report [10]). A computerised physician order entry is a computer-based system for entering and storing medication orders electronically. The fluorouracil incident report does not provide details of the user interface of the computerised physician order entry. However, it highlights that such a system is not networked with the pharmacy information system — the pharmacy staff, hence, had to manually enter the order in the pharmacy information system.

The prepared doses are accompanied by a printed copy of the electronic order and a printed label. The printed label is attached to the bag containing the solution. Figure 1 reproduces the layout of the printed order and label — snapshots of the real-world originals can be found in the fluorouracil report [10] (pages 62 and 72).

3.1   Distributed Cognition Model

Following the constructive procedure described in Section 2.1, we construct step-by-step the distributed cognition model of the system from the contextual data in the report.

5-Fluorouracil 5,250 mg (at 4,000 mg/m2) Intravenous once continuous over 4 days

Cis_5FU_Part2-HN-CC – Cycle – 1, Day – 1
      Substitutions Allowed

      Administration Instructions:
      Continuous infusion via ambulatory infusion pump
      (Baseline regimen dose = 1000 mg/m2/day = 4000 mg/m2/4 days)

```
FLOUROURACIL 50 mg/mL INJ                    5924.48   mg  (118.49 m

In D5W IV   Total Volume: 130 mL
Final Concentration: 45.57 mg/mL
Dose: 5250 mg/4days (1312.5mg/24h)
Rate: 28.8mL/24h (1.2mL/h) Bag will last 4 days
At full usage with 14.8 mL reserve.
Dr.████████████ Rx#ABS19073
Prep: Jul 31 2006  @  905 Exp: 7days
██████████ Pharmacy██████████████
11560 ██████████ Ave.
```

Fig. 1. A reproduction of the printed copy of the electronic order and of the bag label of the fluorouracil incident [10]

Relevant information items. The system under study is a medical day care clinic. Since drugs administration is the main theme of the case study, we consider the "five rights" of drugs administration — administer the right dose, of the right medication, for the right amount of time, to the right patient, via the right route. Such an aim defines five relevant information items: *patient identity, administration route, administration dose, administration time, drug type.*

Observable representations. According to the work-flow described in the report, the following system elements appear to hold one or more observable representations of the five rights: *the patient itself* (holds patient identity), *the printed copy of the electronic order* (holds administration route and drug type), and *the drug label* (holds administration route, dose, time, and drug type). Details on the items used by the bay pharmacist to perform a calculation are not specified in the data available. For the illustrative purpose of this study, we assume that a calculator has been used — hence, the calculator holds a representation of dose and time. Similarly, the details on the electronic order of the computerised physician order entry and the pharmacy system are not reported. We assume that they contain information about all five rights.

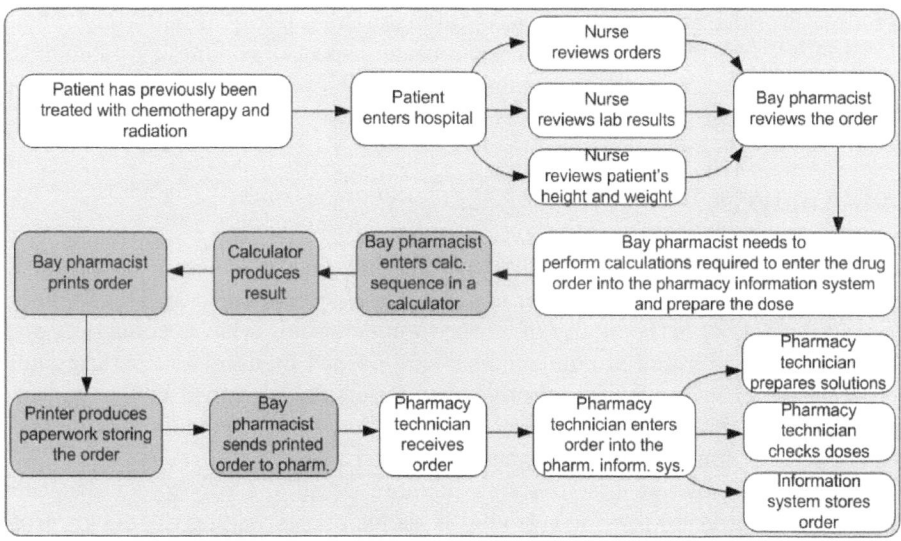

Fig. 2. A distributed cognition model that describes "how the system prepares the doses". Gray boxes represent activities that are not directly mentioned in the ethnographic data of the fluorouracil report.

System behaviour. A diagram showing the system behaviour derived from the contextual data is shown in Figure 2. The diagram uses the syntax of DiCoT information flow models [3]. We use this kind of model because it provides an intuitive semi-formal representation of the distributed cognition model. Briefly, each labelled box in the diagram represents an activity carried out by a system element. Each activity specifies how a system element creates, transforms and propagates the observable representations of information. For instance, the activity *"Patient enters hospital"* models a change of the representational state of the patient (i.e., his or her physical location). Some activities leave all representational states unchanged, e.g., *"Nurse reviews orders"* and *"Nurse reviews lab results"*. Arrows between activities represent explicit dependency relations. In the model, an activity can be performed when all directly connected activities have already been performed, e.g., *"Bay pharmacist reviews the order"* can be performed only when the three activities *"Nurse reviews order"*, *"Nurse reviews lab results"*, and *"Nurse reviews patient's height and weight"* have been performed (in any order). A more complete presentation of the syntax and semantics of the diagram can be found in [18].

In the diagram shown in Figure 2, we use grey boxes to highlight some activities that are not directly mentioned in the fluorouracil report [10]. Such additional information is needed to specify the transformations of the representational state due to the activities carried out by the bay pharmacist. Although this information may be slightly different from that of the system considered in the original study, those we have used are compatible with typical procedures of healthcare systems. Therefore, the diagram represents a plausible description of a real-world system, and it is acceptable for the purpose of our study, which is purely demonstrative. We note that a useful aspect of conducting an analysis such as this is that it could highlight steps that are missing but ought to be described in such an incident report.

4   Analysis

We now use the distributed cognition model for checking selected user-centred design principles related to *situation awareness*. Situation awareness (defined more fully below) is the ability of a user to understand "what is going on", and it is a recognised essential non-technical skill needed by users for operating any critical system in a safe and effective way. Originally identified in the aviation domain, the importance of situation awareness has become evident also in other safety-critical domains, including healthcare [7,13,4,8].

In the following, we first describe in more detail the concept of situation awareness in order to provide a ground basis for understanding the design principles. Then, we use the distributed cognition model constructed in Section 3.1 for checking selected situation awareness design principles.

4.1   Situation Awareness

Situation awareness has been defined by Endsley as *"the perception of the elements in the environment within a volume of time and space, the comprehension of their meaning, and the projection of their status in the near future"* [5].

We consider this definition, which relates situation awareness to a three-stage cognitive process: the ability to identify the critical factors in the environment (stage 1); the ability to deduce the significance of such factors (stage 2); and the ability to anticipate future events on the basis of the identified factors and significance (stage 3). Complete situation awareness is achieved when the user completes all three stages. Partial situation awareness is reached when only some stages are completed: the completion of stage 1 leads to "level 1 situation awareness", whilst the completion of stages 1 and 2 leads to "level 2 situation awareness".

Accurate and complete situation awareness is a *necessary* pre-condition for consistently correct decision making [5,9]: without accurate or complete situation awareness, even the best trained users can make the wrong decision — though, users with perfect situation awareness can still make the wrong decision.

In [5], Endsley discusses the meaning of situation awareness in teamwork systems. She argues that situation awareness for a team member is based on a specific set of elements that are relevant for the member's responsibilities in the team. The set of elements are partially overlapping, and the overlapping set identifies what is relevant for team co-ordination.

Measurement techniques for assessing situation awareness are typically experimental. The techniques rely on structured questionnaires proposed to users during or after their performance in a simulated scenario. The questions aim to collect information about the level of knowledge and understanding of the situation. A discussion of the measurement techniques is beyond the scope of this paper. Readers interested are directed to [6] for an overview of the various approaches and a discussion of the advantages and disadvantages of each.

4.2   Checking Design Principles in Distributed Cognition Systems

Endsley et.al. [6] have shown that a system design can support situation awareness by giving users the right cues at the right moment, and they have identified a series of situation awareness design principles on the basis of a theoretical model of human cognition.

Here, we consider the following two basic design principles: "provide structured information", and "remove extraneous information". Our approach also extends to other design principles. We focus on these in particular here because the contextual data available to us for these rules is sufficient to highlight potential issues not already identified in the original report or in other research concerning the incident.

In the following, for each selected design principle, we briefly introduce its importance in situation awareness, and then check if the principle is satisfied for the activities involving humans in our case study. To this end, we recall that, in our distributed cognition models, the representational state of information is essentially the system state. Hence, assessing the validity of the design principle corresponds to checking specific constraints on the structure and value of the system state.

Principle: provide structured information.   Situation awareness can be facilitated by presenting users with structured information that integrates the meaning of low level cues. Structured information, indeed, can off-load users from juggling (possibly several) different cues from the environment, and therefore enables them to focus on the comprehension of events and the projection of future system states. Also, structured information helps humans to overcome their short-term memory limits. Short term memory can contain only a very limited number of chunks of information, and such a memory is likely to have a central role in situation awareness because it can be used as a cache for storing the information needed for creating a picture of the current situation [6].

Assessment.   We need to check that the observable representational state available to the different users contains structured information reporting the patient identity, the administration route, dose, time, and the drug type. The level of detail of the available contextual data allows us to point out two main issues with the representational state used by the bay pharmacist and the pharmacy staff.

One issue is on the representational state used by the bay pharmacist. The bay pharmacist propagates the representational state from a printed order to a computerised physician order entry and a paper artefact for the pharmacy. We do not have enough details for making a direct comparison between the structure of information contained in those items, but from the report we know that the structured information contained in the order does not match the information needed for the pharmacy. As a consequence of this mismatch, the physician needs to use a calculator. The calculator does not correctly represent either the patient weight and height, or administration doses and time — the calculator knows only numbers, and numbers are not linked to any dimensional unit (Kg, mL, mg, mg/h, ...). Any slip or mistake in typing a number gives a different result, without reporting any error [23]. Also, the calculator helps only with the "easy" part of the calculation problem. The complicated part is that of deciding the calculation sequence [14], and the bay pharmacist is evidently in charge of it. By (unfortunate) chance, there is evidence that the bay pharmacist made a miscalculation in the fluorouracil incident:

> "In reviewing this case, it was learned that a miscalculation occurred when the pharmacist initially reviewed the order in the clinic. [....] The miscalculation was detected by the pharmacy technician when the volume of fluorouracil to be added to the infusion bag calculated by the pharmacist did not match the volume calculated by the computer system." (page 35, fluorouracil incident root cause analysis report [10]).

Another issue is on the representational state used by the pharmacy staff. The pharmacy staff prepares the solutions according to the information stored in the pharmacy information system. Preparing the solutions includes measuring/mixing drugs, selecting a proper container (e.g., a bag), producing a label and attaching it to the container. The pharmacy information system is used for producing the label. Such a label will be the representational media used to transfer information from the pharmacy to the nurse. Such a label, hence, must contain information for deducing the patient identity, the intended route, the dose, the drug, and the amount of administration time. The label used in the fluorouracil incident does not contain the patient identity. Thimbleby, in [23], provides an interesting analysis of the fluorouracil incident report, and he highlights the same omission in the label.

Principle: remove extraneous information. Information that does not contribute to situation awareness should not be presented to users. There is experimental evidence that humans have numerous bottlenecks in performing a simultaneous processing of several pieces of information, especially if the information is gathered from a single channel, e.g., only from the auditive or from the visual channel. A typical failure due to these bottlenecks is known as *attentional tunnelling*, i.e., the user "locks in" on specific information and inadvertently drops other (possibly relevant) information [6].

Assessment. We need to check that the observable representational state contains only the necessary information needed by the user. The level of detail of the contextual data allows to point out one main issue with the representational state generated by the pharmacy staff. The problem lies in the paperwork generated by the computerised physician order system and by the pharmacy information system. Both printed copies of the order and the label contain unnecessary repetitions. For instance, in the printed copy of the order, the name of the drug is reported twice and in two different forms (*"5-Fluorouracil"* on the first line, and *"5FU"* on the second line). Similarly, in the printed label, dose and rate are reported twice, and in two different formats (the dose is reported as *"5250mg/4days"* and *"1312.5mg/24h"*, and the rate is *"28.8mL/24h"* and *"1.2mL/h"*). According to the root cause analysis [10] of the incident, this seems to be a real issue: *"the medication label contained unnecessary information"* (pages 18, 30, and 37), and *"a number of dangerous abbreviations and symbols [...], e.g., 5FU for fluorouracil"* (page 34). The information ideally should be given once and in the representational form needed by the nurses.

5   Discussion

A key lesson that emerged from building and analysing the distributed cognition models is that their main utility is actually not to provide answers, but to raise questions in a systematic way about design choices. This is important not only for understanding how a system works or during investigations of adverse events, but also, for example, for reasoning about system re-design and when making procurement decisions. We give concrete examples below where we report some of the questions that were raised while building and analysing the distributed cognition model of Section 3.1. The last question we report is particularly interesting because it uncovers plausible concerns about a potential issue that was overlooked by the incident report and by other studies.

– *What is the actual procedure if the lab results are not available when the bay pharmacist reviews the order?*
  Laboratory results may take time to be performed, and there are cases in which they are not available when the patient has to start a treatment. A question about the consequences of lab results being unavailable would have uncovered, in this case, that a treatment could start even without lab results. According to the incident report, this seems to be a real issue of the considered system:

  > *"Pharmacists routinely monitor patient laboratory results and will intervene if such results indicate that a patient should not receive chemotherapy, this monitoring is done only if laboratory results are available when the medication order is being reviewed. If laboratory work is pending, the results are not routinely followed up by pharmacy staff."* (page 34, fluorouracil incident report [10]).

– *Why do medication orders have to be manually entered in the information system?*
  This question could trigger a discussion on a simple and inexpensive design change that could help avoid potential number entry errors due to slips and

mistakes (e.g., the use of a visual tag for including a machine-readable representation of the medication order on the paperwork — a similar solution has also been proposed by Thimbleby in [23]). We note that the investigation of the incident revealed at least two documented number entry errors: the bay pharmacist entered the wrong data in the computerised physician order entry system (page 35 of the fluorouracil report [10]), and the nurse entered the wrong rate in the infusion pump (page 18 of the fluorouracil report [10]).

– *What is the actual procedure if the printed version of the electronic order reports different data to the label?.*
  Mismatching pieces of paperwork is a plausible event in the system, since the two pieces of paperwork seem to be generated by two different systems (the computerised physician order entry system and the pharmacy information system). Also, as evidenced during the analysis of the situation awareness design principle on structured information, neither the printed electronic order nor the label report the patient identity. Hence, there is also the possibility that, by mistake, a label is coupled with a wrong printed electronic order. We do not have evidence of such a specific adverse events, but we argue that it is plausible, as other reports have evidenced that misinterpretation of drug labels and confusion between packages are common causes of medication errors [16]. It is therefore worth looking for ways to avoid it happening. This potential issue was not identified in the original report or in other research studies on the incident.

6   Related Work and Conclusions

Previously, distributed cognition models have generally been used for understanding how the system modelled works, and are normally presented in the form of a mixture of narrative descriptions and ad hoc semi-formal diagrams. In the healthcare domain, which is our main concern, Blandford and Furniss [3] have developed various distributed cognition models within their structured methodology (DiCoT) which aims to help ethnographers in the process of understanding the key aspects of a teamwork system. They used DiCoT when studying the London ambulance service [3,11]. Hazlehurst et.al. [13] have used distributed cognition for studying the importance of verbal communications in co-ordinating the teamwork in a heart room. In particular, they investigated how verbal communications support situation awareness. Similarly, Fioratou et. al. [7], used distributed cognition for understanding how anaesthetists gain situation awareness during surgical interventions. Through their analysis, they identified various factors influencing anaesthetists' situation awareness, and they used such factors for explaining the causes of an adverse event.

Our work builds on this earlier work in that we define a constructive procedure for building structured distributed cognition models out of contextual and ethnographic data. Such models can be checked against properties of interest, either manually or within automated reasoning tools. In our previous work [18,2], we demonstrated how such models can be analysed within automated reasoning tools, focusing on completeness and consistency of information flows. In this paper, we have shown the utility of such models for analysing, in a justifiable and we believe repeatable way, if a teamwork system satisfies selected user-centred design principles. In this sense, our work complements experimental user studies, in that it enables reasoning about the situated use of re-designed teamwork system even prior to direct user involvement.

In particular we have applied our procedure to a healthcare case study. We have re-analysed a well-known adverse incident that led to a fatality and for which a comprehensive investigation report is in the public domain. By following our procedure with respect to two situation awareness design rules, we identified an issue that was not addressed in the incident report nor in other subsequent analyses. We have thus demonstrated the potential of the approach.

Although in this study we have used contextual data collected after an adverse event, we argue that the approach extends also to other kinds of studies with different aims. For instance, the analysis can be conveniently used during ethnographic studies for uncovering relevant situations that should be investigated, or in situations involving reasoning about design changes, e.g., during procurement decisions. The investigation of such possibilities is on our research agenda. Further work is required to apply our method to further case studies and also to evaluate our belief that the method really does deliver repeatability. We also intend in future to provide mechanised support for performing the analyses

Acknowledgements. This work is supported by CHI+MED (http://www.chi-med.ac.uk), a flagship project funded by the Engineering and Physical Sciences Research Council (EPSRC) on research agreement EP/G059063/1.

References

1. Baber, C.: Distributed cognition at the crime scene. AI & Society 25, 423–432 (2010), doi:10.1007/s00146-010-0274-6
2. Blandford, A., Cauchi, A., Curzon, P., Eslambolchilar, P., Furniss, D., Gimblett, A., Huang, H., Lee, P., Li, Y., Masci, P., Oladimeji, P., Rajkomar, A., Rukšénas, R., Thimbleby, H.: Comparing actual practice and user manuals: A case study based on programmable infusion pumps. In: Eics4Med, the 1st International Workshop on Engineering Interactive Computing Systems for Medicine and Health Care. ACM Digital Library (2011)
3. Blandford, A., Furniss, D.: DiCoT: A Methodology for Applying Distributed Cognition to the Design of Teamworking Systems. Interactive Systems, 26–38 (2006)
4. Blandford, A., William Wong, B.L.: Situation awareness in emergency medical dispatch. Int. J. Hum.-Comput. Stud. 61, 421–452 (2004)
5. Endsley, M.R.: Toward a theory of situation awareness in dynamic systems: Situation awareness. Human factors 37(1), 32–64 (1995)
6. Endsley, M.R., Bolte, B., Jones, D.G.: Designing for Situation Awareness: An Approach to User-Centered Design. Taylor and Francis (2003)
7. Fioratou, E., Flin, R., Glavin, R., Patey, R.: Beyond monitoring: distributed situation awareness in anaesthesia. British Journal of Anaesthesia 105(1), 83–90 (2010)

8. Fletcher, G., Flin, R., McGeorge, P., Glavin, R., Maran, N., Patey, R.: Anaesthetists' nontechnical skills (ants): evaluation of a behavioural marker system. British Journal of Anesthesia 90(5), 580–588 (2003)

9. Flin, R., Patey, R., Glavin, R., Maran, N.: Anaesthetists' non-technical skills. British Journal of Anaesthesia 105(1), 38–44 (2010)

10. Institute for Safe Medication Practices Canada (ISMP Canada). Fluorouracil incident root cause analysis report (May 2007),
    http://www.ismp-canada.org/download/reports/
    FluorouracilIncidentMay2007.pdf

11. Furniss, D.: Codifying distributed cognition: a case study of emergency medical dispatch. MSc Thesis, UCLIC, UCL Interaction Centre (2004)

12. Han, Y.Y., Carcillo, J.A., Venkataraman, S.T., Clark, R.S.B., Scott Watson, R., Nguyen, T.C., Bayir, H., Orr, R.A.: Unexpected increased mortality after implementation of a commercially sold computerized physician order entry system. Pediatrics 116(6), 1506–1512 (2005)

13. Hazlehurst, B., McMullen, C.K., Gorman, P.N.: Distributed cognition in the heart room: How situation awareness arises from coordinated communications during cardiac surgery. Journal of Biomedical Informatics 40(5), 539–551 (2007)

14. Hutchins, E.: The MIT Press, new edn. The MIT Press (September 1995)

15. Hutchins, E.: How a Cockpit Remembers Its Speed. Cognitive Science 19, 265–288 (1995)

16. Hugh James, R.: 1000 anaesthetic incidents: experience to date. Anaesthesia 58(9), 856–863 (2003)

17. Leveson, N.G.: An investigation of the therac-25 accidents. IEEE Computer 26, 18–41 (1993)

18. Masci, P., Curzon, P., Blandford, A., Furniss, D.: Modelling distributed cognition systems in pvs. In: FMIS 2011, the 4th Intl. Workshop on Formal Methods for Interactive Systems (2011)

19. Nanji, K.C., Rothschild, J.M., Salzberg, C., Keohane, C.A., Zigmont, K., Devita, J., Gandhi, T.K., Dalal, A.K., Bates, D.W., Poon, E.G.: Errors associated with outpatient computerized prescribing systems. Journal of the American Medical Informatics Association (2011)

20. Schmitt, S.M.: Medical device reportings jump to all-time high. The Silver Sheet, Medical Device Quality Control 14(4) (April 2010)

21. Sittig, D.F., Ash, J.S., Zhang, J., Osheroff, J.A., Michael Shabot, M.: Lessons from unexpected increased mortality after implementation of a commercially sold computerized physician order entry system. Pediatrics 118(2), 797–801 (2006)

22. Sittig, D.F., Krall, M., Kaalaas-Sittig, J., Ash, J.S.: Research paper: Emotional aspects of computer-based provider order entry: A qualitative study. Journal of the American Medical Informatics Association 12(5), 561–567 (2005)

23. Thimbleby, H.: Is it a dangerous prescription? BCS Interfaces 84, 5–10 (2010)

Interactive Visualization for Information Analysis in Medical Diagnosis

B.L. William Wong[1], Kai Xu[1], and Andreas Holzinger[2]

[1] Interaction Design Center, School of Engineering and Information Sciences,
Middlesex University, London, UK
{w.wong,k.xu}@mdx.ac.uk
[2] Research Unit Human-Computer Interaction, Institute for Medical Informatics,
Statistics and Documentation (IMI), Medical University Graz, Graz, Austria
andreas.holzinger@medunigraz.at

Abstract. This paper investigates to what extend the findings and solutions of information analysis in intelligence analysis can be applied and transferred into the medical diagnosis domains. Interactive visualization is proposed to address some of the problems faced by both domain. Its design issues related to selected common problems are then discussed in details. Finally, a visual sense making system INVISQUE is used as an example to illustrate how the interactive visualization can be used to support information analysis and medical diagnosis.

Keywords: Visualization, Visual Analytics, Medical Diagnosis.

1 Introduction

In this paper we will briefly compare the similarities between information analysis in intelligence analysis and the medical diagnosis domains, and hence to draw from our work in intelligence and then examine how it might be applied to the medical domain. Our understanding of the cognitive processes in information analysis suggest that it is more than just the process of information search and retrieval, but incorporates a number of other features that is now characterized as *sense-making*. The more frequently cited Pirolli and Card model [15] of intelligence analysis while useful in helping us see the different cycles (i.e., foraging, hypothesis formulation and testing), can be complemented by Klein et al.'s Data-Frame model [11] which describes the process of creating plausible explanations for observed data. This similarity allows us to consider our work in the intelligence, legal investigation and e-discovery domains, in the context of medical diagnostic analysis, particularly in the area of reviewing a patient's medical history for the purpose of developing treatment plans. From our work in designing interactive visualizations for information analysis, we documented a list of 20 design problems [19], and will discuss five problems that we believe have a bearing in designing medical diagnostic displays that can assist in improving the review of a patient's medical history. We will then discuss the design issues and a number of possible designs currently under consideration in the context of a visual sense making system INVISQUE [20].

A. Holzinger and K.-M. Simonic (Eds.): USAB 2011, LNCS 7058, pp. 109–120, 2011.

2   Information Analysis in Intelligence and Medical Domains

In trying to assess the level of maturity of intelligence analysis as a discipline, Fisher and Johnston [1] provide a brief account of the similarities between the process of medical decision-making and clinical judgement, with intelligence analysis. In their review they also reported on the beginnings of evidence-based medicine (EBM) and how EBM, with the use of statistical information, help make clinical judgement and treatment more systematic and able to draw on evidence of past cases, rather than on limited experience or anecdotal information.

But are they really similar? Let's take a look at what makes intelligence analysis difficult. There are many problems, but we'll briefly discuss those that are more relevant to the medical community (e.g. we will not focus on data that has been created for deception and to mislead an analyst).

Fig. 1 is a basic illustration of the information challenges facing intelligence analysts. Analysts often work alone, and are required to make sense out of large data sets that come from different sources and in different formats, and are often of varying quality and reliability. The information may be incomplete, out of sequence, changing as the situation changes, and misleading. For the analyst peering through the tiny viewport of his or her computer display to this very large data space, is like a person peering through the keyhole of a door to an enormous hall. To gain a sense of what the hall is like, the analyst must piece together his or her different views from memory, which can lead to many problems associated with memory and cognitive limitations, attention, and bias. This can lead to errors of re-construction or simply forgetting what was seen previously.

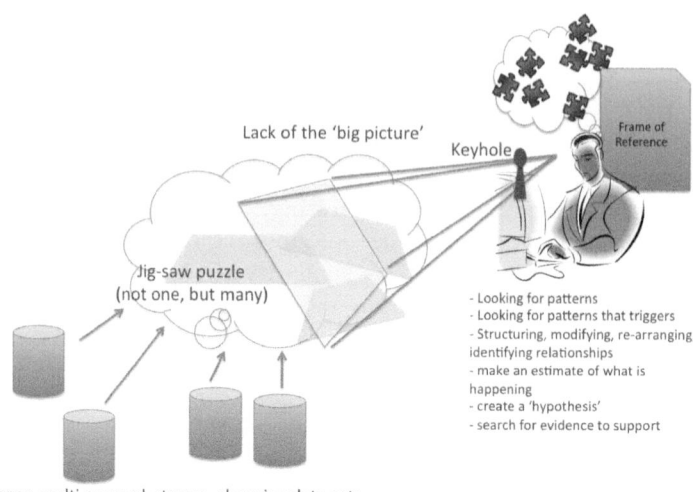

Fig. 1. Illustration of the problems faced by an information analyst

In addition, the data that analysts are often presented with, is akin to a jig-saw puzzle, where the pieces have been emptied onto the table top, and the analyst has to find, organize and join the relevant pieces together. To complicate the problem, the box tops of the jig-saw puzzle, which provides the big picture of the puzzle, are almost always not available, i.e. there is no context in which to view the pieces of information. The analyst instead has to build the picture as he or she carries out the analysis. To further aggravate this already difficult situation, an analyst is often presented with not one jig-saw puzzle, but several at the same time, and each without its box top, where the puzzles may be related or may have absolutely nothing to do with one another.

Then, guided by their training, expectations, beliefs, goals, socio-cultural factors and other background factors, they will create frames that help piece together the information to create explanations or narratives that is able to account for what they have observed [11]. In the process of creating these data-frame relationships that help them make sense of the data, the analysts are looking for patterns, underlying relationships, and triggers in the data, that help them collate evidence to support possible explanations (or 'hypotheses', in the social science, and sometimes in the scientific sense of the word), in order to come to a conclusion.

In a public health context, there is probably a large similarity in trying to identify the source of an outbreak of an infectious disease in a populated area, and depending on various conditions, the situation could evolve very rapidly. Evidence will be collated from different sources such as news items, hospital and doctors reports, laboratory results, and so forth. In order to diagnose a patient's medical situation, it may be necessary for the doctor, or in more complex cases, the medical team to collate and review the patient's medical history, which can be long and complicated, e.g. a geriatric patient with a history of acute glaucoma, hypertension, arthritis and joint pains, liver sclerosis, may require treatment for breathing difficulties. Each of these areas may have been treated separately with records held in different specialist clinics.

3   Sense-Making and the Data-Frame Model

Pirolli and Card [15], based on a cognitive task analysis of intelligence analysts, explains the intelligence process as one primarily of search: searching for information, relationships, evidence to formulate or support a hypothesis; and in the process of searching, the analyst carries out a number of other processing actions as well, such as reading and extracting relevant or meaningful information, indexing and filing away data, creating schema by organizing and re-organizing the data in order to create understanding and insight that can lead further actions for building the case for the formulated hypothesis, and to then subsequently create a narrative that tells a story.

This model has been used and referred to considerably by analysts and researchers. It can however be usefully complemented by Kleins et al. [9] Data-Frame Model of Sense-making. The Data-Frame model basically explains that

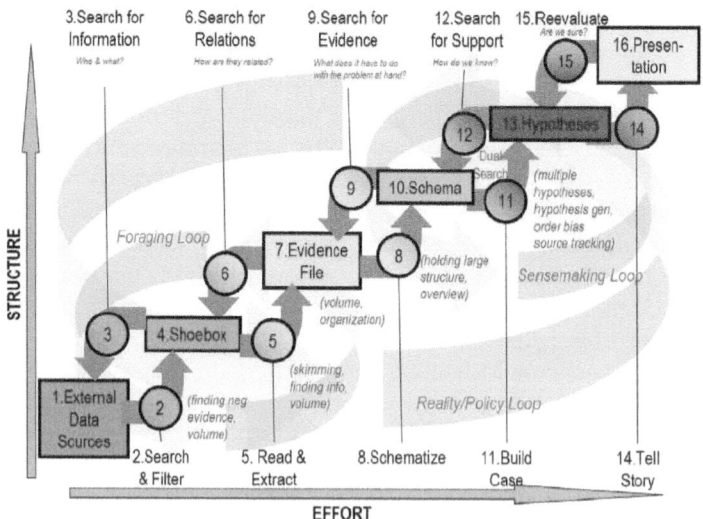

Fig. 2. Sense-making loop for intelligence analysis [15]

an analyst upon observing a set of data, will attempt to create an explanation for this data that they refer to a frame. The creation of this frame is contingent upon the analysts background such as, training and experience, goals and expectancies. Together with the data, this frame will determine how the data is combined and used to explain what has been observed. The frame also determines what the analyst will attend to, what data should be related, or filtered. Klein et al. [9] then describes additional strategies used to help the analyst to gain a deeper understanding by elaborating and filling in gaps or seeking more information, to query one's own assumptions and beliefs and in particular how earlier data has been used to generate the explanations, judging the plausibility of the arguments or narratives, and the quality of the data at the same time. There may be times when the data and the frame are so badly mis-matched that it requires the analyst to re-evaluate his frames, and to possibly revamp these frames or even seek a new frame. There is no real sequence in the process. Instead, it shows the variety of strategies that may be invoked to make sense of the data and one's frame and to assess the plausibility of the offered accounts.

In addition, Klein et al. [10] also explains that people are also engaged in another form of reasoning which they have also observed occurring in naturalistic environments - causal reasoning. While causal reasoning is characterized by the determination of causes for observed effects, this causality can sometimes be confused with correlation as events can co-occur, while not being the cause of the observed effects. Also, another characteristic of causality is mutability, or the ability to engage in a reasoning strategy that allows one to investigate or imagine what might have happened if one or all of the causal factors did not occur or could be reversed, and this can also be used as a test for causality. Josephson and Tanner [8] explain another form of reasoning that is useful: abductive reasoning.

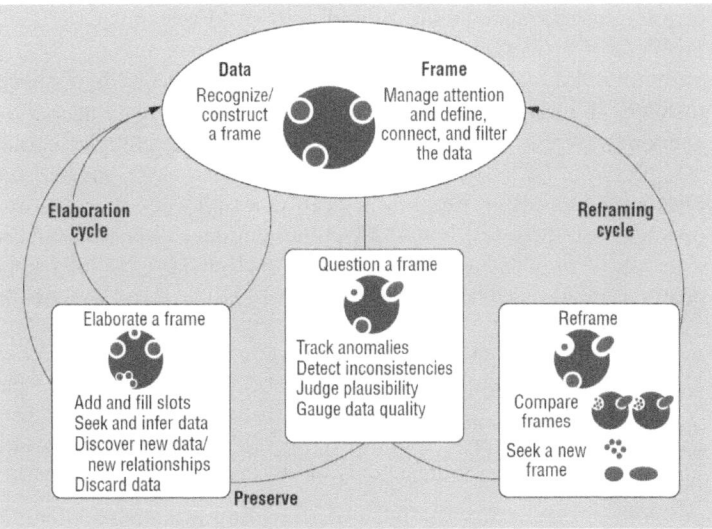

Fig. 3. The Data-Frame Model of Sense-making [11]

Such methods of reasoning is akin to the strategies used by archaeologists, where based on fragments of evidence dug up from the ground, together with other known facts and history, enables them to piece together convincing accounts about life and civilization. This abductive inferencing method is also used in information analysis and medical diagnosis, e.g. given signs and symptoms of a disease, doctors are expected to infer the type of illness and therefore treat it.

4   Interactive Visual Sense-Making Design

In the course of our work in developing visual representations with which to represent datasets, to carry out and to report on analysis carried out on them, and to reason with the data, we have identified a list of 20 user problems that require new or better techniques for their visual representation.

These areas, though described as problems, represent areas where Information Analysts can benefit from more advanced science and technology [19]. The problems have been gathered and condensed from across several studies, and a series of interviews and focus group discussions with researchers and students interacting with library electronic resource systems, legal investigators, and information analysts.

1. The problem of seeing a large data set and reasoning space through a small keyhole.
2. The problem of handling missing data.
3. The problem of handling deceptive / misleading data.
4. The problem of handling contradictory data.
5. The problem of aggregating and reconciling multiple points of view or predictions.

6. The problem of evidence collation and evidential reasoning.
7. The problem of provenance and tracing analytic reasoning.
8. The problem of integrating data space, analytic space and hypothesis spaces.
9. The problem of handling strength of evidence (including subjective and objective measures of strength) + contribution of different pieces of evidence to a conclusion.
10. The problem of handling uncertainty in data and / or information.
11. The problem of representing and handling evidence over time and space.
12. The problem of annotating, remembering, re-visiting, and setting aside.
13. The problem of developing a sense of what is in the data exploring what is there.
14. The problem of predicting and representing emergent behaviour.
15. The problem of Identifying and representing trends.
16. The problem of recognising and representing anomalous changes.
17. The problem of finding the needle in the haystack (or knowing what is chaff i.e. info of no or low value)
18. The problem of predicting the path of cascading failures or effects.
19. The problem or representing the static and dynamic relationship between the data / information.
20. The problem of scalability and reusability.

In the following sections, we hope to explain some of these problems in the context of medical domain.

4.1   Aggregating and Reconciling Multiple Views or Predictions

This problem occurs particularly when analysts have to work together, and where their efforts need to be coordinated, while valuing independent inputs from the respective analysts. Some points of view may be very divergent. What is crucial in representing these differences in opinions or predictions, is not the differences in themselves, but rather the trace of the analytic reasoning process, i.e. how did one get to this conclusion? It should show or reveal how the different analysts have used the data and how the way they used the data contributed to the conclusions. In this way, it then becomes possible for a reviewer to seek out area of potential errors or errors of judgement with the given data.

4.2   Handling Evidence Strength and Contribution to a Conclusion

Unlike intelligence analysis, doctors have access to statistical indicators showing adverse reactions to particular medications or the susceptibility of, say, different types of people to certain diseases. In Evidence Based Medicine, such information is sought to provide a base-line from which to evaluate the likelihood of observed signs and symptoms relating to particular diseases. What is needed in intelligence analysis are schemata (ways in which data may be structured and represented for further analysis) which help make obvious the reliability, quality or likelihood of occurrence in a given context, and their ability to show how their usage can lead them to various logic traps and other flaws such as false positives.

4.3   Annotating, Remembering, Re-visiting and Setting Aside

We are often not able to remember the myriad of small decisions we made along the process of a complicated analysis. There are also times where we use storytelling techniques to fill in missing data in the collection. Analysts as well as doctors (who see many patients often in short period of time), need to annotate for their own remembering purposes, as well as for a trace for other doctors or medical personnel to follow-up on the treatment. Sometimes the data is non-conclusive, or sometimes, data may have some use later, but the analyst or doctor may not want to re-create the search for that piece or collection of data and would like to set it aside, possibly with an annotation, for later use.

Complexity is the main problem in the medical domain, because most of the medical data is weakly structured or even unstructured and there is always the danger of modelling artefacts, which can then lead to wrong decisions. Let us look at standard medical documents for example: The broad application of enterprise hospital information systems amasses large amounts of medical documents, which must be reviewed, observed and analysed by human experts [3] (Kreuzthaler et al., 2011). All essential documents of the patient records contain at least a certain portion of data which has been entered in non-standardized format (wrongly called 'free-text') and has long been in the focus of research. Although such text can be created simply by the end-users, the support of automatic analysis is extremely difficult [2,5,13].

So, it is very likely that some interesting and relevant relationships remain completely undiscovered, due to the fact that the relevant data are scattered and no investigator is able to link them together manually [16,4]. Consequently, there are a lot of relevant open research issues at the intersection of HCI and IR/KDD to help (medical) professionals to identify and extract useful information from data.

4.4   Developing a Sense of What Is in the Data

One problem at the start of any investigation or review occurs when the analyst or doctor is presented with a large set of data, and he or she has to make sense of it. How does one know where to start if one does not know what is in the data set? Or at least, what are the main categories or methods of organization of the data? Tools are needed to summarise the data set in various ways that lend themselves to rapid exploration. Various forms of semantic maps of information clusters have been used to show groups, group densities, group peaks, and relationships between and within groups (e.g. IN-SPIRE, http://in-spire.pnnl.gov/), with software tools that facilitate drill-downs as well as other methods of analysis.

A good example of a data intensive and highly complex microscopic structure is a yeast protein network. Yeasts are eukaryotic micro-organisms (fungi) with 1,500 currently known species, estimated to be only 1% of all yeast species. Yeasts are unicellular, typically measuring 4 μm in diameter. The first protein interaction network was published by [6]. The problem with such structures is that they are very big and that there are so many. A great challenge is to find unknown structures (structural homologies, see e.g. [7]) amongst the enormous set of uncharacterised data. Let us illustrate this process with a typical example from the life sciences: X-ray crystallography is a standard method to analyse the arrangement of objects (atoms, molecules) within a crystal structure. This data contains the mean positions of the entities within the substance, their chemical relationship, and various others and the data is stored in a Protein Data Base (PDB, `http://www.rcsb.org/pdb/`). This database contains vast amounts of data. If a medical professional looks at the data, he or she sees only lengthy tables of numbers.

However, by application of a special visualization method, such structures can be made graphically visible and the medical professionals can understand these data more easily and most of all they can gain knowledge—for instance, it may lead to the discovery of new, unknown structures in order to modify drugs, and consequently to contribute to enhancing human health. The transformation of such information into knowledge is vital for the prevention and treatment of diseases [17,18].

To demonstrate that not only natural processes have such structures there is a nice example (`http://datamining.typepad.com/data_mining/2007/01/the_blogosphere.html`) which shows a visualization of the blogosphere (cf. also with [12]): The larger, denser part of the blogosphere is characterized by socio-political discussion the periphery contains some topical groupings. By showing only the links in the graph, we can get a far better look at the structure than if we include all the nodes.

4.5   The Problem of Identifying and Representing Trends

The final problem is that of identifying and representing patterns in data as well as key trends over time, and whether there are correlating effects of those trends. While it is possible to show trends and patterns in quantitative data relatively easily, how do we reveal patterns in visual forms about qualitative data that the human perceptual system can readily discern?

Maimon & Rokach state in their book [14]: "Knowledge Discovery demonstrates intelligent computing at its best, and is the most desirable and interesting end-product of Information Technology". Whereas this is true, using intelligent computing is necessary but not sufficient: Computers are (still) Von-Neumann machines and not endowed with any insight, and possess little knowledge of the real-world on which to check whether and to what extent the concepts they are examining are worthwhile or useful. Consequently, the challenge is to enable effective human control over powerful intelligent machine services and to integrate statistical methods and information visualization, so as to support human insight, breakthrough discoveries, and bold decisions primary research objectives in the field of Human-Computer Interaction.

A further challenge is based on the fact that only a small percentage of data is structured most of the data is semi-structured, weakly structured or even unstructured. A common misconception is to confuse structure with standardization. While the closely related fields of IR/KDD have developed wonderful intelligent (semi)automatic processes and algorithms to extract useful knowledge

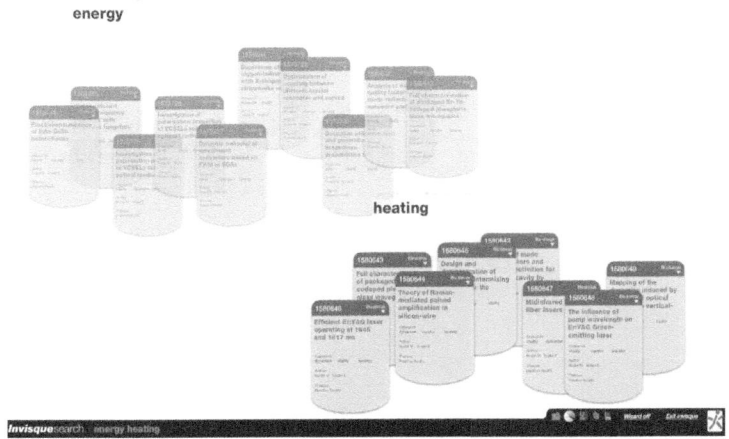

Fig. 4. INVISQUE showing library database search results

from rapidly growing amounts of data, these methods fail when data are weakly structured. The problem is that we are faced with the danger of modelling artifices without being aware of it and this may lead to wrong decisions. One solution is to raise the quality of information, while at the same time make the medical professionals aware of the value of information quality; a possible solution is in a systematic documentation. That means that all treatment relevant data are collected in a quality process oriented manner. Most of all it must be possible to condense the data into information as a function of time to visualize it as longitudinal data; the visible patterns and trends can be used to make decisions and to meet predefined treatment goals e.g. in order to provide individualized treatment.

5   INVISQUE

INVISQUE [20] is an interactive visualization system designed to visual sensemaking. It aims to address the challenges discussed earlier. Presented here are some preliminary results and future features. It is domain independent and can be transferred easily to biomedical domain.

INVISQUE is designed around a metaphor of physical index cards on a two-dimensional infinite canvas workspace. This is a departure from the traditional 1-dimensional list-style interfaces (such as Google), and the cards present basic information about each result. Rather than relying on static text boxes for input, INVIQSUE allows the user to start a new search anywhere on the canvas. This is done simply by clicking on the white space and typing in the search term. Each set of search results are grouped into a cluster. Fig 4 shows an example of INVISQUE working with a library database and displaying the result of two searches: "energy" and "heating".

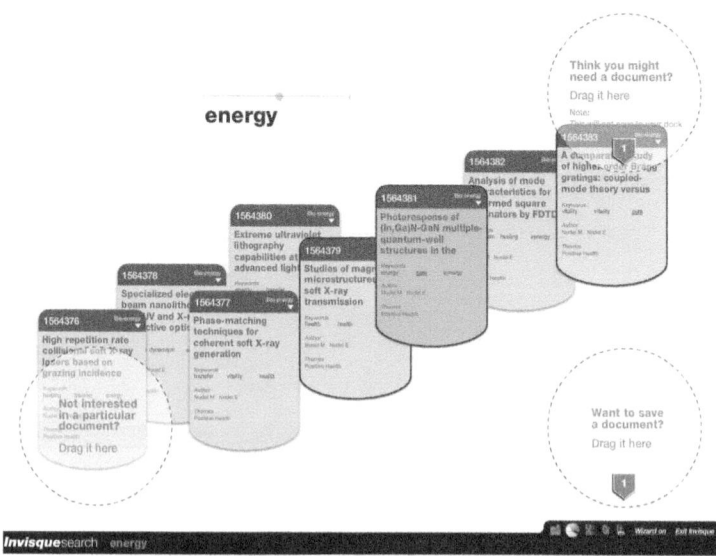

Fig. 5. Marking index cards

By default, the index cards are ordered in both the x and y axes. The ordering attributes are domain dependent and can be set by the user. In the example of searching for journal articles, the y axis can represent the number of citations and the x axis can represent the date of publication. This provides the capability to interactively identify the trend within the data on the selected dimensions. By clicking on an index card, users are able drill down to find more information. In the case of a document search, users can view the content of the document.

The infinite canvas allows users to visualize multiple searches (or clusters) simultaneously (see Fig. 4). This is a step away from traditional tabbed-browsing, and allows users to make visual comparisons between multiple search results. This capability will be further developed to facilitate visually aggregating and reconciling multiple points of view or predictions. Although we are only in a 2D space, the use of transparency creates a series of layers (see Fig. 4). The active search (i.e., 'heating') is opaque, giving it the impression of the closest layer and, therefore, the main focus. Remaining clusters are semi-transparent, giving the impression they are in the background, providing context to the active search.

INVISQUE has a few features to support 'annotating, remembering, re-visiting, and setting aside'. Users can save an index card for later use or mark one as important. These are achieved by dragging the index card to the specific circles in the corners (dashed circles in Fig. 5). Its colour will then change to indicate it is saved (yellow) or marked (green). Users can easily invoke Boolean operations by dragging and dropping. For example, two clusters can be merged by dragging one cluster title on top of the other.

Currently text analysis functions are being integrated into INVISQUES. Once completed, INVISQUE will be able to extract significant phrases (i.e., popular topics) from a collection of documents. This will address the problem of 'developing a sense of what is in the data' by visually presenting the significant topics and their relationships. Another new feature being added to INVISQUE is provenance, which is the conclusion pathway that records the information about the reasoning process from the raw data to final conclusion. Part of the provenance is the information of the strength of evidences and how they contribute to a conclusion, which is another problem discussed earlier.

6   Conclusions

In this paper we demonstrated the similarity between the information analysis during intelligence analysis and medical diagnosis. Based on the Sense-Making Loop and Data-Frame model, we discussed the key issues that need to be addressed when designing an interactive visualization system to support such information analysis. A visual analytics system INVISQUE is used to demonstrate the application of some of these design principles.

References

1. Fisher, R., Johnston, R.: Is intelligence analysis a discipline? In: Analyzing Intelligence, pp. 55–68. Georgetown University Press (2008)
2. Gregory, J., Mattison, J.E., Linde, C.: Naming notes: transitions from free text to structured entry. Methods Inf. Med. 34(1-2), 57–67 (1995)
3. Holzinger, A., Geierhofer, R., Errath, M.: Semantic Information in Medical Information Systems - from Data and Information to Knowledge: Facing Information Overload, pp. 323–330 (2007)
4. Holzinger, A., Geierhofer, R., Mödritscher, F.: Semantic information in medical information systems: Utilization of text mining techniques to analyze medical diagnoses. Journal of Universal Computer Science 14(22), 3781–3795 (2008)
5. Holzinger, A., Kainz, A., Gell, G., Brunold, M., Maurer, H.: Interactive Computer Assisted Formulation of Retrieval Requests for a Medical Information System using an Intelligent Tutoring System, pp. 431–436. AACE, Charlottesville (2000)
6. Jeong, H., Mason, S.P., Barabási, A.L., Oltvai, Z.N.: Lethality and centrality in protein networks. Nature 411(6833), 41–42 (2001)
7. Jornvall, H., Carlstrom, A., Pettersson, T., Jacobsson, B., Persson, M., Mutt, V.: Structural homologies between prealbumin, gastrointestinal prohormones and other proteins. Nature 291(5802), 261–263 (1981),
   http://dx.doi.org/10.1038/291261a0
8. Josephson, J.R., Tanner, M.C.: Conceptual analysis of abduction. In: Abductive Inference: Computation, Philosophy, Technology. Cambridge University Press (1996)
9. Klein, G., Moon, B., Hoffman, R.: Making sense of sensemaking 2: A macrocognitive model. IEEE Intelligent Systems 21(5), 88–92 (2006)
10. Klein, G., Mueller, S., Rasmussen, L., Hoffman, R.: Naturalistic model of causal reasoning: Developing an experiential user guide (eug) to understand fusion algorithms and simulation models. Tech. Rep. AFRL-RH-WP-TR-2011-0018, Air Force Research Laboratory 711th Human Performance Wing, Human Performance Directorate, Wright-Patterson Air Force Base, OH 45433 (2010)

11. Klein, G., Phillips, J.K., Rall, E.L., Peluso, D.A.: A Data/Frame Theory of Sense Making. In: Expertise out of context: Proceedings of the Sixth International Conference on Naturalistic Decision Making, pp. 113–155 (2003)
12. Leskovec, J., McGlohon, M., Faloutsos, C., Glance, N.S., Hurst, M.: Patterns of Cascading Behavior in Large Blog Graphs. In: Proceedings of the Seventh SIAM International Conference on Data Mining (2007)
13. Lovis, C., Baud, R.H., Planche, P.: Power of expression in the electronic patient record: structured data or narrative text? International Journal of Medical Informatics 58-59, 101–110 (2000)
14. Maimon, O., Rokach, L.: Data Mining and Knowledge Discovery Handbook, 2nd edn. Springer, Heidelberg (2010)
15. Pirolli, P., Card, S.: The sensemaking process and leverage points for analyst technology as identified through cognitive task analysis. In: Proceedings of International Conference on Intelligence Analysis (2005)
16. Smalheiser, N.R., Swanson, D.R.: Using arrowsmith: a computer-assisted approach to formulating and assessing scientific hypotheses. Comput Methods Programs Biomed. 57(3), 149–153 (1998)
17. Wiltgen, M., Holzinger, A.: Visualization in bioinformatics: Protein structures with physicochemical and biological annotations. In: Zara, J., Sloup, J. (eds.) Proceedings of Central European Multimedia and Virtual Reality Conference, pp. 69–74 (2005)
18. Wiltgen, M., Holzinger, A., Tilz, G.P.: Interactive Analysis and Visualization of Macromolecular Interfaces Between Proteins. In: Holzinger, A. (ed.) USAB 2007. LNCS, vol. 4799, pp. 199–212. Springer, Heidelberg (2007)
19. Wong, B.W., Varga, M.: Blackholes, keyholes and brownworms: Challenges in sense-making. In: 11th NATO Networks of Expert Workshop, Visual Analytics and Network Operations and Health (2011)
20. Wong, W., Chen, R., Kodagoda, N., Rooney, C., Xu, K.: INVISQUE: intuitive information exploration through interactive visualization. In: Proceedings of the 2011 Annual Conference Extended Abstracts on Human Factors in Computing Systems, CHIEA 2011, pp. 311–316. ACM, Vancouver (2011)

Clinical Data Privacy and Customization via Biometrics Based on ECG Signals

Hugo Silva[1], André Lourenço[1,2], Ana Fred[1], and Joaquim Filipe[3]

[1] Instituto de Telecomunicações
Instituto Superior Técnico
Lisboa, Portugal
{hugo.silva,arlourenco,afred}@lx.it.pt
[2] Instituto Superior de Engenharia de Lisboa
Lisboa, Portugal
[3] Instituto Politécnico de Setúbal
Setúbal, Portugal
j.filipe@est.ips.pt

Abstract. User identity validation is particularly relevant for applications where data privacy is critical, such as Healthcare Information Systems (HIS), where patient records protection and medical acts traceability is extremely important. Current approaches to the problem include biometric solutions, however, traditional modalities only allow momentary verification; readers are generally fixed to a static location, and direct contact or proximity is required. State-of-the-art work has been focusing solutions for continuous, or more frequent assessment in an unobtrusive way. In this paper we present a framework for continuous identity verification, based on knowledge discovery from ECG signals for security enhancement in the HIS context. ECG signals are particularly convenient, as they are frequently already measured in patients, and can also be easily obtained from caregivers interacting with the information system. Experimental results were performed in a population of 32 healthy individuals, and the system attained a $2.75\% \pm 0.29$ EER for the task of identity verification.

Keywords: Healthcare Information Systems, User Authentication, ECG Biometrics, Data Privacy, Human-Computer Interaction.

1 Introduction

Digital information systems have greatly evolved from elementary computational blocks targeted at electronic data processing, to large scale and fully-integrated systems for knowledge management across organizations [20]. This change has had a deep impact in multiple activity sectors, and a special emphasis has been given to the healthcare field. With the advent of Healthcare Information Systems (HIS), caregivers and patients were able to store, access and share clinical information electronically, in an easier and more efficient manner [1].

A. Holzinger and K.-M. Simonic (Eds.): USAB 2011, LNCS 7058, pp. 121–132, 2011.

Due both to the specificity and sensitivity of clinical data managed by current Healthcare Information Systems (HIS), security has always been a major and growing concern [33]. In the context of HIS, two main aspects are particularly important in terms of security, namely: *a) Data Privacy:* ensuring the proper and controlled disclosure of clinical data to authorized individuals; and *b) Identity Verification:* ensuring that a given subject interacting with the system is genuine. A common denominator to both aspects is the authenticity of subjects performing, or intending to perform, some kind of interaction with the HIS.

User authentication is extremely important not only for controlling the access to the clinical data, but also to improve the traceability and quality of care in medical acts, by correctly linking the caregivers to their identity [13,34]. Moreover, in a Human-Computer Interaction (HCI) perspective, enabling the access to the identity of caregivers in a more pervasive manner allows a higher degree of adaptability and customization of the HIS to the role and specific requirements of each subject, leading to more efficient and dedicated processes and services.

Current authentication approaches, as in most systems, are still based on tokens either memorized, or carried by the subject (e.g. passwords, PINs, keys, ID cards), in which transmissibility represents a major security issue. More recently, biometric techniques, such as facial or fingerprint recognition started to be adopted [16]; however, these bind the subject to a specific physical space, and require direct contact or proximity between the subject and the sensing device. Existing biometric recognition techniques may therefore be limiting for continuous and mobile applications [14].

In this paper we present a biometrics framework based on Electrocardiographic (ECG) signals, with the potential to extend current data privacy protection and identity verification systems in the context of HIS. Our approach is especially useful for mobile and continuous biometrics applications [32], as it takes advantage of a signal source that is continuously available, and either already measured on the subject (as the ECG is a commonly measured parameter in patients [26,8]), or easily accessible with minimal intrusiveness for the subject, due to recent advances in biosignal acquisition hardware [11,7].

The remainder of the paper is organized as follows. In Section 2 an overview of state-of-the art and commercial solutions currently in use is presented, together with future trends. In Section 3 we provide an introduction to ECG signals and their application as a biometric trait. In Section 4 a description of the proposed approach is provided. Finally, we outline the main results and conclusions, in Sections 5 and 6, respectively.

2   Subject Authentication Landscape

2.1   Non-biometric Systems

Nowadays, the most common approaches for subject authentication are still mostly based on things that the user memorizes, or objects that the user has, which constitutes potential security threats. To date, the most common technique of personal authentication still consists in the use of an identity card.

Identity cards can have a photo of the owner, name and identity number. They can also have a smart chip, providing space for information storage, and an additional bar code for registration. This kind of identification may be prone to identity theft. Moreover it may represent a security flaw in the access to medical records, since after positive identification all the information becomes available.

Bar codes and radio frequency identification (RFID) solutions are becoming the standard techniques in healthcare applications. Hospitals are using bar coding and RFID to protect the accuracy of critical patient-care processes, including the dispensing and administration of medications and blood products [4], the collection and tracking of specimen tests and x-rays, and the verification of surgical specifications. In [17] RFID technology is used to facilitate automatic streamlining of patient identification processes in health centers, and assist medical practitioners in the quick and accurate diagnosis and treatments.

Patient identification with hospital wristbands is one of the standard techniques for helping hospitals to improve patient identification, providing an automatic, and convenient way to collect and access patient information, attempting to eliminate manual data entry, and the associated opportunity for error. Nevertheless, the scanning of wristband barcodes can lead to misidentification [31], due to operation errors. These types of authentication mechanisms allow the transmissibility of the identification token, resulting in identity fraud or impersonation, in order to access resources or obtain credit and other benefits in another person's name.

2.2 Biometric Systems

Biometric authentication is based on physical or behavioral features, which uniquely characterize humans. Commonly used modalities can be categorized into two main classes: Physiological and Behavioral. Examples of the first include, but are not limited to: fingerprint, palm print, hand geometry, DNA, and iris recognition. The later class is related to the behavior of a person, and examples include voice, gait, keystroke dynamics, and ECG.

Biometric systems are being deployed in several civilian applications, including the context of HIS. With the adoption of electronic medical records in the health care sector, it is becoming more and more common for a health professional to edit and view a patients record digitally [18]. In the United States, governmental regulations require a secure authentication system to access patient records, in order to protect the patients privacy.

The current landscape of biometric systems in the healthcare industry is mainly based on physiological characteristics, and multi-biometrics systems. In [18], a biometric system composed of an on-line signature and voice modalities was tested and seemed convenient for the users, because a tablet PC was equipped with the associated sensing hardware. In [21], a system is proposed based on fingerprint, iris, retina scan, and DNA, to uniquely associate patient biometric characteristics to their medical data. In [5] fingerprint verification is used to ensure that access to the hospital Picture Archiving and Communication System (PACS) is only guaranteed to certified parties.

2.3   Current Biometric Trends

For low security applications, one-time verification systems, which perform authentication before the access to a protected resource, are adequate. However, this type of methods can lead to session "hijacking", in which a different user takes possession of a session in the post-authentication period. Together with the transmissibility and appropriation problems already described, these issues have led the biometrics research community towards developing methods capable of improving current approaches.

A recent trend in the field is continuous biometrics [32,30]; in this approach, the identity of a subject is verified in a periodic way, allowing the system to verify the authenticity of the subject more frequently. A fingerprint verifier, integrated in a mouse and combined with a face verifier is presented in [35], which allows the continuous validation of the presence or participation of a logged-in user.

Another system based on bi-modal Continuous Biometrics Authentication System (CBAS) is devised in [19], combining also fingerprint and facial biometrics to authenticate users, showing that continuous biometric systems are viable in practical scenarios. In [25,24] a new method is proposed for continuous user authentication based on a Webcam, that monitors the face and color of clothing of a logged-in user.

So far, state-of-the-art work in this topic has mostly focused on the combination of more tradicional modalities, such as fingerprint and image recognition. Recent research work has also started to look into the biometric potential of modalities based in biosignals. In a continuous approach, these modalities are quite appealing, as they are accessible and readily available without interfering or limiting the regular tasks performed by the subject. Furthermore, in clinical settings several biosignals are already assessed as part of the patient follow-up process.

3   Identity Verification Using ECG Signals

3.1   Cardiac Activity as a Biometric Modality

The heart possesses a natural pacemaker known as the *sinoatrial node* (SA), which generates periodic electrical impulses, that trigger the depolarization of the heart muscle fibres. The reaction to those impulses is a repolarization and return to the rest state [6]. What the ECG records is then the propagation of these action potentials throughout the different cardiac muscle fibers. Figure 1 depicts a prototypical waveform, labeled with the corresponding complexes. The informative content of ECG recordings is already widely used for clinical applications, traditionally in the assessment and diagnosis of the cardiac function.

Morphologically, the collected signals are directly dependent on multiple physiological properties of the subject, such as tissue conductivity, genetic singularities, a heart condition, constitution of the cardiac muscle and cavity, among others. The fact that there are subject dependent variations enhances its applicability for identity verification. Recent research work has been devoted to the

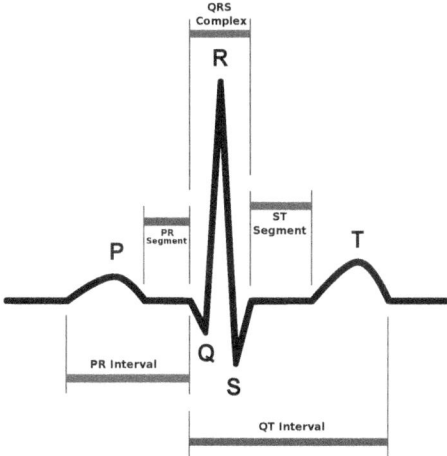

Fig. 1. Prototypical ECG waveform labeled with the corresponding complexes. The P wave corresponds to the SA node triggering impulse, the QRS complex is associated with the depolarization process, and finally the T wave reflects the repolarization process.

characterization of ECG features for human identification, and although further evaluation is necessary, experimental results have highlighted the discriminating capacity of such features [15,28]. Figure 2 illustrates the ECG signal acquired on two different subjects from the PTB-BIH [12] control subjects database. The signals were plotted using the same scale and, as it is easily observed, both waveforms are morphologically quite distinct.

The ECG is quite appealing for biometric applications in terms of desirable properties [16], since nowadays, these signals: a) are continuously available; b) can be easily acquired; c) can only be collected in live subjects; d) are highly correlated with the physical state and condition of the subject; and e) due to their specificity, are not easily spoofed or masqueraded. For identity verification in a clinical setting, an ECG biometric system is particularly advantageous.

3.2   Data Acquisition

The ECG, is a representation of the electrical activity of the heart measured over time, and captured externally through electrodes directly applied on the body surface or on its vicinity. These electrical changes can be detected using different principles; the most common measurement principle is based on the voltage potential between electrodes placed on different parts of the body. Other measurement principles include capacitive [23] and mechanical methods [27].

Conventional clinical grade ECGs are acquired using 12 or more leads mounted on the chest and limbs, using conductive paste or gel to improve the conductivity with the skin. Although this setup has proven to perform accurately for identification purposes [2], one lead has been shown to suffice [29,28]. As pre-gelled

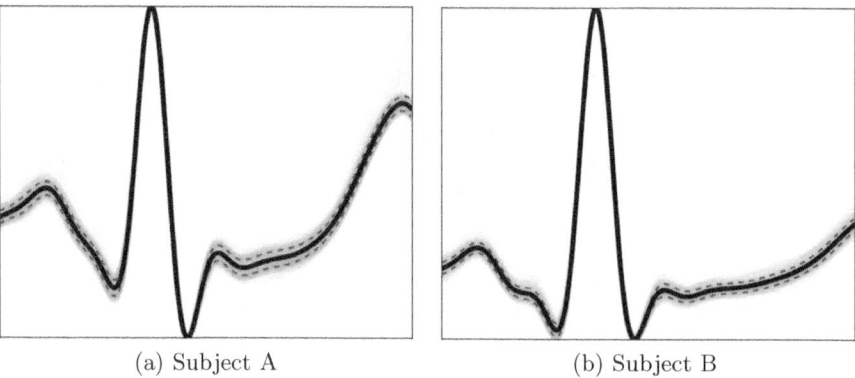

(a) Subject A   (b) Subject B

Fig. 2. ECG readings from two different subjects from the PTB-BIH control subjects database. Both figures have the same vertical scale. The black and gray lines correspond respectively to the mean wave and standard deviation computed from the database.

electrodes mounted at the chest may be limiting in some real world scenarios, state-of-the-art work has been focusing on determining the biometric potential at alternative acquisition points with promising results, namely at the finger level [22,3].

4 Proposed Approach

4.1 System Architecture and Overview

We propose a biometric identity verification framework based on knowledge discovery from ECG signals, which takes as input a raw sensor data from an ECG sensor, and outputs a control signal to a target system validating the subjects identity as a genuine or, as an impostor. Such system is targeted at clinical settings, as a way of guaranteeing data privacy protection through identity verification.

Figure 3 depicts the architecture of the proposed system, which comprises two phases: enrollment and authentication. As depicted in Figure 3(a), in the enrollment phase, the raw signal is acquired, processed using appropriate algorithms, and if the quality of the signal is acceptable, a set of representative templates is stored in a database for future reference. For user authentication, as presented in Figure 3(b), the acquired ECG signal is processed and checked against the templates stored in the database, a decision threshold is then used to accept or reject the user, and the result is sent to the target system as a control signal.

4.2 Sensors for Data Acquisition

In previous work we have shown the validity of a single chest mounted lead from a standard 12-lead electrode placement, for biometric purposes [29]. For

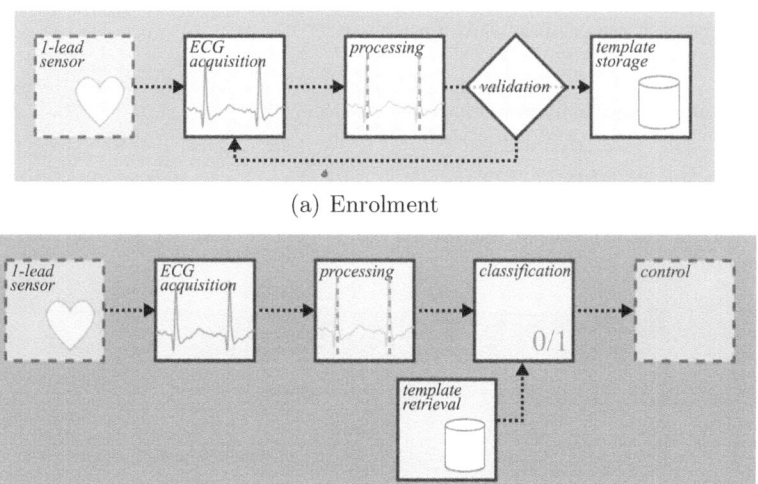

(a) Enrolment

(b) Authentication

Fig. 3. Architecture of the proposed system: user enrolment phase and user authentication phase

the caregivers, we herein propose a setup that integrates an accessory, depicted in Figure 4, that is fitted to a regular computer keyboard or to a tablet PC, over which the user rests his/her hand palms. This apparatus is able to continuously measure the pseudo-V_1 ECG at the hand palms, through a pair of dry Ag/AgCl electrodes. In the scope of our proposed approach for security enhancement in HIS, we will focus on authentication of caregivers through this apparatus.

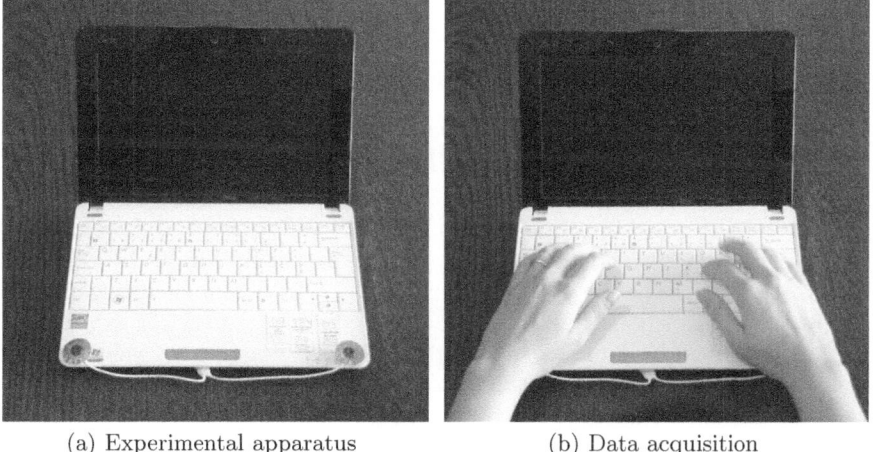

(a) Experimental apparatus   (b) Data acquisition

Fig. 4. Experimental setup for data acquisition

4.3   Signal Processing and Decision Making

After the biosignal data acquisition unit acquires the raw sensor data, they are fed into our system through a secure channel. The raw data, is then band-pass filtered to the 1-30Hz bandwidth, and passed through a R-spike detection block based on the commonly used Englese and Zeelenberg algorithm [9]. Heartbeat waveforms are then segmented, and the mean waves computed in order to obtain a representative wave template pattern of the subjects ECG.

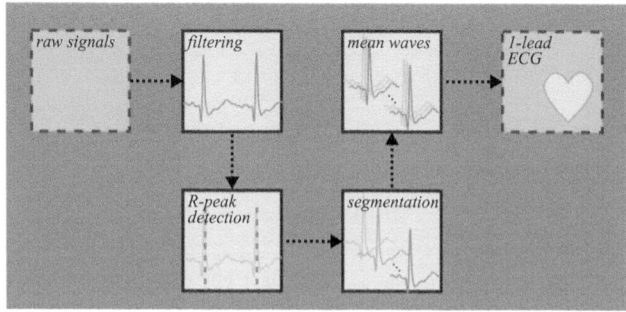

Fig. 5. Signal processing steps block diagram

The classification is performed computing the dissimilarity between wave templates computed in the authentication phase, $a[t]$, with the ones computed on the enrolment phase and stored in a secured database, $e[n]$. The decision on a genuine/impostor is determined verifying if the computed distance, $d(e, a)$ is bellow a given threshold, and the result is sent to the target system as a control signal. This dissimilarity is computed using the Euclidean distance:

$$d(e,a) = \sqrt{\sum_i (e[i] - a[i])^2}. \tag{1}$$

5   Experimental Setup and Results

Tests were performed on 32 healthy individuals (25 males and 7 females); the average age was 31.1±9.46 years. Subjects were asked to rest their left/right hands over the Ag/AgCl electrodes, and data was acquired during a period of approximately 1m30s, during which the experiment supervisor explained the purpose of the study. An ECG sensor with gain 1000 and passing band of 1-30Hz was used for raw data acquisition. To guarantee electrical isolation from other sources, a wireless Bluetooth bioPLUX research acquisition system was used to transmit the data to a base station.

For experimental evaluation purposes, raw signals were processed according to the proposed approach, and two exclusive datasets were created; a training

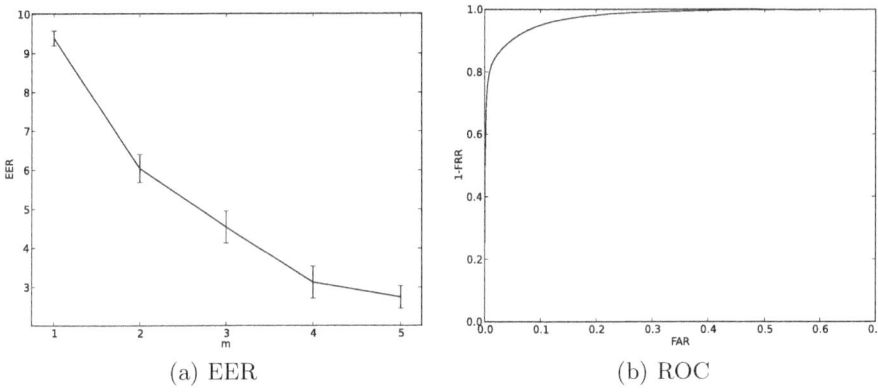

(a) EER   (b) ROC

Fig. 6. Identity verification performance: (a) Equal Error Rate (EER); (b) ROC curve for the $m = 5$ best case scenario. m denotes the number of patterns used to compute the mean wave.

set with 30% of the total collected patterns as the templates database, and a test set with the remaining 70% of the patterns. We evaluated the identity verification potential of ECG signals collected at the hand palms using individual heartbeat waveforms directly, and also mean waves. The template matching technique is extremely lightweight in terms of real-time processing, and the mean waves reduce the pattern variability, establishing the framework for a real-time, continuous biometric system based on ECG signals.

Figure 6(a) shows the Equal Error Rate (EER) for authentication varying the number of patterns m, used on the computation of the mean wave. As summarized in Table 1, if individual heartbeat waveforms are used, a mean EER of $9.39\% \pm 0.19$ is attained, which decreases to $2.75\% \pm 0.29$ when averages of 5 heartbeat waveforms are considered as representative pattern. These correspond respectively to $1s$ and $5s$ of acquired signals approximately. The Receiver Operating Characteristics (ROC) curve for the $m = 5$ best case scenario, is presented in Figure 6(b).

Table 2, outlines the user authentication results typically found in literature for other biosignal based modalities (see [10] and references therein). As we can observe, our results holds comparable performance levels when matched to other modalities; even when compared to previous ECG based approaches. Although the tradicional lead V_2 ECG approaches report higher accuracy levels, our results

Table 1. Equal Error Rate for the proposed approach

m	1	2	3	4	5
EER	$9.39\% \pm 0.19$	$6.05\% \pm 0.36$	$4.55\% \pm 0.41$	$3.13\% \pm 0.41$	$2.75\% \pm 0.29$

Table 2. Equal Error Rate for other biosignal based approaches

Method	Key Stroke	Mouse Pointer	Voice	Gait Analysis	Eye Gaze	EEG	ECG V_2	ECG Fingers
EER	$\sim 4\%$	$\sim 10\%$	$\sim 10\%$	$\sim 5\%$	$\sim 5\%$	$\sim 10\%$	$\sim 5\%$	$\sim 12\%$

improve on the previously reported finger ECG performance levels [22]. Furthermore, our experimental setup enables signal acquisition in a highly convenient way, which does not impact with the users normal activities, potentiating its use in a continuous biometrics framework.

6   Conclusions

In Healthcare Information Systems (HIS), reliable authentication of both patients and caregivers is currently a problem which introduces inefficiencies and reduces the quality of care due to errors resulting from mis-identification. Government agencies and institutions worldwide, have started to recur to biometric modalities as a way of improving current practices; however tradicional biometric systems still present some limitations. Existing systems require the subjects either to be in direct or in close contact with the biometric readers (e.g. fingerprint scanner, webcam or other), which are placed in static positions. A recent trend in biometric research is searching for systems capable of providing continuous biometric methods, that allow periodic validation of the users identity; hence usability in terms of Human-Computer Interaction is a major concern.

In this sense, the research community is starting to turn to biosignals based systems, as these are continuously available and easily accessible. Recently, research has focused on biometric techniques based on ECG signals. In this paper we describe a method and apparatus for identity verification, using ECG signals. We build upon prior work from our group, which validated the biometric potential of ECG signals collected at the chest for identification, and evaluated the authentication performance the ECG signals collected at the hands level for increased usability. Experimental results have revealed that an EER of 2.75%±0.29 is achievable with merely 5s of acquired signal, validating the potential of the proposed approach to increase the security of HIS. Future work will focus on field validation in a real-world scenario, and implementation of a pilot system.

Acknowledgments. This work was partially funded by Fundação para a Ciência e Tecnologia (FCT) under grants PTDC/EIA-CCO/103230/2008, SFRH/BD/65248/2009 and SFRH /PROTEC/49512/2009, by the National Strategic Reference Framework (NSRF-QREN) under the contract no. 3475 "Affective Mouse", and by the Departamento de Engenharia de Electrónica e Telecomunicações e de Computadores from Instituto Superior de Engenharia de Lisboa, whose support the authors gratefully acknowledge.

References

1. Beaver, K.: Healthcare Information Systems (Best Practices), 2nd edn. Auerbach Publications (December 2002)
2. Biel, L., Petterson, O., Phillipson, L., Wide, P.: ECG analysis: A new approach in human identification. IEEE Trans. on Instrum. and Meas. 50(3), 808–812 (2001)
3. Chan, A.D.C., Hamdy, M.M., Badre, A., Badee, V.: Wavelet distance measure for person identification using electrocardiograms. IEEE Trans. on Instrum. and Meas. 57(2), 248–253 (2008)
4. Chan, J.C.W., Chu, R.W., Young, B.W.Y., Chan, F., Chow, C.C., Pang, W.C., Chan, C., Yeung, S.H., Chow, P.K., Lau, J., Leung, P.M.K.: Use of an electronic barcode system for patient identification during blood transfusion: 3-year experience in a regional hospital. Hong Kong Med. J. 10(3), 166–171 (2004)
5. Chen, Y.C.C., Chen, L.K.K., Tsai, M.D.D., Chiu, H.C.C., Chiu, J.S.S., Chong, C.F.F.: Fingerprint verification on medical image reporting system. Computer Methods and Programs in Biomedicine 89(3), 282–288 (2008)
6. Chung, E.K.: Pocketguide to ECG Diagnosis. Blackwell Publishing (2000)
7. Cunha, J., Cunha, B., Xavier, W., Ferreira, N., Pereira, A.: Vital-Jacket: A wearable wireless vital signs monitor for patients' mobility. In: Avantex Symp. (2007)
8. Drew, B.J., Califf, R.M., Funk, M., Kaufman, E.S., Krucoff, M.W., Laks, M.M., Macfarlane, P.W., Sommargren, C., Swiryn, S., Van Hare, G.F.: Practice standards for electrocardiographic monitoring in hospital settings. Circulation 110(17), 2721–2746 (2004)
9. Engelse, W.A.H., Zeelenberg, C.: A single scan algorithm for QRS-detection and feature extraction. Computers in Cardiology 6, 37–42 (1979)
10. Gamboa, H.: Multi-Modal Behavioural Biometrics Based on HCI and Electrophysiology. Ph.D. thesis, Instituto Superior Técnico (2008)
11. Gamboa, H., Silva, F., Silva, H.: Patient tracking system. In: Pervasive Computing Technologies for Healthcare (Pervasive Health), pp. 1–2 (March 2010)
12. Goldberger, A., Amaral, L., Glass, L., Hausdorff, J., Ivanov, P., Marck, R., Mietus, J., Moody, G., Peng, C., Stanley, H.: PhysioBank, physiotoolkit, and physionet: Components of a new research resource for complex physiologic signals (2000)
13. Hillestad, R., Bigelow, J.H., Chaudhry, B., Dreyer, P., Greenberg, M.D., Meili, R.C., Ridgely, M.S., Rothenberg, J., Taylor, R.: Identity Crisis: An Examination of the Costs and Benefits of a Unique Patient Identifier for the U.S. Health Care System. RAND Corporation (2008)
14. Holzinger, A., Geierhofer, R., Searle, G.: Biometrical signatures in practice: A challenge for improving human-computer interaction in clinical workflows. In: Heinecke, A.M., Paul, H. (eds.) Proc. Mensch und Computer, pp. 339–347 (2006)
15. Israel, S., Irvine, J., Cheng, A., Wiederhold, M., Wiederhold, B.: ECG to identify individuals. Pattern Recognition 38(1), 133–142 (2005)
16. Jain, A., Flynn, P., Ross, A.: Handbook of Biometrics. Springer, Heidelberg (2007)
17. Khosla, R., Chowdhury, B.: Real-Time RFID-Based Intelligent Healthcare Diagnosis System. In: Zhang, D. (ed.) ICMB 2008. LNCS, vol. 4901, pp. 184–191. Springer, Heidelberg (2007)
18. Krawczyk, S., Jain, A.K.: Securing Electronic Medical Records Using Biometric Authentication. In: Kanade, T., Jain, A., Ratha, N.K. (eds.) AVBPA 2005. LNCS, vol. 3546, pp. 1110–1119. Springer, Heidelberg (2005)
19. Kwang, G., Yap, R., Sim, T., Ramnath, R.: An usability study of continuous biometrics authentication. In: Tistarelli, M., Nixon, M.S. (eds.) ICB 2009. LNCS, vol. 5558, pp. 828–837. Springer, Heidelberg (2009)

20. Laudon, K., Laudon, J.: Management Information Systems, 11th edn. Prentice Hall (January 2009)
21. Leonard, D.C., Pons, A.P., Asfour, S.S.: Realization of a universal patient identifier for electronic medical records through biometric technology. IEEE Trans. on Information Technology in Biomedicine 13(4), 494–500 (2009)
22. Lourenço, A., Silva, H., Fred, A.: Unveiling the biometric potential of Finger-Based ECG signals. Computational Intelligence and Neuroscience (2011)
23. Martins, R., Primor, D., Paiva, T.: High-Performance groundless EEG/ECG capacitive electrodes. In: Proceedings of the IEEE International Symposium on Medical Measurements and Applications - MeMeA, vol. 1, pp. 503–506 (2011)
24. Niinuma, K., Park, U., Jain, A.K.: Soft biometric traits for continuous user authentication. IEEE Trans. on Inf. Forensics and Security 5(4), 771–780 (2010)
25. Niinuma, K., Jain, A.K.: Continuous user authentication using temporal information. In: Defense, Security, and Sensing, vol. 7667, p. 76670L+. The International Society for Optical Engineering (April 2010)
26. Olson, J.A., Fouts, A.M., Padanilam, B.J., Prystowsky, E.N.: Utility of mobile cardiac outpatient telemetry for the diagnosis of palpitations, presyncope, syncope, and the assessment of therapy efficacy. Journal of Cardiovascular Electrophysiology 18(5), 473–477 (2007)
27. Postolache, O.A., Girao, P.M.B.S., Mendes, J., Pinheiro, E.C., Postolache, G.: Physiological parameters measurement based on wheelchair embedded sensors and advanced signal processing. IEEE Trans. on Instrum. and Meas. 59(10) (2010)
28. Shen, T.W., Tompkins, W.J., Hu, Y.H.: One-lead ECG for identity verification. In: Proc. of the 2nd Joint Conf. of the IEEE Eng. in Medicine and Biology Soc. and the 24th Annual Fall Meeting of the Biomedical Eng. Soc., vol. 1, pp. 62–63 (2002)
29. Silva, H., Gamboa, H., Fred, A.: Applicability of lead v2 ECG measurements in biometrics. In: Med-e-Tel Proceedings (2007)
30. Sim, T., Zhang, S., Janakiraman, R., Kumar, S.: Continuous verification using multimodal biometrics. IEEE Trans. on Pattern Analysis and Machine Intelligence 29, 687–700 (2007)
31. Snyder, M.L., Carter, A., Jenkins, K., Fantz, C.R.: Patient misidentifications caused by errors in standard bar code technology. Clin. Chem. 56(10) (2010)
32. Traore, I., Ahmed, A.: Continuous Authentication Using Biometrics: Data, Models, and Metrics. IGI Global (2011)
33. Van de Velde, R., Degoulet, P.: Clinical Information Systems: A Component-Based Approach (Health Informatics). Springer, Heidelberg (December 2010)
34. WHO: Patient identification. In: Patient Safety Solutions, vol. 1. World Health Organization (May 2007)
35. Zhang, S., Janakiraman, R., Sim, T., Kumar, S.: Continuous verification using multimodal biometrics. In: Proceeding of the Int'l. Conf. on Biometrics (January 2006)

Usability Evaluation of Digital Dictation Procedure – An Interaction Analysis Approach

Johanna Viitanen and Marko Nieminen

Strategic Usability Research Group, Department of Computer Science and Engineering,
Aalto University School of Science, P.O. Box 19210, FIN-00076 Aalto, Finland
{Johanna.Viitanen,Marko.Nieminen}@aalto.fi

Abstract. This paper introduces a usability study of digital dictation procedure in which a task-originating modelling method, called interaction sequence illustration (ISI), was used for analysing interaction steps and stages. The analysis was conducted from the physician's viewpoint in a real-life clinical environment. Study results showed that the observed process of digital dictation is inefficient and unnecessarily lengthy. The analysis also revealed a number of interaction design failures and complex interaction sequences. In the study the ISI approach is suitable for providing concrete and detailed information about the steps and stages of interaction, the usability of user interfaces, and the success of interaction design.

Keywords: Usability, interaction sequence illustration analysis, digital dictation, evaluation.

1   Introduction

Empirical results regarding the use of current healthcare information technology (IT) systems have pointed out serious challenges to clinicians' abilities to effectively and satisfactory utilise these applications in their everyday work. Recent literature reviews have indicated numerous barriers concerning the uptake of healthcare IT interventions, and few of their results indicate any benefit from the systems [1,2]. Several researchers have reported numerous usability flaws [e.g. 3-6]. Specifically, time taken up by clinical documentation seems to be one of the most challenging bottlenecks of information system use and adaptation [7-10]. These findings raise the question of what makes the design of interactive systems for healthcare purposes especially challenging and vulnerable to shortcomings compared to other domains in which software applications are widely deployed. They also inquire as to what kind of enhancements to methodology approaches have been suggested by researchers in order to overcome these challenges.

This paper focuses on the research of usability and user interfaces of dictation solutions and related IT systems at the level of interaction analysis from the viewpoint of physicians in clinical contexts. Earlier studies have explored the use of documentation systems from other perspectives. For example, Poissant et al. [7] conducted a systematic literature review, whereas Holden [8] and Reuss et al. [9] applied a qualitative approach and interview methods to study physicians' beliefs and

A. Holzinger and K.-M. Simonic (Eds.): USAB 2011, LNCS 7058, pp. 133–149, 2011.
© Springer-Verlag Berlin Heidelberg 2011

experiences pertaining to electronic documentation. Braun et al. [10] investigated how physicians' information needs can be modelled on a general level. Holzinger et al. [11] explored the use of speech recognition in daily hospital practise from human-computer interaction (HCI) perspective. All these studies provide important findings about the documentation practices and needs of physicians' regarding future applications. However, little information can be found that pertains to judging the success of digital dictation from the viewpoint of physicians in a detailed and practical level. This kind of approach would be beneficial in order to increase the understanding of the current challenges and problems in electronic documentation as experienced by end-users.

2   Background: Usability Evaluation in Health Informatics Field

In HCI field methods for conducting user-centred evaluations fall into two categories: inspection-based evaluation using usability and accessibility guidelines and user-based testing [12].

The advantages of *inspection methods* relate to their abilities to take into account of a wide range of users and tasks and to emphasise obvious usability problems [12]. In contrast to user-based testing methods, these methods are often simpler and quicker to carry out and for these reasons also more cost effective. On the other hand, inspection methods have several weaknesses, which is why they should compliment user-based methods. Results from the inspections tend to be highly influenced by the knowledge and skills of the expert reviewers. Additionally, findings have indicated that the inspection methods might not scale well for complex or novel interfaces [12]. Therefore, they are suggested to be carried out in conjunction with application domain experts [12].

A *user-centred evaluation* is said to be useful at all stages in the project, from the early concept of the design to its long-term usage, which can then provide input for future versions of the system [12]. Variations of user testing involve field validations, i.e. testing design concepts and prototypes in real environments as well as techniques that are more interview- and observation-based [12]. One such technique is contextual inquiry, which is an often-used method for gathering data to support the design of products, systems, and services [13]. In contextual inquiry, a researcher typically conducts field interviews with four to eight users, one at a time, in the working environment and, while observing the user at work, asks about the user's actions in order to understand his or her motivation and strategy [13].

The significance of evaluation studies has grown during the past decade in the health informatics field as a consequence of IT adoption and use-related problems and contradictory findings. As an illustration of this, several papers have focused on methodology aspects and described how to evaluate the usability of healthcare IT systems. These include approaches and methodologies such as: cognitive and usability engineering methods (e.g. [14,15,16,17,18]), the introduction of formative versus summative evaluation methods [19] remote usability testing [20], cooperative usability testing [21], qualitative usability testing enhanced with data mining techniques [22], and evaluation of mobile in healthcare settings [20,23]. Alongside, several researchers have reported challenges in applying these evaluation methods.

According to Jaspers [16], each of the widely known usability evaluation methods (heuristic evaluation, cognitive walkthrough, and think-aloud or usability testing) has its own disadvantages and advantages. This is illustrated by Edwards et al. [4], who stated that several challenges with heuristic walkthrough resulted from the complex nature of the clinical work domain and the limitations of the predictive evaluation method. Therefore, special attention should be paid to reflecting on the realism and concreteness of healthcare contexts [24] and evaluating system usability in collaborative tasks [4]. These findings and experiences from empirical studies have caused researchers to suggest that field study methods are more suitable for informing conceptual problems and developing an understanding of the wider context in which clinical ICT systems are used [23,25].

3   Aim of the Study

This paper has two objectives. First, we investigate the process of conducting digital dictation from a physician's viewpoint. This includes comparing the interaction stages with other dictation techniques and processes: cassette dictation and speech recognition dictation. In addition, we apply task-oriented approach in evaluating the usability of digital dictation procedure and related user interfaces.

Second, this paper aims at contributing to the discussions of usability methods in healthcare. We report an experimental employment of the interaction sequence illustration (ISI) method using the digital dictation study as an example. The motivation for this objective derives from the following observations. Usability evaluation studies in the health informatics field seem to share several characteristics: they focus on a single healthcare information system, apply traditional evaluation methods (user testing, heuristic evaluation, or cognitive walkthrough), are conducted in one specified context, and involve one end-user group perspective. However, challenges in the field as well as worrying findings about the usability of currently used systems demonstrate the need for developing new approaches to evaluating usability and for supporting the redesign and user-centred development of healthcare IT systems.

4   Introduction of Interaction Sequence Illustration (ISI) Method

The widely known methods for conducting inspections in HCI field are *cognitive walkthrough* [26] and *heuristic evaluation* [27]. Variations of these methods include, among others, *low-level interaction walkthrough*, introduced by Ryu and Monk [28], and *interaction walkthrough* for the evaluation of safety-critical interactive systems, described by Thimbleby [29].

Typically, inspection methods emphasise the evaluation of one system or a piece of software in isolation from the system's real-use environment and focus on a selected set of user interfaces. In the HCI research field, these methods have often been criticised for not sufficiently addressing the interaction issues in a real-use context. Additionally, the widely known inspection methods are targeted for designer and evaluator use. Little attention has been paid to considering the advantages or limitations of these methods from the viewpoint of collaborative (usability researcher – software developer) development activities. How well the results and findings from the usability studies can be communicated to developers? Do the study results illustrate the findings in a way that (a) increases the shared understanding of the reasons behind the problems and (b) describes how failures in the interaction design of the user interface design should be improved.

This paper introduces and discusses and experimental task- and context-originating modelling approach, called *interaction sequence illustration (ISI),* for the analysis of interaction steps and stages in the healthcare context. The idea behind the method is to document and analyse activities– those between a user and computer-based systems– that take place during a predetermined sequence of tasks. The modelling of interaction stages and interaction steps is conducted from the user's viewpoint with an objective to (a) illustrate how the use of information systems appears from the end-user's perspective, (b) identify and report interaction steps and related insufficiencies in the user interface and interaction design, and (c) thereby support the user-centred design and development of healthcare applications. The ISI method focuses on user interface issues and low-level analysis of human-computer interaction. In this paper, we present two types of analysis: analysis of interaction stages and step-by-step illustration of a sequence of tasks.

The approach is different from traditional inspection methods in the following ways: 1) the modelling is conducted in a real-life environment, and 2) the analysis does not focus on one system but instead of those systems that are used to accomplish a set of tasks – in our case to perform digital dictations.

5   Case Study: Evaluation of Digital Dictation Procedure from a Physician's Viewpoint

5.1   Objectives of the Study

The digital dictation study [6] was carried out in the spring of 2008 in a large hospital in Finland. At that time, various dictation techniques, procedures, and equipment were used in the hospital. Three pilot units had already been using a digital dictation solution for several years. From the administration's viewpoint the digital dictation method was seen as the most promising solution for replacing the traditional cassette dictation method in the near future. The hospital also had experiences in using the speech recognition technology for dictation in radiology unit. This emerging technology seemed well suited to the radiology context.

The digital dictation study had three objectives [6]: (1) To describe the digital dictation processes from the physician's viewpoint; (2) To compare the currently used other dictation techniques; (3) To determine physicians' opinions concerning mobile dictation solutions. In our earlier paper [6], we described the process of conducting dictations and the context of use at a general level: we presented the identified needs, wants, and desires of physicians as well as constrains as user requirements for a dictation solution. We also used the described seven requirements as criteria for evaluating the currently used techniques, and describe the physicians' views of future dictation solutions [6]. In this paper, we present complementary analysis and findings: we compare the currently used dictation techniques in interaction stages level and report step-by-step analysis and illustration of digital dictation procedure.

5.2   Methods and Data Gathering

The study incorporated two usability research methods: contextual inquiry enhanced with interaction sequence illustration (ISI). The *contextual inquiry* followed the established principles of the method [13]. The contextual inquiry was seen as a suitable approach for exploring the currently used dictation techniques in their real context of use (clinical work in wards, clinics, and offices) because the flexible structure of the semi-structured interview would allow the researcher to generate questions during the interview based on what the interviewee had said or done. The aim of the inquiries was to gather data about the users' needs, documenting practices, and procedures as well as users' experiences in using various techniques.

Contextual inquiries were conducted with seven physicians who were accustomed to using a variety of dictating methods and tools in their daily working environments. The physicians were asked to perform a dictation sequence as they normally would and, while working, describe and give reasoning for their actions. In the inquiries, two of the physicians used cassette dictation, three used digital dictation, and two used speech recognition dictation technique. An audio recorder and a digital camera were used to record interviews for later analysis.

The *ISI analysis* focused on interaction steps and stages in digital dictation procedure. For the purposes of low-level interaction analysis, inquiry data was supplemented by documenting all interaction steps in the digital dictation procedure that occurred between a user and the dictating tools. This data was gathered after all seven inquiries were conducted with the physicians. Based on the inquiries, the researchers developed an understanding of the process and main phases of conducting dictations using digital dictation techniques. The collection of data was done in collaboration with a chief physician who daily dictated using digital techniques but who did not participate in the inquiries. While gathering the data, taking screen captures of all the interaction steps that occur in the dictation process, the chief physician was asked to slowly conduct a realistic case (with real patient data) from the very first stages until the end. Meanwhile, the researcher observed the process and captured screenshots after every interaction step.

5.3   Analysis of the Data

Research data consisted of two sets of documented information: 1) typed notes and photographs from the seven contextual inquiry sessions and 2) a set of screenshots from the digital dictation procedure. Based on data from seven inquires, the researchers aimed at providing answers to the first two study objectives: to describe the dictation processes from the physician's viewpoint and to compare the three currently used dictation techniques with each other. The ISI analysis was conducted to outline as well as to describe the stages of interaction specific to each of the three dictation techniques: digital, cassette, and speech recognition dictation.

The interaction analysis of screenshots taken during the digital dictation walkthrough with the chief physician included arranging the screenshots in the right order and removing duplicates and other extraneous data captured. In this work, the researchers utilised their knowledge of the real-life dictation procedures and practices gathered during the seven inquiries. The number of interaction steps in the digital dictation process was counted based on the analysis of the screenshots and the activities performed by the physicians. The screenshot analysis included organising and modifying the pictures as well as highlighting the details of conducted interactions in such a way that the transitions between screenshots would be understandable and reasonable. Individuals' private information was removed from the pictures in order to guarantee both the patients' and the physicians' anonymity. In addition, each of the screenshots was marked with consecutive numbers and enhanced with short descriptive texts.

6   Results

6.1   Comparison of Dictation Techniques: Illustrating Stages of Interaction

The digital dictation procedure consists of nine stages of interaction, whereas cassette dictation process consists of six, and speech recognition consists of four. The stages are presented in Table 1.

Digital dictation. The main disparity between the cassette and the digital dictation techniques is the format in which the signal is recorded and transmitted. In brief, the digital dictation procedure consists of nine stages, which are illustrated in Table 1. First, the physician starts up the computer, logs in, and opens the electronic health record (EHR) system. Then, he or she finds the right patient and related information in the system with the help of a social security number. The third stage closely resembles that of cassette dictation: the physician searches for relevant patient information using the paper records, the EHR system, and other electronic resources; opens those; and becomes familiar with patient's earlier health records. After the preparatory stages, the physician is ready to start the dictation using the software. While dictating, the physician mainly operates with the handset and, now and then, searches for relevant information from various sources. At the end, he or she saves the dictation, and thereafter the audio file is automatically sent to a dictation centre (stage 5). After being converted from speech to text by transcriptionists, the dictation is usually returned to the physician for approval within several days. The approval process includes the following activities: finding the notification about the transcribed dictation from the physician's personal checklist (stage 6); based on the patient information in the notification, searching for the dictation in the EHR system (stage 7); reviewing the text, making possible corrections following the text-editing process; saving the approved dictation (stage 8); and marking the notification as having been checked (stage 9).

Cassette dictation. Cassette and digital dictation processes resemble each other closely: the dictation is first recorded and then converted from speech to text. From the physician's point of view, the cassette dictation process is characterised by simplicity and concreteness. The preparatory actions include filling in a dictation form (stage 1), sticking a note to a cassette indicating the patient's social security number, and inserting the cassette into a recorder (stage 2).

Table 1. Stages of interaction during digital, cassette, and speech recognition dictation

Stage of interaction	Digital dictation	Cassette dictation	Speech recognition dictation (radiology)
1.	Start up the computer, log in, and open electronic health record (EHR) system.	Fill in the dictation paper form (patient identification information).	Open the CRIS radiology information system.
2.	Find the target patient information in the EHR system (using his/her social security number).	Other preparatory actions e.g. stick a note to a cassette and insert the cassette into a recorder.	Select the target patient from the list (→ the patient's pictures will open).
3.	Open up and become familiar with previous documentation using electronic health records and other related systems.	Become familiar with patient documentation using papers and electronic information systems.	Dictate (while modifying the pictures) using a handset. The dictated text appears on screen in almost real time.
4.	Dictate (including identification information and dictated message) using a handset.	Dictation (including identification information and dictated message) using a handset and a recorder.	Edit (using the keyboard) and save the dictation (using the handset).
5.	End and save dictation.	Put cassette and papers into an envelope. (Nurses will deliver the envelope from the physician's desk further.)	
	Dictation is converted from voice to text by transcriptionists and is returned to the physician within several days.		
6.	Find the notification about the transcribed dictation.	Review, and if necessary, make revisions with paper and pen; deliver paper to nurses.	
7.	Search for the dictation using the EHR system.		
8.	Review and, in necessary, make corrections; save the approved dictation.		
9.	Mark the notification as having been checked.		

Speech recognition dictation. The observed process of speech recognition dictation was in use in the radiology unit and consists of five stages (Table 1). First, the radiology physician starts the computer, logs in, and opens up the radiology information solution (CRIS system). Then, from a list, the physician selects the patient and the related radiological materials to be utilised in dictation. Most often, the procedure can be started from the second stage, since performing dictations is a continuous process and one of the main activities in radiology work. The dictation stage includes looking up and reviewing x-rays as well as dictating with a handset. The speech recognition dictation technique enables the dictated text to appear on a screen almost in real time and thereby supports the physicians in continuously structuring the dictation message. The fourth stage includes making necessary changes using text-editing functionalities, and the last stage consists of saving the dictation and closing the patient information file and pictures using the handset.

6.2   Step-by-Step Illustration of the Digital Dictation Procedure

As described earlier, the low-level analysis of interaction between the user and user interfaces concentrated on examining the digital dictation procedure. The total number of screenshots taken from the digital dictation process was 58. Furthermore, the number of interaction steps was 61. The numbers of screenshots and interaction steps are presented in Table 2. As an example, figures 1-4 illustrate the set of screenshots and interaction steps relating to stages four "Dictate (including identification information and dictated message) using a handset" and five "End and save dictation".

Table 2. Total number of interaction steps in the digital dictation procedure shown together with the stages of interaction and the number of screenshots

Stage of interaction	Number of screenshots	Number of interaction
1	10	13
2	2	3
3	3	5
4	12	11
5	4	3
6	4	6
7	4	4
8	12	10
9	5	6
Total:	56	61

Results from the step-by-step analysis indicate that a high number of steps are required to perform the activities after the dictation is returned for approval (stages six to nine). Analysis of the screenshots reveals the following reasons for this: the notification of a transcribed dictation waiting for confirmation appears in the physician's "personal checklist". The notification does not include a link to the dictation text; instead, the physician needs to copy and paste the patient's social security number when seeking the dictation text from the EHR system. Similarly, several interaction steps need to be taken when marking the notification about the transcribed dictation as having been checked.

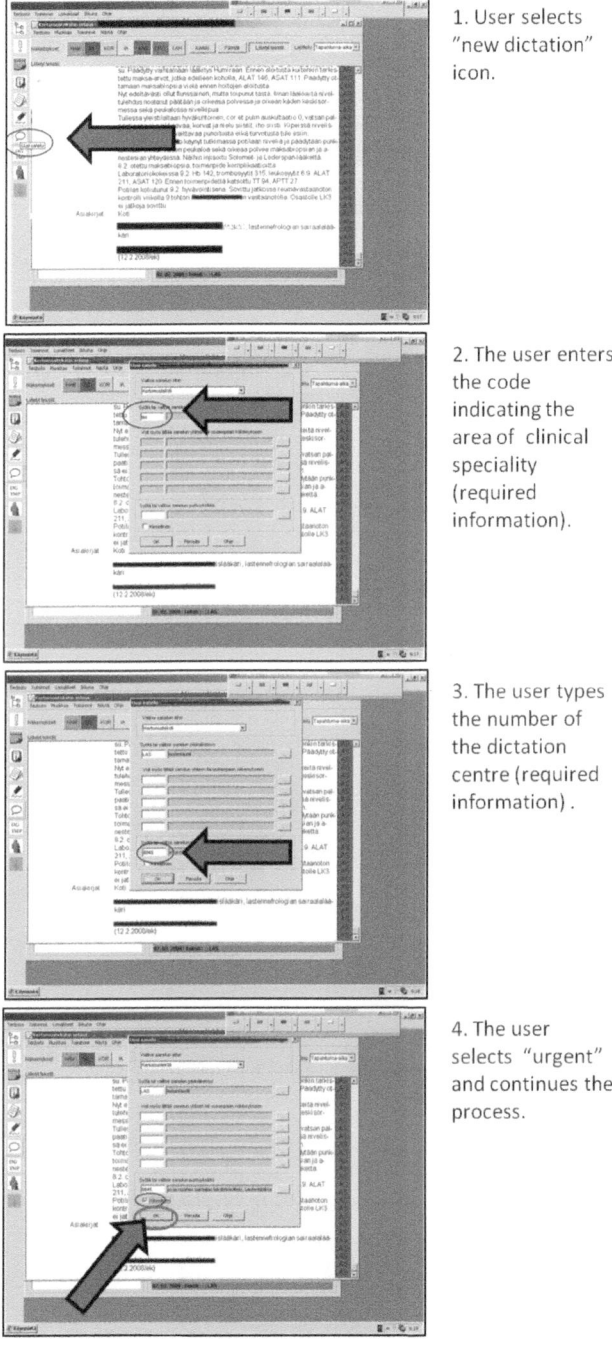

Fig. 1. An example of the interaction steps illustration (steps one to four, i.e. stage 4 of the digital process in Table 1). First four screenshots and descriptions of action from the digital dictation process.

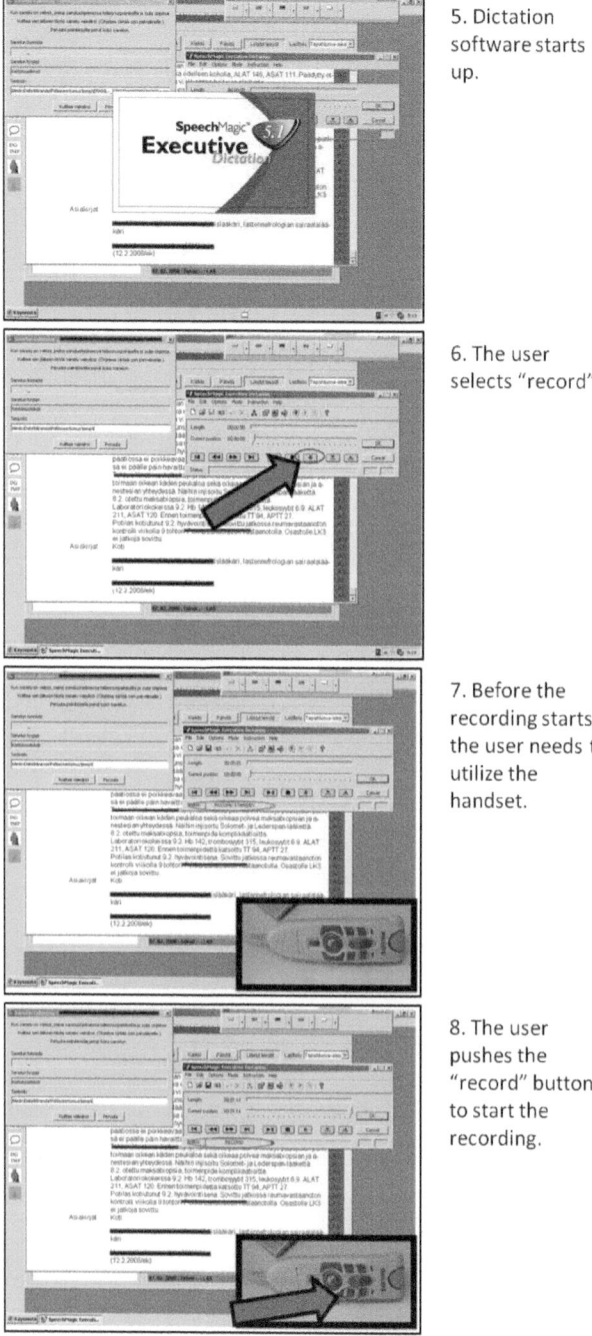

5. Dictation software starts up.

6. The user selects "record".

7. Before the recording starts, the user needs to utilize the handset.

8. The user pushes the "record" button to start the recording.

Fig. 2. An example of the interaction steps illustration (steps five to eight). Four screenshots and descriptions of action from the digital dictation process enhanced with pictures of actions performed using a handset.

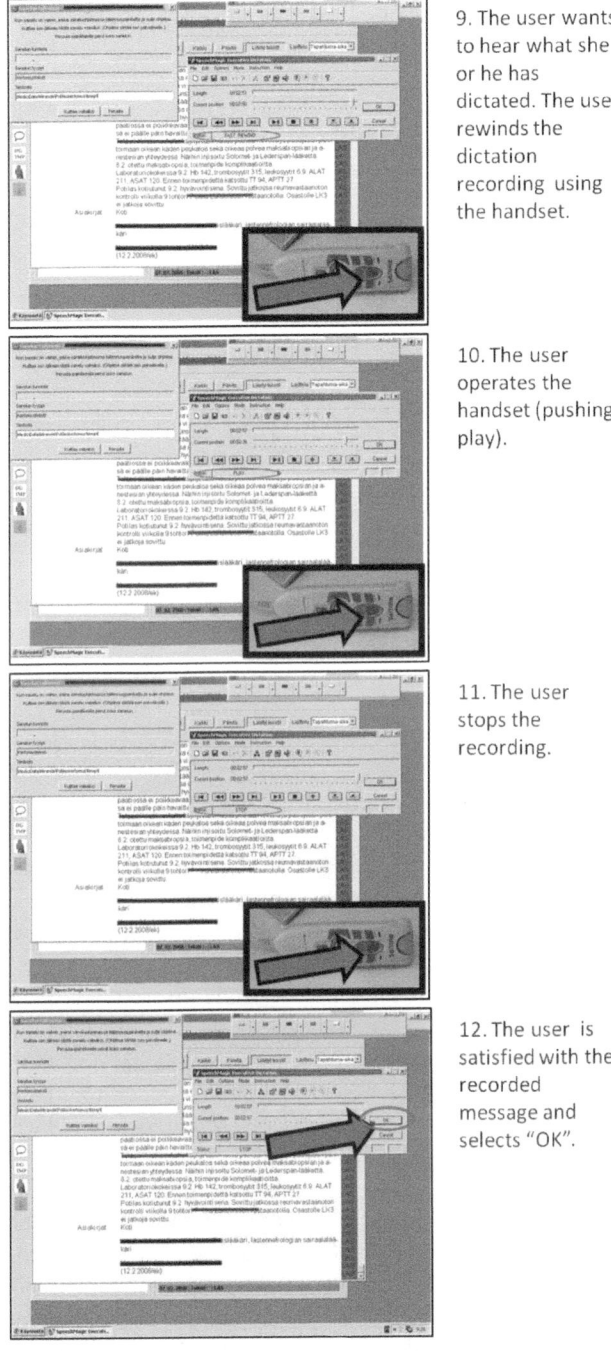

Fig. 3. An example of the interaction steps illustration (steps 9 to 12). Four screenshots and descriptions of action from the digital dictation process enhanced with pictures of actions performed using a handset.

144 J. Viitanen and M. Nieminen

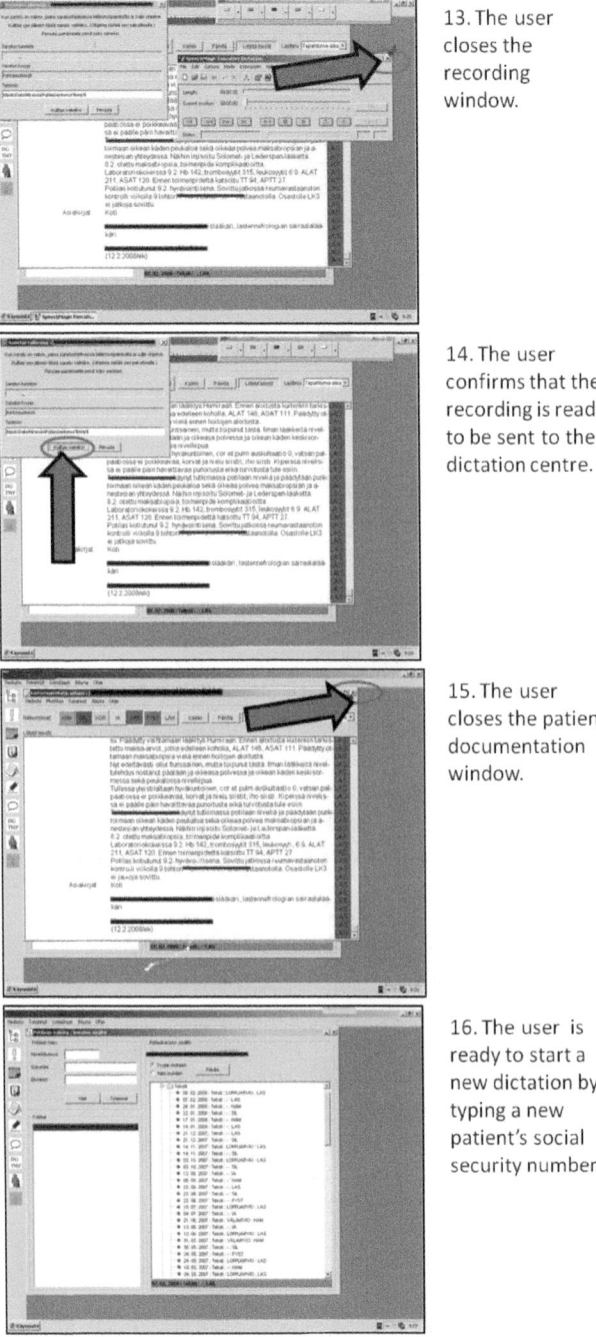

Fig. 4. An example of the interaction steps illustration (steps 13 to 16). Four screenshots and descriptions of action from the digital dictation process.

7   Discussion

7.1   On the Results of the Study

This paper continued the earlier research concerning user-centred evaluation of digital dictation solution [6]. The outcomes of the interaction analysis consisted of two sets of data and documentation: 1) illustrations of interaction stages in three dictation procedures that utilise digital, analogue, and speech recognition recording techniques, and 2) step-by-step illustrations of user-computer interaction focusing on the sequence of events in the digital dictation process.

The outcomes of the ISI method and related analysis provide practical and hands-on data about the interaction stages and steps. The observed process of digital dictation consists of nine stages of interaction and involves several complicated steps. Compared to both conventional cassette dictation and advanced speech recognition techniques, the number of steps and stages is considerably higher. Findings from the step-by-step analysis showed that in total, the amount of required interaction steps in a simplified digital dictation process was found to be 61. What is more, this does not include steps involved in searching for patient information from various resources or dictating lengthy messages, during which interruptions are common and considerably complicate the continuity of dictation.

The observed digital dictation software was closely integrated into the EHR system. Thus, any problems related to the information system were also attributed to the dictation process. The interaction analysis indicated dozens of apparent usability problems, including unnecessary codes and verifications, ambiguous terminology, and additional but superfluous clicking, to mention only a few examples. The detailed evaluation of the user interface characteristics was not the focus of this study; however, these findings partly explain the high number of interaction stages and steps.

Based on the study results, one can easily argue that the problems found in the digital dictation process and procedure derive from poor usability and insufficiencies in the interaction design. The number of unnecessary clicks required, and thus resources wasted, considerably hinder clinical work. Earlier studies have shown challenges in documenting and retrieving patient information using electronic systems [7-10]. Our findings are consistent with these. In addition, our study provided concrete and detailed findings that can be utilised in the further development of digital dictation application.

Dictation is a time-consuming tasks of physicians within modern hospitals, but a necessary task. The study findings suggest for choosing speech recognition dictation due to the reported benefits, e.g. less interaction stages. However, it should be noted that the in the target hospital, the speech recognition solutions had been developed and tested for radiology purposes in close collaboration with the physicians and software provider for about three years. Experience had indicated that there were many challenges to overcome, before similar solution could be utilised in other clinical contexts.

7.2   Experiences with the ISI Analysis

In the clinical context, the technology environment consists of many IT applications, of which several are used simultaneously. From the viewpoint of clinicians, research on the usability of a single system can be claimed as contradictory, perhaps irrelevant, when their daily work environment and the nature of their jobs are taken into account. Traditional usability inspection methods concentrate on the evaluation of a single system with little emphasis on context of use considerations. The introduced task- and context-originated analysis aimed at addressing the challenges of evaluating healthcare IT systems in clinical contexts and thereby contributing to ongoing discussions about methodology challenges in health informatics field. Our work with interaction analysis, continued the earlier work and the development of HCI inspection methods established by Ruy and Monk [28] and Thimbleby [29].

Findings from the experimental study indicated that the analysis approach that was introduced and the ISI method that was used are suitable for providing concrete and detailed information about the steps of interaction, the usability of user interface, the effectiveness of use, and the success of interaction design. Such a remote analysis enables thorough walkthroughs that can be conducted not only by usability specialists and by developers but also by the users of the system. The possibility for remote analysis is especially important in the healthcare domain because: 1) conducting on-site analyses may be difficult due to sensitive topics being discussed between the physicians and the patients, 2) the evaluation of information systems that include real patient data is not usually possible, and 3) involving end-users into intensive data capturing sessions might be difficult due to the hectic and critical nature of clinical work. When working with user interface screenshots, modifications to the visible data in screenshots can be made with authorised personnel so that patient privacy will not be compromised.

Based on our experiences, however, determining the criteria for defining stages of interaction is not a straightforward or strictly guided process. In our case, stages were defined based on the number of user actions and interaction steps between the user and the system as well as on time taken up by performing these in a realistic work context. Such a methodology approach was seen as useful when comparing dictation techniques to each other from the end-user's viewpoint. When applied for these kinds of purposes, it is important throughout the study to follow the agreed-upon principles or criteria. It is worth noticing that for the sake of simplicity, issues of complex medical details in dictated messages and contents of patient documentation were intentionally reduced as being minimal (depending on the patient situation, the contents of the dictation may be complex and the physician may use numerous information systems and applications during dictation). Often, physicians seek patient information from several information systems (e.g. laboratory system) and from numerous entries documented in EHR systems. Therefore, the described step-by-step process only accounted for those steps that users are required to perform in each and every digital dictation process.

Furthermore, our study pointed out that considering issues of patient privacy is essential when applying methods like ISI in healthcare contexts. Access to real environments in which clinical systems are used is crucial in order to gather reliable and rich data for research and development purposes. Nevertheless, getting access and permission to record audio data might not be easy. At the very least pictures and other data need to be carefully modified in the analysis phase in such a way that the anonymity of both the patient and healthcare professionals is guaranteed.

7.3   Future Work

It seems that healthcare technology failures often derive from misunderstandings and poor collaboration between developers, users, administrators, and other stakeholders. The approach introduced for analysing human-computer interaction in healthcare may provide new opportunities and concrete tools for supporting collaborative activities during technology development. Future research should address the questions of how this data and these illustrations of stages and steps could be utilised in development work and how software developers perceive the usefulness of such a method. In addition, more work needs to be conducted to understand and to evaluate the ISI method. Such an assessment should describe its advantages and disadvantages when employed in usability evaluations, in user interface design, and for interaction design purposes.

8   Conclusion

This paper introduced an analysis approach, interaction sequence illustration (ISI), for documenting and analysing users' actions with interactive systems – a method thereby studying the successfulness and failures of interaction design and user interface aspects. The study showed that at present, the process of digital dictation is inefficient and unnecessarily lengthy from the physician's viewpoint. The analysis of digital dictation procedure revealed a number of interaction design failures and complex interaction sequences, the improvement of which is essential.

References

1. Khangura, S., Grimsha, J., Mohe, D.: Evidence Summary: Electronic Health Records (EHRs). Ottawa Hospital Research Institute,
   http://www.ohri.ca/kta/docs/KTA-EHR-Evidence-Review.pdf
   (accessed July 01, 2011)
2. Black, A.D., Car, J., Pagliari, C., Anandan, C., Cresswell, K., Bokun, T., McKinstry, B., Procter, R., Majeed, A., Sheikh, A.: The Impact of eHealth on the Quality and Safety of Health Care: A Systematic Overview. PLoS Med. 18 (2011),
   http://www.plosmedicine.org/article/info%3Adoi%2F10.1371%2Fjournal.pmed.1000387 (accessed July 01, 2011)
3. Kjeldskov, J., Skov, M.B., Stage, J.A.: Longitudinal Study of Usability in Health Care: Does Time Heal? Studies in Health Technology and Informatics 130, 181–191 (2007)
4. Edwards, P.J., Moloney, K.P., Jacko, J.A., Sainfort, F.: Evaluating Usability of a Commercial Electronic Health Record: A Case Study. International Journal of Human-Computer Studies 66, 718–728 (2008)
5. Peute, L.W.P., Jaspers, M.W.M.: The Significance of a Usability Evaluation of an Emerging Laboratory Order Entry System. International Journal of Medical Informatics 76, 157–168 (2007)
6. Viitanen, J.: Redesigning Digital Dictation for Physicians: A User-centred Approach. Health Informatics Journal 15, 179–190 (2009)

7. Poissant, L., Pereira, J., Tamblyn, R., Kawasumi, Y.: The Impact of Electronic Health Records on Time Efficiency of Physicians and Nurses: A Systematic Review. Journal of the American Medical Information Association 12(5), 505–516 (2005)
8. Holden, R.J.: Physicians' Beliefs about Using EMR and CPOE: In Pursuit of a Contextual Understanding of Health IT Use Behavior. International Journal of Medical Informatics 79, 71–80 (2010)
9. Reuss, E., Naef, P., Keller, R., Norrie, M.: Physicians' and Nurses' Documenting Practices and Implications for Electronic Patient Record Design. In: Holzinger, A. (ed.) USAB 2007. LNCS, vol. 4799, pp. 113–118. Springer, Heidelberg (2007)
10. Braun, L.M.M., Wiesman, F., van der Herik, H.J., Hasman, A., Korsten, E.: Towards Patient-related Information Needs. International Journal of Medical Informatics 76, 246–251 (2007)
11. Holzinger, A., Ackerl, S., Searle, G., Sorantin, E.: Speech Recognition in Daily Hospital Practice: Human-computer Interaction Lessons Learned. In: Lanyi, S. (ed.) Central European Multimedia and Virtual Reality Conference CEMVRC 2004, pp. 125–134. University of Veszprém Press (2004)
12. ISO 9241-210. International standard: Ergonomics of human-system interaction, Part 210: Human-centred design for interactive systems. First edition 2010-03-15. Reference number ISO 9241-210:2010(E)
13. Beyer, H., Holzblatt, K.: Contextual Design: Defining Customer-centered Systems. Academic Press, San Diego (1998)
14. Beuscart-Zéphir, M.C., Brender, J., Beuscart, R., Ménager-Depriester, I.: Cognitive Evaluation: How to Assess the Usability of Information Technology in Healthcare. Computer Methods and Programs in Biomedicine 54, 19–28 (1997)
15. Kushniruk, A.W., Patel, V.L.: Cognitive and Usability Engineering Methods for the Evaluation of Clinical Information Systems. Journal of Biomedical Informatics 37, 56–76 (2004)
16. Jaspers, M.W.M.: A Comparison of Usability Methods for Testing Interactive Technologies: Methodological Aspects and Empirical Evidence. International Journal of Medical Informatics 78, 340–353 (2009)
17. Janß, A., Lauer, W., Radermacher, K.: Cognitive Task Analysis for Prospective Usability Evaluation in Computer-Assisted Surgery. In: Holzinger, A. (ed.) USAB 2007. LNCS, vol. 4799, pp. 349–356. Springer, Heidelberg (2007)
18. Horsky, J., Kaufman, D.R., Oppenheim, M.I., Patel, V.L.: A Framework for Analyzing the Cognitive Complexity of Computer-assisted Clinical Ordering. Journal of Biomedical Informatics 4, 4–22 (2003)
19. Belden, J.L., Grayson, R., Barnes, J.: Defining and Testing EMR Usability: Principles and Proposed Methods of EMR Usability Evaluation and Rating. Healthcare Information and Management Systems Society (HIMSS) EHR Task Force (June 2009), http://www.himss.org/content/files/HIMSS_DefiningandTestingE MRUsability.pdf (accessed July 01, 2011)
20. Bastien, J.M.C.: Usability Testing: A Review of Some Methodological and Technical Aspects of the Method. International Journal of Medical Informatics 79, e18–e23 (2010)
21. Følstad, A., Hornbæk, K.: Work-domain Knowledge in Usability Evaluation: Experiences with Cooperative Usability Testing. The Journal of Systems and Software 83, 2019–2030 (2010)
22. González, M.P., Lorés, J., Granollers, A.: Enhancing Usability Testing through Datamining Techniques: A Novel Approach to Detecting Usability Problem Patterns for a Context of Use. Information and Software Technology 50, 547–568 (2008)

23. Alsos, O.A., Dahl, Y.: Towards a Best Practice for Laboratory-based Usability Evaluations of Mobile ICT for Hospitals. In: NordiHCI 2008, Lund, Sweden, pp. 3–12. ACM Press (2008)
24. Svanæs, D., Alsos, O.A., Dahl, Y.: Usability Testing of Mobile ICT for Clinical Settings: Methodological and Practical Challenges. International Journal of Medical Informatics 79, e24–e34 (2010)
25. Horsky, J., McColgan, K., Pang, J.E., Melnikas, A.J., Linder, J.-A., Schinipper, J.L., Middleton, B.: Complementary Methods of System Usability Evaluation: Surveys and Observations During Software Design and Development Cycles. Journal of Biomedical Informatics 43, 782–790 (2010)
26. Wharton, C., Rieman, J., Lewis, C., Polson, P.: The Cognitive Walkthrough Method: A Practitioner's Guide. In: Nielsen, J., Mack, R. (eds.) Usability Inspection Methods. John Wiley & Sons, Inc., New York (1994)
27. Nielsen, J.: Usability Engineering. Academic Press, Inc., San Diego (1993)
28. Ryu, H., Monk, A.: Analysing Interaction Problems with Cyclic Interaction Theory: Low-level Interaction Walkthrough. PsychNology Journal 2, 304–330 (2004)
29. Thimbleby, H.: Interaction Walkthrough: Evaluation of Safety Critical Interactive Systems. In: Doherty, G., Blandford, A. (eds.) DSVIS 2006. LNCS, vol. 4323, pp. 52–66. Springer, Heidelberg (2007)

Openness to Accept Medical Technology – A Cultural View

Firat Alagöz, Martina Ziefle,
Wiktoria Wilkowska, and André Calero Valdez

RWTH Aachen University, D-52056 Aachen, Human Technology Centre (Humtec)
alagoez@humtec.rwth-aachen.de

Abstract. Technology acceptance is a widely acknowledged key player in explaining technology adoption. However, there is a notable knowledge gap concerning the impact of cultural factors on technology acceptance, especially in the medical sector. It is evident though that countries differ greatly regarding their technical proneness, development and usage habits what should have considerable impact on acceptance. This study compares the openness to accept medical technology in Germany, Poland and Turkey. 300 respondents (19-85 years, 56% women, 38% chronically ill) participated in a survey, in which the pros and cons for using medical technologies were examined as well as the underlying acceptance motives and utilization barriers. The effects of different cultures, but also of age, gender and health status were analyzed regarding their impact on acceptance patterns. Results reveal both, culturally insensitive as well culturally sensitive acceptance, with strong effects of gender and exercising frequency. Overall, the study corroborates the importance of cultural views on technology acceptance.

Keywords: cross-cultural survey, technology acceptance, medical technology, cardiac illness, acceptance barriers.

1   Introduction

The last decades were characterized by a rapid development of new technical systems, accompanied by fast changing technology cycles, area-wide penetrations of information and communication technologies (ICT), and their pervasive implementation in many fields of social living. The latter development has profound socio-technical consequences. Technology use in private spheres is affected by and is also affecting societal structures and organizational procedures. Different from former times, where only small portions of people were factually working with specific technology in a professional context, today, a diverse user group is confronted with the use of a myriad of technical devices across all fields of professional and private concerns. In the next decennia new generations of technologies, services, and products based on computer technologies will have to master fundamental global societal and technological challenges: the graying society with an increasingly aged work force, the raising need for medical technology for the aged to be continuously

A. Holzinger and K.-M. Simonic (Eds.): USAB 2011, LNCS 7058, pp. 151–170, 2011.
© Springer-Verlag Berlin Heidelberg 2011

integrated in the social environments of persons and an increase in the complexity of technologies to be handled by diversely skilled persons. More than ever, usable interfaces, a broad understanding of these technologies as well as slick user experience will be critical success factors for acceptance, sustainability and competitive capacity of any technical system.

1.1   Technology Acceptance

Technology acceptance and technology adoption, respectively, describes the approval, favorable reception and ongoing use of newly introduced devices and systems. The first model of technology acceptance model (TAM) had been formulated and empirically validated by Davies et al. [1]. It refers to *the ease of using a system* (the degree to which a person believes that using a particular system would be free of effort) and *the perceived usefulness* (the degree to which a person thinks that a technical system increases job performance) as the two main determinants.

Even though the TAM was confirmed by many studies, one of the main criticisms of the TAM was that external factors such as the influence of individual user variables on technology acceptance were almost completely disregarded. In later refinements of the model (e.g. [2]), social and cognitive processes of users interacting with technology were added, which influence technology adoption behaviors (performance expectancy, effort expectancy, social influence, and facilitating conditions). Also, individual factors received attention to impact the technology acceptance. Although the vital importance of ensuring that the technology produced is both usable and appropriate for a diverse user group, recognition of the importance of diversity is only slowly influencing mainstream acceptance studies [3, 4, 5]. Design approaches thus have to undergo a radical change taking current societal trends into account, which have considerable impact for the inclusion of a diverse user group. Yet, only few studies concentrated on the diversity of users and their acceptance patterns [6, 7, 8, 9, 43, 44], even though it is clear from daily life experience that people may have different adoption behaviors due to individual characteristics.

1.2   Cultural Impact on Technology Acceptance

Another blind spot of existing models of technology acceptance is their cultural neutrality or, still worse, their ignorance to cultural impacts on acceptance. Still, the development of technology seems to be tailored to predominately young, technology experienced, Western, middle- and upper class males [5, 10, 11, 12]. Up to now there is a notable lack of knowledge on how society and culture affect the technology acceptance and the underlying reasons for or against technology usage [13, 14]. Comparably few studies have been concerned with the investigation of technology acceptance across national boundaries [15, 16, 17, 18]. Undoubtedly, existing knowledge about technology acceptance – mostly referring to highly-developed western countries – cannot be simply transferred to other cultures, as the cultural beliefs and values form a cultural mental model [19], which definitively impacts technology acceptance in a differential way [13, 20, 21, 22].

Persons do not use a single technology in isolation, but within a social and cultural context. These contextual factors are influencing how humans are acting with technology; the use of technology modifies the embedding context [5]. Social taboos, legal and political constraints as well as ethics, religious traditions and values differ across cultures. Thus, users around the world may differ in perception, cognition and style of thinking, cultural assumptions and values. This especially applies to underdeveloped countries, but also to countries, which experienced a quick technology change over the last years, striving for economic welfare and closing the technological gap to highly developed countries [23].

Culturally informed medical technology acceptance is another prominent issue [24, 25]. Whether medical technology is accepted in different cultures depends to a large extent on cultural mindsets of family caring, as well as on cultural ageing concepts [4] and prevailing health-care structures [25], which might imply a different form of social and societal responsibility of others. Also, the cultural handling of illness and the acceptance of end of life decisions are highly culturally sensitive [26, 27, 28].

1.3   The Specificity of Acceptance Towards Medical Technology

In most of the studies, technology acceptance had been examined and validated for ICT, predominantly in a job-related context. This is due to the context in which the TAM had been developed. In the 1980ies, when personal computers entered the offices national wide, there was a considerable need to understand technology adoption behaviors in the working context. A transfer of its assumptions on medical technology acceptance is highly disputable though [3, 7, 9]. Rather, it is reasonable to assume that the acceptance of medical technology distinctly differs from acceptance patterns of ICT technologies: First, medical devices are used not just for fun, but out of (critical) health states and vital medical reasons. Second, beyond its importance for patients' safety and the feeling of being safe, medical technology touch on "taboo" areas associated with disease and illness [4], which has an intricate impact on acceptance. Third, recent studies report that medical technical assistance is often perceived as breaking into persons' intimacy and privacy spheres and leads to a feeling of being permanently controlled [4, 29]. Recently it had been found that users – in case of using a medical device – reported to fear to be continuously controlled, while this was not ascribed to a device in the ICT context (mobile phone) [30]. Finally, a higher heterogeneity in user groups and an even stronger impact of individual factors on acceptance is expected for medical technologies, as users/patients might be far older than "typical ICT-users" and they might additionally suffer from multiple physical and psychological restraints in comparison to healthy user groups.

1.4   Questions Addressed and Logic of Research Procedure

If we want to recognize the impact of technology adoption on persons' social lives, a deeper understanding of technology acceptance is needed. Yet, hardly any study so far considered cultural factors on the acceptance of medical technologies. This was undertaken in the current study. Users in three different countries (Germany, Poland and Turkey) were examined regarding the extent of medical technology acceptance, thereby learning the specificity of pro-using arguments as well as usage barriers. The intention of the recruitment procedure of respondents was to reach a healthy mix of all ages, genders and health conditions, as well as diverse education and income levels across the three countries. This was done primarily on a "best-effort" basis, starting from face-to-face visits to cardiology departments of several different hospitals with the help and/or by selected members of the author's extended social networks. A small handful of younger and middle-aged participants were reached by online advertisements in medical forums. Special care was taken to not primarily employ the author's networks to recruit "the usual suspects" of university students for the younger aged group, as it is widely known that external validity is low in participants' which do not represent the whole target group [31, 32].

2   Methodology

The following section presents the methodology and research model of this study.

2.1   Research Model

The acceptance of and intention to use medical technology was measured with 19 items in total, divided into nine pro items and ten contra items (depicted in Table 1), each on a 4-point Likert scale ranging from 4 ("agree") to 1 ("do not agree"). The items were developed and tested in earlier studies [15, 42], based on interviews and focus-groups with participants suffering from chronic cardiovascular diseases.

Table 1. Pro items (Cronbach's α = .903) and Contra items (α = .864) used in three surveys. English translations were done for illustration purposes and did not undergo revision.

PRO	CON
Yes, I use / would use medical technology, because …	No, I do not use / I would not use medical technology ,because
I would feel safer.	I do not want to be ruled by technology.
I could see the doctor less often.	I do not want to be annoyed by technology with bad usability.
I would be able to live independently at home.	I do not need it.
I would be relieved of my health responsibilities.	It is too complicated for me.
I find it convenient to not have to remember everything myself (drugs, doctor appointments, measuring vitals...)	I think it is unreliable.
	It can't change my health status.
I would stay mobile in spite of illness.	I cannot stand total supervision.
I would not be a burden for others.	I do not want others to learn of my illness.
I would stay mentally fit in spite of old age and illness.	I do not want to be constantly reminded of my illness.
My health would improve.	I am afraid of false information.

Pro arguments, measuring the perceived benefits and motives to use medical technology, were summed up to a scale ranging from minimum 4 points to a maximum of 36 points (full acceptance and intention to use medical technology). Contra arguments, measuring utilization barriers and motives against the use of medical technology, were also summed up to a scale from 5 to 40 (40 = full rejection and distrust regarding medical technology). Reliability analysis with standardized Cronbach's alpha reached excellent values for Pro (.903) and Con (.864).

In Figure 1, the research model is illustrated. The Pro and Con scales were the *two dependent variables* in this study, each analyzed according to *seven independent variables*: (1) country, (2) age, (3) gender, (4) heart disease, (5) exercise frequency and (6) ICT technology acceptance, measured via 9 items each for (6a) perceived ease of use (PEU) and (6b) perceived usefulness (PU) of mobile phones, chosen based on previous research for the three countries under study [15]. PEU mobile and PU mobile were each measured with 9 items and summed up to a scale with maximum 36 (easy to use / very useful). Standardized Cronbach's alpha values for PEU mobile (.886) and PU mobile (.860) were also very high.

To maintain groups of satisfactory sample size during analysis, median-splits had to be employed for age (50 years), exercise frequency (once per week), PEU mobile (25 out of max 36) and PU mobile (24 out of max. 36). This furthermore kept the analysis complexity manageable. "Best guess" tests without median-split (where appropriate) showed that loss of power was tolerable.

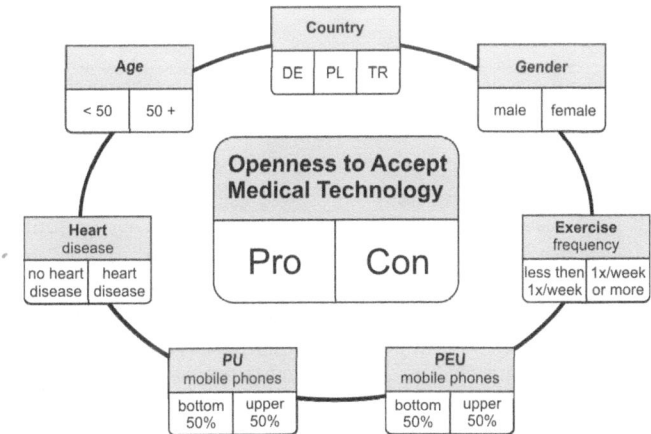

Fig. 1. Research model: dependent variables Pro and Con surrounded by independent variables

2.2   Questionnaire

In order to reach a large number of participants from three different countries and with respect to the diversities in culture, age and health status, the questionnaire-method was employed. The questionnaire was designed to obtain specific data of four main categories: (a) demographic data (country, age, gender, education, profession, income), (b) health status and related variables (chronic cardiovascular condition, risk factors, coping styles, exercise frequency), (c) technology experience (PEU and usability of ICT), and (d) acceptance and intention to use medical technology (pro / contra arguments). Whether participants suffer from a chronic cardiovascular condition (henceforth "heart disease") was self-reported and ranged from having chronic high blood pressure over coronary heart disease to having a heart transplant. The questionnaire was first developed in German during earlier studies [15, 42] and revised by a sample of older adults (n = 10) as well as two usability experts with respect to issues of comprehensibility and wording of items. After passing this quality control step, the questionnaire was translated into Polish and Turkish by professional translators. The final version of the questionnaire consisted of closed multiple-choice questions, using a four-point Likert scale to help force a choice and reduce complexity. The items ranged from "agree" (4) to "do not agree" (1). Every item-block further had a field for additional remarks. The total time to fill in the questionnaire took 20-30 minutes, depending on the health status of the participants.

2.3   Participants

The data of N = 300 respondents were analyzed in this study (see Fig. 2). Of these, 72 (24%) live in Germany, 111 (37%) in Poland and 117 (39%) in Turkey. There were 114 (38%) participants with heart disease, of which 67 (59%) were female.

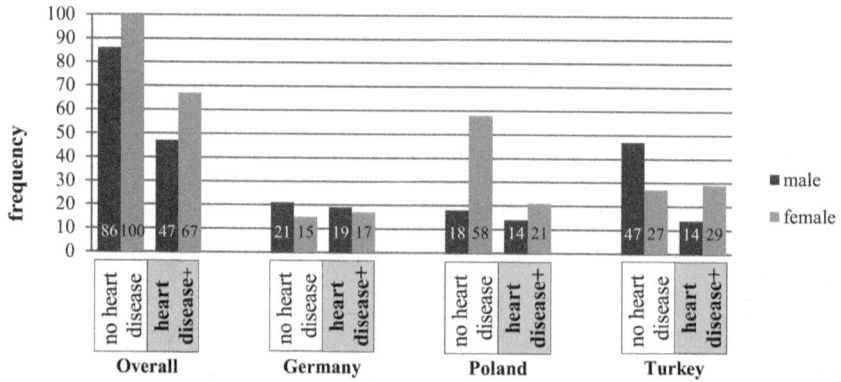

Fig. 2. Frequency distribution of study participants (N = 300)

Participant's age ranged from 19 to 85 (m=50.7; SE=.891). The age distribution is depicted in Fig. 3. An age analysis via three-way independent ANOVA (sig. p=.05) revealed significant main effects of country (F(2, 288) = 11.608; p < .000), showing that Polish participants were the youngest (m_{PL}=44.7), followed by German participants (m_{DE}=50.2). Turkish participants were the oldest group (m_{TR}=56.5). Participants with heart disease also significantly differed by age across countries (F(1, 288) = 68.216; p < .000), with participants without heart disease being younger ($m_{no\ heart\ d.}$=45.4) than those with heart disease (m_{heart}=59.2). Furthermore, there was an interaction of country * gender * heart disease (F(2, 288) = 3.265; p = .040). No further interactions were found.

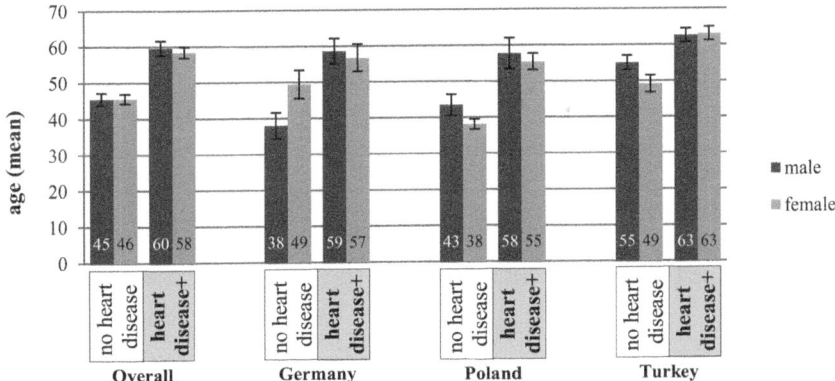

Fig. 3. Age distribution by country, gender and heart disease. Error bars show 95% CI

3   Results

Results are presented in a top-down fashion, first describing effects in the overall study sample, and then analyzing more specific effects, like e.g. effects in-between countries. Beforehand, the employed statistical tests are introduced.

3.1   Employed Statistical Tests

Results were analyzed by Spearman's rank correlations, t-tests and analysis of variance (ANOVA) with Games-Howell post-hoc tests to control type I error rates. Type I error rates were set to $\alpha = 5\%$ (two-tailed), i.e. the chance to have a false positive result is at most 5%. Type II error rates were set to $(1-\beta) = 80\%$, i.e. the chance to detect a genuine effect (if one exists) is at least 80%. Due to the exploratory nature of this study, some results are presented which did not reach the defined error rates. For these results, the exact error rates are computed and reported with the help of the software G*Power 3.1.3 [33].

Games-Howell post-hoc tests for ANOVAs were all re-run and reported via t-tests, as long as they yielded the same results. For effect sizes, Cohen's d was chosen, where $d = .2$ is referred to as a small effect, $d = .5$ as a medium effect and $d = .8$ as a large effect [34]. Effect sizes for nonparametric tests are reported via Pearson's r, with .1, .3 and .5 referred to as small, medium and large effects respectively.

If assumptions of the parametric tests were violated, the nonparametric equivalent test was run and reported. Overall, t-tests and ANOVAs proved very robust with respect to violations of normality, but often parametric tests showed increased effects sizes, albeit very small increases. Only very different variances led to poor type II errors in parametric tests. In those cases, the appropriate nonparametric results are reported.

3.2   Comparing Overall Pro/Con Totals

First, the motives for using medical technology, divided into Pro and Con arguments, were compared overall and by country. For clarity, results were scaled to percent, with 100% representing the maximum (36 points for pro, 40 points for con) and values greater 50% acceptance. Results show that there is a greater tendency towards using medical technology, as depicted by the increased pro results compared to con (see Fig. 4). The countries differed significantly in their pro scores (Welch's F(2,170) = 3.251; p = .41). On average, polish participants had higher Pro scores than Turkish participants (t(226) = 2.459; p = .015), representing a small effect (d = .331; (1-β) = .70). Con arguments also differed across countries (Kruskall-Walis: H(2) = 6.037; p = .049), showing less Con for Germany than Turkey, but the small effect missed a satisfactory type II error rate (t(187) = 2.066; p = .040; d = .300; (1-β) = .50).

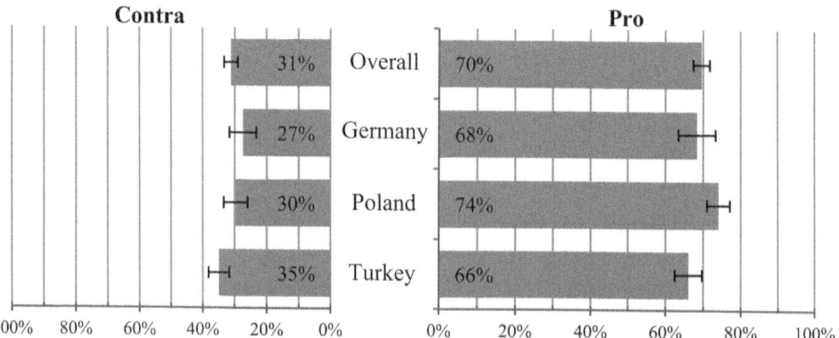

Fig. 4. Pro and Con for medical technology scores by country, scaled to percent, all participants (N = 300). Values >50% equal agreement, 100% is full agreement. Error bars show 95% CI.

3.3 Correlation Analysis between Variables

To guide the following analyses, Spearman's rank correlations were computed (see Table 2). While Con only had one small negative correlation with Pro (r = -.209; p < .001), Pro had three more small correlations with: females (r =.147; p < .01), exercise frequency (r =.177; p < .001) and PU (r = .132; p <. 05).

Table 2. Intercorrelations (Spearman's rank, 2 tailed) of research variables with all participants (N = 300). Only significant values p< .05 are shown (*p< .01; ***p< .001).

N = 300	Pro	Con	age	gender	heart d.	exercise	PEU
Pro							
Contra	-.209***						
Age							
gender	.147*						
heart disease			.442***				
exercise	.177***		-.133		-.150*		
PEU mobile			-.516***	-.175***	-.345***	.192***	
PU mobile	.132		-.358***	-.173***	-.294***	.154*	.785***

Age has a medium-to-large correlation with heart disease (r = .442; p < .001) and medium-to-large negative correlations with the technology dimensions PEU and PU. These findings conform to earlier research [3, 4, 6, 35] and show that younger adults and males relate to higher technology experience even across countries.

3.4   Comparing Pro/Con Overall

Detailed effects of the independent variables on Pro and Con are shown in Fig. 5. Overall, when splitting participants into low-Con and high-Con groups via median-split (mdn$_{Con}$ = 16) and comparing differences in Pro scores, the low-Con group (m=29.04; SE=.572) scored higher on Pro than the high-Con group (m=26.72; SE=.542), which is a highly significant difference (t(298) = 2.948; p = .003), representing a small effect (d = .342). This result was alluded to from earlier correlation analysis. For Pro (max 36 points), there was a very significant difference for gender (t(298) = 2.751; p = .006), with females scoring higher (m=28.75; SE=.491) then men (m=26.57; SE=.640), representing a small effect (d = .319; (1-β) = 79%). Also, exercising frequency had a very significant effect on Pro (t(298) = 3.340; p = .001), with participants exercising once per week or more scoring higher (m=28.84; SE=.477) then participants exercising less frequently (m=26.16; SE=.673), representing a small-to-medium effect (d = .387; (1-β)= 92%).

Effects of perceived usability of mobile phones (PU mobile) on Pro missed statistical significance (t(298) = 1.810; p = .071) and was of small size (d = .210). With N = 300 participants, this small effect can only be detected with (1-β) = 44% probability, suggesting a false positive effect of PU on Pro. No statistically significant differences were found on Con by independent values.

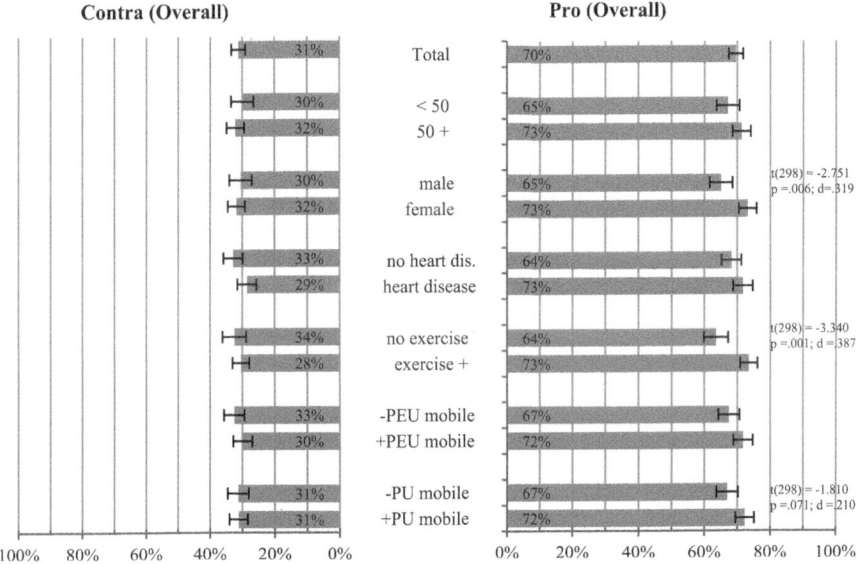

Fig. 5. Pro and Con for medical technology scores, compared by median-splits of independent variables, scaled to percent, all participants (N = 300). Error bars show 95% CI.

There was a significant interaction effect (see Fig. 6 (left)) between age and exercise on Pro scores (F(1, 296) = 10.324; p = .001), indicating that older adults had significantly higher Pro scores when exercising at least once per week (m=30.33; SE=.506) compared to older participants that do not exercise that often (m=25.43; SE=.866). There was no significant effect of exercise frequency on younger adult's Pro scores. The same interaction between age and exercise frequency was also found for Con scores (see Fig. 6 (middle)), but missed statistical significance (F(1, 296) = 3.210; p = .074). A mirror interaction effect of said effect of age and exercise frequency on Pro scores was found for heart disease and exercise frequency on Pro, but missed statistical significance (F(1, 296) = 2.776; p = .097).

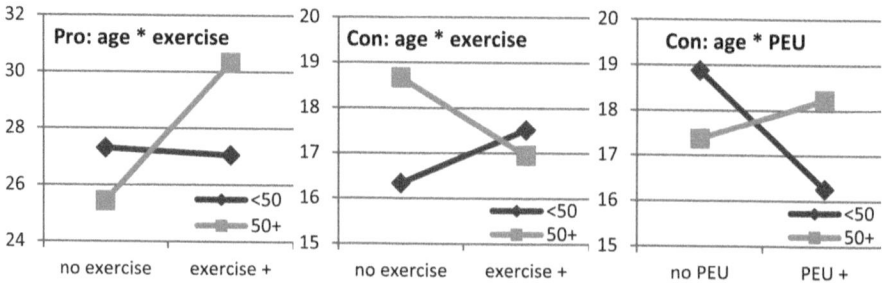

Fig. 6. (Left): interaction graph of age * exercise on Pro. (Middle): interaction graph of age * exercise on Con. (Right): interaction graph of age * PEU on Con.

For Con, there was an interaction of age * PEU (F(1, 296) = 4.340; p = .038) (see Fig. 6 (right)). While older adult's Con scores remained unaffected by PEU, younger adults with low PEU (m=18.88; SE=1.120) scored higher on Con than younger adults with high PEU (m=16.26; SE=.651).

3.5   Pro/Con in Germany

The distribution of Pro and Con values in Germany is depicted in Fig. 7. No statistically significant effects were found. German participants who exercise less than once per week (m=25.80; SE=1.382) scored lower compared to those that exercise at least once per week (m=29.03; SE=1.135), but this effect missed statistical significance (t(70) = 1.814; p = .074) and was too small to be reliably detected in a group of this size (N = 72; d = .434; (1–β) = 44%).

3.6   Pro/Con in Poland

The distribution of Pro and Con values in Poland is depicted in Fig. 8. On the Pro scale, younger Polish adults (m=27.81; SE=.760) scored significantly lower compared to older adults (m=30.93; SE=.697), which was highly significant result (t(109) = 2.792; p = .006) of medium size (d = .535;). Polish participants with heart disease (m_Pro=30.80; SE_Pro=.803; m_Con=15.11; SE_Con=1.207), compared to those without (m_Pro =28.16;

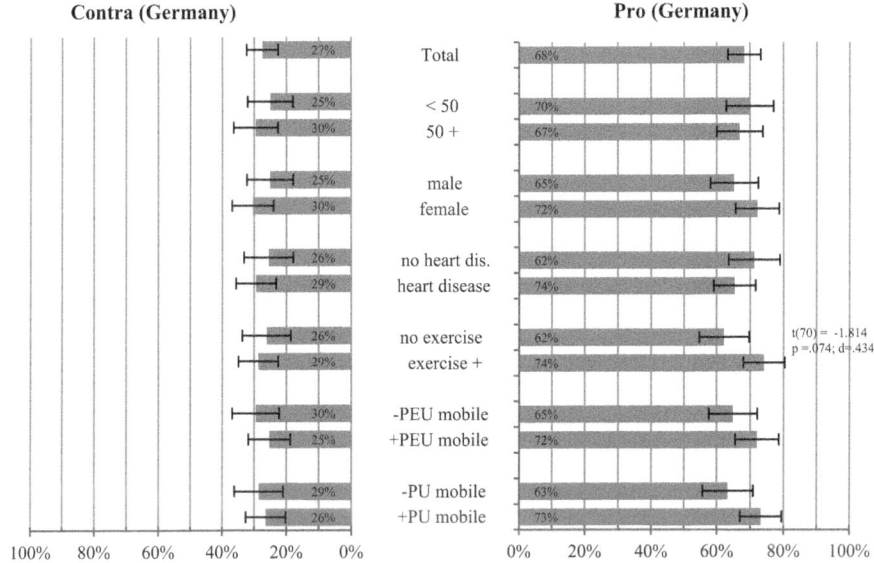

Fig. 7. Pro and Con for medical technology scores in Germany (N = 72), compared by median-splits of independent variables, scaled to percent. Error bars show 95% CI.

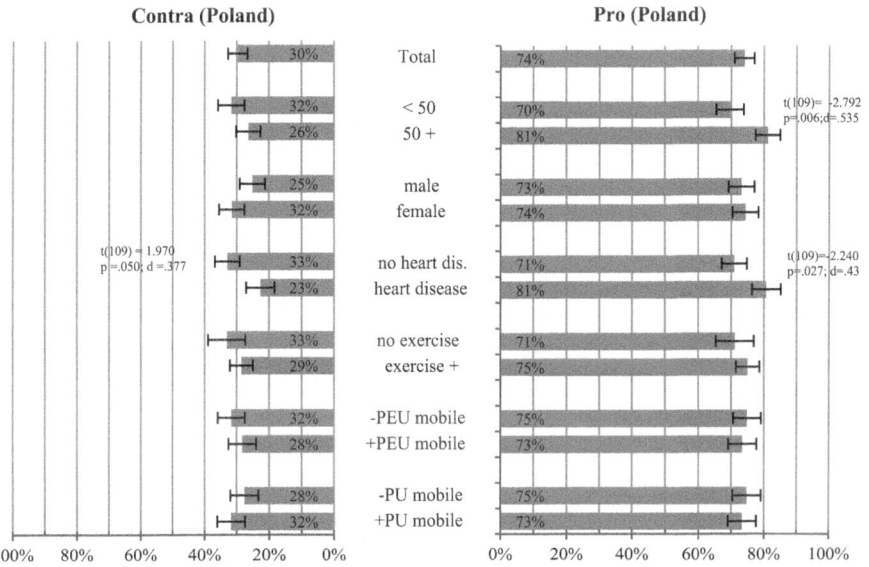

Fig. 8. Pro and Con for medical technology scores in Poland (N = 111), compared by median-splits of independent variables, scaled to percent. Error bars show 95% CI.

SE_{Pro}=.709; m_{Con}=17.89; SE_{Con}=.803), showed higher acceptance of medical technology on both Pro (t_{Pro}(109) = 2.240; p_{Pro} = .027) and Con (t_{Con}(109) = 1.970; p_{Con} = .05) scales. The small-to-medium sized Pro effect (N = 111; d = .429; (1–β) = 60%) and Con effect (d = .377; (1–β) = 50%) did not fully reach the desired power of 80%, but the higher prevalence of heart disease in older adults (see Chapter 3.3) and the significant age effect that was found increase the likelihood of a genuine effect.

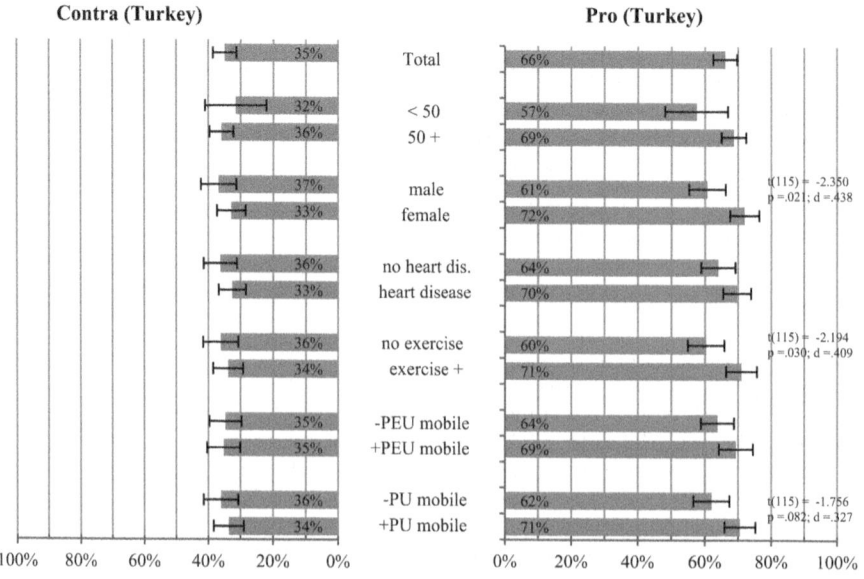

Fig. 9. Pro and Con for medical technology scores in Turkey (N = 117), compared by median-splits of independent variables, scaled to percent. Error bars show 95% CI.

3.7   Pro/Con in Turkey

The distribution of Pro and Con values in Turkey is depicted in Fig. 9. The effects mimic the effects found in the overall sample (see 3.4), although less pronounced. Older adults in Turkey (m=28.43; SE=.806), compared to younger adults (m=25.39; SE=1.009), showed higher Pro scores overall (t(115) = 2.35; p = .021), representing a small-to-medium effect, but did not achieve enough power (d = .438; (1–β) = 65%). Participants that exercised regularly (m=28.17; SE=.857) also showed higher Pro scores (t(115) = 2.194; p = .030) compared to less frequently exercising adults (m=25.30; SE=.1004), revealing a small-to-medium effect, again missing the type II error mark (d = .409; (1–β) = 59%). As in the overall sample, perceived usefulness also increased Pro scores, but missed significance criteria as well (t(115) = 1.756; p = .082; d = .327; (1–β) = 42%).

3.8   Differences in Pro/Con in between Countries

Countries differed in several variables (see Fig. 10). Gender analysis revealed significant differences across countries (Welch's F(2, 81) = 3.841; p = .025), with Turkish males (m=25.39: SE=1.009) scoring lower than Polish males (m=28.75; SE=.727). This effect was mirrored on Con scores as well (F(2, 130) = 4.493; p = .013), with higher Con scores in Turkish males (m=18.93; SE=.808) and more reservation against medical technology than Polish (m=15.78; SE=.960) or German males (m=15.78; SE=.966), as alluded to by correlation analysis in Chapter 3.3.

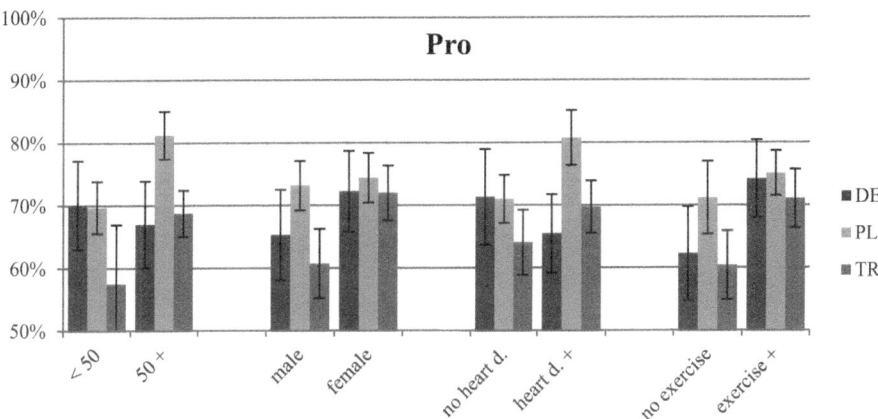

Fig. 10. Pro scores for medical technology (percent) by country (N_{DE}=72; N_{PL}=111; N_{TR}=117), compared by median-split of age, gender, heart disease and exercise. Error bars show 95% CI.

Of the two technology experience scales PEU and PU, only low PU had a difference across countries on Pro scores (Welch's F(2, 82) = 4.330; p = .016). Here, participants within the lower group of PU scores from Germany (m=26.09; SE=1.393) and Turkey (m=25.74; SE=.987) scored lower than participants in Poland (m=29.18; SE=.791).

Analysis of age by country showed significant main effects of age (F(1, 294) = 4.309; p = .39) and country (F(2, 294) = 5.699; p < .000). Fig. 11 shows that older adults alone differed very significantly in their Pro scores across countries (F(2, 168) = 4.851; p = .009), with older adults from Poland (m=30.93; SE=.697) scoring higher than those from Germany (m=27.08; SE=1.269) and Turkey (m=27.54; SE=.679). Participants with heart disease across countries showed the same effect (F(2, 111) = 5.144; p = .007), which may be due to the higher prevalence of heart disease in older adults (see Chapter 3.3). It is interesting to note that the apparent trend of participants in Poland and Turkey, to increase in Pro scores from younger to older adults, did not occur in Germany, although this interaction effect did not reach statistical significance (country*age: F(2, 294) = 2.152; p = .118). The same trend was observable in participants with heart disease, but the interaction also did not reach significance (country*heart disease: F(2, 294) = 2.057; p = .130).

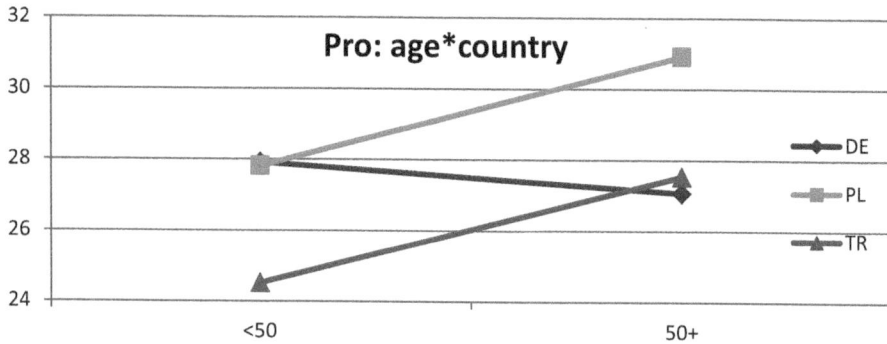

Fig. 11. Differences in Pro scores (absolute) for medical technology by country, compared by median-split of age (N_{DE}=72; N_{PL}=111; N_{TR}=117)

3.9   A Special Look at Gender and Heart Disease

As the previous results suggested that gender and chronic heart disease have significant effects on medical technology acceptance, a more detailed analysis is warranted. An analysis of gender and the technology variables PEU (Fig. 12, left) and PU (Fig. 12, right) again revealed significant main effects of gender ($F(1, 296)$ = 11.385; $p < .000$), but this time also PEU ($F(1, 296)$ = 6.446; $p = .012$), as well as a significant interactions of gender * PEU ($F(1, 296)$ = 6.491; $p = .011$). When graphing the results, it interesting to note that PEU had no effect on women's pro scores, but pro scores of males with low PEU ($m = 23.98$; $SE = 1.180$) were significantly lower than the scores of males with high PEU ($m = 28.76$; $SE = .599$). The exact duplicate effect was found when analyzing gender and PU, although the interaction of gender * PU was only marginally significant ($F(1, 296)$ = 2.931; $p = .088$).

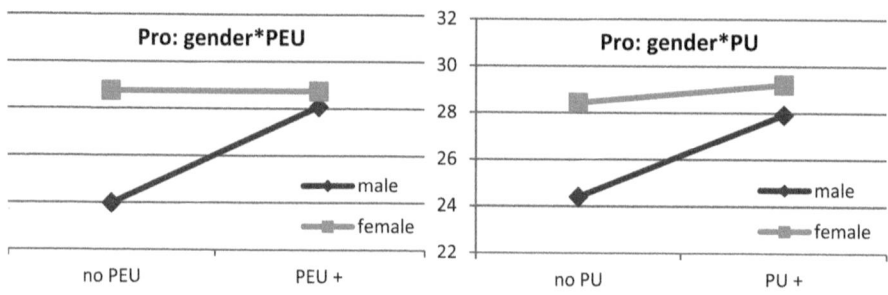

Fig. 12. Interaction graphs of (left) gender * PEU on Pro, and (right) of gender*PU on Pro

Exercising frequency also has an interesting gender component (Fig. 13, right). Again, both gender ($F(1, 296)$ = 6.920; $p = .009$) and exercise ($F(1, 296)$ = 9.725; $p = .002$) show significant main effects where again male's pro scores increased significantly from no exercise ($m = 24.55$; $SE = 1.012$) to exercising at least once per week ($m = 28.34$; $SE = .752$). The interaction gender * exercise missed marginal significance ($F(1, 296)$ = 2.572; $p = .110$). Comparing exercise and heart disease

(Fig. 13, left), exercising showed a significant main effect (F(1, 296) = 13.989; p < .000), but while there was no significant main effect of heart disease and only a marginally significant interaction heart disease * exercise (F(1, 296) = 2.776; p = .097), t-tests revealed (t(112) = 3.349; p < .000) that participants with heart disease that exercised regularly had significantly higher (m = 25.92; SE = .820) pro scores than those that exercised less than once per week (m = 30.35 ; SE = .632), revealing a large effect (d = .821; (1–β) = 99%).

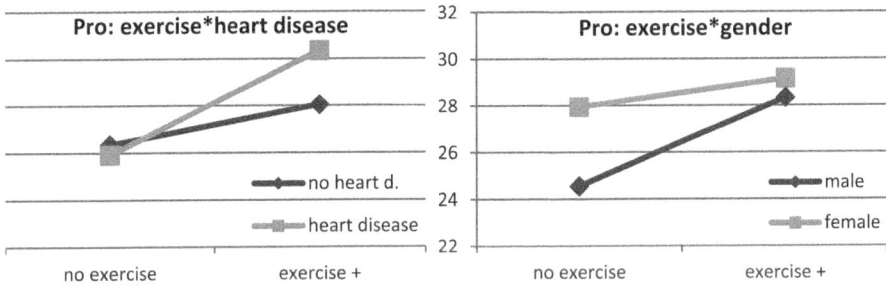

Fig. 13. Interactions of (left): exercise*heart disease on Pro, (right): exercise*gender on Pro

4 Discussion

The present study aimed to investigate the different acceptance factors for medical technology across countries from Europe to the Middle East. Differentiated by motives for use (Pro arguments) and usage barriers (Con arguments), the study analyzed the contributions of individual factors, such as age, gender, exercising frequency, as well as technology experience and chronic cardiovascular disease, on motives for using medical technology. Overall, a quite large group of 300 participants in all countries took part, with a wide age range (19-85 years) and gender equality (56% women). Also, 38% of participants (across countries) were reached in order to analyze the impact of health states on medical technology acceptance.

Before discussing the results, including the study's limitations and implications for future research, it is worthy to note that the acceptance of medical technology is a highly sensitive topic, touching on intimate and personal aspects, and is in many ways different from the usage and acceptance of ICT from the perspective of users, even though the underlying technology might be the very same [30]. Participants showed high interest in the topic as well as high willingness to participate and contribute to the understanding of medical technology, which was valid for all three countries. There was an increased awareness for the societal needs of medical technology and significant motivation to share one's opinions and fears. Apparently, questions about one's individual aging and potential confrontation with medical technology are topics that people are aware of and with which they are dealing thoroughly.

A first insight refers to an overall evaluation of the extent of medical technology acceptance. Results reveal a considerably higher willingness to use medical technology compared to perceived usage barriers, as is reflected by the Pro scores outweighing the Con scores about 7:3, independently of country of origin (even though the absolute extent of pro vs. con differed across cultures). Thus, the weighing of "more pro" than "con" using motivation can be referred to as a culture-unspecific and universal, respectively. It was furthermore reassuring to find that older participants scored equally well as younger participants. This may be due to the fact that older participants may need medical technology more than younger participants, increasing the perceived usefulness of medical technology [7], which in turn might positively influence acceptance scores. This was especially true in this study sample, since heart disease was more prevalent in older participants, and can be summarized in one participant's commentary:

"Having to cope with my chronic illnesses, I would like to point out that I'm looking forward to every device that could help ease my life."
- Turkish female, 74, suffering from diabetes and multiple heart diseases

In all results obtained in this study, most striking were the effects of gender and exercise on acceptance patterns. Women in particular displayed much higher acceptance of medical technology, although utilization barriers showed no gender effects. This suggests that while both males and females seem to share the same doubts, women are generally more open to medical technology than males. Male participant's acceptance (pro) scores did only catch up to women's scores when a) males exercise at least once per week, although exercising had a positive effect on women's pro scores as well, or b) when males, especially in Turkey, have high scores in PEU and PU. Generally, the effects of PEU and PU were weak overall, especially for women, mostly just affecting only young males. Even though the ender effect in this study was clear and showed a higher openness to use medical technology in female users, a cautionary note regards the "simplicity" of this outcome. Recent studies showed [3, 9] that women's higher openness to medical technology tilts over when not the general usage of medical technology but the acceptance of a specific medical technology has to be evaluated Women's positive attitude towards medical technology declines considerably when it comes to the question of accepting body near or even invasive medical technology (e.g. [9]), in which the perceived risk of physical harm is high. The same applies if a smart robot supporting medial care at home has to be evaluated ([3]): Whereas for both gender the usage motives as well as the usage barriers play an important role for explaining the intention to use a smart robot, women showed an overall lower acceptance to accept a technical device in the caring context at all. In addition, women's acceptance was moderated by age, showing that there is a greater difference in acceptance between younger and older women than it is within the group of men. Thus, gender effects seem to be a highly complex in the medical technology context, torn between gendered differences in social role taking, reluctance to take risks and technology affinity.

This again confirms that traditional acceptance models, like e.g. the TAM, cannot simply be translated and adopted for health related technologies [3, 4, 5, 6, 7, 8, 9].

Furthermore, it was quite unexpected to find such a profound impact of exercising frequency. With participants older than 50 years of age, or those participants suffering from a chronic heart disease, an exercising frequency of at least once per week significantly increased acceptance (pro) scores and reduced barriers (con). It would be interesting to study if this increase in pro and decrease in con scores is connected to a) the increase in mental capacity in older patients who exercise regularly [36], b) increased health awareness and consequently higher perceived usefulness of health related applications, c) personality traits, such as higher conscientiousness in the "big five" [37], or a mixture of all.

Based on these findings, the most receptive target demographic for medical technology products seem to be older women with a chronic cardiovascular condition that exercise regularly, especially in Poland.

Of the three countries studied, each has a unique history and current economical standing, and Poland and Turkey each show a special motivation towards technology, possibly due to wanting to close the economical gap to more developed countries [23], such as Germany. This difference might be reflected in the trend displayed in Fig. 11, where Polish and Turkish participants significantly increased in their acceptance of medical technology as they aged, which was absent in Germany. It is also interesting to note that Turkish participants generally show lower acceptance and more utilization barriers. It would be interesting to see if this might be based on religious aspects [14, 16], as in the following unique commentary (Turkish male, 57):

"I am a 57 year old Imam, who was ill only once in his life and who is still carrying the hepatitis B virus (1978). Since then I've always been healthy and have not visited a doctor ever again. I believe that an Imam has to be his own best doctor."

We should be aware that the claim for "universal access" and the overcoming of the "digital divide" always implies a specific cultural system. Since technology development and designs across countries are highly desirable but intricate on global markets, a deep understanding and appreciation of factors underlying technology acceptance, beyond national boundaries and cultural contexts, is of high importance.

5   Limitations of the Approach and Future Research Duties

Even though the present study revealed interesting insights into cultural facets of technology acceptance patterns, it - of course – can be only a glimpse into medical technology acceptance. We are definitely aware that, strictly speaking, "cultural effects" have been treated quite superficial in this study and this applies to the conceptualization, operationalization and analysis of cultural acceptance, given the many facts of underlying drivers within culture and technology utilization behaviors. Future studies will have to scrutinize the nature of the culturally formed acceptance, and some of the future research duties are shortly outlined here.

- So far, we only divided the sample according to "health" and a generic category of "heart diseased". Next studies will have to differentiate different forms and extents of heart diseases, and compare the acceptance patterns of heart-affected people to people suffering from other chronic illnesses. This would allow a deeper understanding if acceptance and coping strategies do follow a more universal "illness" pattern or, whether kind and form of chronic disease might impact acceptance differentially [38, 39].
- Another shortcoming regards the selection of countries and culture, respectively. Due to the personal family background of authors we selected these three

countries. We learned that there are large differences regarding the impact and value of family responsibility, commitment and care for the aged and chronically ill across the three countries [15]. Beyond the comparison of these three countries, a more detailed approach would be welcome that informs about the country specific ageing policy, ethical and societal values regarding illness and end of lives and the acceptance of medical technology as part of it.

- Also, the impact of the technical standard and technical development of a country is assumed to form acceptance for medical technology in addition [23]. Here, it would be insightful to include other countries that differ in their technical development (e.g. Nigeria [40] or Japan [41]).

- A next point addresses the type of medical technology, which was not yet differentially investigated in this study. Rather, "medical technology" was used quite generic. However, kind, type and specific characteristics of medical technology differ grossly, ranging from invasive medical technology (e.g. stent, [9]), medical technology implemented in clothes [9] up to mobile devices used in a medical context [30, 38, 39].

- The impact of gender [3,9] and religion [14, 16] with respect to the handling of body-related ethics are distinctive factors that should be further addressed.

Acknowledgements. Many thanks to the international respondents in Poland, Turkey, and Germany to openly participate in this research. Thanks also to three anonymous reviewers for their critical and constructive comments on an earlier version of this manuscript. This work was funded by the Excellence Initiative of German State and Federal Government.

References

1. Davis, F.D.: Perceived Usefulness, Perceived Ease of Use, and User Acceptance of Information Technology. MIS Quarterly 13, 319–337 (1989)
2. Venkatesh, V., Morris, M.G., Davis, G.B., Davis, F.D.: User acceptance of information technology: Toward a unified view. MIS Quarterly 27(3), 425–478 (2003)
3. Wilkowska, W., Gaul, S., Ziefle, M.: A Small but Significant Difference – The Role of Gender on Acceptance of Medical Assistive Technologies. In: Leitner, G., Hitz, M., Holzinger, A. (eds.) USAB 2010. LNCS, vol. 6389, pp. 82–100. Springer, Heidelberg (2010)
4. Wilkowska, W., Ziefle, M.: User diversity as a challenge for the integration of medical technology into future home environments. In: Ziefle, M., Röcker, C. (eds.) Human-Centred Design of eHealth Technologies, pp. 95–126. IGI Global, Hershey (2011)
5. Ziefle, M., Jakobs, E.-M.: New challenges in Human Computer Interaction: Strategic Directions and Interdisciplinary Trends. In: 4th International Conference on Competitive Manufacturing Technologies, pp. 389–398. University of Stellenbosch, South Africa (2010)
6. Arning, K., Ziefle, M.: Understanding differences in PDA acceptance and performance. Computers in Human Behaviour 23(6), 2904–2927 (2007)
7. Arning, K., Ziefle, M.: Different Perspectives on Technology Acceptance: The Role of Technology Type and Age. In: Holzinger, A., Miesenberger, K. (eds.) USAB 2009. LNCS, vol. 5889, pp. 20–41. Springer, Heidelberg (2009)
8. Gaul, S., Ziefle, M.: Smart Home Technologies: Insights into Generation-Specific Acceptance Motives. In: Holzinger, A., Miesenberger, K. (eds.) USAB 2009. LNCS, vol. 5889, pp. 312–332. Springer, Heidelberg (2009)

9. Ziefle, M., Schaar, A.K.: Gender differences in acceptance and attitudes towards an invasive medical stent. Electronic Journal of Health Informatics 6(2), e13, 1–18 (2011)
10. Tedre, M., Sutinen, E., Kähkönen, E., Kommers, P.: Ethnocomputing: ICT in cultural and social context. Communications of the ACM 49(1), 126–130 (2006)
11. Rogers, Y.: The Changing Face of Human-Computer Interaction in the Age of Ubiquitous Computing. In: Holzinger, A., Miesenberger, K. (eds.) USAB 2009. LNCS, vol. 5889, pp. 1–19. Springer, Heidelberg (2009)
12. Maguire, M., Osman, Z.: Designing for older and inexperienced mobile phone users. In: Stephanidis, C. (ed.) Universal Access in HCI: Inclusive Design in the Information Society, pp. 439–443. LEA, Mahwah (2003)
13. Straub, D., Keil, M., Brenner, W.: Testing the technology acceptance model across cultures: A three country study. Information & Management 33(1), 1–11 (1997)
14. Straub, D., Loch, K., Hill, C.: Transfer of Information technology to the Arab World: A test of Cultural influence modeling. In: Dadashuadeh, M. (ed.) Information Technology Management in Developing Countries, pp. 92–151. IRM Press, Hershey (2002)
15. Alagöz, F., Calero Valdez, A., Wilkowska, W., Ziefle, M., Dorner, S., Holzinger, A.: From Cloud Computing to Mobile Internet, From User Focus to Culture and Hedonism: The Crucible of Mobile Health Care and Wellness Applications. In: IEEE 5th International Conference on Pervasive Computing and Applications, pp. 38–45 (2010)
16. Teo, T., Su Luan, W., Sing, C.C.: A cross-cultural examination of the intention to use technology between Singaporean and Malaysian pre-service teachers: an application of the TAM. Educational Technology & Society 11(4), 265–280 (2008)
17. Arenas-Gaitána, J., Ramírez-Correab, P., Rondán-Cataluñaa, F.: Cross cultural analysis of the use and perceptions of web Based learning systems. Computers & Education 57(2), 1762–1774 (2011)
18. Srite, M., Karahanna, E.: The Role of Espoused National Cultural Values in Technology Acceptance. MIS Quarterly 30, 3 (2006)
19. Hofstede, G.: Culture's Consequences. In: International Differences in Work-Related Values. Sage, Beverly-Hills (1980)
20. Leidner, D., Kayworth, T.: A Review of Culture in Information Systems Research: Toward a Theory of Information Technology Culture Conflict. MIS Quarterly 30, 2 (2006)
21. Kedia, B., Bhagat, R.: Cultural Constraints on Transfer of Technology across Nations. Academy of Management Review 13(4), 471–559 (1988)
22. Choon, Y.-Y.: Cross-Cultural Issues in Human-Computer Interaction. In: Karwowski, W. (ed.) International Encyclopedia of Ergonomics and Human Factors, pp. 1063–1069. Taylor & Francis, London (2005)
23. Anandarajan, M., Igbaria, M., Anakwe, U.: IT acceptance in a less-developed country: a motivational factor perspective. International Journal of Information Management 22(1), 47–65 (2002)
24. Pai, F.-Y., Huang, K.: Applying the Technology Acceptance Model to the introduction of healthcare information systems. Technological Forecasting and Social Change 78(4), 650–660 (2011)
25. Campiniha-Bacote, J.: The Process of Cultural Competence in the delivery of Health care Services: A Model of Care. Journal of Transcultural Nursing 13(3), 181–184 (2002)
26. Klessig, J.: Cross-cultural Medicine A Decade Later. The Effect of Values and Culture on Life-Support Decisions. The Western Journal of Medicine 157, 316–322 (1992)
27. Searight, H., Gafford, J.: Cultural Diversity at the End of Life: Issues and Guidelines for Family Physicians. American Family Physician 71(3), 515–525 (2005)

28. Berger, J.T.: Cultural discrimination in mechanisms for health decisions: a view from New York. Journal of Clinical Ethics 9, 127–131 (1998)
29. Ziefle, M., Röcker, C., Holzinger, A.: Medical Technology in Smart Homes: Exploring the User's Perspective on Privacy, Intimacy and Trust. In: Proc. of the 3rd International IEEE Workshop on Security Aspects of Process and Services Engineering (SAPSE 2011), 35th Annual IEEE Computer Software and Applications Conference, Munich, Germany (2011)
30. Arning, K., Gaul, S., Ziefle, M.: "Same Same But Different". How Service Contexts of Mobile Technologies Shape Usage Motives and Barriers. In: Leitner, G., Hitz, M., Holzinger, A. (eds.) USAB 2010. LNCS, vol. 6389, pp. 34–54. Springer, Heidelberg (2010)
31. Oakes, W.: External validity and the use of real people as subjects. American Psychologist 27(7), 959–962 (1972)
32. Peterson, R.A.: On the use of college students in social science research: insights from a second-order meta-analysis. Journal of Consumer Research 28(3), 450–461 (2001)
33. Faul, F., Erdfelder, E., Buchner, A., Lang, A.-G.: Statistical power analyses using G*Power 3.1: Tests for correlation and regression analyses. Behavior Research Methods 41, 1149–1160 (2009)
34. Cohen, J.: Statistical Power Analysis for the Behavioral Sciences, 2nd edn. Lawrence Erlbaum Associates, Hillsdale (1988)
35. Ziefle, M.: The influence of user expertise and phone complexity on performance, ease of use and learnability of different mobile phones. Behaviour & Information Technology 21(5), 303–311 (2002)
36. Khatri, P., Blumenthal, J.A., Babyak, M.A., Craighead, W.E., Herman, S., Baldewicz, T., Madden, D.J., Doraiswamy, M., Waugh, R., Krishnan, K.R.: Effects of exercise training on cognitive functioning among depressed older men and women. Journal of Aging and Physical Activity 9(1), 43–57 (2001)
37. Digman, J.M.: Personality structure: Emergence of the five-factor model. Annual Review of Psychology 41, 417–440 (1990)
38. Calero Valdez, A., Ziefle, M., Alagöz, F., Holzinger, A.: Mental Models of Menu Structures in Diabetes Assistants. In: Miesenberger, K., Klaus, J., Zagler, W., Karshmer, A. (eds.) ICCHP 2010. LNCS, vol. 6180, pp. 584–591. Springer, Heidelberg (2010)
39. Calero Valdez, A., Ziefle, M., Horstmann, A., Herding, D., Schroeder, U.: Effects of Aging and Domain Knowledge on Usability in Small Screen Devices for Diabetes Patients. In: Holzinger, A., Miesenberger, K. (eds.) USAB 2009. LNCS, vol. 5889, pp. 366–386. Springer, Heidelberg (2009)
40. Chau, P.Y.K., Hu, P.J.H.: Investigating healthcare professionals' decisions to accept telemedicine technology: an empirical test of competing theories. Information & Management 39(4), 297–311 (2002)
41. Hassink, R.: Technology transfer infrastructures: Some lessons from experiences in Europe, the US and Japan. European Planning Studies 5(3), 351–370 (1997)
42. Alagöz, F., Wilkowska, W., Roefe, D., Klack, L., Ziefle, M., Schmitz-Rode, T.: Technik ohne Herz? Nutzungsmotive und Akzeptanzbarrieren medizintechnischer Systeme aus der Sicht von Kunstherzpatienten. In: Proceedings of the Third Ambient Assisted Living Conference (AAL 2010), January 26-27. VDE Verlag, Berlin, CD-ROM (2010)
43. Holzinger, A., Baernthaler, M., Pammer, W., Katz, H., Bjelic-Radisic, V., Ziefle, M.: Investigating paper vs. screen in real-life hospital workflows: Performance contradicts perceived superiority of paper in the user experience. Int. J. Hum.-Comput. Stud. 69(9), 563–570 (2011)
44. Holzinger, A., Searle, G., Wernbacher, M.: The effect of previous exposure to technology on acceptance and its importance in usability and accessibility engineering. Universal Access in the Information Society 10(3), 245–260 (2011)

Need for Usability and Wish for Mobility: Case Study of Client End Applications for Primary Healthcare Providers in Croatia

Mihael Kukec[1], Sandi Ljubic[2], and Vlado Glavinic[3]

[1] Polytechnic of Varazdin,
Jurja Krizanica 33, HR-42000 Varazdin, Croatia
`mihael.kukec@velv.hr`
[2] Faculty of Engineering, University of Rijeka,
Vukovarska 58, HR-51000 Rijeka, Croatia
`sandi.ljubic@riteh.hr`
[3] Faculty of Electrical Engineering and Computing, University of Zagreb,
Unska 3, HR-10000 Zagreb, Croatia
`vlado.glavinic@fer.hr`

Abstract. In the Croatian e-Health system, client end applications for primary healthcare providers must undergo the process of official approval. This process is based on verifying both content and format of messages used in client software for data exchange with the central part of the integral information system. However, there are no formal specifications, nor design guidelines concerning usability and overall user experience. In this paper, we reveal a number of UI usability issues in existing client applications that represent the source of enlarged interaction burden and user displeasure when working with client software. Furthermore, we propose a UI lightweight prototype model, based on both conducted investigation and well known usability guidelines, adding the value of its potentiality for usage in the mobile domain. End users supported our model design, by emphasizing its simplicity and better usability, as well as by showing eagerness for prototype implementation for mobile devices such as smartphones and/or tablets.

Keywords: e-health applications, usability, mobile applications.

1 Introduction

Rapid development of the communication-information infrastructure, along with the need for health record data exchange in both horizontal and vertical organizational direction, has made it possible to introduce new initiatives for the integrated health information systems. In the Republic of Croatia, the first comprehensive initiative related to such project implementation involved primary healthcare (PHC) offices only (dispensaries of general practitioners, pediatricians, and gynecologists).

A. Holzinger and K.-M. Simonic (Eds.): USAB 2011, LNCS 7058, pp. 171–190, 2011.
© Springer-Verlag Berlin Heidelberg 2011

As a result, the first version of the Croatian Primary Healthcare Information System (PHCIS) was developed, incorporating specifications and widely accepted standards for medical data logging, exchanging and securing, in a form of Electronic Health Records – EHRs [1, 2, 3]. This project represents the beginning of the era of applying e-health concepts in Croatian health data management.

Introducing e-health concepts is an ongoing procedure, with many business entities and partners gradually integrating into central system. Currently, alongside PHC practitioners and nurses, relevant applications are actively used within parties such as the National Health Insurance Company (HZZO) and the Public Health Institution (HZJZ), while pharmacies (e-prescriptions) and laboratories (e-ordering) represent recent and upcoming objectives (Figure 1).

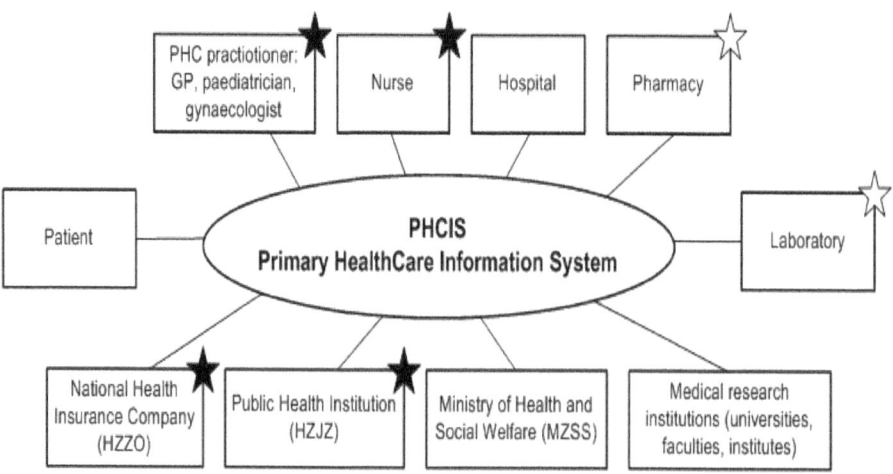

Fig. 1. Overview of possible users (business entities and partners) within the PHCIS system in the Republic of Croatia. Full stars represent entities involved in the first phase of system integration, while hollow ones represent units that are currently being introduced.

Figure 2 shows the PHCIS basic component and communication layout. The complete solution consists of the G1 system (PHCIS central part, including the PHC portal, the message management system and the relative registries), (a number of) G2 applications (which are the software for PHC practitioners), and the HL7v3 [4] international standard for medical data format and message exchange protocol. The company *Ericsson – Nikola Tesla* (ETK) was awarded the G1 component realization, while the implementation of G2 software(s) was offered to independent software providers on the Croatian market. In order to ease the implementation efforts of the autonomous providers, and to ensure HL7v3 compatibility, ETK released a special software interface for communication with the G1 infrastructure.

G2 applications (client-end applications for primary healthcare providers) must undergo the process of certification, where the final approval is granted by the Croatian Ministry of Health and Social Welfare (MZSS).

Certification criteria are focused on several issues, such as: (i) appropriate data structures associated to Reference Information Model (RIM) of the HL7 standard, (ii) suitable communication requirements for private data security, (iii) adequate XML messages format for data exchange, according to the relevant HL7-based XML schema, and (iv) satisfactory programming form and task flow adjusted with typical usage in medical domain [5, 6].

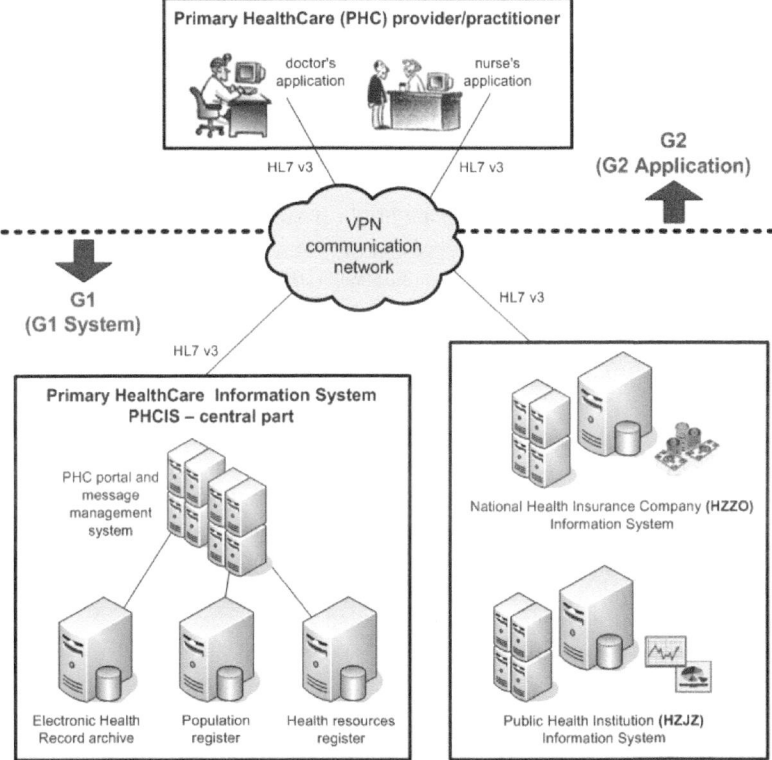

Fig. 2. Primary HealthCare Information System: the complete solution consists of the G1 system, a number of G2 applications, and the HL7v3 standard defining both data formats and the message exchange protocol.

However, there are no formal specifications, nor design guidelines concerning usability and overall user experience for G2 client end applications. Ergonomic factors, user interface design, interaction design, and usability in general are not encompassed by the certification procedure. This represents a big shortcoming in the overall process of e-health introduction, as end users are often left struggling with inconsistent interfaces and bad interaction designs.

Moreover, the current system is obviously undersupplied with respect to a suitable mobile context support. Although nowadays mobile technology upgrowth promises the introduction of a variety of mobile services, actual e-health system specifications are not dealing with the possibilities of involving m-health activities.

As personal mobile devices are becoming more pervasive and more powerful application platforms, it could be very useful and valuable to use them in particular primary healthcare procedures. A typical example of such a procedure is the doctor's home visit to a patient. Usually in such kind of context, every action in the characteristic task flow (opening patient's record, diagnosis recording, treatment and/or medication prescribing) is performed via paperwork, thus subsequently requiring the doctor to carry out some data synchronization with the software application (generally done by retyping some manual annotations). In such cases, appropriate mobile applications for smartphone and/or tablet devices, with data auto-synchronization feature, would be a great time-saver tool for efficiency enhancement. Certainly, the mobile application UI, as well as the overall mobile interaction design, should be implemented according the general principles of good usability and taking into consideration typical mobile device limitations.

In the following sections, we will highlight a number of UI usability issues in a typical client (G2) application that represent the source of enlarged interaction burden and user displeasure for the user. Alongside usability evaluation and analysis of such an application, we propose a lightweight prototype model of a mobile UI for a doctor's home visits (mobile) application.

2   Usability Issues in a G2 Application: Heuristic Evaluation

Usability is a term that collectively describes multiple components of user contentment in the course of interaction with the interface of computer software. A well known definition of usability by Nielsen explains usability as a multidimensional property of a user interface comprising the following five generally accepted attributes: (i) *learnability*, (ii) *efficiency*, (iii) *memorability*, (iv) *errors*, and (v) *satisfaction* [7]. A system that is "acceptable and easy to use for a particular class of users carrying out specific task in a specific environment" [8] should be very easy to learn, with a very steep learning curve (*learnability*), thus enabling the user to start producing results with the system in the earliest moment possible. Acquired knowledge of UI metaphors, symbols, and expected action results should be easy to recall after some period of time without the need to repeat the learning process (*memorability*). After the initial learning process has ended, the user must be able to achieve a high level of productivity (*efficiency*) and low error rate in the course of interaction with the system using the UI. If errors are made, the system must enable an easy recovery (*errors*). Overall, the system should give the user the impression of subjective *satisfaction*.

To ensure that a software project has an appropriate level of these essential usability characteristics, we can use methods that can be divided into two general groups: inspection methods (involving expert users) and test methods (involving test users in carefully prepared experiments) [8]. Following the concept of discount usability assessment [9, 10], we decided to perform a heuristic evaluation of a typical G2 application, including both domain experts (doctors and nurses that use this application on a regular basis) and usability/HCI experts. In this way, we intended to achieve a synergetic effect of multidimensional insight into existing usability issues within application representative use cases.

Final results of a heuristic evaluation always depend on a few experts' judgment of the application/system compliance with a particular set of generally formulated design guidelines (heuristics) in the specific context of use. Conclusions are therefore determined according to evaluators' experience and intuition. However, there is no unique consensus on general usability guidelines, resulting in many different sets of recommendations for designing systems with high level of usability. Consequently, a heuristic usability evaluation can be based on various well-known design principles, e.g. Hansen's (*principles for the design of interactive graphics systems*) [11], Shneiderman's (*eight golden rules of interface design*) [12], Nielsen's (*ten usability heuristics*) [13], Polson and Lewis' (*design for successful guessing*) [14], Gould's (*four principles of system design*) [15] or Norman's (*seven principles for transforming difficult tasks into simple ones*) [16]. Each one of these principle sets deals with particular characteristics of the target system/application (see Table 1).

Table 1. Well known design/usability heuristics and application/system characteristics that are covered by corresponding sets of principles

Application/system characteristic	Principle set (heuristics)					
	Hansen	Shneiderman	Nielsen	Polson & Lewis	Gould	Norman
Consistency	✓	✓	✓		✓	✓
Presentation convenience		✓	✓	✓	✓	✓
Error handling	✓	✓	✓	✓	✓	✓
Memory load reduction	✓	✓	✓		✓	✓
Task adequacy			✓	✓		✓
Shortcuts/accelerators		✓	✓			
Back way redirection		✓	✓		✓	
Help			✓		✓	

We decided to use Nielsen's usability heuristics, as it covers all of the significant aspects of application UI usability. The corresponding set of principles represents general guidelines for UI design, and thus can, without any restriction, be applied as an evaluation base for e-health application software.

As for the number of evaluators included in the application analysis, we used a relatively small set of experts (end users). According to [17], no less than 85% of all usability problems can be detected with only 5 users, while more recent research denote "10±2" as a general rule for the number of people required in a usability evaluation [18]. Therefore in our case, a total of 8 evaluators were included in the application inspection procedure, 5 of them being domain experts (familiar with medical terminology and usual primary healthcare datasets) and 3 of them being HCI professionals (with thorough understanding of usability matters). The latter were introduced with some basic task flow in the primary healthcare practice.

Evaluators were asked to fulfill several typical tasks via the application UI that correspond to real use cases: opening a health record database, finding the record for a particular patient, logging (writing) the examination outcomes - diagnosis, prescribing a medication, and ordering a laboratory test. Unlike domain professionals (doctors and nurses), usability experts are explicitly told to do some additional explanatory UI inspection. Upon completion of the application tasks, all users were presented with a heuristic evaluation questionnaire, containing altogether 17 questions derived from Nielsen's usability guidelines (Table 2). Discrete values (from 1 to 5) were expected as assigned answers on the semantic differential scale. In order to insure consistency throughout the questionnaire, each question started with same prefix ("In what extent..."). There was no time limit to complete the survey, but all evaluators managed to finish it within 30 minutes.

Table 2. Nielsen's ten usability heuristics - general principles for user interface design (H1-H10) along with questions for the evaluation survey (Q1-Q17) derived therefrom

H1 - Visibility of system status	The system should always keep users informed about what is going on, through appropriate feedback within reasonable time.
Q1: In what extent the user feels to have full control over the application behavior?	
H2 - Match between system and the real world	The system should speak the users' language, with words, phrases and concepts familiar to the user, rather than system-oriented terms. Follow real-world conventions, making information appear in a natural and logical order.
Q2: In what extent the user can understand phrases and messages shown within application interface? **Q3:** In what extent the used terminology is more computer-oriented than medicine-oriented?	
H3 - User control and freedom	Users often choose system functions by mistake and will need a clearly marked "emergency exit" to leave the unwanted state without having to go through an extended dialogue. Support undo and redo.
Q4: In what extent the user can easily (i.e. in a consistent way, and without unexpected consequences) abort the current activity through UI dialogues? **Q5:** In what extent the user can be redirected without trouble to a former abort point?	
H4 - Consistency and standards	Users should not have to wonder whether different words, situations, or actions mean the same thing. Follow platform conventions.
Q6: In what extent the application interface contains different terms and phrases for the same concept? **Q7:** In what extent the different application actions result with the same outcome?	
H5 - Error prevention	Even better than good error messages is a careful design which prevents a problem from occurring in the first place. Either eliminate error-prone conditions or check for them and present users with a confirmation option before they commit to the action.
Q8: In what extent the application help system supports the user by both indicating possible errors and trying to resolve them? **Q9:** In what extent the application can help the user to follow well-known procedures in primary healthcare tasks, without introducing unexpected errors?	
H6 - Recognition rather than recall	Minimize the user's memory load by making objects, actions, and options visible. The user should not have to remember information from one part of the dialogue to another. Instructions for use of the system should be visible or easily retrievable whenever appropriate.
Q10: In what extent the user has to temporarily stop and (re)consider the UI action/control to be activated? **Q11:** In what extent the application provides additional relevant information about the meaning of a particular UI element (e.g. through tooltip use)?	
H7 - Flexibility and efficiency of use	Accelerators -- unseen by the novice user -- may often speed up the interaction for the expert user such that the system can cater to both inexperienced and experienced users. Allow users to tailor frequent actions.

Table 2. (*continued*)

Q12: In what extent the user can use interface shortcuts (accelerator keys, automatic procedures) for frequently performed actions?	
H8 - Aesthetic and minimalist design	Dialogues should not contain information which is irrelevant or rarely needed. Every extra unit of information in a dialogue competes with the relevant units of information and diminishes their relative visibility.
Q13: In what extent the user interface increases visual complexity by imposing rarely required and irrelevant controls?	
H9 - Help users recognize, diagnose, and recover from errors	Error messages should be expressed in plain language (no codes), precisely indicate the problem, and constructively suggest a solution.
Q14: In what extent the user can understand the real meaning of the error messages? **Q15:** In what extent UI actions can result with unexpected outcomes with no error/warning messages?	
H10 - Help and documentation	Even though it is better if the system can be used without documentation, it may be necessary to provide help and documentation. Any such information should be easy to search, focused on the user's task, list concrete steps to be carried out, and not be too large.
Q16: In what extent the application can be used without any help (sub)system and/or user manuals? **Q17:** In what extent the user can easily find task-oriented information within available manuals and/or help system?	

Results thus obtained are shown in Table 3, where the last column marks questions whose answers indicate a higher discrepancy from "good usability". In general, we can infer that application usability is considered rather low, with distinguished flaws in the area of aesthetic and minimalist design, user control and freedom, flexibility and efficiency of use, metaphors, and help and documentation.

Table 3. Results of usability heuristics evaluation survey. Examinees 6, 7 and 8 are the HCI/usability experts, hence the extent of their overall application usage is not relevant. Up-arrows denote records where a higher value indicates better compliance to the usability guideline. Down-arrows indicate that a lower value conforms better to the particular principle.

Examinee	1	2	3	4	5	6	7	8	
Age	45	29	44	35	58	41	31	33	AVG = 39,50
Time period of overall application usage (months)	11	18	31	30	28	-	-	-	AVG = 23,60
Gender	F	F	F	F	M	F	M	M	

Question	Individual answers								AVG	↑↓	
Q1	2	4	3	4	3	3	2	3	**3,00**	↑	
Q2	3	4	3	4	4	4	3	4	**3,63**	↑	
Q3	3	3	4	5	5	4	5	3	**4,00**	↓	✗
Q4	2	2	3	2	3	2	2	1	**2,13**	↑	✗
Q5	3	2	4	2	3	2	2	2	**2,50**	↑	✗
Q6	2	3	4	3	2	2	3	2	**2,63**	↓	
Q7	1	2	2	2	1	2	2	3	**1,88**	↓	
Q8	3	3	3	2	3	4	5	4	**3,38**	↑	

Table 3. (*continued*)

Q9	2	3	2	3	3	3	4	4	3,00	↑	
Q10	3	3	3	3	3	3	4	3	3,13	↓	
Q11	1	2	2	2	2	2	3	2	2,00	↑	✗
Q12	2	2	3	3	2	1	2	1	2,00	↑	✗
Q13	3	2	1	2	3	1	2	1	1,89	↑	✗
Q14	3	3	3	2	4	3	2	3	2,88	↑	
Q15	3	3	4	2	3	3	4	2	3,00	↓	
Q16	2	3	2	2	3	2	2	2	2,25	↑	✗
Q17	2	2	3	3	2	2	2	2	2,25	↑	✗

Informal conversations with application end users (carried out after the evaluation) revealed general displeasure with the respective UI. While domain experts emphasized "fuzziness" in the UI layout, along with overwhelming window dialogues (especially at the beginning of the application usage), HCI experts were able to strictly point out some examples of bad design. In the next section, these application issues are explained in more detail, highlighting the main causes of poor usability as exposed by heuristic evaluation results.

3   Usability Issues in a G2 Application: Problem Analysis

In the evaluated application we can assume that problems related with usability are mainly inherited from the implementation approach. Since the G2 application certification process is primarily focused on data format (and data exchange) compliance, most of the UI dialog layouts appear like auto-generated entry forms and/or reports extracted from programmed dataset structures. Some UI elements (visual controls) even look identically to those used in database management systems. Obviously, such a data-driven approach (which binds complete datasets to a large number of UI controls) outweighs user-centered design principles if any at all were used. In such circumstances, there exists a considerable possibility for introduction of severe usability problems.

Regarding aesthetic and minimalist design (H8 – Q13), the related usability guidelines are consistently violated throughout the majority of UI dialogues. The example illustrated in Fig. 3 shows a UI dialogue snapshot within the process of generating medication prescription. A large number of very rarely used controls (labels, textboxes, and combo boxes) is always imaged on the screen, unnecessarily increasing the UI visual complexity. Domain experts claim that these controls are used in no more than 5% of all use cases. The related usability issue can easily be avoided by simple hiding the control set, and exposing only one "activate command" (e.g. a button) for displaying rarely used forms. Also, using the separate tab control for infrequently used fields would be an appropriate solution in this case.

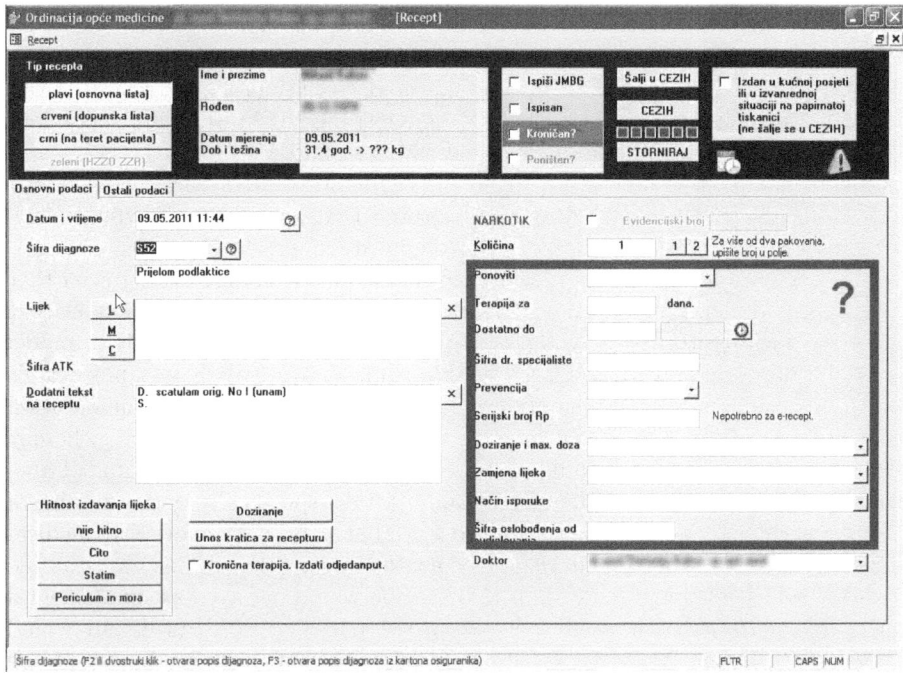

Fig. 3. Violation of aesthetic and minimalist design guidelines: snapshot of application UI dialogue for generating medication prescription

When it comes to user control and freedom (H3 – Q4, Q5), the application sometimes holds an inconsequent way of using the "exit" command. In general, the "emergency exit" should be used for leaving an unwanted state, and should additionally be clearly marked. However, Fig. 4 presents the case when the user has to confirm (save) the changes she/he made in the dialogue form, by explicitly calling the "exit" command. Absence of some kind of "save button" is unclear enough, but having to call from the context menu (otherwise not visible on the screen until an explicit mouse right-click) the "exit" command for saving changes furthermore spoils the situation. Such a procedure for an otherwise simple task is very confusing, leaving the user with a sense of loosing control over the application behavior. This especially holds when it comes to UI consistency since other dialogues use "exit" as a well-known action, without implicitly saving user data.

Concerning flexibility and efficiency of use (H7 – Q12), the application UI is lacking any shortcut commands. There exist no embedded procedures for distinguishing experienced and inexperienced users' interaction patterns. As a result, a more proficient user has no possibility to speed up the dialogue flow, nor she/he can customize any part of the user interface. A typical example where valuable efficiency enhancements could be obtained is shown in Fig. 5. Very often the user is required to

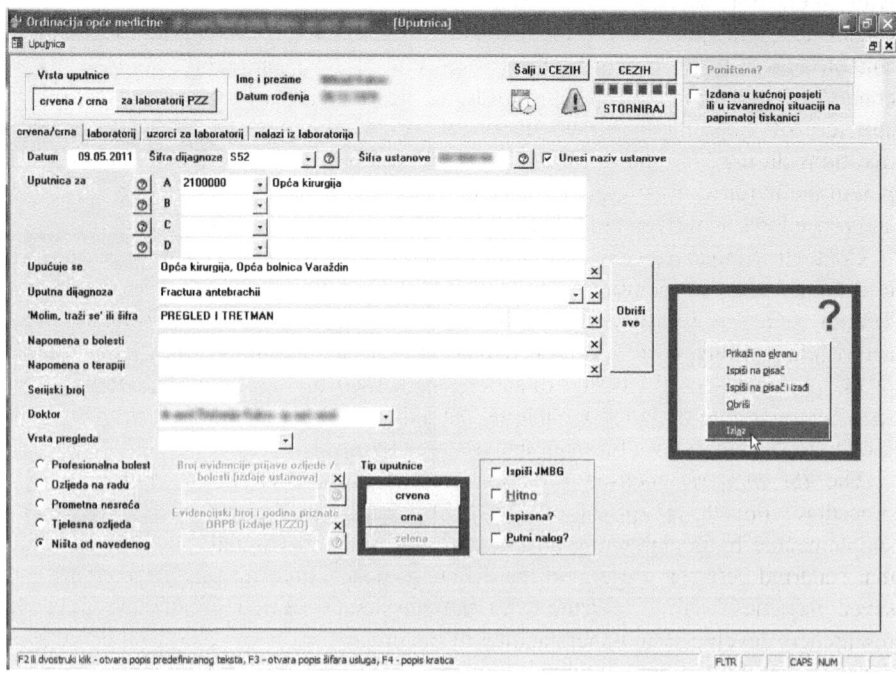

Fig. 4. Violation of user control and freedom guidelines: inconsequent use of the context menu "exit" command for input confirmation. This application snapshot shows the use case of ordering a patient for specialist treatment.

browse for a distinct item within extremely large drop-down lists and/or combo-boxes. This is regularly related to with searching through various medical registries (primary healthcare service types, diagnosis descriptions, medication codes etc.). Related tasks are time-consuming, as the user is distracted by a complete set of numerous options. For this purpose, involving algorithms for automatic menus personalization would be a great choice. Using both frequency-based and recency-based adaptive approaches, a user's prior navigation behavior can be taken into account, thus resulting with optimal items arrangement within large lists [19]. In this way, each individual user could easily find and activate her/his commonly used selections and could become much more efficient in comparison with currently implemented solutions.

Poor icon metaphors represent another application limitation in the terms of usability, where a number of principles is undermined (H2 – Q3, H6 – Q11). Since clear communication between the application and end user is critical to usability, the user needs to be able to immediately know what the icon represents. However, this is not the case in the example presented on Fig. 6.

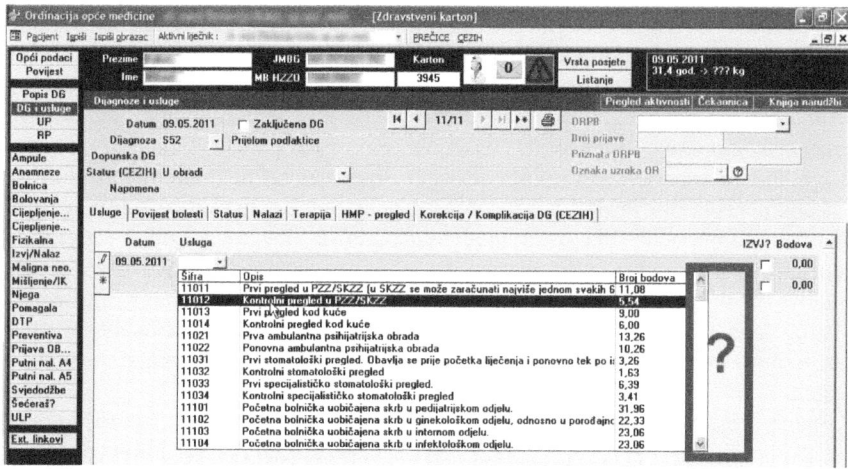

Fig. 5. Violation of flexibility and efficiency of use guidelines: there is no possibility (at all) for UI customization and/or adaptation. This snapshot presents the selection of primary healthcare service type provided to the patient.

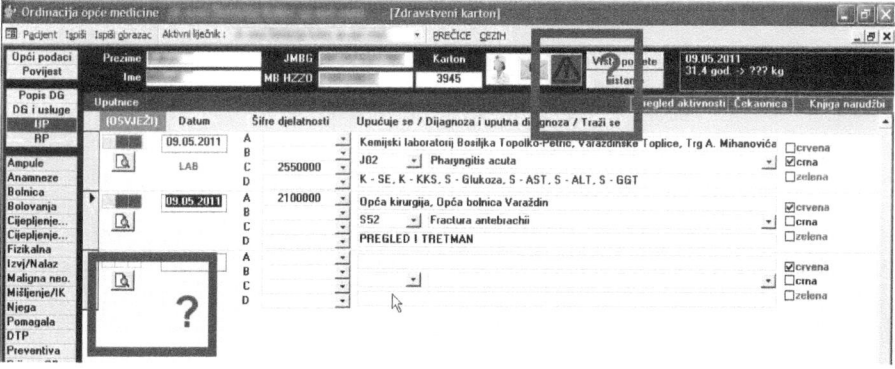

Fig. 6. Examples of poor icon metaphors and insufficient emphasis of significant information. The snapshot shows the use case of referring a patient to laboratory testing.

Although the magnifier icon usually stands for searching and/or zooming (at least in the majority of modern software interfaces), within the tested application it is unexpectedly used for starting a new record entry (in the process of referring the patient to laboratory test or specialist treatment). All of the domain experts highlighted this as a special distraction, especially at the beginning of the application usage. According to heuristic evaluation results, application's UI terminology (words, phrases, concepts) is often too computer-oriented, and when this terminology is furthermore used in a wrong way (as the magnifier icon case tackled above), usability can downsize rapidly. Obviously, the guidelines about matching the application presentation with real world concepts were not consistently applied.

The same UI dialogue can be additionally criticized from the standpoint of highlighting a very important information. The red warning icon (placed at the top of the window) indicates that a certain patient can have allergic reaction to some kind of medication substances. Wrong interpretation of this iconic symbol, or missing to perceive it, can have tremendous consequences for the patient. In such a case, the UI design should be oriented to put a stronger emphasis on related crucial information. Just another symbol in the three-icon toolbar is not a satisfactory solution, as there exist better approaches like using modal dialogs (for blocking all other activities until the user confirms a displayed warning message) or changing the palette of the entire window (background color and foreground font color). What is more surprising, the existing icon is not supplemented with any kind of additional relevant information (e.g. tooltip), hence users were forced to learn and recall the associated meaning from scratch.

Finally, results obtained from the heuristic evaluation revealed the need for a much better application help (sub)system. Even experienced users admitted that they sometimes have problems using the application without manual, underlining the rather low support for specific task-oriented questions.

System response time is another issue which is not closely related to UI design, but can also be a significant parameter of overall usability. Domain experts, who use the evaluated application on a regular basis, are very often irritated by the slow and time-consuming process of data synchronization with the central PHCIS server. Data exchange can last for more than half an hour, what results with end user's displeasure ranging from minor annoyance to severe frustration. However, this problem cannot be resolved on the interface design level because it concerns hardware and network issues, as well as the implementation of the central message management system.

Basing on both formal heuristic evaluation and informal discussions with application users, we can conclude that all of the abovementioned usability issues have a deep impact on users' dissatisfaction. The results obtained expose a low usability level of the G2 application, which can be directly related to the lack of user-centered design/implementation principles. Following well known usability guidelines, a number of issues thus discovered could be easily solved, making e-health software support more usable and, at the same time, also making end users more efficient, self-confident and satisfied.

4   Doctor's Home Visit: A Special Mobile Context

Home visits are an important part of general practitioners' (GPs) work as they can get more insight into a patient's general social and economic status, the status of her/his family, and the people that take care of him or her. Knowledge of surroundings and living conditions is an important factor in the general care of a patient. Moreover, home visits can be a part of necessary care for patients with mobility impairments or in situations when home surroundings can have positive effects on patients' health status. However, home visits are a specific part of GPs' work requiring them to use their knowledge and skills without support of instruments and technology possibly at disposal at their institution. In order to analyze this problem we have asked GPs and their supporting nurses and technicians about the general workflow of a home visit.

We have also especially investigated the role of the desktop computer stationed at their desks during preparations for home visit and after their return to the office. Before performing a home visit, GPs use the software system to access data about patients: they browse through patients' records and try to get a general picture of their latest status, prescribed treatments and medications. For many of their patients, a short overview of their records is sufficient to recollect important data. (Having, however, more than two thousand patients, GPs admit that as humans they are just not capable of being at any time fully aware of every patient's status [20].) During the home visit, GPs recall data gathered at their desks or use complementary aids in the form of additional printed documentation and their personal notes. Data collected during home visits and further records of prescribed treatments and medicaments is annotated as some kind of paper documentation. These notes are carried back to the desktop computer where everything has to be retyped/stored in the software system. Occasionally, although quite rarely, GPs memorize data produced during home visits, afterward inputting it without written notes, which are then created "post festum".

Considering all data and facts gathered from the interview with GPs we have carefully hinted them the possibility of using some kind of electronic device during the home visit, which will enable the access to (subsets of) data normally available only at the desktop level. At the first mention we have been faced with utter rejection of the notion: it was fully unacceptable to them to have a portable computer such as a laptop by their side during home visits. Laptops where described as heavy, awkward and slow, which GPs commented could just get in the way and slow them down. This latter is certainly true when waiting for the boot and loading processes to successfully conclude, in order to have just a glance at some small portion of data. Other than laptop form factor and the related loss of time, GPs were in general not very fond of the idea of having yet another system they must learn and use. However, they were intrigued by the possibility to have some important subset of patients' data readily available to them without previous preparation whenever they have to visit a patient at home. It was mentioned that a very helpful feature of such a system could be the exemption of having to retype data into stationary computer systems once back in the GP clinic.

Dismissing the idea of laptops as a support device during home visit, we have, yet again, very cautiously noted that there are devices that would much less get in the way but could nevertheless provide the necessary data, naturally hinting at touchscreen devices like mobile (smart)phones and tablets. This suggestion was partially accepted, in the first place because of the reduced form factor these devices exhibit, but raising anyway a number of questions and starting a vivid debate.

One part of our examinees have been instructed that the software they use at their desk computers is part of a complex system which includes many areas of computing technology; but the question of fitting such an elaborate system into the devices such as mobile phones was promptly answered by the other part of them which are incidentally happy smartphone users. These latter have promptly demonstrated how fast and easy is to use modern smartphones e.g. to find data on the Web, being additionally aware of mobile applications for personal use that enable health record management (e.g. Elevate Mobile's Online Health Portfolio service [21]). The overall conclusion of the group was that although such a solution appears to be technically possible, it needs further thorough investigation. I.e. the idea of having at hand a smartphone and/or tablet application enabling GPs to access patient records during home visit was interesting, however it was very hard for them to make any conclusion without actually using one in a real workset.

5   UI Prototype for GP Mobile Application

In this section we outline a user interface prototype intended to provide GPs with IT support when on a home visit. This prototype naturally follows from the information gathered in the brainstorming session, and is developed using some well-known HCI techniques for software and user interface validation [7, 8, 12, 22]: user interface mock-ups, paper prototyping [23] and storyboard scenario [24]. We reviewed similar cases as reported in the literature [25, 26, 27], concluding that these techniques would produce valuable data in a very resource efficient and time preserving way.

The most probable general scenario of a possible mobile application use during a home visit thus devised consists of the following tasks: (i) finding the patient in the patients list, (ii) opening and reviewing her/his latest medical records, (iii) finding and noting the current diagnosis in the list of World Health Organization International Statistical Classification of Diseases and Related Health Problems (WHO ICD) [28], (v) finding and noting the prescribed medicaments from WHO Anatomical Therapeutic Chemical Classification System (ATC) index [29], and (vi) reviewing the records created. Having defined the general user tasks, we have created six mock-ups, one for each defined task (Fig. 7 – Fig. 9), which we used as faithful representations for possible solutions to the above mentioned problems.

The prototype examinees were members of the group previously involved in the brainstorming session. We asked them, each separately, to set aside about 45 minutes for one final session where they will be presented the idea of a mobile client application supporting home visits.

5.1   Mobile Application UI Storyboard

The story presented to the examinees consists of tasks devised through analysis of data gathered from former evaluation sessions. The first task to be carried out in a real situation is to find the patient in consideration, which is explained in the first figure in the storyboard (Fig. 7 – left).

The user interface in this first mock-up (Fig. 7 – left) consists of three vertically placed parts: (i) buttons for selecting the age group, (ii) input boxes for entering the first name/surname, (iii) list of names sorted alphabetically. As previously already noted, GPs in Croatia can have more than two thousand patients, the UI for selecting the right patient has to support the user in narrowing down the list. During our previous interviews it came to our attention that doctors typically use age groups to

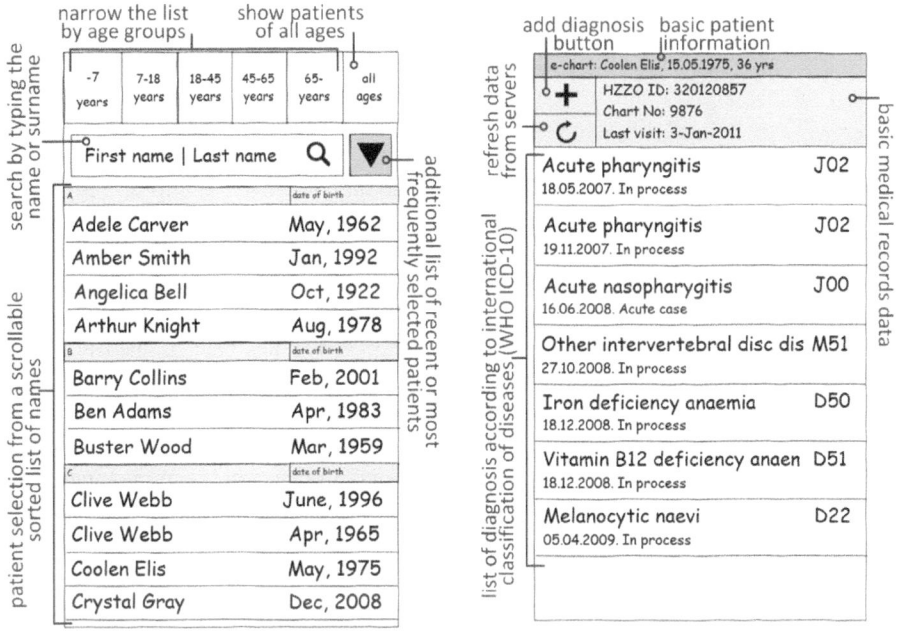

Fig. 7. LEFT: *Patient search screen* prototype. RIGHT: Screen showing patient's record.

distinguish between patients groups, and this almost intuitively, leading us to include UI elements to narrow the list of patients according to the age group. After this first step, the user can select a patient either from an alphabetically sorted list or it can further narrow down the list by typing the first letters of a patient's first name or surname. To be able to distinguish between patients with the same name, year and month of birth where included in the patients list. For cases where a doctor has to revisit patient records in the short time after having closed the list, there is a control which will open the list of both the recent and the most frequent patients. Names of selected patients are stored on a stack-like structure, where the latest selected name is put to the front of the list.

Selection of patient name is followed by the screen showing records consisting of patient's diagnosis, date of diagnosis and status of the case (Fig. 7 – right). This screen can be used to swiftly review a patient's status and her/his former diagnosis. The *Add Diagnosis* button is positioned in the upper left corner on the screen of the application; it is denoted with the plus icon which resembles the Red Cross sign and in the same time symbolizing addition of a new diagnosis.

The activation of the *Add Diagnosis* button opens the *Diagnosis search screen* (Fig. 8 – left); here the user (doctor) can select the code of the established diagnosis according to the WHO ICD index. The *Diagnosis search screen* consists of text entry fields enabling the user to enter keywords for finding both the appropriate diagnosis

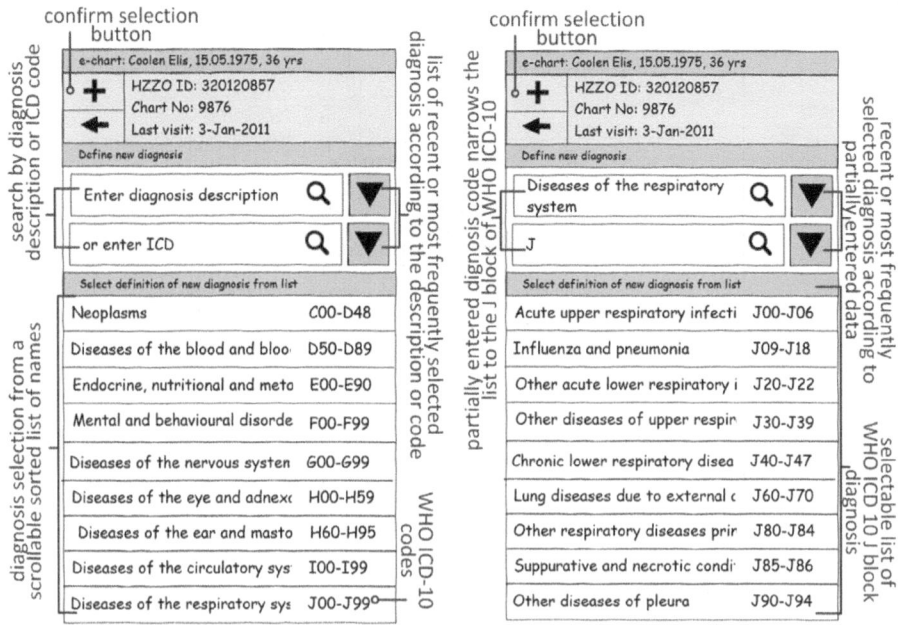

Fig. 8. LEFT: *Diagnosis search screen* showing top level of WHO ICD. RIGHT: *Diagnosis search screen*, ICD J level.

and the filtered list of possible diagnosis, which is displayed below the keyword entry fields. At the beginning, *Diagnosis search screen* shows the top level of the WHO ICD index, with every subsequently performed action leading to diagnosis refinement through a deeper "dive" into the WHO ICD index hierarchy, see Fig. 8 (right). Here the user entered the letter "J" as the diagnosis code, resulting in a narrowed view of the WHO ICD index localized to the J block. Furthermore, the user can select the first entry in the list ("Acute upper respiratory infections J00-J06") from the same screen, and eventually "Acute pharyngitis J02" thus completely defining the diagnosis. If in the process the user makes a mistake, the *Back button* represented by the back ("left") arrow icon can revert this action.

The next task in the storyboard is defining and annotating the prescribed medicament. The respective *Medicament search screen* (Fig. 9 – left) is very similar to the *Diagnosis search screen* as both have an identical layout, with UI elements used in the same way, thus following the UI development guideline of providing the user with consistent way to perform analogous actions. Finding the suitable medicament follows a series of actions as previously described in the process of finding the appropriate diagnosis. The difference between these screens consists in the latter displaying a filtered list of medicaments, with each entry comprising the WHO International Nonproprietary Name (INN), the defined daily dose (DDD), routes of administration (O – oral, P – parenteral, R – rectal, N – nasal, …) and the WHO ATC code.

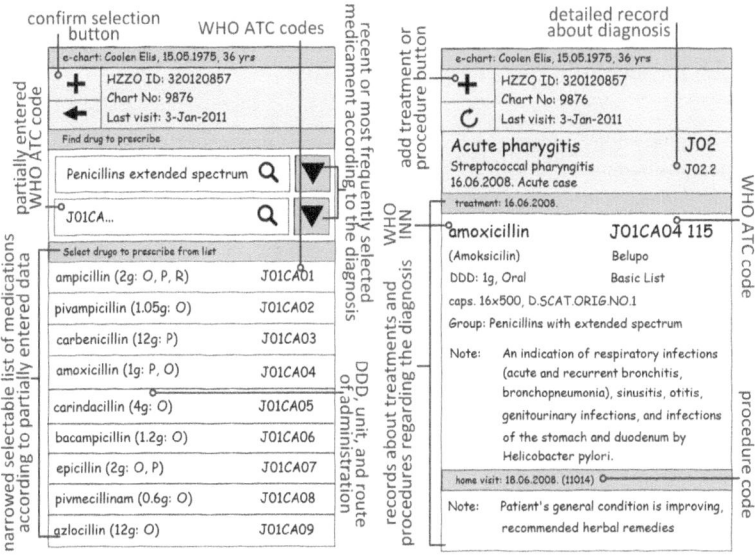

Fig. 9. LEFT: *Medicament search screen* with list of INNs, DDD and administration routes for every medicine. RIGHT: Overview of treatments for specific diagnosis.

Reviewing the created records is the final step in the storyboard. To give the user both the sense of control over the process and the chance to ponder on the changes made, the final storyboard screen (Fig. 9 – right) shows both data about the diagnosis defined and the medicaments prescribed.

5.2   Prototype Evaluation

Completing the storyboard, at the end of session with every of our examinees (GPs) we asked them to answer questions (listed in Table 4) about their general satisfaction with the demonstrated prototype. These questions were aiming at evaluating usefulness and efficiency of the prototype (Q1, Q5), its memorability and learnability (Q3) and examine the willingness to test (Q2) and use the real application (Q4).

Table 4. List of questions for the mobile GP prototype evaluation

Q1: Grade you perceived overall usefulness of the proposed solution.
Q2: Grade your willingness to test mobile application in real usage scenarios.
Q3: In what extent do you feel confident to repeat the demonstrated scenarios without any help?
Q4: Grade the possibility of mobile application replacing completely the notes written during home visits.
Q5: In what extent do you believe that this prototype implementation could raise your overall efficiency during home visits?

Results thus obtained (see Table 5) show general acceptance of the prototype, and even better, they demonstrate an almost full approval of the notion of mobile application for supporting GPs during home visits.

Table 5. Results obtained from prototype evaluation. Examinees responded to the question list with grades in the range of 1 to 5. Grade 1 denotes poor agreement with suggested statement, while grade 5 denotes full agreement with it.

Examinee		1	2	3	4	5	
Age		45	29	44	35	58	AVG = 42,20
Gender		F	F	F	F	M	
Previous experience with smartphones		Y	Y	Y	Y	Y	
Previous experience with touchscreen smartphones		Y	Y	Y	N	N	
Previous experience with tablet computers		N	N	N	Y	N	
Question	Individual answers						AVG
Q1	4	5	5	4	3		**4,20**
Q2	4	5	5	4	4		**4,40**
Q3	5	4	5	3	3		**4,00**
Q4	4	4	4	5	3		**4,00**
Q5	4	5	4	5	3		**4,20**
				AVG =			**4,16**

Although our examinee group cannot be regarded as a representative sample that would grant conclusive data on the introduction of mobile applications into the PHC software ecosystem, our evaluation shows a clear and positive attitude towards it, along with a willingness to proceed with further investigation of the matter.

It must be noted that thoughtful design of the prototype following the many usability guidelines has brought us positive results. All of the appointed grades in the final prototype evaluation are above 4.0, with the overall grade of 4.16 out of 5, thus backing our claim to consider the prototype a successful one.

6   Conclusion

In the process of introducing the e-health infrastructure together with its related services in the Republic of Croatia, disregard of user interface, interaction design as well as usability issues in both the official specifications and the G2 client application certification process resulted with implementations which are not based on the user-centered approach. Valuable benefits of the e-health concept are therefore diminished, as primary healthcare end users (especially general practitioners and nurses) must interact with software packages that are not fully tailored to their context and to their needs. Formal evaluation of an existing application for PHC providers, through assessing compliance to Nielsen's heuristics, shows that the related usability level is far from being ideal, hence justifying end users' general dissatisfaction with the provided software support. A number of usability issues (high visual complexity, inefficient selections, poor metaphors, confusing dialogue flow) has been identified as salient application features, forcing users to cope with inappropriate application interface on a daily basis.

Along with the need for much better usability in e-health solutions, PHC providers would benefit from a corresponding set of mobile services. Such an ambition for m-health support especially refers to doctors in the specific context of house visits, where there exists the possibility to employ to a full advantage existing powerful mobile devices such as smartphones and/or tablets. According to domain experts, an appropriate mobile application for managing patients' electronic records "on the move" would be a real efficiency booster.

Our lightweight mobile application UI prototype model is built using well-known usability guidelines, with special care to avoid typical bad design examples found within the desktop solution. Outcomes of the previously performed desktop software heuristic evaluation were very helpful in this process, along with our decision to perform participatory design by including end users in the prototyping process. The final version was considered as very promising, with a high level of simplicity and usability, hence making it a strong candidate to become one of the first initiatives for m-health support for PHC providers in our country.

Acknowledgments. This paper describes the results of research being carried out within the project 036-0361994-1995, as well as within the program 036-1994, both funded by the Ministry of Science, Education and Sports of the Republic of Croatia.

References

1. Erricson – Nikola Tesla, HR PCIS Functional Specification, http://www.cezih.hr/
2. Erricson – Nikola Tesla, HR PCIS Data Specification, http://www.cezih.hr/
3. Erricson – Nikola Tesla, HR PCIS Business Process, http://www.cezih.hr/
4. Health Level Seven International, HL7 Standards, http://www.hl7.org/
5. Erricson – Nikola Tesla, G2 System Requirements, http://www.cezih.hr/
6. Erricson – Nikola Tesla, G1 User Certification, http://www.cezih.hr/
7. Nielsen, J.: Usability Engineering. Morgan Kaufmann, San Francisco (1994)
8. Holzinger, A.: Usability Engineering for Software Developers. ACM Communications 48, 71–74 (2005)
9. Curtis, B., Nielsen, J.: Applying Discount Usability Engineering. IEEE Software 12, 98–100 (1995)
10. Nielsen, J.: Guerrilla HCI: Using Discount Usability Engineering to Penetrate the Intimidation Barrier. useit.com: Jakob Nielsen's Website (1994), http://www.useit.com/papers/guerrilla_hci.html
11. Hansen, W.J.: User Engineering Principles for Interactive Systems. In: Proc. Fall Joint Computer Conf (AFIPS 1971), pp. 523–532. ACM Press, NY (1971)
12. Shneiderman, B.: Designing the User Interface: Strategies for Effective Human-Computer Interaction, 3rd edn. Addison-Wesley, Boston (1997)
13. Nielsen, J.: Ten Usability Heuristics. useit.com: Jakob Nielsen's Website, http://www.useit.com/papers/heuristic/heuristic_list.html
14. Poison, P.G., Lewis, C.H.: Theory-based Design for Easily Learned Interfaces. Human-Computer Interaction 5, 191–220 (1990)

15. Gould, J.: How to Design Usable Systems. In: Helander, M. (ed.) Handbook of Human-Computer Interaction, Elsevier Science, Amsterdam (1988)
16. Norman, D.A.: The Psychology of Everyday Things. Basic Books, NY (1988)
17. Nielsen, J.: Why You Only Need to Test with 5 Users. Jakob Nielsen's Website (Alertbox), http://www.useit.com/alertbox/20000319.html
18. Hwang, W., Salvendy, G.: Number of People Required for Usability Evaluation; The 10±2 Rule. ACM Communication 53, 130–133 (2010)
19. Glavinic, V., Ljubic, S., Kukec, M.: On Efficiency of Adaptation Algorithms for Mobile Interfaces Navigation. In: Stephanidis, C. (ed.) UAHCI 2009. LNCS, vol. 5615, pp. 307–316. Springer, Heidelberg (2009)
20. Miller, G.A.: The Magical Number Seven, Plus or Minus Two: Some Limits on our Capacity for Processing Information. Psychological Review 63(2), 81–97 (1956)
21. Elevate Mobile Online Health Portfolio Web site, http://www.elevatemobile.com/products/products.html
22. Dumas, J., Redish, J.: A Practical Guide to Usability Testing. Intellect, Bristol (1999)
23. Snyder, C.: Paper Prototyping: The Fast and Easy Way to Design and Refine User Interfaces. Morgan Kaufmann, San Francisco (2003)
24. Quesenbery, W., Brooks, K.: Storytelling for User Experience: Crafting Stories for Better Design. Rosenfeld Media, New York (2010)
25. Holzinger, A., Hoeller, M., Bloice, M., Urlesberger, B.: Typical Problems with Developing Mobile Applications for Health Care: Some Lessons Learned from Developing User-Centered Mobile Applications in a Hospital Environment. In: Filipe, J., Marca, D.A., Shishkov, B., Sinderen, M. (eds.) International Conference on E-Business (ICE-B 2008), pp. 235–240. IEEE, Los Alamitos (2008)
26. Holzinger, A., Dorner, S., Födinger, M., Valdez, A.C., Ziefle, M.: Chances of Increasing Youth Health Awareness through Mobile Wellness Applications. In: Leitner, G., Hitz, M., Holzinger, A. (eds.) USAB 2010. LNCS, vol. 6389, pp. 71–81. Springer, Heidelberg (2010)
27. Verhoeven, F., van Gemert-Pijnen, J.: Discount User-Centered e-Health Design: A Quick-but-not-Dirty Method. In: Leitner, G., Hitz, M., Holzinger, A. (eds.) USAB 2010. LNCS, vol. 6389, pp. 101–123. Springer, Heidelberg (2010)
28. World Health Organization - International Classification of Diseases, http://www.who.int/classifications/icd/en/
29. World Health Organization – Collaborating Centre for Drug Statistics Methodology: ATC/DDD Index, http://www.whocc.no/atc_ddd_index/

The Prepared Partner: Can a Video Game Teach Labor and Childbirth Support Techniques?

Alexandra Holloway and Sri Kurniawan

Assistive Technology Lab, University of California, Santa Cruz
Santa Cruz, CA 95064, USA
{fire,srikur}@soe.ucsc.edu

Abstract. The experience of childbirth is highly individualized. Proper preparation and support before, during, and after the onset of labor is key to shortening labor, decreasing the need for interventions during labor, and ultimately increasing maternal happiness. This paper reports the evaluation of The Prepared Partner, a simple game with goals to introduce natural ways to help a woman in labor, and their effects on labor; to introduce the mechanics of labor and childbirth; to practice interacting with a woman in labor; and to simulate the stages of labor. The user evaluation of The Prepared Partner showed an overwhelming majority of positive responses to the subjective portion of the study, and showed participants performed significantly better on a post-test about labor and childbirth than on a pre-test ($p < 0.01$). Furthermore, labor support was a major theme in a write-in question about childbirth, thus highlighting the effectiveness of The Prepared Partner in introducing the profound need for supporting a woman throughout birth.

Keywords: games for health, childbirth, user study.

1 Motivation and Background

Childbirth is a subjective and multidimensional experience. No single specific technique or combination of interventions can help all women, or even the same woman throughout the entire labor experience [5]. Therefore, it can be difficult to learn all of these techniques through reading books and watching videos alone. Face-to-face childbirth preparation sessions can provide a more thorough education to help future parents increase their confidence and learn strategies to reduce stress and anxiety and to manage pain during the childbirth event [6]. However, at least 15% of parents do not attend these classes, and are at an increased risk for having a more complicated labor and delivery [16,23].

The experience of childbirth is affected by a woman's emotional, motivational, cognitive, social, and cultural circumstance [1]. Maternal anxiety is associated with a less positive childbirth experience, whereas maternal comfort and preparedness can lead to a positive experience [29]. One source of anxiety is that parents are often forced to make uninformed or poorly-informed decisions at critical times (e.g., method of labor induction, whether to perform a C-section,

A. Holzinger and K.-M. Simonic (Eds.): USAB 2011, LNCS 7058, pp. 191–210, 2011.

epidural administration) without understanding the risks and benefits of the various options. This is particularly dangerous when stress and pain can impede decision making ability. Unfortunately, inappropriate decisions, made by the parents or by medical personnel, can lead to issues as mild as frustration and discomfort and as severe as short- and long-term morbidity or even mortality for the mother and the baby [24]. Proper preparation and support before, during, and after the onset of labor is key to increasing the chance of a spontaneous labor [16], shortening the length of labor, decreasing the need for interventions during labor, and ultimately increasing maternal happiness [21].

To address the issue of the preparedness of first time parents, we developed The Prepared Partner, an educational video game about labor and childbirth.

Because The Prepared Partner is an online video game, it can be distributed to a much larger area and thereby can minimize the cost of sending human trainers, or the cost that the parents incur from paying for and traveling to conventional preparation classes. Additionally, the system is available 24 hours a day and thus allows single parents and parents with irregular work schedules to access the information at any time.

This paper presents The Prepared Partner, an educational video game about labor and childbirth. We evaluate results of a study assessing whether the system supports learning. Because literature suggests that fathers and birth partners need more support in labor and childbirth than was previously assumed [13], we target anyone with an interest in childbirth, including future mothers and birth partners.

We started The Prepared Partner with five main goals for the system. They are as follows [18,17].

1. To introduce natural coping mechanisms and their effects on labor,
2. To introduce the mechanics of labor and childbirth,
3. To train birth partners to help women in childbirth,
4. To practice interacting with a woman in labor, and
5. To simulate the stages of labor.

The focus of The Prepared Partner is not to advocate for natural childbirth. Instead, we only wish to prepare mothers and birth partners by providing a set of techniques that can be used during childbirth to help the mother through any pain and discomfort. Childbirth is a pivotal moment in many women's lives; women value a positive experience. Because women tend to feel more satisfied after a spontaneous, drug-free delivery [7], we aim to provide information about different natural techniques to help a woman in labor.

Childbirth is a sequence of unpredictable natural events, it is impossible to determine in advance how to help a woman in labor. Unlike reading a book or attending a childbirth class, The Prepared Partner rapidly exposes the player to an evolving, replayable simulation of the experience of labor and many different coping techniques. More scenarios are experienced in a dynamic way through The Prepared Partner gameplay than through reading books, watching videos, or attending childbirth class.

To assess the success of The Prepared Partner in achieving its intended goal, we performed a preliminary pilot study followed by a full study to measure whether players learned several key things about labor and childbirth and about natural coping mechanisms. Data were collected through an online survey. Closed- and open-ended questions were asked before and after the participants used the designed system. Due to the positive response of the pilot study, a full study of the learning assessment of the system was conducted.

The overwhelming majority of positive survey responses speaks to the success of The Prepared Partner as an enjoyable learning aid. We attribute its success to the close ties we had to both the childbirth professionals and the usability and game design experts during all stages of design and development of The Prepared Partner.

Several types of system evaluations were performed to assess the design of the system as well as the effectiveness of the system in informing the participants about natural coping mechanisms.

2   Relevant Work

Although a myriad of books is available on labor and childbirth [9,11,12,30], and childbirth preparation classes exist to educate and inform expectant parents and birth partners, childbirth-themed interactive media is limited in diversity and scope. Books have the advantage of being complete references, but they lack sensory immersion. With a book, the reader must split her mental efforts between learning the content and imagining the described scenario. In a video game, the scenario is described; the player no longer needs to imagine the scenario and is free to concentrate on the necessary action [10]. Furthermore, books, videos, and childbirth preparation classes are linear references. They show the same information each time the material is experienced; each time a book is re-read or a video is re-watched, the same information is presented in the same order. The Prepared Partner provides a different simulated childbirth experience and presentation of information with each invocation of the system.

Childbirth preparation classes are commonly used by expectant parents; however, parents under 25 years of age, parents who have not completed secondary education, single parents, parents coming from low income families and with no health insurance, parents living in rural areas, and public hospital clinic patients [23] are less likely to attend childbirth preparation classes and yet are at an increased risk for having a more complicated labor and delivery. Childbirth classes differ by instructor, setting, and method (e.g., Lamaze [22], Bradley [4], and Mongan methods [26]). Classes can be inaccessible for parents due to work schedule, travel, and finance reasons [16]; yet the Internet is one of the most influential resources for expectant parents [15]. For these reasons, we chose to deploy The Prepared Partner on the Internet.

Before designing and developing The Prepared Partner, we conducted thorough domain background research – an integral part of usability engineering as research must be completed before prototyping [19]. We read accounts of childbirth, or birth stories, in popular books suggested to expectant parents, and paid particular attention to information about the stages of labor, relaxation to reduce anxiety, natural techniques to deal with pain and discomfort associated with childbirth, and information about pharmacological options available to mothers in a hospital or birth center [9,11,12,30]. We attended a class for training doulas for their work in continuous support of women throughout labor, birth, and breastfeeding initiation. This class was a thorough introduction to the mechanics of labor, the emotional implications and effects on the woman in labor and her partner, the options available to the parents, and involved hands-on practice of dozens of natural coping mechanisms. We experienced childbirth first-hand and assisted one other woman in the birth of her child, and used these experiences to fuel our research.

Video games aimed at health-related change have produced desirable outcomes in players, from knowledge increase to behavior change [2], yet they should augment, not replace, clinical oversight [20]. Moreover, electronic games for health education produce positive results, including results related to health education [28]. Although books and other static media have the advantage of being complete references, they lack sensory immersion. With a book, the reader must split her mental efforts between learning the content and imagining the described scenario. In an electronic game, the scenario is described; the player no longer needs to imagine the scenario and is free to concentrate on the necessary action [10]. Furthermore, books, videos, and childbirth preparation classes are linear references. They show the same information each time the material is experienced; each time a book is re-read or a video is re-watched, the same information is presented in the same order. Serious games, which are video games with a specific purpose: to educate, train, inform [25], or persuade the player, on the other hand, provide a different simulated childbirth experience and presentation of information with each invocation of the system.

The constructivist view of player learning in games, which is frequently adopted by serious-games' designers and evaluators, postulates that games teach ideas rather than particular behaviors, and rules of play rather than principles [3]. Therefore, we believe that presenting an educational intervention about childbirth and labor through a video game, which teaches the rules and mechanics of the game's purpose (namely, childbirth mechanics and support), can result in desirable outcomes regarding the preparedness of mothers and their partners. Those playing the game can learn, as a result of interacting with the game mechanics, the progression of labor, the meaning of contractions, and the simple things one can do to support a woman in labor.

3   Game Mechanics

The game, shown in Figure 1, depicts Amanda in labor. The stages of labor progress in unpredictable ways and are generated procedurally, by a simple mathematical formula tying Amanda's overall well-being to her cervical dilation and other factors [18,17]. As the labor progresses, Amanda's overall well-being decreases at a rate proportional to her energy, physical support, cognitive support, and other internal factors. The player must keep her well-being level high by showing her coping mechanisms, altering her environment, and making educated choices about medical pain relief. The player is shown three action cards at a time. Each action card has a chance to increase or decrease the character's sense of emotional support, physical support, cognitive support, and the strength of her contractions; and these four attributes determine the character's hit-points, which are steadily decreasing. If the hit-points reach zero, the character is taken by the doctor and the player's role in supporting the mother is terminated. Otherwise, if the character passes through the pushing stage of labor successfully, she delivers her baby normally. The player's score increases with the character's dilation and with the help he or she offers her. There is a score bonus for delivering the baby normally.

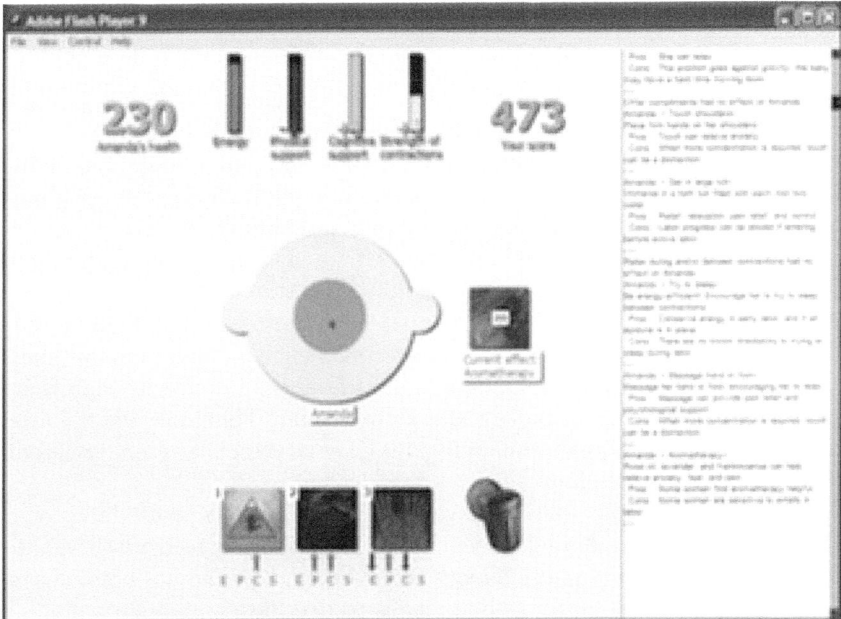

Fig. 1. Amanda is using aromatherapy in active labor as a natural pain relief measure. Available actions are visualization, stroking, and counting breaths.

4   Heuristic Evaluation

To receive early feedback about the system design, we conducted heuristics evaluation with five independent expert evaluators. We used an early version of the system for the heuristic evaluation, and modified the system in response to the evaluation results. A set of heuristics specifically designed for games and their playability was used [8]. The categories under evaluation were game play, game story, mechanics, and usability. Severity ratings were used as in Nielsen's heuristics method [27]. The minimum rating was 0, and the maximum rating was 4. The heuristic evaluation found a total of 73 issues; these are summarized in Table 1 and the highest scoring (worst) issues are reported below.

Table 1. Issues found by category and severity through five independent heuristic evaluations

Severity rating	Game play	Game story	Mechanics	Usability	Total
(1) Cosmetic, trivial	11 (40.74%)	5 (35.71%)	4 (44.44%)	10 (43.48%)	30 (41.10%)
(2) Minor	11 (40.74%)	6 (42.86%)	5 (55.56%)	6 (26.09%)	28 (38.36%)
(3) Major	2 (7.41%)	2 (14.29%)	0 (0.00%)	4 (17.39%)	8 (10.96%)
(4) Critical	3 (11.11%)	1 (7.14%)	0 (0.00%)	3 (13.04%)	7 (9.59%)
Total	27 (100%)	14 (100%)	9 (100%)	23 (100%)	73 (100%)

Game play. Game play heuristics include issues such as scoring, winning conditions, goals of the game, out-of-the-box experience, and challenges.

The game should give rewards that immerse the player more deeply in the game by increasing their capabilities (power-up), and expanding their ability to customize:(Score: 1.75) Evaluators were concerned that there were no power-ups in the game, nor any ability to customize. Mini-achievements were proposed but not implemented in the interests of time.

Pace the game to apply pressure but not frustrate the player. Vary the difficulty level so that the player has greater challenge as they develop mastery. Easy to learn, hard to master: (Score: 1.60) Evaluator concerns were that the game was easy to learn, but also too easy to master. This issue was resolved by tuning the game variables to quicken game play later in the game, yet leave the slow pace earlier in the game.

Player is taught skills early that you expect the players to use later, or right before the new skill is needed: (Score: 1.50) Evaluators agreed that the tutorial was effective in teaching the skills, but argued that skills did not provide enough information in how to accomplish the skills in real life.

Game story. The game story category assesses the player's mental and emotional involvement in the game.

The game transports the player into a level of personal involvement emotionally (e.g., scare, threat, thrill, reward, punishment) and viscerally (e.g., sounds of environment). (Score: 1.40) Comments from the evaluators listed an threat-to-reward imbalance, and a lack of immersion. To address this, we added a congratulatory reward screen at the end of the game which listed the player's accomplishments, score, and in-game statistics. We also added sounds — the name of the action is read aloud, and when the action is applied, the character in labor vocalizes a response to the action — and visual effects, such as bath tub water.

The Player has a sense of control over their character and is able to use tactics and strategies: (Score: 1.25) Comments from the evaluators listed an threat-to-reward imbalance, and a lack of immersion. Two of the five evaluators were concerned about the sense of strategy component of this heuristic. Initially, the player must experiment with the actions until the corresponding game mechanic is understood. We did not address this issue because we felt it to be more realistic. When helping a woman in labor, it is difficult to know in advance which actions will have a positive effect. We wanted to mimic this uncertainty in the game.

Player is interested in the characters because (1) they are like me; (2) they are interesting to me, (3) the characters develop as action occurs: (Score: 1.25) Two of the five evaluators felt no connection to the character in the game. Players of the game should have some interest in childbirth to really connect with the character.

Mechanics. The set of mechanics heuristics refers to the controls for the game, the learning curve, and underlying mechanics including score reporting.

Game should react in a consistent, challenging, and exciting way to the player's actions (e.g., appropriate music with the action). (Score: 1.20) As with the corresponding Game Story heuristic, sound was added to the game. Mousing-over the actions caused the action name to be read, and applying the action to the character caused the character to respond vocally (e.g., the *sing* action caused the character to sing). Visual assets were added where appropriate (e.g., *take a bath* filled the screen with water for the duration of the action; *dim lights* darkened the screen's background).

Usability. The usability heuristics refer to the non-game aspects of the player experience, including menus, manuals and help, feedback, art, and generally how easy it is to understand and interact with the game.

The Player can easily turn the game off and on, and be able to save games in different states. (Score: 2.60) Evaluators were concerned that there was no way to pause; the only way to turn the game off was to close the browser or Flash Player window; the only way to turn the game on was to reload the browser window or reload the Flash file. In response, we implemented a replay option after the game is over. We did not add pausing capabilities.

Players should be given context sensitive help while playing so that they do not get stuck or have to rely on a manual. (Score: 1.60) Although help was available on the action cards (including the pro and con of applying each action and its effect on each of the character's stats), evaluators were concerned that it was not clear how to help the woman, and certain game assets (such as the trash can) were not explained. We added the unexplained items to the tutorial.

Make the menu layers well-organized and minimalist to the extent the menu options are intuitive. (Score: 1.60) Initially, there was no menu option; we added a menu with a large *Play* button to make the only option very clear.

5   Learning Assessment

To test the efficacy of the system in teaching about ways to support a woman in childbirth, as well as whether the player learned some key facts about the mechanics of labor and birth, we recruited participants for a remote play-test of the system. We used a standard pre-test—intervention—post-test format for the assessment, and included a survey to gauge the player's playing and learning experience in interacting with The Prepared Partner.

Although we did not state any age restriction, if participants were under age 18, their data were deleted (as our Human Subjects approval did not cover those under 18 years old). We purposely did not limit the age as the study had a drawing for a US$25 gift card, and we did not want participants to lie about their age for the purpose of participating in the drawing.

5.1   Pilot Study Summary

We recruited seven participants for a pilot study of the system. The participants were recruited from a liberal arts college. All participants were females between the ages of 19 and 26 years old.

The pilot study was conducted over the Internet. In this study, the participants first answered a demographics survey, followed by a survey about video game habits and preferences. They then took a brief pre-test about labor and childbirth (for all the subsequent analysis, this test is referred to as pre-test). Next, the participants played The Prepared Partner at least twice. At the conclusion of the play, the participants took a brief post-test, where questions were either identical to the pre-test with answer choices randomized, or of similar difficulty and subject matter to pre-test questions. Finally, participants answered exit survey questions. The study took between 30 to 45 minutes.

One of the reasons for the pilot study was to determine the effectiveness of the test questions in gauging learning. Each portion of the test (pre and post) was split into three parts: multiple-choice questions about the mechanics of labor, a short-answer question asking for five ways to help a woman in labor without using drugs, and long-answer questions tying the game mechanic to natural support methods.

Pilot study results indicated that the second part of the test (the short-answer question) failed to measure learning. However, the test as a whole, as well as the first and third parts individually, did show a difference that we considered would be statistically significant given a large enough sample set. Hence, for the full study, we modified the second portion of the test.

Due to the positive results in the pilot study, we conducted a full study to assess The Prepared Partner as an enjoyable learning experience. The following sections describe the full study.

5.2   Participants

Participants were recruited for the study by e-mail announcement, through social networking sites, with online communication aids, and through a video game online community called Quarter To Three forums[1].

Though 90 participants began the survey (including completing the pre-test), 24 did not complete The Prepared Partner playthrough. Of these 66, 15 did not complete the post-test. Hence, only 51 participants completed all portions of the study, including the pre-test, the game, and the post-test and survey.

Ages ranged from 19 to 43 years with a mean age of 30. More than half (54%) of the participants identified as being married and/or a member of an unmarried couple. The remaining 46% were single, separated, or divorced. The median education level among participants was four-year college graduate (43% of participants). Less than a quarter (23%) of participants had either given birth, or helped wife or partner give birth. About half (47%) of participants stated no prior experience with childbirth. Finally, more than half (51%) of the participants marked that they play video games daily with the most common duration of gameplay between one and three hours.

Because of the nature of the advertisement for the study, 80% (N=36) of the participants were male, 25% (N=13) were female, and two participants declined to state their gender.

The large sample of male participants is not a problem because The Prepared Partner aims to reach future birth partners; in today's birthing climate, most birth partners are the expectant fathers and hence the large sample of male participants captures the target audience. However, more participants in this study have a four-year college degree than the average American. According to the US Census data from 2009, only 27.7% of people in the US attaining a Bachelor's degree. Hence, our sample set was not representative of the general population.

5.3   Stimulus and Procedure

The stimulus was The Prepared Partner: a game in Macromedia Flash and requiring Macromedia Flash Player 9 or higher. The learning assessment was conducted remotely. Estimated time from beginning to end of the study was 30 to 45 minutes.

Participants first answered a demographic survey, followed by a survey about video game habits and preferences. Participants took a brief pre-test about labor and childbirth. The pre-test consisted of multiple-choice questions, a long-answer question, and a series of short-answer questions tying the game mechanic to the player's understanding of labor support. Next, participants were instructed to play The Prepared Partner at least twice. Participants took another brief test (post-test) about labor and childbirth. Questions were either identical to the pre-test with answer choices randomized, or of similar difficulty and subject matter

---

[1] Quarter To Three: http://quartertothree.com

to pre-test questions. Finally, participants answered exit survey questions about their learning and playing experience.

Long-answer survey questions provided qualitative results. Quantitative performance measurements included each player's game score, number of successful and failed actions, and amount of time spent in each stage of labor, as reported by The Prepared Partner. Survey responses were on a 5-point Likert scale. Quantitative measures were linked to qualitative measures by a unique invitation code identifier.

5.4   Hypothesis

We state the hypothesis for the study below.

H1/0 There is no difference in aggregate pre-test and post-test scores.
H1 Aggregate post-test scores are different than the pre-test scores.

5.5   Test Scoring

The pre- and post-tests were scored both human and machine-scored. Multiple-choice answers were machine-scored and write-in answers were human-scored by a professional birth doula who has extensive domain knowledge, having undergone approved childbirth education and specific workshops dedicated to labor support. Write-in answers were scored liberally, with almost any answer accepted. Answers which expressed not understanding the question or not knowing the answer (such as "I don't know") were not accepted. Each correct answer was awarded one point.

For the long answer question, *How can you help a woman in labor without using drugs? Name as many ways as you can. Please separate each answer with a comma (,)* a computer counted the number of distinct answers separated by commas and awarded the number of points equal to the number of answers. This is because one could argue that nearly anything can be helpful, given the appropriate circumstance.

For the short answer questions, the scoring was as follows.

What is one thing you can do as birth partner to speed up labor, or increase the strength of labor contractions? Almost any answer was accepted, including clearly correct answers such as "walk around," "change position," and "have sex with your partner." Questionable answers such as "tickling" and "tell her to push" were accepted as well. Clearly incorrect answers such as "scare her witless" and "You can't do anything to speed up labor" were not accepted.

What is one thing you can do as a birth partner to help a woman in labor gain energy? Clearly correct answers included "feed her," "Make sure she is eating and drinking, allowing her to rest and sleep as much as possible," and "hold her up." All answers were accepted; there were no clearly incorrect answers.

What is one thing you can do as a birth partner to help a woman in labor feel more physically supported? Any answer was accepted, including clearly correct answers such as "hold her hand," "push on her back during contractions," "sit behind her," and answers such as "make sure she has clean sheets." Only one person answered, on the post-test, "give her pain killers." This answer was accepted, though it was contrary to the goal of the exercise, which was to name natural support methods.

What is one thing you can do as a birth partner to help a woman in labor feel mentally, or cognitively, supported? Any answer was accepted, including clearly correct answers such as "talk to her," "encourage her," and "meditation or hypnosis."

6   Results and Discussion

The following sections describe the result of the learning assessment of The Prepared Partner, and the discussion surrounding the data.

Learning outcomes. The Prepared Partner was formally evaluated by the 51 participants who participated in the study in its entirety: a combination of mothers, birth partners, and those that have never had children. The average score on the pre-test was 7.49 ($s = 7.13$), while the mean score on the post-test was 11.08 ($s = 7.50$). That is, participants had an average of 3.59 more correct answers to the questions on the post-test compared to the pre-test. Paired-samples t-test showed that the difference between the pre-and post-scores was significant ($t = 3.622$, df= 50, $p = 0.001$, two-tailed), and this result is depicted graphically in Figure 2. This significant difference indicates rejection of the null hypothesis **H1/0**, indicating that the increase in test scores is not due to chance variation, but can be attributed to playing The Prepared Partner.

Pre-test scores were normally distributed but skewed towards lower scores. Post-test scores were close to bimodal with modes at around 5 and 17. A difference of 3.59 correct answers gives an effect size of about 0.5, which is considered a large difference effect.

Interestingly, there was a difference in pre-test score by gender, with women outperforming men ($t = -2.185$, df= 16.276, $p = 0.044$, two-tailed). In fact, women scored 5.7 points higher than men on the pre-test, with a large difference effect (0.6). For the post-test, although women's scores were higher than men's, here was no significant difference. The reader is encouraged to study Figure 3.

Players of The Prepared Partner answered with more breadth and confidence in the short-answer portion of the test. When asked how to speed up labor naturally, participants answered with more concrete actions such as "intimacy," "take a bath," "apply pressure to the lower back," and "acupressure." On the pre-test answers were generally more vague and several participants included question marks in their answers, indicating uncertainty. When asked how to help a mother re-energize in labor, on the post-test, most participants answered with a variation of "feed her" and far fewer respondents left the question blank. Finally, participants answered with a broader range of cognitive support methods on the post-test than the pre-test, most of which were presented in the game.

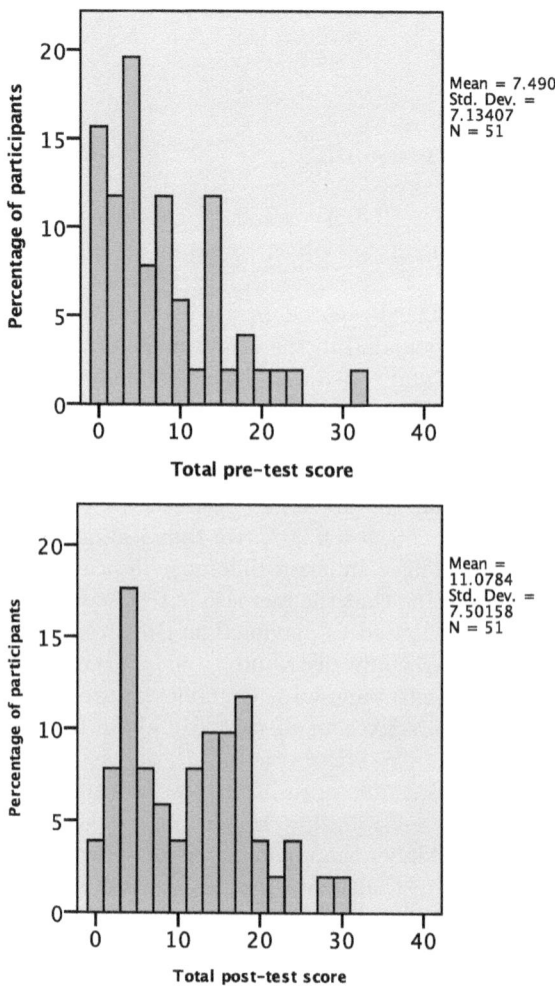

Fig. 2. Pre-test score and post-test score distributions: Difference in mean scores was 3.59 ($p < 0.01$) with a large difference effect. A score of zero implies either all incorrect answers, or all pre-test answers left blank.

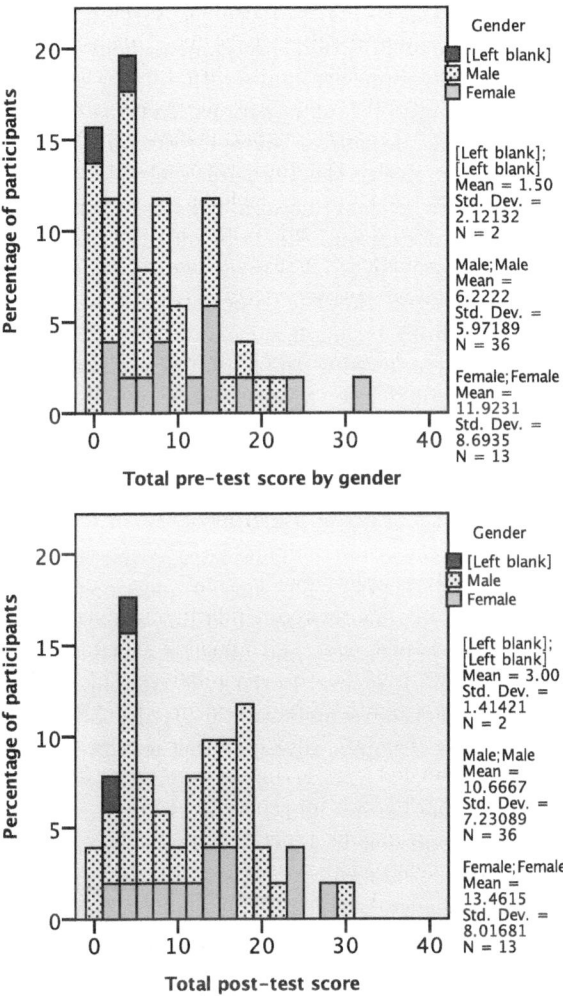

Fig. 3. Pre-test score distributions by gender. Two participants declined to state their gender. A score of zero implies either all incorrect answers, or all answers left blank.

Game results. Participants were instructed to play The Prepared Partner at least twice, thus leaving the total number of games played up to the individual participant. As the study was remote, it was impossible to control for the number of games played, though we did keep track of this number per participant. The 51 respondents that played and correctly completed the post-test played a grand total of 122 games; the mean number of games played was 2.08, with a minimum of 1 and maximum of 7 games.

Players used an average of 20 actions per game to help the character in labor, thus exploring 40% of the actions available to the player by the game mechanic, as the game afforded around 50 unique actions. Actions included massage, hydrotherapy (immersion in the tub or shower), distraction, visualization, and position change. In all but five of the 122 games' births, the player was present for the delivery of the baby. In the remaining five (less than 5% of all games), the mother was taken by the doctor and the game ended with a birth by C-section. As the average C-section rate in the US is over 30% [14], our game results may indicate one of the following. Either the game was perceived as too easy, and the game metrics need fine-tuning to increase the difficulty of delivering a baby normally (though this is contradicted in the survey responses), or the game shows that helping a woman through the stages of labor greatly decreases her risk of C-section. This is corroborated by research; Klaus, et al. found that having a doula, or a woman in a role of professional support for the woman in labor, can decrease the C-section rate by up to 50% [21].

Survey responses. We asked participants survey questions about their experience with The Prepared Partner. The survey questions were split into three sections: questions about the participant's learning experience, questions about the participant's playing experience, and questions about the player's view of the game mechanics in The Prepared Partner. Participants were asked to mark their level of agreement or disagreement on a five-point Likert scale to questions in each category (strongly disagree, disagree, neither agree nor disagree, agree, strongly agree).

Ten participants left the survey blank altogether. The remaining 41 participants' answers are summarized in Figure 4, Figure 5, and Figure 6, for the learning, playing, and mechanics questions, respectively.

For the learning experience (Figure 4), 69% (N=35) participants agreed or strongly agreed that they learned about labor and childbirth by participating in this study, 61% (N=31) participants agreed or strongly agreed that they learned five natural ways to help a woman in labor, and a majority (53%, N=27) of participants agreed or strongly agreed that they felt more prepared for childbirth than before participating in the study. The positive replies corroborate the quantitative evidence of learning on the labor and childbirth test as well as the qualitative evidence given by the write-in questions. That the majority of respondents both felt that they learned something, and actually learned something as measured on a test, is encouraging for The Prepared Partner.

A low percentage (37% N=19) of participants agreed or strongly agreed that they understood the stages of labor. This may be explained by the large percentage (47%) of the participants claiming no prior experience with childbirth, and corroborated by the conflicting feelings in the describing birth portion of the survey (see below). Those that have not had any prior exposure to childbirth may have found the game educational yet insufficient to thoroughly prepare them for what they may know of childbirth from other sources.

Finally, 67% (N=34) of participants agreed or strongly agreed that they had a positive learning experience as a result of playing The Prepared Partner. One participant wrote:

> My own childbirth experience involved induced labor, an epidural and a c-section, so I do feel like I learned about something that I know very little about (i.e. natural childbirth).

Another participant added, "I now know how very unprepared I am!"

For the playing experience (Figure 5), participants agreed or strongly agreed that The Prepared Partner was enjoyable and fun (63%, N=32), engaging (67%, N=34), interesting (64%, N=33), enjoyable to replay (55%, N=27), and 61% (N=31) of the participants would recommend The Prepared Partner to a friend. Most (62%, N=32) participants agreed or strongly agreed that they had a positive overall playing experience.

To gauge participant reactions to the game's mechanics, we asked five questions about perceptions of the game (Figure 6). Unfortunately, only 30% of participants (N=15) felt some degree of connection to the character representing the woman in labor, whereas 25% of participants neither agreed nor disagreed with their sense of connection, and 22% disagreed or strongly disagreed about feeling connected. This result was expected based on earlier heuristic evaluation results and may be a consequence of the abstract, conceptual representation of the woman [17]. Next, 45% (N=23) of participants agreed or strongly agreed that there were multiple ways to win the game, which highlights the emergent, non-scripted gameplay experience. Regarding the pace of the game, 34% (N=18) disagreed or strongly disagreed that the game went too fast, and 43% (N=22) agreed or strongly agreed that the pace of the game was varied.

Describing birth. Finally, we asked participants, *How would you describe the process of labor and childbirth to a friend?* To explore the topic, two independent researchers extracted themes from the written answers. Common themes were labor support, with sub-themes methods of support and the mother's need for support in labor; a description of the stages of labor, with sub-themes natural process and medical description of birth; and conflicting emotions as felt by the birth partner. Responses were evenly mixed between describing birth as a natural process and one that requires a doctor-led medical influence. An example of the *conflicting emotions* and *labor support* themes is found in the following response.

> I would describe it as long, arduous, painful, possibly verging on torture for both mother and child. Also exciting. Also potentially wonderful. Also something for which the mother needs a great deal of support.

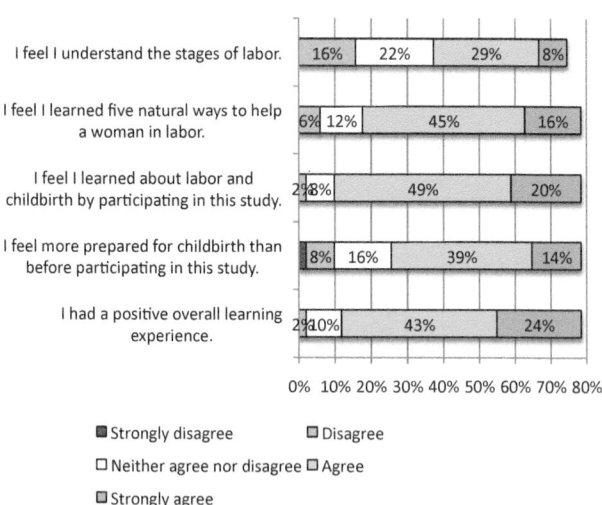

Fig. 4. Participants' answers for the learning experience portion of the survey

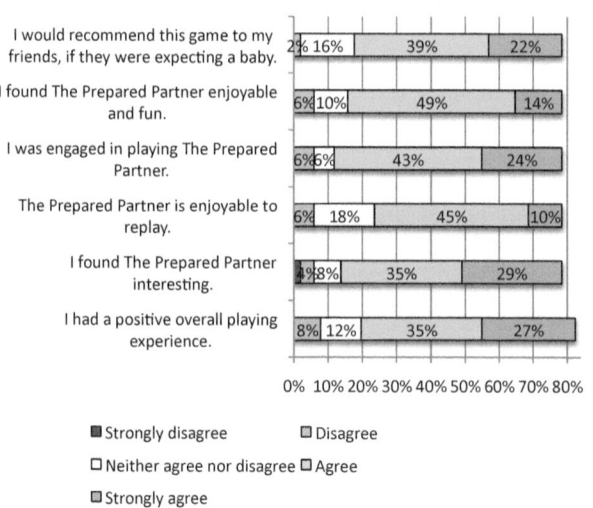

Fig. 5. Participants' answers for the playing experience portion of the survey

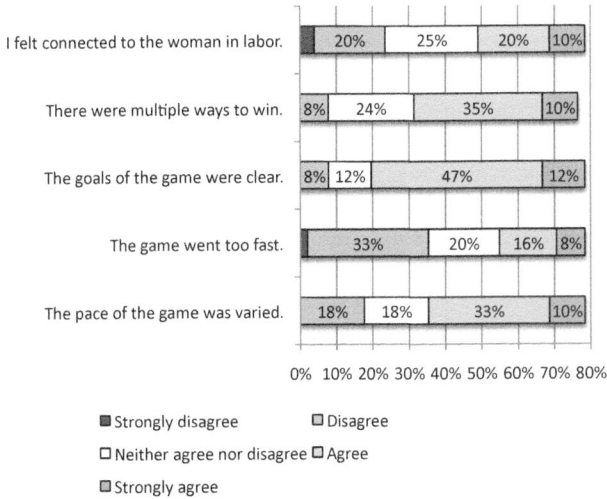

I felt connected to the woman in labor.   20%   25%   20%   10%

There were multiple ways to win.   8%   24%   35%   10%

The goals of the game were clear.   8%   12%   47%   12%

The game went too fast.   33%   20%   16%   8%

The pace of the game was varied.   18%   18%   33%   10%

0% 10% 20% 30% 40% 50% 60% 70% 80%

■ Strongly disagree   □ Disagree
□ Neither agree nor disagree □ Agree
■ Strongly agree

Fig. 6. Participants' answers for the game mechanics portion of the survey

Thus, given the large number of respondents that mentioned labor support after playing The Prepared Partner (22 participants out of 51), the game was successful in highlighting the need for continuous support for a woman throughout labor and childbirth. Moreover, as 12 participants mentioned specific methods of supporting a mother throughout her birth experience, corroborating the results from the childbirth test as well as the survey results asking about participant learning.

7 Conclusion

We presented the evolution of the system design of The Prepared Partner, an educational video game about labor and childbirth. In the game, we implemented a novel approach to modeling a woman in labor, and a game model for actions taken to help her through her labor. The Prepared Partner is the first game of its kind. Although the models The Prepared Partner uses to simulate a woman through the stages of labor are simple, our learning assessment and other studies show the methods are effective in teaching players about the stages of labor and natural ways to help a woman in labor. The game presents about 50 natural ways to help a woman in labor, and allows the player to explore these different options by trying them on the simulated woman in labor.

We showed that The Prepared Partner teaches players about the importance of supporting a mother through labor as well as several techniques of natural support. Objective evidence from a childbirth test was paired with subjective Likert-scaled data on a survey as well as a long-answer question about childbirth; all three measures showed that participants both believed The Prepared Partner to be an effective and fun teaching aid and that The Prepared Partner was effective at teaching about labor support.

The overwhelming majority of positive survey responses spoke to the success of The Prepared Partner as an interesting, enjoyable, replayable, and fun learning aid. The game encourages learning through an engaging, interactive interface designed through tight, interdisciplinary collaboration. We attribute its success to the close ties we had to childbirth professionals and usability and game design experts during all stages of design and development of The Prepared Partner.

Our study showed that we met our goals of introducing natural coping mechanisms and their effects on labor, introducing the mechanics of labor and childbirth, training birth partners to help women in childbirth, allowing the player to practice interacting with a woman in labor, and simulating the stages of labor. The Prepared Partner is the first game of its kind, and uses a simple, novel approach to simulating a woman in labor.

8   Future Work

Work on The Prepared Partner can be further improved by exploiting different pedagogical strategies based on the on-line game functionalities. The game could be enhanced to be a game engine that can develop different scenarios and thus implement different pedagogical strategies. This can lead to further investigations on the effect of the pedagogical strategy adopted to the achievement of the anticipated learning outcomes.

Appendix A   Test Questions

1. Which of the following are stages of labor?
   (a) Latent phase, hyperactive labor, pushing, delivery
   (b) First stage, second stage, third stage, fourth stage
   (c) Early labor, active labor, transition, pushing
   (d) Active labor, translational phase, pushing, delivery
   (e) Other (please specify)
2. When is a woman considered to be in active labor?
   (a) Between 1cm and 10cm dilation
   (b) Between 3cm and 5cm dilation
   (c) Between 4cm and 8cm dilation
   (d) Between 7cm and 10cm dilation
   (e) Above 10cm dilation
   (f) Other (please specify)
3. Which cervical dilation is required in order to allow the baby to pass through the cervix?
   (a) Less than 5cm dilation   (d) 10cm dilation
   (b) Between 5cm and 8cm dilation   (e) Between 11cm and 12cm dilation
   (c) 10cm dilation
4. When is it most appropriate to do something distracting, like play a card game, with a woman in labor?
   (a) Early labor   (d) Pushing
   (b) Active labor   (e) All of the above
   (c) Transition   (f) None of the above

5. Please name five ways you can help a woman in labor without using drugs.
6. What is one thing you can do as a birth partner to speed up labor, or increase the strength of labor contractions?
7. What is one thing you can do as a birth partner to help a woman in labor gain energy?
8. What is one thing you can do as a birth partner to help a woman in labor feel more physically supported?
9. What is one thing you can do as a birth partner to help a woman in labor feel mentally, or cognitively, supported?

References

1. Alehagen, S., Wijma, B., Lundberg, U., Wijma, K.: Fear, pain and stress hormones during childbirth. Journal of Psychosomatic Obstetrics & Gynecology 26(3), 153–165 (2005)
2. Baranowski, T., Buday, R., Thompson, D., Baranowski, J.: Playing for real: Video games and stories for health-related behavior change. American Journal of Preventive Medicine 34(1), 74–82.e10 (2008)
3. Bogost, I.: Persuasive games: The expressive power of videogames. The MIT Press (2007)
4. Bradley, R., Hathaway, M., Hathaway, J., Hathaway, J.: Husband-Coached Childbirth: The Bradley Method of Natural Childbirth. Bantam (2008)
5. Brown, S., Douglas, C., Flood, L.P.: Women's evaluation of intrapartum nonpharmacological pain relief methods used during labor. Journal of Perinatal Education 10(3), 1–8 (2001)
6. Cheung, W., Ip, W., Chan, D.: Maternal anxiety and feelings of control during labour: A study of chinese first-time pregnant women. Midwifery 23(2), 123–130 (2007)
7. Cooper, G., MacArthur, C., Wilson, M., Moore, P., Shennan, A.: Satisfaction, control and pain relief: short-and long-term assessments in a randomised controlled trial of low-dose and traditional epidurals and a non-epidural comparison group. International Journal of Obstetric Anesthesia 19(1), 31–37 (2010)
8. Desurvire, H., Caplan, M., Toth, J.: Using heuristics to evaluate the playability of games. In: CHI 2004 Extended Abstracts on Human Factors in Computing Systems, p. 1512. ACM (2004)
9. England, P., Horowitz, R.: Birthing From Within: An Extra-Ordinary Guide to Childbirth Preparation. Partera Press, Albuquerque (1998)
10. Ermi, L., Mäyrä, F.: Fundamental components of the gameplay experience: Analysing immersion. In: Proceedings of the DiGRA Conference, Citeseer (2005)
11. Gaskin, I.: Ina May's Guide to Childbirth. Bantam Books (2003)
12. Goer, H.: The Thinking Woman's Guide to a Better Birth. Perigee (1999)
13. Hallgren, A., Kilhgren, M., Forslin, L., Norberg, A.: Swedish fathers' involvement in and experiences of childbirth preparation and childbirth. Midwifery 15(1), 6–15 (1999)
14. Hamilton, B., Martin, J., Ventura, S., et al.: Births: preliminary data for 2006. National Vital Statistics Reports 56(7), 1–18 (2007)
15. Handfield, B., Turnbull, S., et al.: What do obstetricians think about media inuences on their patients? Australian and New Zealand Journal of Obstetrics and Gynaecology 46(5), 379–383 (2006)

16. Hetherington, S.: A controlled study of the effect of prepared childbirth classes on obstetric outcomes. Birth 17(2), 86–90 (1990)
17. Holloway, A.: System design and evaluation of The Prepared Partner: a labor and childbirth game. Master's thesis, University of California, Santa Cruz, 1156 High Street, Santa Cruz, CA 95064 (August 2010)
18. Holloway, A., Kurniawan, S.: System design evolution of The Prepared Partner: How a labor and childbirth game came to term. In: Meaningful Play (October 2010)
19. Holzinger, A.: Usability engineering methods for software developers. Communications of the ACM 48(1), 71–74 (2005)
20. Holzinger, A., Kickmeier-Rust, M., Wassertheurer, S., Hessinger, M.: Learning performance with interactive simulations in medical education: Lessons learned from results of learning complex physiological models with the haemodynamics simulator. Computers & Education 52(2), 292–301 (2009)
21. Klaus, M., Kennell, J., Klaus, P.: The Doula Book. Da Capo Press (2002)
22. Lamaze, F.: Painless Childbirth: The Lamaze Method. McGraw-Hill/Contemporary (1984)
23. Lumley, J., Brown, S.: Attenders and nonattenders at childbirth education classes in Australia: how do they and their births differ? Birth 20(3), 123–130 (1993)
24. MacCorkle, J.: Fighting VBAC-lash: Critiquing current research. Mothering (110) (January-February 2002),
    http://www.mothering.com/pregnancy-birth/fighting-vbac-lash-critiquing-current-research
25. Michael, D., Chen, S.: Serious games: Games that educate, train, and inform. Muska & Lipman/Premier-Trade (2005)
26. Mongan, M.: Hypnobirthing: The Mongan Method: A Natural Approach to a Safe, Easier, More Comfortable Birthing. In: HCI (2005)
27. Nielse, J.: Usability inspection methods. In: Conference Companion on Human Factors in Computing Systems, pp. 413–414. ACM (1994)
28. Papastergiou, M.: Exploring the potential of computer and video games for health and physical education: A literature review. Computers & Education 53(3), 603–622 (2009)
29. Romano, A., Lothian, J.: Promoting, protecting, and supporting normal birth: A look at the evidence. Journal of Obstetric, Gynecologic, and Neonatal Nursing 37(1), 94–105 (2008)
30. Simkin, P.: The Birth Partner, Third Edition: A Complete Guide To Childbirth For Dads, Doulas, and All Other Labor Companions. Harvard Common Press (2008)

Development of an Interactive Application for Learning Medical Procedures and Clinical Decision Making

Marcus Bloice, Klaus-Martin Simonic, Markus Kreuzthaler,
and Andreas Holzinger

Institute for Medical Informatics, Medical University of Graz,
Auenbruggerplatz 2, 8036, Graz, Austria

Abstract. This paper outlines the development of a Virtual Patient
style tablet application for the purpose of teaching decision making to undergraduate students of medicine. In order to objectively compare some
of the various technologies available, the application was written using
two different languages: one as a native iPad app written in Objective-C,
the other as a web-based app written in HTML5, CSS3, and JavaScript.
The requirements for both applications were identical, and this paper will
discuss the relative advantages and disadvantages of both technologies
from both a HCI point of view and from a technological point of view.
Application deployment, user-computer interaction, usability, security,
and cross-platform interoperability are also discussed. The motivation
for developing this application, entitled *Casebook*, was to create a platform to test the novel approach of using real patient records to teach
undergraduate students. These medical records form patient cases, and
these cases are navigated using the Casebook application with the goal
of teaching decision making and clinical reasoning; the pretext being
that real cases more closely match the context of the hospital ward and
thereby increase *authentic activity*. Of course, patient cases must possess
a certain level of quality to be useful. Therefore, the quality of documentation and, most importantly, quality's impact on healthcare is also
discussed.

Keywords: Virtual Patients, Patient Records, Decision Making.

1 Introduction

The term *Virtual Patient* is an umbrella term for a type of interactive medical system used for teaching and learning medicine, especially clinical reasoning.
According to the electronic Virtual Patients (eViP) project website a Virtual Patient can be formally defined as "an interactive computer simulation of real-life
clinical scenarios for the purpose of medical training, education or assessment
[8]". These systems exist in many forms, and range from physical robotic patients, entire hospital simulation systems, to online accessible interactive patient
cases. The application presented in this paper takes a slightly different approach,

A. Holzinger and K.-M. Simonic (Eds.): USAB 2011, LNCS 7058, pp. 211–224, 2011.

using real electronic patient records to display patient cases to students. Using this application, users can interact with the case and make decisions based on the information contained within the case itself. Cases are presented linearly (this early version of Casebook supports linear cases only), and students assume the role of the physician examining a patient's history. At strategic points throughout the case, the student is asked what their next course of action would be based on the information known to them up to that point, thereby mimicking the context of a hospital ward. This is known as the authentic activity of learning. The full requirements of the application are described in Section 1.1 below.

Of interest to the HCI community are the experiences that were gained when developing two versions of the same application using two distinctly different technologies. Specifically, to what degree does the choice of technology affect the usability of Casebook? The application itself employs a multi-touch, gesture-based approach, and the feasibility of using HTML to implement this is also outlined. Therefore, the question of whether a web-based application can compare to a native application in terms of the user experience is the main focus of Section 2.

After the development stage of Casebook is described, the motivation and reasoning behind creating a Virtual Patient based on patient data are discussed. Section 3 addresses the motivation behind creating a Virtual Patient application using patient cases based on real medical records. First, it is argued that patient cases that consist of electronic medical records more closely match the context of the hospital ward. Second, it provides an opportunity to analyze the impact of the quality of documentation on its usefulness as teaching material.

1.1 Requirements

As stated previously, the requirements were identical for both the HTML and Objective-C versions of Casebook. Namely, the application should allow a student to view and browse patient cases, comprising of electronic health records, where at certain points stipulated by the case creator the student must answer questions as to what their course of action might be. Records can be physician notes, sonographies, radiological images, and so on. Students begin by opening a case and viewing the first patient record available (this is usually the patient presentation). Using gestures, the students can navigate through the case from left to right using a linear timeline of the patient records. Upon reaching a question, students are asked about their next course of action, and are given a choice of four answers. Upon answering, the next medical record is displayed, revealing the correct answer. At the end of the case, the student is given a summary of how they scored. Cases themselves are created manually by the teacher and bundled as a ZIP archive before being uploaded and read by the Casebook application. These ZIP files must follow a strict structure so that they can be correctly read by Casebook.

Each case consists of a number PDF files linearly named from 1 to n (e.g. `1.pdf`, `2.pdf`, ..., `n.pdf`). Any questions that should appear between patient records for the student to answer are stored in XML files, where each question is represented by one XML file. Question XML files are named according to where they are positioned between PDF documents, with the first part of the file name denoting the previous document and a second part denoting the subsequent document, separated by a dash. For example the file 2-3.xml denotes a question that appears between documents 2.pdf and 3.pdf. An example question XML file is shown just below. All PDFs must be portrait oriented and A4 in size to ensure design consistency. Each individual case is contained within a single ZIP archive.

```
<question previousFile="2.pdf" nextFile="3.pdf">
    <headerText>
        What is the your next course of action?
    </headerText>
    <text>
        After seeing the Befundbericht and Status,
        what is the next course of action?
    </text>
    <option>
        Request an ECG
    </option>
    <option correct="true">
        Request a Sonography
    </option>
    <option>
        Transfer Patient
    </option>
    <option>
        Request a Lab
    </option>
</question>
```

Concerning the usability requirements, the application was designed to be operated on tablet devices, specifically the iPad. Cases should be navigable through the use of swipe gestures, allowing for the case to be traversed both forwards and backwards. Zooming is accomplished using a standard pinch gesture. An overview of the case's timeline can also be viewed at any time (see Figures 2b and 4a). It was also a requirement that the transitions between documents be animated to emphasize the timeline-based view of the case, progressing from left to right.

2 Development

Two versions of Casebook were created in parallel, both targeting the iPad. One version was developed as a standard, native Objective-C iPad application while the other was written in HTML as a web-based solution. The HTML version

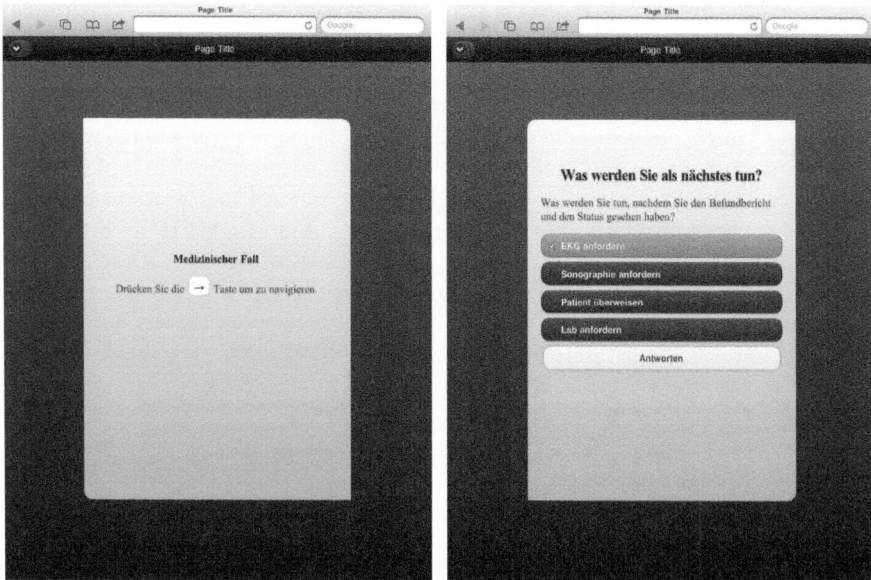

(a) The opening screen of a case. Notice that the case can be navigated using a keyboard as well as with a swipe gesture.

(b) Answering a question. Students are presented with questions at strategic points throughout a case, but can progress further whether they answer correctly or not.

Fig. 1. Casebook HTML application in use

aimed to mimic the look and feel of a native application, as is shown in Figure 1a and Figure 2.

In order to mimic a native application's look and feel, the jQuery Mobile framework was used. This is a "touch-optimized framework for smartphones and tablets [17]" that allows advanced interfaces to be built targeting multiple platforms. Although Casebook was developed specifically with iOS in mind (iOS being the iPad operating system), the jQuery framework also supports Android, BlackBerry, Samsung bada, Windows Phone, Palm webOS, Symbian, MeeGo, and even the Amazon Kindle. Our development focused primarily on targeting the WebKit browser engine, the rendering engine used by both iOS and the Android OS—an iPad was used for testing purposes.

The goal of developing Casebook in HTML as well as Objective-C was to be able to judge HTML's applicability in creating a touch screen, gesture-based application for viewing medical records. Optimized views of many websites exist for touch screen tablets, and several HTML applications rival native applications in terms of their usability and look & feel (see for example the Financial Times Web App: http://app.ft.com). Also, showcase demonstrations such as Sencha's TouchSolitaire application (see http://www.touchsolitaire.mobi) highlight just what is possible using HTML, CSS, and JavaScript. Having said that,

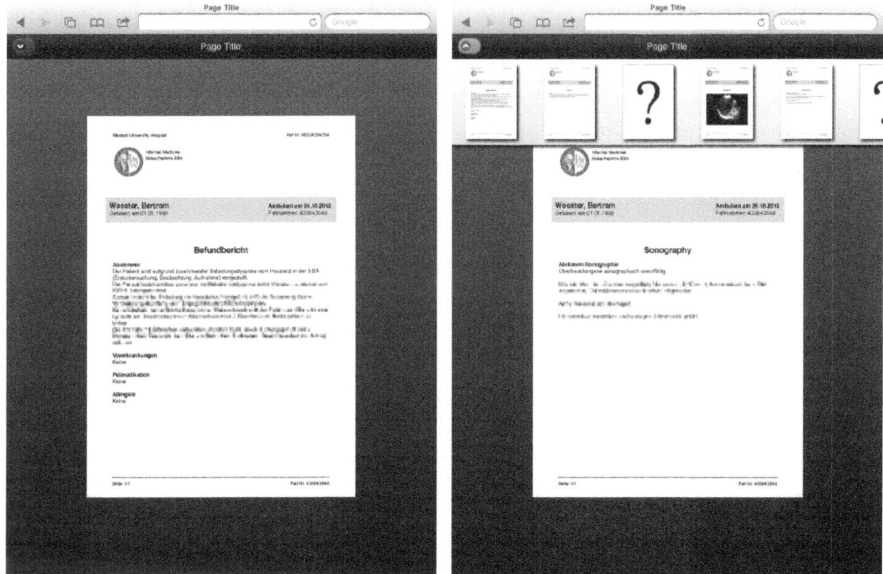

(a) Viewing a single patient record   (b) Viewing the timeline of the case

Fig. 2. Casebook HTML application in use, using the timeline

our main concern before development began was performance. Due to the nature of patient records and their large file size and high resolution, it was questionable whether a browser would be able to handle large cases containing 30 to 40 patient records.

Nonetheless, there are a number of advantages inherent to web-based application development that made the idea of using it as a basis for Casebook compelling, especially considering that Casebook was intended for in-house use within the hospital campus and not for worldwide deployment. However, developers must also be aware of a number of compromises if deciding to write software for the iPad, or any other tablet, in HTML. This section will discuss the development of Casebook in both HTML and Objective-C and will emphasize the advantages and disadvantages of each. First, some general observations regarding both technologies will be made, followed by a discussion of some issues that were encountered during development that were specific to Casebook.

2.1   HTML

The following list of observations were made in favor of HTML for iPad or tablet development:

App Store. Perhaps the most obvious advantage in developing web-based applications is that the Apple App Store is avoided. This bypasses the need for paying Apple a developer fee, and also means the application is not at the mercy of the approval process.

Integrated Development Environment. When writing web applications, there is far more freedom in terms of what IDE or OS one can use for development—when writing native apps for iOS an Intel Macintosh is required, and realistically Xcode is the only IDE that can be used (although technically speaking any editor could be used in conjunction with the apple-darwin9-gcc-4.2.1 compiler).

Device Independence. Using a framework such as the aforementioned jQuery Mobile, or Sencha Touch, multiple devices can be targeted. This potentially means a higher customer base and there is certainly more flexibility in terms of what hardware can be purchased.

Updates. Updates made on the server side are instantly propagated by subsequent client requests. Fragmentation of client versions is avoided.

In-house Distribution. By controlling access to within your LAN or WAN, the distribution of web-based applications can be tightly managed. iOS applications can also be distributed in-house, but an enterprise developer account is required to do so.

Development Platform. A dual core Intel-based Apple Mac computer is required for iOS development. Almost any computer can be used to develop web-based applications.

Device Specific. HTML applications can be designed to accept keyboard input and therefore can also function on standard PCs. Google Chrome and Apple Safari are both based on the WebKit rendering engine, the same engine used by the iPad and Android browsers.

2.2   Objective-C

A number of advantages that exist when developing in HTML that may make it convenient for certain types of deployment, especially for in-house applications and applications that must run on a range of devices. At the same time, web-based applications are not ideal for all situations. During the development of Casebook, the following list of general observations were made in favor of writing programs natively (i.e., in Objective-C):

Monetization. Apple has paid out over $2 billion to developers since opening the App Store, allowing publishers to charge users anything from between $0.99 and $999.99 for their applications. Web-based applications, on the other hand, must rely on advertising schemes such as Google's Adsense for revenue. It is worth noting that reliable information concerning the click through rate (CTR) for mobile advertisements is difficult to find, and would warrant further study. It is certainly conceivable to suggest that the CTR is lower for mobile devices such as the iPhone than for desktop machines, especially when one considers the interruption incurred when a new browser window is opened in iOS.

Hardware Access. Native applications have access to the complete array of sensors on the iPhone or iPad, including the GPS device, magnetometer, accelerometer, and gyroscope. Conversely, HTML applications have no access to a device's hardware. There are efforts to help reduce this deficit, such as the HTML5 `geolocation` API which can resolve the user's location based on their IP address, although with a far lower accuracy than that of GPS.

iOS API. The iOS API is large and mature, with extensive documentation available from directly within the Xcode IDE. While the HTML5 specification has been finalized, implementation of this specification is incomplete and differs from engine to engine. Documentation is therefore fragmented and sparely distributed. JavaScript also suffers from the lack of a centralized point of access for documentation and this is compounded by the fact that JavaScript code is interpreted differently from browser to browser. By all accounts, using a single, officially supported API has definite benefits for the developer.

Xcode. The Xcode IDE itself is a powerful platform on which to work, complete with a debugger, code completion, as well as the aforementioned inline help, automatic error detection, and an interface builder. Developing HTML applications requires more effort on the part of the programmer, with many editors offering no more than syntax highlighting. Writing complex HTML and JavaScript without the aid of a debugger is an error prone and difficult process. That said, IDEs designed specifically for HTML5 development, such as Aptana, are becoming more common, and Ext Designer even includes an interface builder.

Security. By deploying apps to your users via the App Store, you mitigate the risk of a malicious attack on your own servers or hardware. HTML applications must be hosted, at both your expense and your risk. Web servers are potential targets for attacks, including denial-of-service exploits and outright theft of confidential data.

Notifications. Native applications can make use of Apple's notification framework to send messages to users, even when the app is closed. As of yet, there is no way in which a HTML application can do this, although there is a draft specification that aims to address this (WebKit's `webkitNotifications` is one implementation of this draft, for example).

Multi-touch. Multi-touch is an inherent part of the Objective-C framework for developing mobile applications. As described previously, advanced touch-enabled applications can be built using frameworks such as Sencha Touch or jQuery Mobile. Sencha, for example, comes with a gesture library [11]. However, these are third party libraries that could disappear at any time, or change their terms of service or license agreements to be incompatible with your project.

If your application requires specific iOS features such as the ability to send notifications, or requires access to the hardware of the device on which it is running, there is no choice but to develop natively. If not, however, there is little reason to dismiss HTML. There are also some caveats that must be considered, such as the reliance on third party frameworks, the lack of a definitive and comprehensive IDE and debugger, and somewhat fragmented help. But this is certainly changing; more robust and mature IDEs are appearing, and there are even projects being developed that convert HTML applications into their native equivalents (for example PhoneGap, see `http://www.phonegap.com`)[20].

2.3 Lessons Learned during Development

Once two working prototypes were developed and preliminarily tested, it was ultimately decided to continue further development of the Objective-C application only. The main reason for this was performance; while it was possible to entirely duplicate the functionality of the Objective-C application, the performance of the HTML application deteriorated rapidly when displaying cases consisting of more than about 5 or 6 patient records. Part of the requirements for the project was that the cases themselves consist of individual A4-sized PDF files in portrait orientation. This was to ensure that no unrecognized filetypes would be encountered and that all patient records were the same size and orientation on the screen. Text within PDFs is vector based, which allows for close up zooming. Patient records that consist solely of scans, such as sonographic images, are wrapped in PDF files, as seen in Figure 4b. Unfortunately, WebKit cannot natively display PDFs meaning that all PDFs had to be rasterized as PNG images for the web-based Casebook application. This meant that when zooming into text the PNG images would become blocky and unreadable and the zoom functionality was eventually deactivated.

This led to the next problem that was encountered: because all the patient records had to be rasterized as PNG images, the performance of the transition animation between documents would become unacceptably slow as more PNG files load into the browser's memory. To compensate for this, files in the patient cases are dynamically loaded only when needed. In other words, after a question is answered the next group of records is loaded into memory. This method worked well, but as cases progress increasingly larger amounts of memory is required. Because there is no way to deallocate memory once it has been loaded, long cases would result in the user experiencing progressively slower response times to their swipe gestures, to the point where the application would be become all but unusable.

Furthermore, it was observed that the development time for the native application was shorter than that of the HTML application. The main reason for this being the iOS API, which has been designed from the ground up to make it easy to create multi-touch and gesture-based applications. While Sencha Touch and jQuery are impressive in their own right, they are based on technology that was arguably never intended for such application development. The result is that workarounds must often be used to emulate trivial features of the iOS API. From the point of view of the Casebook project, all subsequent development time will concentrate on the native application, and further work on the HTML application will cease.

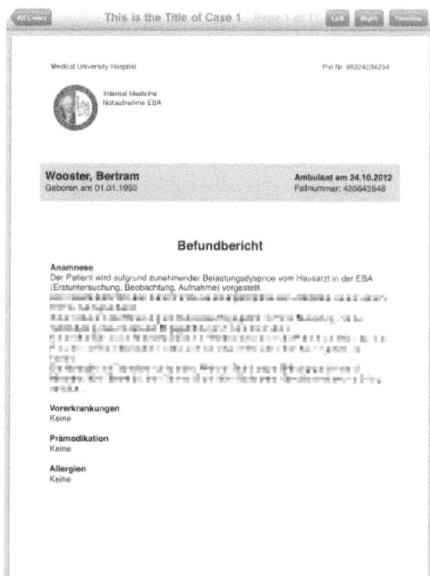

Fig. 3. Casebook Objective-C application, viewing a single patient record

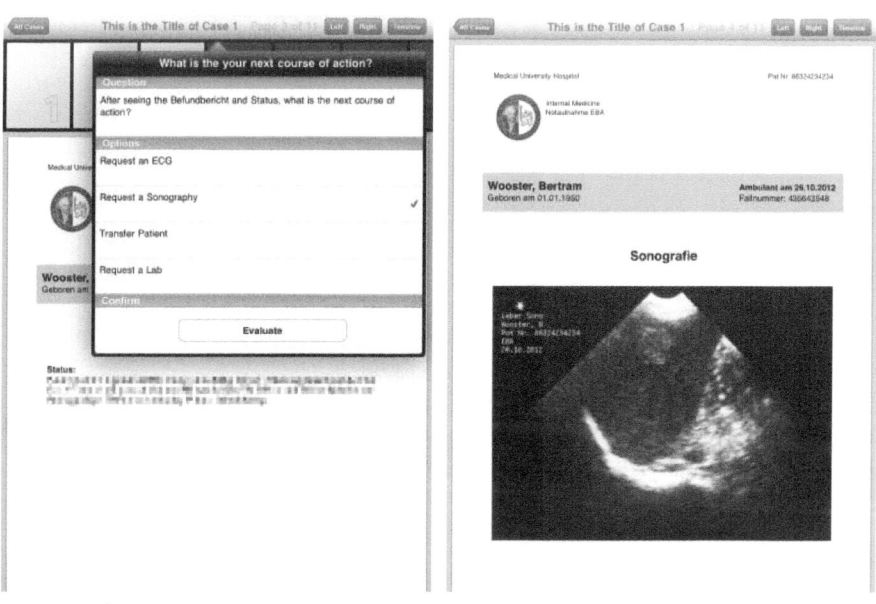

(a) Answering a question

(b) Viewing a sonograph. Images are wrapped in a PDF template to ensure design consistency.

Fig. 4. Objective-C Casebook Application

3   Motivation and Theory

Upon reaching the point of graduation, students of medicine must embark on a new challenge when they start working as doctors during their internships. This is the point where students must now apply what they have learned during their studies to real world situations that require quick thinking in time critical situations. However, recent work has outlined that as many as 40% of students do not feel they are prepared for their first medical positions, and this perceived lack of preparedness is attributed to a number of factors such as students' level of knowledge of communications skills, paperwork, and ward work [12][14]. Crucially however, according to Illing, et al., student exposure to clinical processes and practice is directly correlated to their preparedness or perceived preparedness. Illing, et al. relate their work to the ideas outlined in Lave and Wenger's book Situated Learning, where preparedness increases with authentic activity [16]. The theory of authentic activity ties in closely to that of context, which stipulates that information learned in the context of where it will be used increases information retention, facilitates learning, and improves the transfer of knowledge [1]. Currently Virtual Patient applications and Case-Based Learning tools attempt to increase this authentic activity by simulating the environment and situation in which medical students will eventually work. Many Virtual Patients are case based—they consist of cases that can be interacted with and the student learns clinical reasoning and decision making by examining and working with these cases. Nonetheless, studies indicate that rule-based diagnoses are frequently made due to skills that students gain from both Case-Based Learning and Problem Based Learning, thus confirming their legitimacy as a teaching method[7][4][22].

However, Case-Based Learning, in its current form at least, suffers from a number of detrimental issues that have recently been identified. Research has shown that Case-Based Learning can actually encourage adverse student performance, such as the phenomenon of premature closure—a situation where a diagnosis is made before all alternative diagnostic paths have been explored [2][3]. As well as this, developing cases for Virtual Patients can be an expensive and time consuming process. In 2007, Huang et al. reviewed over 100 virtual patient applications and found that in 34% of the cases, development costs were over $50,000 and a staggering 85% of the cases cost over $10,000 to develop (this was due, mostly, to the very nature of virtual patients that are built from scratch—they are generally rich in media and incur extensive production costs)[13].

It is the opinion of the authors that a new approach could address many of these issues at once. This novel approach uses real medical data as the basis for the cases within the Virtual Patient. This has several advantages over Virtual Patient cases that are based on fictitious data and must be manufactured. First, we believe that the trend towards more and more interactive and media rich cases actually decreases the authentic activity perceived by the students. On the other hand using real medical records will increase this perception of authentic activity and more closely mimic the context of the ward. This idea was touched upon by Dammers et al., who used real patients to teach problem solving [6].

Second, cases based on real patient records can be collected from modern hospital information systems with ease—this mitigates premature closure by ensuring there is a large pool of cases on which students can base their learning and diagnostic reasoning [18]. Hospital information systems contain millions of patient records and potentially thousands of suitable cases. Third, the cost and time effort involved in producing a case is reduced dramatically as cases do not need to be produced or manufactured from scratch. As mentioned previously, cases can be extremely costly to produce, limiting their suitability for small institutions that do not have the time or monetary resources required for the development of case-based Virtual Patients. Such costs also inhibit the feasibility of introducing case-based Virtual Patients in to institutions based in less developed countries.

3.1   Teaching Using Medical Records

Using real patient data makes possible a unique way of teaching the procedure of documentation to students of medicine. Analyzing cases that were written by medical professionals provides important insight into how this crucial task is undertaken. Not only can students learn good documentation practice, but they can also experience examples of badly written documentation or poorly documented cases. This has multiple benefits: first, students learn how to document well by example and second, students learn first hand the impact of good documentation on the understandability of a patient's history. The more students realize the importance of good documentation, the better they understand the impact of good documentation on the quality of care. Therefore, Casebook is an attempt to promote the need for good documentation standards and methods, teach documentation skills, prep students for real life documentation work, and emphasize the importance of thorough and well written patient history taking. This will also allow students to learn the importance of documentation in the wider clinical context—this is becoming more important as patient records are being used in an ever increasingly varied number of situations. This has been observed by Ganslandt et al. where they found uses of electronic patient records in areas such as clinical research, clinical management, and quality management [10]. Also, physicians already spend a disproportionate amount of time writing medical reports, and making the most use of these records after they have been documented is surely logical. According to preliminary work by Oxentenko, et al., 67.9% of physicians spend up to 4 hours per day writing documentation, while only 38.9% spend this amount on time in direct patient contact [19]. Therefore, because of the increasing variety of use of medical records, and the effort that must be invested in to writing patient reports in the first place, it is essential that students realize that good documentation is beneficial for many areas of medicine.

As mentioned previously, premature closure is one source of diagnostic error that is known to cause adverse conditions in patient outcomes. Other sources of diagnostic error include aggregate bias, anchoring, ascertainment bias, base-rate neglect, confirmation bias, diagnostic momentum, overconfidence bias, representative error, and search satisfying [5]. By using real patient data, cases where such errors are known to have occurred can be shown to the students and the point at which the diagnostic error manifested can be discussed. Students can learn a great deal about the pitfalls of diagnostic error by examining previous examples of when they happened in real world situations.

This leads on to a final point regarding the annotation of patient records by physicians. Work by Eva, K.W. (2005), stated that properly conveying knowledge and reasoning strategies to novice diagnosticians is fundamental to a student's understanding of the procedure of a case [9]. Eva's work recognized that this task is difficult as the clinical teacher must understand the strategies that expert clinicians use to make their diagnostic decisions. Interestingly, a model formulation described by Johnson, et al. outlines a system where a physician's thought processes can be documented along with the standard documentation and history taking [15]. As future work, we propose a similar system, whereby diagnostic reasoning notes could be added to patient records at the time of documentation in the form of meta-data annotations specifically with the aim of using these records for teaching purposes. That way, physicians and medical professionals could document their reasons for making certain decisions at the point at which they are made. This information would be saved as supplemental meta-information not normally visible on the patient record itself, but would be used by Casebook when the patient records are viewed by students who are observing the case. Students viewing the cases themselves can earn credits for comments, questions, and discussion regarding the case. The case creator's task would be to act as moderator for the discussion and offer help, pointers, and feedback regarding any questions or issues that may arise.

4   Future Work

Due to time constraints, Casebook has so far only been tested on a small amount of users. The winter semester of 2011 will provide the opportunity to test the application on a large amount of students who will use Casebook as part of their seminar on Decision Support. Their feedback will be used to decide on further development directions and serve as a constant testing environment for the application. Future work will also entail annotating a number of cases with meta-information to provide the students insight into decision making criteria. In other words, cases will be supplemented with information outlining the reasoning and criteria physicians had for making certain diagnostic decisions. The question being, when cases are supplemented with information on the clinical reasoning of physicians, do students gain more useful insight into the mind's of doctors and how they think and make diagnostic decisions? Do they then learn more about reasoning strategies? These are extremely pertinent questions in the field of medical education, documentation, and health information systems. Once a collection of annotated cases has been assembled, we will also be able to ascertain the granularity of annotation required.

User feedback aside, Casebook will nonetheless be further developed to support non-linear cases. The static and linear approach currently employed has its limitations when several branches occur within one case at the same time.

Currently, it is possible to order patient records logically in a linear fashion, but this is not optimal from our point of view.

In the long term, a case repository will be built to collect cases developed by teachers. Cases themselves will have to be tagged with keywords from the National Library of Medicine's controlled vocabularies to ensure that they can more easily be found and that similar cases can be logically grouped together[21].

5   Conclusion

This paper outlined the development of a Virtual Patient application that uses real patient data to teach students. The application itself was developed using two different technologies in parallel; one as a standard iPad application running on iOS, the other as a web-based HTML application designed to be accessed using tablet browsers. Tablets were chosen as the platform on which to develop Casebook for a number of reasons. The multi-touch metaphor utilized by tablets emphasizes the perception of navigating through a timeline, revealing more of the patient's case as the records are traversed from left to right. In the environment of a classroom or seminar, tablets make ideal devices to view patient cases. They can be readily passed around a classroom, and encourage team work and discussion within groups of students in a seminar session. Not only this, but tablets are increasingly being used as replacements for workstations in hospital wards, thus further increasing the authentic activity and learning context. Ultimately, performance issues led to the abandonment of the web-based application, due mainly to the fact that PDFs must be rasterized before being displayed within a browser window.

The motivation for using real patient data as the basis for a Virtual Patient was also described in this paper, and several advantages for both the learner and the teaching institution were outlined. First, hospital information systems contain huge pools of medical cases allowing for collections of case-based Virtual Patients to be compiled. This can help to avoid premature closure as mentioned throughout the paper, but is also very cost effective. Second, due to the real world nature of the cases, the perception of authentic activity can be increased better preparing students for their internships upon graduation. Third, good documentation practice can be learned and its importance appreciated, thus increasing the quality of the documentation that the students will eventually write as junior doctors. With so many students expressing concerns about their preparedness for clinical work, it was felt that their exposure to clinical practice could be increased by allowing them to analyze actual patient cases and learn from the real world work of clinicians.

References

1. Bergman, E.M., Van Der Vleuten, C.P.M., Scherpbier, A.J.J.A.: Why don't they know enough about anatomy? A narrative review. Medical Teacher 33(5), 403–409 (2011)
2. Bowen, J.L.: Educational strategies to promote clinical diagnostic reasoning. New England Journal of Medicine 355(21), 2217–2225 (2006)

3. Colliver, J.: Effectiveness of problem-based learning curricula: research and theory. Academic Medicine 75(3), 259–266 (2000)
4. Cook, D., Erwin, P., Triola, M.: Computerized virtual patients in health professions education: A systematic review and meta-analysis. Academic Medicine 85(10), 1589–1602 (2010)
5. Croskerry, P.: The importance of cognitive errors in diagnosis and strategies to minimize them. Academic Medicine 78(8), 775–780 (2003)
6. Dammers, J., Spencer, J., Thomas, M.: Using real patients in problem-based learning: students' comments on the value of using real, as opposed to paper cases, in a problem-based learning module in general practice. Medical Education 35(1), 27–34 (2001)
7. Dolmans, D., Schmidt, H.: The advantages of problem-based curricula. Postgraduate Medical Journal 72(851), 535–538 (1996)
8. eViP Electronic Virtual Patients: About Virtual Patients, http://www.virtual patients.eu/about/about-virtual-patients/ (accessed July 2011)
9. Eva, K.W.: What every teacher needs to know about clinical reasoning. Medical Education 39(1), 98–106 (2005)
10. Ganslandt, T., Krieglstein, C., Mueller, M., Senninger, N., Prokosch, H.: Electronic documentation in medicine; flexible concepts versus isolated solutions. Zentralblatt fuer Gynaekologie 122(8), 445–451 (2000)
11. Garcia, J., De Moss, A.: Sencha Touch in Action, 1st edn. Manning Publications (2011)
12. Goldacre, M., Lambert, I., Evans, J., Turner, G.: PRHOs' views on whether their experience at medical school prepared them well for heir jobs: national questionnaire survey. BMJ 326, 1011–1101 (2003)
13. Huang, G., Reynolds, R., Candler, C.: Virtual patient simulation at US and Canadian medical schools. Academic Medicine 82(5), 446 (2007)
14. Illing, J., Morrow, G., Kergon, C., Burford, B., Davies, C., Baldauf, B., Morrison, G., Allen, M., Spencer, J., Peile, E., Johnson, N.: Do medical graduates need more on-the-job experience? A prospective qualitative study comparing three diverse UK medical schools. Medical Education 43, 39 (2009)
15. Johnson, S., Bakken, S., Dine, D., Hyun, S., Mendonça, E., Morrison, F., Bright, T., Van Vleck, T., Wrenn, J., Stetson, P.: An electronic health record based on structured narrative. Journal of the American Medical Informatics Association 15(1), 54–64 (2008)
16. Lave, J., Wenger, E.: Situated Learning. Cambridge University Press (1991)
17. jQuery Mobile Framework: jQuery Mobile, http://jquerymobile.com/ (accessed July 2011)
18. Norman, G.: Research in clinical reasoning: past history and current trends. Medical Education 39(4), 418–427 (2005)
19. Oxentenko, A.S., West, C.P., Popkave, C., Weinberger, S.E., Kolars, J.C.: Time spent on clinical documentation, a survey of internal medicine residents and program directors. Archives of Internal Medicine 170(4), 377–380 (2010)
20. Stark, J.: Building iPhone Apps with HTML, CSS, and JavaScript, Making App Store Apps Without Objective-C or Cocoa, 1st edn. O'Reilly (2010)
21. Stead, W., Searle, J., Fessler, H., Smith, J., Shortliffe, E.: Biomedical informatics: changing what physicians need to know and how they learn. Academic Medicine 86(4), 429–434 (2011)
22. Williams, B.: Case based learning—a review of the literature: is there scope for this educational paradigm in prehospital education? Emergency Medicine Journal 22(8), 577–581 (2005)

Enhancing Collaboration in ASD-Centric Treatment Environments: A Proposed Architecture[*]

Panagiotis Germanakos[1], Dimosthenis Georgiadis[2], Marina Buzzi[1],
Maria Claudia Buzzi[1], and Claudia Fenili[3]

[1] Institute of Informatics and Telematics (IIT), CNR, Via Giuseppe Moruzzi 1,
56124, Pisa, Italy
pgerman@cs.ucy.ac.cy, {marina.buzzi,claudia.buzzi}@iit.cnr.it
[2] Department of Management & MIS, University of Nicosia,
46 Makedonitissas Ave., 1700 Nicosia, Cyprus
georgiadis.d@unic.ac.cy
[3] ASA (Associazione Sindromi Autistiche), Sesto Fiorentino (FI), Italy
claudiafenili14@libero.it

Abstract. There is a growing body of evidence that people diagnosed with Autistic Spectrum Disorder (ASD) is increasing each year. ASD is a neurodevelopmental spectrum disorder with overarching characteristics the abnormal social interaction, communication ability, patterns of interests, and patterns of behavior. Individuals with ASD are characterized by unique and divergent needs and requirements which make a generalized treatment approach obsolete. Early diagnosis and interventions in persons with ASD, along with a consistent and continuous monitoring of their situation by the dedicated care team may increase their learning abilities and social inclusion. In this respect, we propose an ASD-centric Computer Supported Collaborative Treatment Architecture which employs the notion of Virtual Care Teams and dynamic workflows. We analyze its various components and outline a set of services that have been adjusted on the qualities and limitations of the ASD sector. Through this architecture a continuous treatment with updated exchange of information, effective communication, prompt error handling, and improved decision making, can be achieved within and between the members of a care team. Finally, we present a real life case scenario which employs the particular architecture, encapsulating the arisen benefits of the proposed approach.

Keywords: eHealth, Autistic Spectrum Disorder, Collaboration, Virtual Care Teams.

1   Introduction

Autistic Spectrum Disorder (ASD) is an overarching term that describes a group of developmental disabilities that include Autistic Disorder, Rett's Disorder, Childhood Disintegrative Disorder, Asperger's Syndrome, Pervasive Developmental Disorder,

---

[*] This work was carried out during the tenure of an ERCIM fellowship.

A. Holzinger and K.-M. Simonic (Eds.): USAB 2011, LNCS 7058, pp. 225–244, 2011.

and Not Otherwise Specified (PDD-NOS) [1]. These neurodevelopmental disorders are characterized by severe and pervasive impairments that involve problems with social interactions, trouble in communication, and repeating patterns of behavior, interests and activities. ASD affect different people during their development and to different degrees. Symptoms and behaviors can vary, ranging from mild to severe. Although people with autism share some common characteristics (such as abnormal communication and social interaction, unusual behavior, unusual patterns of attention and learning qualities), no two individuals are the same. In addition, the pattern and extent of difficulties may change with development. Given this dynamic nature of diagnoses over time for autistic persons as well as the unpredicted behaviors and responses on particular sensor stimuli the treatment method should be dynamic and adapted always in their current state. It is generally agreed that no single intervention will suit all people with autism, and in addition any intervention can have negative as well as positive effects. No one approach is appropriate for all individuals on the autism spectrum or even for the same individual across his/her lifespan [2]. A range of interventions have been developed [3], and examples include those based on behavioral methods, education-based approaches and non-verbal communication systems. Choosing an intervention can be a difficult task as there are many different options available, they can be costly, and it is often difficult to determine which interventions will best suit a person with autism. Persons with ASD need individually designed interventions and supports and not rather what is available that may not meet their needs, which is sometimes the case [2].

Nevertheless, no intervention can have an actual effect, if there is not a comprehensive and continuous synergy among the involved care parties around the autistic person's treatment approach (i.e. family, teacher, therapist, psychologist, social worker, etc.) In other words, the collaboration among the social entities in which the autistic person lives and functions (that is Family, School and Community) should be well-coordinated, pragmatic, consistent, contingent, with a continuous exchange and update of related information and ASD-centric services.

Computer-mediated platforms have been shown to be a catalyst for increased social interaction in persons with ASD, even though that effect requires further study to be effectively employed as a therapeutic intervention [4]. Similarly, technology-based collaborative environments and systems could be proofed a profound solution and to have indisputable effects on an ASD person's development. In recent years, there is an increasing number of researches, studies and projects in Computer Supported Cooperative Work (CSCW) applications and systems in the eHealth [29] and Ambient Assisted Living [5] domains with successful and encouraging results with regards to treatment and social inclusion of patients and elderly people accordingly. In this respect, main purpose of this work is to propose an ASD-centric Computer Supported Collaborative Treatment Architecture (ASD-centric CSCTA). The particular architecture aims to identify the components and collaboration dynamics that enhance the services provision by an assigned Virtual Care Team (VCT) for the treatment of persons with ASD. Given the one-to-one treatment and therapy applied in such cases collaborative system will enhance decision-making through collaboration and a continuous update of the person with ASD state. This will enable the error-free efficient development and control of its situation.

2   The Importance of Collaboration and CSCW in ASD and eHealth

ASD is a complex lifelong disorder that has an intense impact on a person's development and is more common in males than females. Individuals with ASD, predominantly demonstrate strong deficiencies in many types of social behavior, social imagination and communication; also known as the "Triad of Impairments" [6]. Furthermore, they might indicate difficulties with self-motivation, severe deficits in turn-taking, joint attention and pointing, play, imitation, and self-initiated behavior [7]; impairments in reciprocal social interaction and communication, and restricted and stereotyped patterns of interests and activities as well as repetitive movements and resistance to change [8]; poor eye-contact and lack of face and body understanding, and difficulties on using verbal and non-verbal communication [6]; learning difficulties or learning disabilities [9]; and difficulties in creating and producing emotional understanding and expressions while they are unconscious of being able to exert control over their surroundings environments and obtaining coherent response, even in the cases when they themselves causing the events [10]. The complexity of these disorders necessitates a range of services that are tailored to the needs of an individual with ASD and his/her family, from screening and referral services through diagnosis, assessment for intervention planning, and treatment. Specific standardized instruments are available that aid the clinician in gathering relevant information and evaluating specific ASD impairments [11]. The comprehensive evaluation of a child with a suspected ASD may include speech, language, and communication assessments, cognitive testing, behavioral assessments, academic assessments, and a medical evaluation [12]. It is critical that these are identified so that appropriate treatment and services can be initiated based on the strengths of a person with ASD. These strengths and personality traits are considered vital to be identified, since based on these the intervention planning that will be applied for the treatment of the individual will be formulated [13]. Studies have shown that early identification of individuals with ASD can lead to earlier entry into intervention programs that support improved developmental outcomes [14]. Early intervention has been associated with gains in verbal and nonverbal communication, higher intelligence test scores, improved peer interactions, more effective learning and development of social abilities, and improved quality of life [15]. A substantial benefit also of early intervention is the positive impact on the family's ability to interact in a manner that facilitates and copes with their child's developmental concerns, and the greater understanding of their child's disability and how it interacts with family life [16].

It is widely acknowledged in the research community that generalization of methods and approaches in the individuals' with ASD treatment is neither feasible nor effective. A personalized (ASD-centric) and intensive treatment could be considered to have the most positive impact on the abilities of an individual with autism, applied on a continuous basis and with high synergy among the involved care parties [17]. Hence, families have to work collaboratively with professionals from i.e. school, community and special education, to integrate the various multidisciplinary assessment findings into a comprehensive profile of the individual's strengths and concerns. This profile becomes the family's basis for planning for the selection of specific interventions. This synergy can promote discussion among the involved parties and add value to the collective expertise and the broad perspective of the interdisciplinary team, to ensure that the many needs of these individuals are met across multiple settings, and the identification of the best course of action has been framed [17]. Although a variety of service models have been described that focus on collaboration among medical and educational service professionals [18], one important component that should unite all these models is the reliance on the exchanged updated data and continuous support; in order to revise decision making and treatment planning. This collaboration and involvement allows for management and modification of treatment plans over time [19] and the provision of more accurate and comprehensive set of services.

The existing technological advancements, either Web based, desktop and/or wireless/mobile, are numerous; with several applications to offer synchronous and asynchronous (tele-) cooperation among the members of a dedicated care team. These efforts are lying mostly under the overarching research area of Computer Supported Cooperative Work (CSCW). Even though there is still no commonly accepted definition of CSCW [20], we could say that is an "umbrella term" that allow people from a variety of disciplines, with partially overlapping concerns, to cooperate and research issues of how to use computers to support activities of people working together. Suchman [21] describes CSCW as the design of computer-based technologies with explicit concern for the socially organized practices of their intended users. CSCW approaches have been in recent years extensively applied in the research domains of eHealth and Ambient Assisted Living (AAL), with a significant success. In this respect, an alternative term that has been proposed by Consolvo et al. [22], that is Computer Supported Cooperative Care (CSCC), includes the broad range of care-giving activities that a group does using technology, having in the center patients and/or elderly people.

The increasing number of different efforts that have been undertaken, in the fields of eHealth and AAL (as compared to ASD related attempts where, to the best of our knowledge, are more stand-alone and fragmented), are mainly interested in the in-house "independent living" [23]; the development of specific technologies for disabilities, i.e. dementia [24], and for addressing the needs of the users and lifestyle considerations [25]; the design of distributed integrated innovative services for elderly at home [26]; the investigation of technology that could enhance social and health care [26]; the socialization and daily monitoring of needs and requirements of the elderly in an outdoor environment [5]; and the support of the dynamic creation, management and co-ordination of virtual collaborative medical teams, for the continuous treatment of patients with chronic diseases (i.e. cancer) at home and specialist healthcare centres [28].

The particular considerations and applications are of extreme importance in our case, since many of the characteristics and the context of these areas, are similar to the ASD domain. Our main research concentration is to propose an architecture that supports active participation, communication, socialization, mutual assistance and self-organization; promoting seamless integration and interaction of different people (family members, education and community) at any time and any place and providing daily ASD-centric monitoring activity.

3   A Proposed ASD-Centric Computer Supported Collaborative Treatment Architecture

Considering the different requirements, needs and demands of the ASD domain this section outlines an ASD-centric Computer Supported Collaborative Treatment Architecture (ASD-centric CSCTA). It has its grounds on a CSCW system which has been successfully implemented in the domains of eHealth and AAL with significant acceptance and value to the use cases that has been applied (i.e. home care for cancer patients and socialization of elderly people) [28, 27, 5]. The main innovation of the proposed architecture lies at the services layer since it employs notions and techniques based on the specificities and contextual characteristics of the collaborative environment around a person with ASD (in section 4 we will analyze the notion of the ASD-centric Virtual Care Teams which supports the dynamicity of the workflows for the provision of services during a treatment session to an individual with ASD). Furthermore, it is based on IBM's reference architecture for Service-Oriented Architecture[1] (SOA). The goal of using SOA is to liberate the logic from the constraints of technology and to achieve reusability of components. Our technical approach combines Agile Software Development (ASD) and Model Driven Architectures (MDA). Agile software development focuses on optimizing quality of both software and documentation by facilitating a high level of interaction between members of the development teams and the end-users. Our system architecture is divided into 5 layers (see Figure 1): (a) *Presentation Layer*, hosts the Graphical User Interfaces (GUIs), that are personalized according to user's preferences and adaptable to any client (e.g. Mobile Device, Web browser, Desktop, etc.) according to the individual's needs maximizing the added value of the system; (b) *Interoperability Layer*, a toolset that enables the development of system components and services that use the same syntax and semantics, by utilizing information models and concepts from the underlying Information Middleware with application programming interfaces (API) and interface description languages (IDL); (c) *Service Layer*, figures as the primal innovation of the proposed architecture; implemented with the notion of ASD-centric Virtual Care Teams, dynamic workflows and a set of services that enhance collaboration dynamics among the prospective bodies that involved in the treatment of persons with ASD (it is further

---

[1] "Service-oriented modeling and architecture - How to identify, specify, and realize services for your SOA", Ali Arsanjani, SOA and Web services Center of Excellence, IBM. 09 Nov 2004: http://www-128.ibm.com/ developerworks/webservices/library/ws-soa-design1/

analyzed in section 4 of this paper); (d) *Information Layer*, hosts the Database Management System of the system (DBMS), that all the data are stored for the user management, profiling, collaboration features, virtual care teams, dynamic workflows, actions, questionnaires, etc. In our architecture, any DBMS can be utilized such as Oracle, Microsoft SQL Server and MySQL as long as all basic database functionalities are provided; and (e) *Security Layer*, ensures that the end user applications can be trusted with respect to confidentiality, integrity and availability. These three aspects are imperative to the personal information privacy and safety of the users. The security layer is designed to fulfill the domain requirements. It uses current and emerging security standards in order to create a platform that will reduce the time to market for software providers.

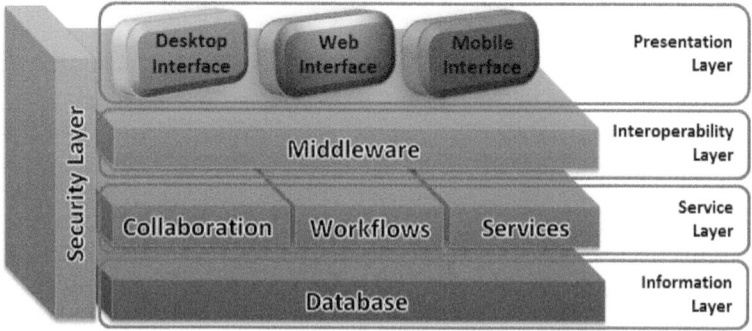

Fig. 1. An ASD-centric Computer Supported Collaborative Treatment Architecture

This layer constitutes a framework that supports PKI (X.509), ebXML framework (ISO 15000) and interoperability support for existing middleware security architectures.

4   The Enhanced *Service Layer* of the ASD-Centric CSCTA

As it is clearly perceived so far the importance of one-to-one treatment for persons with ASD is of paramount significance. Hence, efficient approaches presuppose the formulation of multidisciplinary care teams that will combine knowledge and expertise towards the application of various interventions on an individual with ASD. However, formulating such an effective care team is not an easy task. Apart from the individualistic characteristics of a person with ASD, other issues i.e., concerning the services, communication patterns and the context of a unique case have to be analyzed and well defined in order to decide which members will finally constitute such a care team. Henceforth, embracing these needs and requirements, the "Service Layer" of the proposed ASD-centric CSCTA has been designed by utilizing the notions of ASD-centric Virtual Care Teams (in "Collaboration" component), the dynamic workflows (in "Workflows" component), and a set of ASD-centric services (in "Services" component), that are continuously exchanging vital information for the most efficient and effective provision of treatment to an individual with ASD (see Figure 2). The *Collaboration* component is responsible to provide all the collaboration mechanisms between the Virtual Care Team members. Such mechanisms are emails, SMS, messages, etc. The *Workflows* component is responsible to provide mechanisms for business process automation and business intelligence. It resembles the business processes layer in the SOA architecture, having an orchestration and coordination of the basic system services, but in a more dynamic and ad-hoc manner. The *Services* component hosts the basic services that provide all the functionality of the system [33]. These services can be called directly from the application or from a workflow, and even more from another service.

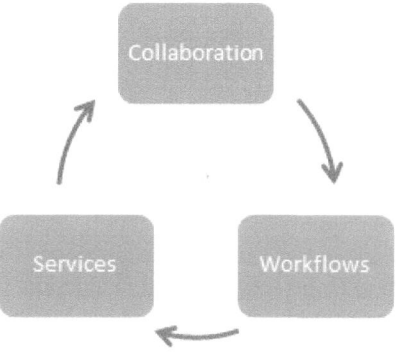

Fig. 2. The Enhanced Service Layer

Due to the peculiarity of the ASD domain, the arising contextual concepts and constraints infer to a specialized approach based on which the appropriate services will be devised for covering the needs of an ASD care team. In this regards, such an ASD-centric CSCTA should adhere to: (a) *Availability awareness*, the ASD-centric CSCTA must be aware of the user status (availability), in order to manage better any critical situations; (b) *Expandability*, an ASD-centric CSCTA has to be able to expand easily with new workflows and collaboration schemas; (c) *Easy information sharing*, users must be able to share the information they want (and nothing more) with other users, with minimum effort; (d) *Flexible messaging methods*, care team members are not always computer literate and the environment has to adapt to their communication skills. Some of them prefer the use of emails and others prefer the use of SMS text messages. The environment should be able to provide all means of communication; (e) *Availability*, an ASD-centric CSCTA has to be available 24/7 from anyplace and by any means. This brings in the wireless requirement as mandatory; (f) *Confidentiality*, collaboration messages must be confidential and only available to the intended recipients; and (g*) Security*, all collaboration messages must be secured (at least at a level acceptable to the ASD domain, given the National and/or EU policies and regulations). Most of these requirements/characteristics have been positively evaluated in the eHealth sector [28], and it is considered a motivating challenge to be applied in the ASD sector.

4.1   The "Collaboration" Component

It has been shown, in the eHealth (and more specifically in the chronic patients care) and Ambient Assisted Living (AAL) sectors, that the integration of all the aforementioned concerns under a common dynamic collaborative technological framework can be acceptable, successful and competent with the employment of Virtual Care Teams (VCT) [29]. Collaboration and virtual teams, abstractly, refer to the notion that a team of professionals decides to collaborate over the Internet and thus create a virtual team that eliminates the need of physical presence [28]. During the last few years there has been an increasing volume of literature on virtual organizations and virtual teams. This body of research generally agrees that virtual teams consist of a collection of geographically dispersed individuals who work on a joint project or common tasks and communicate electronically. For example, Lipnack and Stamps [30] define a virtual team as "a group of people who interact through inter-dependent tasks guided by a common purpose" that "works across space, time and organizational boundaries with links strengthened by webs of communication technologies". The main benefit is that in a virtual team you can do what you can't do alone. The challenge of our time is to learn to work in virtual teams and networks while retaining the benefits of earlier forms. In time, virtual teams will become the natural way to work. Since many virtual teams do occasionally meet physically on predefined time intervals, they find themselves in the conventional face-to-face setting. It is generally agreed that a good virtual team is, in a way, a good team. Four words capture the essence of virtual teams: *people, purpose, links, and time. People* populate and lead small groups and teams of every kind at every level, from the executive suite to the subcommittees of the local school's parent association. *Purpose* holds groups together, which for teams mean a focus on tasks that makes work progressing from goals to results. *Links* are the channels, interactions, and relationships. The greatest difference between in-the-same-place teams and virtual ones lies in the nature and variety of their links. *Time* is a dimension common to schedules, milestones, calendars, processes, and life cycles [30].

Adapting the term into the context, needs and requirements of the ASD domain, we are suggesting the notion of ASD-Virtual Care Teams (ASD-VCT), that are focusing on treatment objectives for a person with ASD and consisted of members coming mainly from the three more important contextual-fields for such a person, the family, school and community. It is interesting to note that the physical distance among these team members define the urgency of the collaboration and the need for dynamicity. Indeed, virtual teams have been presented in the research literature as a communication intensive and a computer-mediated linked type of group. Electronic data interchange, computer-supported cooperative work, group support systems, as well as email, videoconferencing and teleconferencing facilities, to name but a few, enable people based in different locations to communicate and coordinate their actions with great speed and effectiveness [31].

4.2   The "Workflows" Component

Nowadays, utilization of workflows in CSCW environments is a trend, that handle the abovementioned requirements through the application of specialized techniques such as ad-hoc, recursive, event driven and time triggered [32]. Workflows are mainly used to determine the sequence of an operation in order to speed up procedures, enabling better handling of resources and reorganizing energy and information flows. In the ASD-centric CSCTA context, given the current evolution of wireless technologies, workflows application mainly aim to provide end users with an easier way to orchestrate or describe complex processing of data. Moreover, they establish the need for providing dynamic working environments (dynamic workflows) of different actors (VCT members) promoting effective collaboration among them, including the person with ASD, at any time, and any context (place). Furthermore, ASD-centric CSCTA that supports workflows should not have their syntactic and contextual rules and processes hardcoded and predefined, but rather dynamic. By syntactic dynamicity (i.e configurable), we mean the ability of the workflow to change on demand during a task's execution (according to new requirements, i.e. some specialists might change rules based on a given situation).

4.3   The "Services" Component

Given the multidisciplinarity, dynamicity and constraints of the ASD sector, main objective is to comprehensively identify a number of services that could be successfully communicated within and between a specific ASD-centric Computer Supported Collaborative Treatment Environment on a continuous and consistent manner for maximizing, among others, communication efficiency and decision making in terms of time and accuracy. In this regards, a particular services model has been discussed by authors in [33], which has investigated the real user needs that are referring to an ASD-centric social community level, as well as the innovative cost-effective technologies which integrate personalized socialization services. Based on an extensive research on the individualistic and contextual characteristics of persons with ASD, literature review and interviews with specialists it has been proposed a set of services that utilize the basic notions of CSCW environments and are classified under five main categories: i) ASD Continuing Monitoring, ii) Collaboration Services, iii) Care & Wellness Services, iv) Socialization Services and v) Intervention Treatment Approach. The particular services are expressing the main outputs of the "Services Layer" and provide an added value to the communication among care parties, monitoring and error handling, decision making and social inclusion, improving the quality of life of the person with ASD.

5   A Conceptual Real Life Case Scenario: Marco

In this section we will present a real life scenario of an individual with ASD. We will elaborate on an instance of the intervention treatment approach that has been decided to be followed based on its initial diagnosis with the use of the proposed ASD-centric

CSCTA and the formulation of the dedicated VCT around it. It has to be mentioned that, for ethical and confidentiality issues, the name, age and/or any other characteristics that could reveal the real identity of this person have been altered, without though deteriorating the validity of the case.

5.1   Marco's Short Profile Description

Marco is a 5 ½ years-old boy who was diagnosed with a Pervasive Developmental Disorder; he is receptive but not verbal (i.e. he understands but he cannot speak). He is hypotonic in the vocal apparatus and mouth, he has several verbal self-stimuli (sounds like howl) and flicker/flapping hands reactions.

Parents were unable to change Marco's behaviors and to communicate with him, with great frustration of the child and his family. The exact diagnosis received only 1 year later when social, speech and communication were totally degraded and the child had become not verbal. Doctors evaluated the clinical aspects while the speech, language, and communication assessments carried out by a psychologist specialized in autism evaluations using ad-hoc test and rate scales (Vineland Adaptive Behaviour Scales, PsychoEducational Profile (PEP 3) for the functional evaluation, etc.)

5.2   Marco's Intervention Approach

The beginning of the treatment was made through training programs that were functional to his age and living environments, for the development of his verbal speech. The programs aimed at creating the basic prerequisites for school learning, like: oral motor imitation, verbal imitation, matching letters, matching numbers, matching similar words (even not "real" words), matching word/word, receptive labels, expressive labels (reading and writing), and academic sequence of letters (once acquired: numbers, seasons, days, weeks, months). Such programs include *procedures for settle/remove the howling* through strategies such as: make the discrete trials faster (i.e. increasing the teaching pace) and provide a different "powerful" reinforcement (particularly interesting for the child) for trials without howling, and *procedures for settle/remove the flicker* through strategies such as: the teaching of an alternative answer which is incompatible with the flicker (i.e. teaching the child how to put his hands into his pockets; do cycling, if necessary teaching him to ride a bicycle).

A useful tool for monitoring problem behavior (used in Marco's treatment) is the *Antecedent-Behavior-Consequence (ABC)* Analysis (Table 1). *Antecedent* is the event or activity that immediately precedes a problem behavior; *Behavior* refers to an observed behavior; and *Consequence* refers to the event that immediately follows a response. This tool allows an observer to record descriptive information about a child in a systematic and organized way, recognizing emerging predictable patterns and then studying the strategy for modifying the behavior. The idea is that when problem behavior appears, there is an antecedent that triggers the behavior and a consequence that "maintains" the behavior. The therapists/caregivers may act on the environment for avoiding the antecedent to take place, eliminating the problem behavior.

Table 1. The ABC tool

Date/Time	Activity	Antecedent	Behavior	Consequence

Furthermore, consequences increase or decrease the probability that the analyzed behavior will occur again in the future. Hence, reshaping consequences allows to model the behavior, fading out inappropriate behaviors (even though this may be difficult at some point since usually requires the change of the response by the therapists/caregivers to a problem behavior).

5.3   Marco's Typical Treatment Scenario and Concerns

A typical treatment scenario for Marco, involves 5 team members plus the parents. The team members that are participating in this scenario are the Senior Therapist, Therapist A, Therapist B, Therapist C, and a Consultant, together with the child's parents. In this scenario (see Figure 3), Senior Therapist (ST) initiate Marco's therapy program, decided and prepared by the Consultant, and assign tasks to the Therapist A (TA), Therapist B (TB) and Therapist C (TC). TA carries out a training program called "Sequence of imitation with Blocks".

TA uses ABC analysis (see Table 1) in order to monitor any problem behavior and tries to reduce/eliminate it. The therapist monitors the problem behavior spending an additional time for filling the ABC (paper) form that has to be delivered to the ST for reviewing the results. During another therapy session, TB gives a discriminative stimulus (DS) that is not coherent with the DS Marco previously received by the TA. As a result, the child fails, the program does not progress and the child do not collaborate since there was not coherence. TB monitors the problem behavior spending an additional time for filling the ABC (paper) form. Furthermore, TB spends some time to advice the child's parents on their future behavior in order to advance child's progress. TB then also delivers the results to the ST for revision. When ST gathers all results, he analyses them and conducts a cross check on the findings.

ST identifies that the DS of the TB is not coherent with the DS previously the child received (from TA). He decides to suspend the program "Blocks" and schedules a meeting with all team members in order to find an optimum solution for this problem. ST calls all team members to inform them for the updated program and tries to schedule an appropriate time for the meeting. Later, ST calls the Consultant to update him on child's program and progress. During the meeting, team members gather and observe videos of various program executions on Marco and try to analyze his behavior. ST provides corrections and resumes the program. Finally, ST prepares a report based on the meeting, referring to the changes on the program and child's progress, and disseminates the results to the Consultant.

Observing the traditional treatment scenario above, we can distinguish some limitations on the existing operational workflow of the care team members. These limitations include communication restrictions, data integrity issues, data availability and

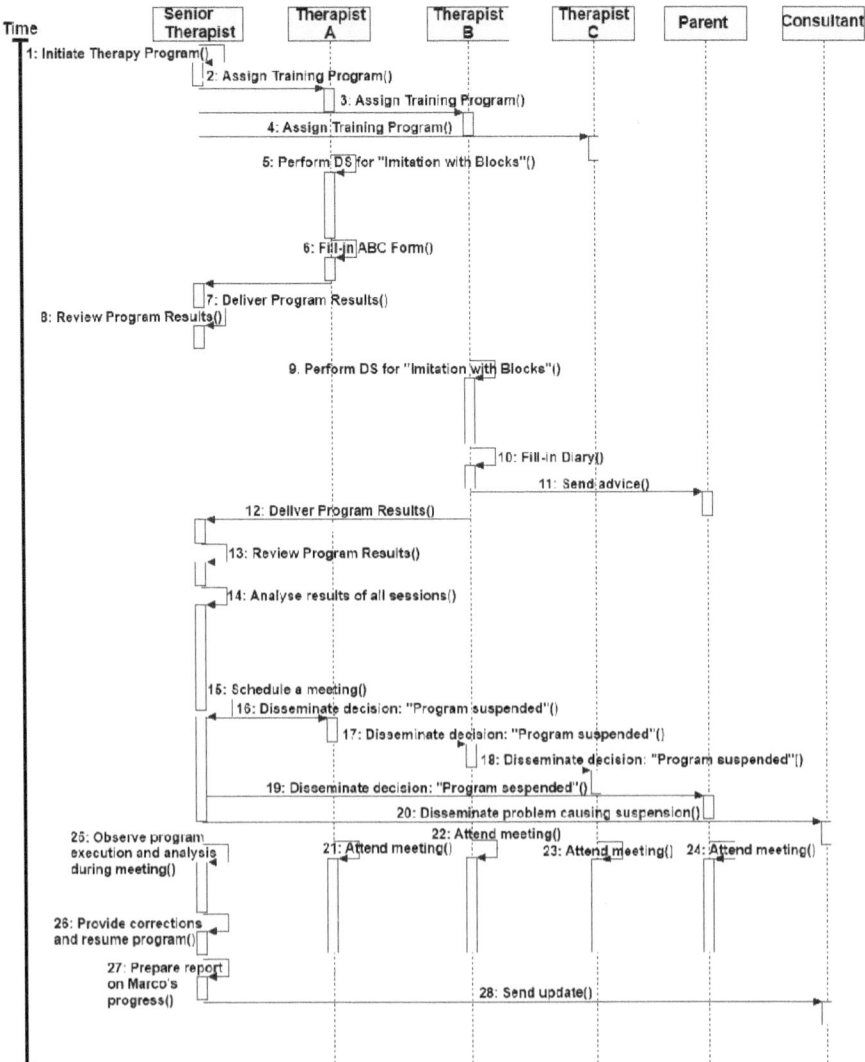

Fig. 3. Marco's Treatment Scenario UML

data sharing problems. We can easily notice that each team member has to dissemi-nate each session's results to the rest of the members via telephone or email, spending unnecessary time for propagating the results. Also, there are real life cases where the dissemination of results was not identical due to human error or mishaps and typos. Furthermore, another time consuming event is the meeting scheduling by the senior therapist. ST has to call all team members separately, in order to check their availabil-ity for each meeting. Many times, ST has to call back to rearrange the meeting and finally has to call each team member again to finalize the meeting. Such a task could be proofed frustrating and time consuming for the ST. In addition, therapists are attending sessions without the proper knowledge on previous sessions and thus the complete picture of child's progress. In our case, TB would have had consulted the ST before attempting to give a DS that is not coherent with previously DS of TA. Numerous cases show that a proper circulation of results could speed up children's progress. Through the implementation of the proposed ASD-centric CSCTA we tackle these limitations with the utilization of VCTs, a centralized knowledge base and a bouquet of ASD-centric services.

5.4   Optimizing Marco's Typical Treatment Scenario and Evaluation

In Figure 4, we illustrate the abovementioned scenario using the proposed ASD-CSCTA. For each individual with ASD we formulate a VCT by assigning users with roles that will participate in that specific team. All team members are equipped with mobile devices (i.e. iPhones, iPads, Android phones, HTC windows mobile enabled, laptops, etc.) VCT members can access and update all information about their caring individual easily from anywhere and anytime (24/7) with the utilization of mobile technologies (i.e. GPRS, 3G, WIFI, etc.), depending on their authentication rights.

In our case, the ST instead of assigning separately the initiation of the program to each therapist, logs into the system (currently we are evaluating the proposed architecture with the use of a pilot system) and initiates Marco's therapy program (called "Sequence of imitation with Blocks"), where all the therapists (TA, TB, TC) are notified automatically. At a later stage, TA monitors the Marco's problem behavior that has been noticed and fills-in online the ABC form, which is available from the system under the child's diary. As expected, the results are instantly available to ST and he reviews the results without having to wait for the TA to deliver them in person. Similarly, during another session, TB gives a DS which was not coherent with the one the child previously received by the TA. As a result, the child fails (do not collaborate), and the program does not progress as planned. TB monitors the problem behavior and updates the ABC (online) form. The results are instantly available to the ST through the system, who reviews the outcome without having to wait for the TB to deliver them in person. In addition, ST easily gathers and analyses all results and conducts a cross check on the findings since they are all available to him through the system. The derived consensus with regards to the case progression is better supported and documented. We notice that by utilizing the messaging service of the proposed treatment environment, we save valuable time and effort (as it can also be observed by comparing the two Figures, 3 and 4).

The ST decides to update the program and the system alerts TA, TB, TC and child's parents about this change. The system also makes the ST's findings available to the Consultant. ST decides to schedule a meeting with the team members and he can do this easily since he can review each team member's schedule online. Their schedule is automatically updated by the system. During the meeting session, all team members observe videos of various program executions and try to analyze Marco's behavior. ST provides corrections and resumes the program. Finally, ST prepares a report on the meeting, with the changes on the program, and child's progress and uploads it to the system. The system makes also the updates available to the Consultant.

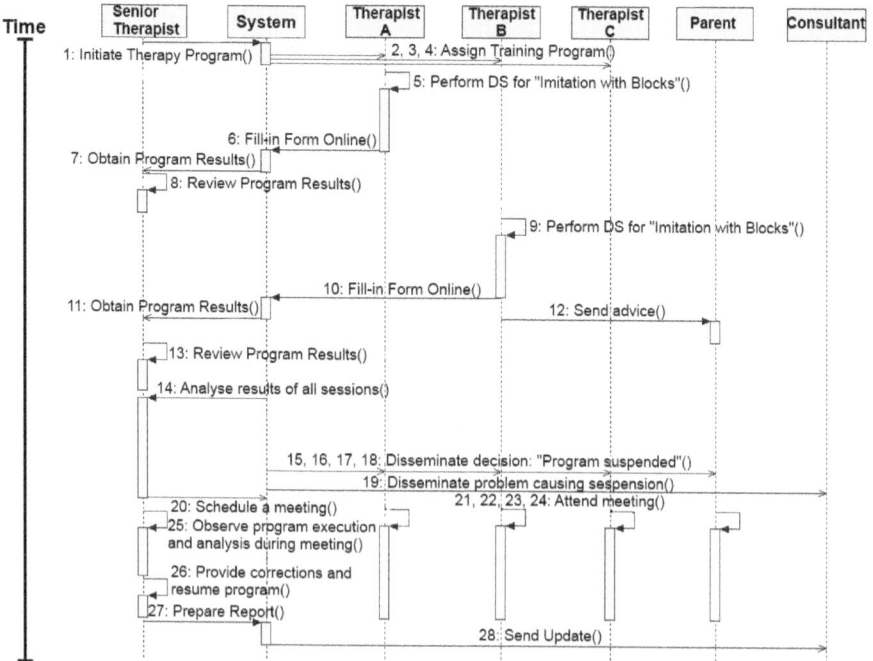

Fig. 4. Marco's Treatment Scenario UML using the ASD-centric CSCTA

Comparing the two scenarios, we can easily identify an upgrade in the Quality of Data (QoD), Quality of Service (QoS) and security in the optimized version. This is achieved through the enhanced communication and coordination among the ASD-VCT's members, with the use of the pilot system and the functionalities: Schedule updates, messaging service between users, reminders and alerts. In a more detail, QoD has been enhanced due to the continuous real-time update of information, accuracy, completeness, constancy and relevancy. QoS has been advanced since the users are collaborating in more effective and efficient manner; while security is supported by the CIA triad (Confidentiality, Integrity and Availability), which describes the fundamental security principles in a sustainable information security framework [34].

Using the system in the second optimized scenario, we identify savings in Program Management, Schedule Management and Information retrieval, which can be estimated in terms of time savings and consequently cost savings. More specifically, it has been identified that (see Figure 4) there are:

(i)   3 savings in assigning the program to the therapists (steps 2, 3 and 4).
(ii) 2 savings in information retrieval from the system (steps 7 and 11).
(iii) 2 savings in informing the consultant on updates (steps 19 and 28)
(iv) 4 savings in updates on the program to the therapists (steps 15, 16, 17 and 18)
(v)   1 saving on scheduling a meeting and 4 saving on updating therapists' schedule.

A rough diagonal estimation shows that there is a significant average saving time of the total process. In order to have a more precise estimation, we have calculated the cost for each one of these 5 groups of savings. Lying on the valuable insight of the Marco's ASD-VCT, with regards to time and cost spent in each process-step, we were able to estimate the values for these groups, based on the formulas shown in Table 2.

Table 2. Marco's Treatment Scenario Groups of Savings: Estimated Time and Cost for each Process-Step

Groups of Savings	Formula for Calculating Estimation
(i) Program assignment by the senior therapist it takes on average 15 minutes through GSM telephony.	– Total saving time = $15_{minutes}$ * number of assignments – Total cost saving = Total saving time * (cost of GSM call$_{per\ minute}$ + rate of the senior therapist$_{per\ minute}$ + rate of the therapist$_{per\ minute}$)
(ii) In order for the senior therapist to get the result, all other therapists had to return the results (ABC paper form) in the headquarters. This procedure demanded a travelling time of 30 minutes and 20 Km on average.	– Total saving time = $30_{minutes}$ * trips to headquarters – Total cost saving = (Total saving time * rate of the senior therapist$_{per\ minute}$) + (Traveling cost for 20 Km * trips to headquarters)
(iii) The update of the consultant usually takes 30 minutes and usually with the use of GSM telephony.	– Total saving time = $30_{minutes}$ * calls to the consultant – Total cost saving = Total saving time * (cost of GSM call$_{per\ minute}$ + rate of the senior therapist$_{per\ minute}$ + rate of the consultant$_{per\ minute}$)
(iv) Each therapist's update on the program by the senior therapist takes an average time of 20 minutes, again through GSM telephony.	– Total saving time = $20_{minutes}$ * calls to therapists – Total cost saving = Total saving time * (cost of GSM call$_{per\ minute}$ + rate of the senior therapist$_{per\ minute}$ + rate of the therapist$_{per\ minute}$)
(v) The scheduling of a meeting is the most time consuming task. The senior therapist has to call each participant separately in order to arrange the time that is suitable for all. After the agreement (sometimes more than one phone calls is needed) he has to call again each one of them in order to notify them about the agreed time for the meeting. This task needs 30 minutes on average for each participant through GSM telephony.	– Total saving time = $30_{minutes}$ * number of participants – Total cost saving = Total saving time * (cost of GSM call$_{per\ minute}$ + rate of the senior therapist$_{per\ minute}$ + rate of the therapist$_{per\ minute}$)

Henceforth, applying this conceptualization, in Italy, the estimated cost for the senior therapist is 18€/h, for the therapist is 12€/h, and for the consultant is 90€/h. We can also estimate the costs of supporting services, such as, telephone calls (average cost of 15c/min for GSM phone calls) and trips to visits (average cost of 10c/min or

15c/Km for gas). Furthermore, based on the team members experience the average phone call duration is 20 min and the average travel time is 30 min (approximately 20Km in urban areas). Most of the times in order for the team members to provide the above services a preparatory work has to be undertaken, as shown in Table 3.

Table 3. Cost (in EUROS) of preparatory work prior or after visit

Task	Duration (in minutes)	Cost for senior therapist	Cost for therapist	Cost for consultant
Office, discussion on patient issues, read patient notes, communication book entry	10	3€	2€	15€
Phone call to patient or his family	5	1.5€	1€	7.5€
Phone calls to other health professionals	5	1.5€	1€	7.5€
organize equipment	5	1.5€	1€	7.5€
Office work including updating patient notes, briefing team, communication book etc	15	4.5€	3€	22.5€

Finally, we calculated all other costs like traveling from/to persons' with ASD houses, from/to team members' houses and from/to headquarters, telephone costs, travel to obtain special equipment, etc. Therefore, in Marco's case, we have estimated (using the formulas in Table 2) the cost for each scenario (without and with the proposed system). In Table 4 we can view the costs in more detail for both versions of this scenario.

Table 4. Cost (in EUROS) of each scenario

Without the System				
Communication Costs	Travelling Costs	Visits Costs	Other Costs	Total
10 Calls (Steps: 2,3,4,11,16, 17,18,19,20,28)	2 trips to deliver the results (Steps:7,12)	2 Visits (Steps: 5,6,9,10)	3 reviews and a meeting (Steps: 1,8,13,14,15,21, 22,23,24,25,26,27)	
84,75€	18€	60€	351€	513.75€
With the System				
Communication Costs	Travelling Costs	Visits Costs	Other Costs	Total
1 Advice Parents (Steps: 2)	0 trips to deliver the results	2 Visits (Steps: 5,6,9,10)	3 reviews and a meeting (Steps: 1,8,13,14,21, 22,23,24,25,26,27)	
6€	0	60€	351€	417€ (≈19,5% Savings)

The calculated costs are divided into 4 categories. The Communication Costs, Traveling Costs, Visits Costs and Other Costs. The Visiting and Other Costs are not affected by the use of the system. As we can observe, the majority of the savings are mainly in Communication Costs where our system organizes all actions and speeds up communications and information sharing resulting to a cost decrease of 93%. In addition, the Traveling Costs for reporting back to the headquarters are eliminated with the use of the system. Finally, for this simple scenario, the total estimation is around 19.5% savings.

It can be easily noticed that these savings are of great importance, since the scenario instance we have used in this paper is small in scale. A normal full scale scenario consists of at least 3 therapists that are having 3-6 sessions per week each, for every child. The saving for communications only, for a sample of 50 children, can be escalated up to 20.000€ per month. In addition, there are many indirect and hidden cost savings such as traveling of trainers back to headquarters in order to obtain session of other trainers on the child that he is going to visit. There are also cases that therapists did not return the results to the headquarters on time and as a result all other therapists went to a session without proper knowledge on child's progress.

6   Conclusion and Discussion

In this paper we have underlined the significance of continuous collaborative treatment provision to individuals with ASD. Given the differences, particularities and abnormal progression of ASD a personalized multidisciplinary collaborative intervention approach for persons with ASD is considered vital for their most effective development. It has been realized that early one-to-one treatment interventions, accurate exchange of information and prompt delivery of services to such persons increase their intellectual and social abilities and make them feel more comfortable and adapted to their contextual environment. Furthermore, the rapid advancement of desktop, Web-based and mobile / wireless technologies have created new opportunities and possibilities of designing sophisticated environments and systems that can capture the needs and requirements of these persons, since they are able to improve drastically the synergy and communication within and between the ASD-centric care teams. In this respect we have proposed an ASD-centric Computer Supported Collaborative Treatment Architecture which employs the notion of Virtual Care Teams and the provision of ASD-centric services over dynamic workflows. VCTs can significantly enhance the main strategies used by all care parties that are emphasized on collaboration in the sharing of information for data-based decisions regarding diagnosis, treatment planning, and intervention and ongoing monitoring in order to meet the medical and educational needs of persons with ASD. The latter conceptualization benefits are also grounded from the ongoing positive evaluation of VCTs in the eHealth sector.

More specifically, we have applied the proposed architecture in a real life case scenario instance, with the use of a pilot system, in order to initially evaluate its effectiveness and efficiency during a treatment process which is based on ABC analysis. It has been identified an upgrade in the QoD, QoS and security in the optimized version. This is achieved through the enhanced communication and coordination recognizing savings in Program Management, Schedule Management and Information retrieval, which have been interpreted in terms of time savings and consequently cost savings on an average of 19.5% of the total process.

Limitations of this study in terms of evaluation at the various levels of interest include not only the common problems of adopting information and communication collaborative technologies in the dynamic ASD environment (i.e. reorganization working process, phobia of technology, lack of trust, limited budget) but also to a missing universal legal ASD framework. In the ASD sector legal issues are essential due to the sensitivity of the individuals' with ASD data (health / medical records, diagnostic reports, etc.) Furthermore, factors like the need to full time personnel to manage IT problems, regular retraining users to constantly changing technologies and the high cost of wireless medium lead to enormous budgets that hampers most of the times the adequate adoption of such systems.

Nevertheless, the anticipated impact on the attitudes and benefits of persons with ASD could be perceived as multifold. Indicatively, we could say that it is expected that the treatment will be more direct and sufficient since the person with ASD will feel safe and secure with the care team being around it on a 24/7 basis; the decision making with regards to the progression of this person will be enhanced and will be more accurate since there will be a live update of the exchanged information; the communication among the care team members will be more sound and prompt avoiding any delays in the whole treatment process while at the same time a more effective timely error handling will be achieved; the cost and effort of the care team members will be reduced, especially if they are in dispersed areas, without though jeopardizing the quality of the treatment.

Future work includes the extensive evaluation of the effectiveness and efficiency of the architecture at a conceptual (proof-of-concept) and as an application at a system level. Key research issues that need to be further addressed, among others, include: the support of continuity of care, by the VCTs to persons with ASD, at any given time, irrespective of locality, or cross country movement; improvement of communication within (virtual) care team members that constitute the context of the individual with ASD (home, school, community); improvement of the security and timely access to information, in accordance to the authorization roles' levels, through a unified information space (centralized database) centered around the person with ASD; improvement of the flexible collection of statistical data for further audit and research within the VCTs setting; improvement of decisions' making evaluation in terms of time and accuracy; improvement of cost effectiveness through improved communications and better planning services; etc.

References

1. American Psychiatric Association: DSM-IV-TR. Diagnostic and Statistical Manual of Mental Disorders, 4th edn., Text Revision (2000)
2. National Research Council: Educating children with autism (Committee on Educational Interventions for Children with Autism, Division of Behavioral and Social Sciences and Education). National Academy Press, Washington, DC (2001)

3. Koegel, R.L., Koegel, L.K., Frea Smith, A.E.: Emerging interventions for children with autism: Longitudinal and lifestyle applications. In: Koegel, R.L., Koegel, L.K. (eds.) Teaching Children With Autism: Strategies for Initiating Positive Interactions and Improving Learning Opportunities, pp. 1–15. Paul H. Brookes Publishing Co., Baltimore (1995)
4. Moore, D.: Computers and people with autism/Asperger syndrome. Communication (The Magazine of The National Autistic Society), 20–21 (1998)
5. Christodoulou, E., Samaras, G., Polydorou, E., Tsiourti, C., Belk, M.: Building Virtual Care Communities Supporting Elderly Socialization and Independent Living by integrating mobile wireless ICT based services. In: Conference Proceedings of Med-e-Tel, Luxenburg, April 14-16 (2010)
6. Wing, L.: The Autism Spectrum: A Guide for Parents and Professionals, London, Constable (1996)
7. Koegel, L., Carter, C., Koegel, R.: Teaching children with autism self-initiations as a pivotal response. Topics in Language Disorders 23, 134–145 (2003)
8. Rapin, I., Tuchman, R. F.: Autism: Definition, neurobiology, screening, diagnosis. Pediatric Clinics of North America 55(5), 1129–1146 (2008)
9. Jordan, P., Jones, G., Morgan, H.: The Foundation for People with Learning Disabilities (2001)
10. Happe, F.: Autism: cognitive deficit or cognitive style? Trends in Cognitive Neurosciences 3(6), 216–222 (1999)
11. Bryson, E.S., Rogers, S.J., Fombonne, E.: Autism Spectrum Disorders: Early Detection, Intervention, Education, and Psychopharmacological Management. Canadian Journal of Psychiatry 48(8) (2003)
12. Filipek, P.A., Accardo, P.J., Ashwal, S., Baranek, G.T., Cook, E.H., Dawson, G., Volkmar, F.R.: Practice parameter: Screening and diagnosis of autism. Report of the quality standards subcommittee of the American Academy of Neurology and the Child Neurology Society. Neurology 55, 468–479 (2000)
13. Volkmar, F.R., Cook Jr., E.H., Pomeroy, J., Realmuto, G., Tanquay, P.: Practice parameters for the assessment and treatment of children, adolescents, and adults with autism and other pervasive developmental disorders. Journal of the American Academy of Child and Adolescent Psychiatry 38(12 suppl.), 32S–54S (1999)
14. Sallows, G.O., Graupner, T.D.: Intensive behavioral treatment for children with autism: Four-year outcome and predictors. American Journal on Mental Retardation 110(6), 417–438 (2005)
15. Rogers, S.J., Vismara, L.: Evidence-based comprehensive treatments for early autism. Journal of Clinical Child and Adolescent Psychology 37(1), 8–38 (2008)
16. Committee on Children with Disabilities: American Academy of Pediatrics: Screening infants and young children for developmental disabilities. Pediatrics 93, 863–865 (1994)
17. Power, T., DuPaul, G.J., Shapiro, E.S., Kazak, A.E.: Promoting children's health: Integrating school, family, and community. Guilford Press, New York (2003)
18. Drotar, D., Palermo, T., Barry, C.: Collaboration with schools: Models and methods in pediatric psychology and pediatrics. In: Brown, R.T. (ed.) Handbook of Pediatric Psychology in School Settings, pp. 21–36. Erlbaum, Mahwah (2004)
19. Shellenberger, S., Couch, K.W.: The school psychologist's pivotal role in promoting the health and well-being of children. School Psychology Review 13, 211–215 (1984)
20. Wilson, P.: Computer Supported Cooperative Work (CSCW): Origins, concepts and research initiatives. Comp. Networks ISDN Syst. 23(1-3), 91–95 (1991)
21. Suchman, L.: Notes on Computer Support for Cooperative Work. Working Paper WP-12, Dept. of Computer Science, University of Jyvaskyla, SF-40100, Jyvaskyla, Finland (1989)

22. Consolvo, S., Roessler, P., Shelton, B.E., LaMarca, A., Schilit, B., Bly, S.: Technology for Care Networks of Elders. IEEE Pervasive Computing Mobile and Ubiquitous Systems: Successful Aging, 22–29 (2004)
23. Berlo, A.: Smart Houses and Smart Living for Older People: Lessons Learnt from 10 Years Experience in the Netherlands. In: Med-e-Tel 2007, Luxexpo, Luxembourg, April 18-20 (2007)
24. Hagen, I., Bjørneby, S.: User and carer involvement in the development of assistive technology for people with dementia in Challenges for Assistive Technology. In: Enzmendi, G., et al. (eds.), pp. 809–814. IOS Press (2007)
25. Dickinson, R., Eisma, A., Syme, G.P.: UTOPIA: Usable Technology for Older People: Inclusive and Appropriate. In: Brewster, S., Zajicek, M. (eds.) A New Research Agenda for Older Adults BCS HCI 2002, London, pp. 38–39 (2002)
26. Cabral, J.P., Renals, S., Richmond, K., Yamagishi, J.: Towards An Improved Modeling of the Glottal Source in Statistical Parametric Speech Synthesis. In: Proc. 6th ISCA Speech Synthesis Workshop, Bonn, Germany (2007)
27. Mikalsen, M., Hanke, S., Fuxreiter, T., Walderhaug, S., Wienhofen, L.: Interoperability Services in the MPOWER Ambient Assisted Living Platform. In: Medical Informatics Europe (MIE) Conference 2009, Sarajevo, August 30-September 2 (2009)
28. Pitsillides, A., Samaras, G., Georgiadis, D., Andreou, P., Christodoulou, E., Pitsillides, B.: Tele-homecare supported by the DITIS collaborative platform. In: IST Africa, Maputo, Mozambique, Africa, May 09-11 (2007)
29. Georgiadis, D., Germanakos, P., Mourlas, C., Samaras, G., Christodoulou, E.: Dynamic Business Processes and Virtual Communities in Wireless eHealth Environments. In: Mohammed, S., Fiaidhi, J. (eds.) A Chapter to Appear in: Ubiquitous Health and Medical Informatics: the Ubiquity 2.0 Trend and Beyond. IGI Global, Hershey (2010) ISBN: 978-1-61520-777-0
30. Lipnack, J., Stamps, J.: VIRTUAL TEAMS: People Working Across Boundaries with Technology, 2nd edn. John Wiley & Sons, NY (2000)
31. Samaras, G., Georgiades, D., Pitsillides, A.: Computational and Wireless Modeling for Collaborative Virtual Medical Teams. In: Istepanian, R.H., Laxminarayan, S., Pattichis, C.S. (eds.) M-Health: Emerging Mobile Health Systems, pp. 107–132. Kluwer Academic/Plenum Publishers (2005)
32. Georgiadis, D., Germanakos, P., Samaras, G., Mourlas, C., Christodoulou, E.: An Intelligent Web-based Healthcare System: The Case of DYMOS. In: Lazakidou, A. (ed.) Web-based Applications in Health Care and Biomedicine of the Annals of Information Systems Series (AoIS), pp. 19–46. Springer, Heidelberg (2010), doi:10.1007/978-1-4419-1274-9_3
33. Germanakos, P., Georgiadis, D., Buzzi, M., Buzzi, M.C., Fenili, C.: A Proposed ASD-Centric Collaborative Treatment Environment: The Underlying Role of Virtual Care Teams. In: Proceedings of the 6th Mediterranean Conference on Information Systems (MCIS 2011), Limassol, Cyprus, September 3-5 (2011)
34. Merkow, M., Breithaupt, J.: Information Security: Principles and Practices. Prentice Hall (2006) ISBN:0131547291

Home-Healthcare-Network (H2N): An Autonomous Care-Giving System for Elderly People

Rezwan Islam[1], Sheikh Iqbal Ahamed[2], Chowdhury S. Hasan[3], and Casey O'Brien[4]

[1] Marshfield Clinic, 3501 Cranberry Blvd, weston, WI 54476, Wisconsin, USA
islam.rezwan@marshfieldclinic.org
[2] MSCS Dept., Marquette University, 1313 W Wisconsin Ave., Milwaukee, WI, USA
iq@mscs.mu.edu
[3] Dept. of Computer Science, University of Calfornia, Irvine, CA, USA
cshasan@ics.uci.edu
[4] MSCS Dept., Marquette University, 1313 W Wisconsin Ave., Milwaukee, Wisconsin, USA
casey.obrien@mu.edu

Abstract. As the world's population ages, the number of elderly people suffering from various diseases increases. Due to a variety of reasons such as convenience or a need for security and privacy these elderly people generally prefer to avail healthcare facilities at their home. Advances in ubiquitous computing and wireless sensor networking have opened up new opportunities in healthcare systems. In-home pervasive networks may assist residents by providing memory enhancement, remote control of home appliances, medical data lookup and emergency communication. This is time to break through the physical boundaries of hospitals and bring healthcare facilities to the homes. Wireless and internet-based healthcare devices can play a vital role in this regard given that reliable, individualized systems with user-friendly interfaces are developed to enable elderly people feel comfortable with making use of novel technology. This paper presents Home Healthcare Network (H2N), a complete system integrating the abundance of existing sensor nodes and other devices with pervasive, wireless networks. Our approach focuses on improving social aspects of elderly care besides the conventional care-giving functionalities. Finally, we talk about the importance of preserving privacy of such a system and propose a primitive solution for the inclusion of privacy awareness in the system. Although H2N is basically designed to function as a healthcare aide for the elderly people, with little customization it can be used to accommodate other user groups as well.

Keywords: Home monitoring, Smart home, Assisted living, Elderly people, TinyOS.

1 Introduction

During the last decade, the size of elderly population has shown noteworthy growth, especially in the developed countries. Carrying out daily tasks at home becomes difficult or impossible for elderly persons with restricted mobility capabilities.

A. Holzinger and K.-M. Simonic (Eds.): USAB 2011, LNCS 7058, pp. 245–262, 2011.

Besides, movement in (out)-doors requires a third-party's assistance [18, 19]. Yet, these elderly people clearly prefer independent living to institutionalization [16, 17]. At same time, they exhibit ever-increasing tendency towards leading an isolated life away from their offspring. In this context, conceiving technologies for increasing their autonomy, so as to enable them to self-manage their life is of utmost importance. Furthermore, a safe, convenient, sound and healthy living environment is the prerequisite for a good house for the elderly people with special needs.

Recent progresses in wireless sensor networking have created huge opportunities in healthcare systems. There seems to exist immense possibility for the integration of the abundance of existing specialized medical technology with pervasive, wireless networks. These will co-exist with the installed infrastructure, real-time data collection and augmenting response. Examples of areas in which current medical systems can be promoted the most from wireless sensor networks are in-home assistance, smart nursing homes, and clinical trial.

The number of elderly people increases as the world's population ages. Residents may be assisted by in-home pervasive networks through providing memory enhancement, remote control of home appliances, medical data lookup and emergency communication. Unobtrusive, wearable sensors will allow vast amounts of data to be collected and mined for long-term historical analysis. Data will be collected and reported automatically, reducing the cost and inconvenience of regular visits to the physician.

The well-being of elderly people depends greatly on proper care and treatment. Their physical status needs to be monitored regularly on a continuous basis. Normally this can be accomplished with the help of a human assistant. In modern days people are rarely available to take care of their elderly relatives. Due to that, design and development of automated care-giving system is an important issue. This is a complicated process as it involves numerous concerns. The design and development of an effective full-featured automated care-giving system is a challenging task. Taking proper care of elderly people differs from generic care-giving systems in various ways because of diverse nature of problems experienced by people at old age. At the core of any attempt to build an automated system, we see the identification of required features and characteristics based on the functionalities to be performed. We have conducted extensive analysis and practical survey to properly find out the requirements of an effective automated care-giving system. Our analysis exhibits that such a system which targets elderly people should incorporate a number of exclusive functionalities in addition to the standard in-home healthcare facilities. Such requirement makes us face novel challenges which should be handled properly. In this paper, we have listed all the required functionalities of an automated in-home healthcare system and mentioned which ones among them should obviously be included for elderly care management. We also come up with the challenging research issues we need to consider. Then we propose an automated system featured with all those facilities solving the challenges arisen.

The whole care-giving process for elderly people can be divided into two parts. Primarily we should concern about the physical health and wellbeing of the body. This requires continuous monitoring of physical condition, movement of the subject and the status of the environment where he stays along with the option of control when necessary. In reality, numerous parameters and conditions are related to the health status of a person. Among those we have chosen fall detection and sleep monitoring as the most significant for elderly people and built systems for continuously monitoring those two aspects. Aside from this system, we have developed another module which facilitates remote monitoring and control of home electronic devices. This tool can contribute significantly to the elderly care-giving process. Using this module an elderly user can see the status of a number of electric devices belonging to his house while he is away from his residence. This type of application should be of great help for a person suffering from memory deficiency which is very common at old age. As an additional advantage, by using this application friends and relatives of an elderly person can monitor and control the status of certain electronic appliances of his home. This sort of interesting service will surely have some sort of psychological impact on the subject and eventually tend to boost his social interaction. In order to maintain good health performing regular physical exercise is a must. Very often it becomes troublesome for elderly people to maintain regularity of the tasks. Sometimes conducting regular exercise is required as part of medical treatment. We have built an enhanced game glove system which can either be used as a joystick to play computer games or as a therapy tool. While playing games using the game glove detailed movements of different parts of the user's hand is captured automatically. The performance of the user in the game also measures the fitness of different parts of hand. This data is later used for analysis and treatment is suggested based on that. Thus the game glove system can be used as a therapy tool side by side providing entertainment and in this way it will eliminate the boredom of performing regular hand exercise.

Reluctance to social interaction is another major aspect of problems common in elderly people. Most of them show tendency to remain secluded as they do not feel comfortable to meet people and participate into social gatherings. In our research we find that improving the quality of social life should be considered with importance. We have proposed an application which aims at monitoring the level of social activity from online chat history and then providing relevant suggestions to enhance social interaction. We have shown how this application can cooperate with the other modules. For this, we propose a central integration unit which supervises functions of different components and ensures proper synchronization among them in a systematic way.

The rest of the paper is organized as follows. Section 2 discusses the required features of an ideal elderly care system. Section 3 focuses on the related works. Then we propose our system in Section 4 and describe its core functionalities. Section 5 walks through the necessary details of the major components related to different subsystems. We talk about the prototype developed so far in Section 6. This section also contains results of our survey regarding user experience. Finally, we conclude the paper in Section 7.

2   Essential Features

The home healthcare network which we propose possesses a number of special features which make it novel and unique. These features are discussed below.

Cost effective: Elderly care is typically a very costly process, especially when done at a clinic or nursing home. Our system uses inexpensive, readily available sensors, electrical devices and takes advantage of the existing technology a user would already have at her home, such as computer, cell phone or PDA. In addition, the system can handle multiple users simultaneously.

Accurate: In order to be comparable to the diagnosis a nursing home would give, a portable solution must keep accuracy as an important goal. To balance cost and accuracy, the chosen sensors and other tools, instruments are in some cases multifunctional (the pulse oximeter) and in all cases deliver the best results as compared to the price. Also, because our approach can be used as a long-term monitoring solution, extreme readings from the automated system will average out over the longer period of time which will produce a more accurate assessment.

Reliable: Because we have designed our home healthcare system with long-term monitoring as an objective, the system itself must be reliable. It should be able to be used consistently for weeks or even months continuously without degrading in accuracy or requiring any maintenance on the part of the user. Although it is impossible to prepare for all situations that may occur, the system is easily customizable for any age of the user, allowing it to respond to unique needs more effectively than a "one size fits all" solution could do.

Privacy aware: Our proposed system monitors daily activities, health status and collects lifestyle data. So, it is quite natural that users would want to control the use of their confidential information. Our solution allows the user to customize how their information is shared and who can have access to it. By default, only the doctor who will diagnose the user or any close relative will have access to the information and data on the system itself will be restricted to the specific user who collected it.

Simple yet meaningful GUI: The major target age group of our home care-giving system is the elderly. With the passage of time the older age groups are becoming more and more familiar with computers and mobile devices. Still in order to accommodate everyone now and in the future the user interface of our application is very simple. Text is easy to read and most importantly a new user should have little problems utilizing the full potential of the system. For the completely trained user it can be nearly autonomous, requiring the user to simply wear the sensors and then visit the doctor when collection is complete. However, it will also accommodate to the other end of the spectrum by being very customizable and revealing more options to more experienced users.

Easy and noninvasive to setup and use: A user will be expected to use the system throughout the whole day in order to get an accurate assessment of her daily life patterns. For this reason, the entire system must be easy to setup not interfere with normally used household objects. Emerging pervasive technologies make this especially easy but present some challenges as well. The communication between devices is wireless, so the user does not need to worry about many wires being tangled up. However, the number of wireless motes and other devices needs to be balanced as well, because the more parts a system contains the less easy it is to setup and use. Because of the expandability of the system, it is easy to incorporate many wireless nodes or stick to fewer nodes with more sensors attached to each one.

Safety of the User: A major part of the application deals with remote handling of electrical appliances, so ensuring safety of the environment is of utmost importance. The process of distant regulation of a device should be safe enough for the home environment such that it does not cause electrical shocks, short-circuits, fires etc. Besides, immediate actions should be taken regarding any malfunctioning behavior of a device to safeguard major mishaps.

Security, Authenticity and Integrity of Data: In order to avoid false data all tiny sensors must be authenticated before data can be treated as reliable. Security and reliability of the data are highly dependent on the authentication mechanism. There should be integrity among all these data and by checking this integrity the system will be able to detect any anomalous situation such as faulty/malfunctioning device, erroneous information from any source.

Universal and Ceaseless Access: The entire system must provide uninterrupted connectivity between the remote PC or handheld device of the users and the home monitoring system.

3   Related Work

Telemedicine and remote monitoring of patients at home are gaining higher urgency and importance [3, 4]. In [2], the in-house movements of elderly people are monitored by placing infrared sensors in each room of their homes. While such a method may not be as obviously intrusive as using cameras, still it intrudes into the privacy of the person. Ahamed et al. discusses the challenges of developing Wellness Assistant (WA) [10], software which can be used by people with obesity, diabetes, or high blood pressure, conditions which need constant monitoring. In [13] they provide the details of another application 'Healthcare Aide'. A similar software called Wellness Monitor (WM) is presented in [11] which facilitates continuous follow-up of cancer patients.

In [3] the new possibilities for home care and monitoring are described using wireless micro sensors. Regular patient monitoring using personal area networks of wireless intelligent sensors is reported in [4]. The development of care support system to monitor the overall health of residents who need constant care has been reported in [5]. The Home Heartbeat [6] is commercial product developed by Eaton [6] with assistance from MAYA design [7]. Home Heartbeat uses wireless sensors to determine if windows or doors are open, which devices/appliances are on, if there is water in the basement, and so forth. Gaddam et al. proposed the development of a wireless sensors based home monitoring system especially for elder people [8]. All these systems have the purpose of monitoring a patient remotely or taking care of elderly people. These systems do not facilitate universal access as they target a particular user group. Most of these systems are not even affordable by common people.

The relationship between services, spaces and users in the context of a smart home is analyzed in [9]. Then they propose a framework as well as a corresponding algorithm to model their interaction. In [14] an omnipresent customizable service is presented which can be used by different types of users from different fields such as education, healthcare, marketing, or business, at any time, and at any place. In [15] Mileo et al. describe an intelligent home environment in which modern wireless sensor network technologies allow constant monitoring of a patient in a context-aware setting.

Some recent works in relation to ambient assisted living is reported in [16] which refer to electronic environments that are sensitive and responsive to the presence of people and provide assistive propositions for maintaining an independent lifestyle. Similar works presented in [17] aims at producing technological and media support to help elderly people to stay at their homes longer. These works propose advanced interface mechanisms and other techniques to assist lifestyle. In [22-24] Holzinger et al. discusses some usability metrics ascertained on the basis of experiments made with applications for elderly people and investigates achievable metrics for the evaluation of passive technology, trustworthiness and usability while categorizing them according to applicability for usability testing.

4   Our Approach: H2N (Home-Healthcare-Network)

We present the concept of a complete and autonomous system for providing in-home healthcare services to the elderly people. A central control unit supervises the components and integrates their functionalities. Our system makes use of easily available devices and technologies to build the sub-systems. They include PDA, smart phone, RFID, mote sensors, iRobot, webcam etc. Most of these are frequently used by modern people.

A group of services are essential for taking proper care of elderly people. There exist numerous systems which provide some common services. But here we mention some services which will provide extra facilities to the elderly people. These services are discussed in brief below. Prior to that, we have depicted an overview of the overall architecture of our proposed system in Figure 1. It should be noted that several components comprise the entire H2N system and each component is responsible for one or more services.

4.1   Continuous Patient Monitoring

This is a common feature for any elderly care system. Due to its inevitability we include this service into our system. There should be an automated system for monitoring the health status of the elderly residents on a continuous basis. Old people most

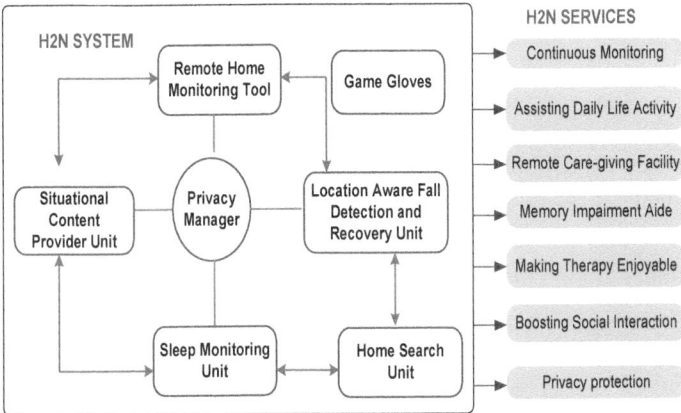

Fig. 1. H2N Architecture and Its Services

often suffer from restricted mobility. Such people are vulnerable to sudden fall down which may cause serious injury or even death due to severe stroke or heart failure. For this a fall detection unit should be a significant part of the continuous monitoring system. Another aspect which we focus on is sleep monitoring as disturbance in regular sleep habit is common at old age and it causes a number of other complicacies. So, our proposed system includes a fall detection unit and a sleep monitoring unit as part of the continuous patient monitoring. These units monitor the patients, collect data and send to a central unit. The central unit later analyses the data and takes decision regarding emergency situation.

4.2   Assisting Daily Life Activity

In modern age elderly people are smart enough to make use of advanced electronic devices. In fact, these devices have become part and parcel of their life. The more they get accustomed to using these devices, the more they face the problem of properly handling them. As memory deficit is common in most elderly people, proper maintenance of home electronic devices becomes more difficult. Keeping this in mind we provide the facility of controlling the electronic devices remotely. Using this advanced feature relatives of the elderly people will be able to check the status of the devices and control them. Even the elderly people themselves will be able to do that while they are out of home.

4.3   Remote Care-Giving Facility

The remote device monitoring tool incorporated in our system will facilitate taking care of elderly people from distant places. There are a lot of people staying away from their old-aged parents. They can monitor status of the place where their parents are living through the remote home monitoring tool. After viewing the status they can control some devices as well if needed. This can be done periodically or on an emergency basis. There might arise some emergency situation due to malfunctioning of some of the devices which will trigger an alarm and the alarm will be immediately informed to some of the friends or relatives of the residents. This sort of facility will enable prompt action against any emergency situation to avoid any potential danger.

Moreover, a deep insight into such facility reveals another indirect benefit which has emotional impact on the elderly people. Using this remote device monitoring tool their relatives will be able to keep in continuous touch with them which will show more deep concern regarding them.

4.4   Memory Impairment Aide

As we have already mentioned, memory impairment is very common to elderly people. This syndrome interrupts the normal flow of life in many ways. They forget the locations of household objects very frequently. We consider this problem and provide a solution to this.

Our system makes use of a moving object which can be a simple iRobot and RFID tags attached with it. The most frequently used objects of daily life are attached with RFID tags. Whenever any object is being searched for the iRobot starts travelling throughout the home environment and as soon as it receives signal from the RFID tag attached with the object it reports the location. Thus it takes the user to the nearest possible location of the object being looked for.

4.5   Making Therapy Enjoyable

Elderly people go through various types of regular treatments and therapies. Some of these involve regular physical exercise which is a bit cumbersome task. Most people consider the task of regular exercise as monotonous and so they show reluctance to conduct that. Moreover, many patients even cannot remember to do that regularly. We propose a game glove module which intends to provide therapy in an entertaining way. We have focused on the therapy needed for people suffering from restricted hand movement or other problem at any parts of the hand. The therapy system involves movement of every individual part of the hand while playing a computer game. The game glove system functions just like a standard joystick. The patients will play games wearing the game glove which will facilitate the task of doing regular exercise. Thus we aim at providing enjoyable therapy system.

4.6   Boosting Social Interaction

Social aspect of elderly people should be considered as an important issue. Many people at their older age feel reluctant to maintain social attachment. They intend to keep themselves aloof from others even from their close relatives. This tendency hampers the quality of their life a lot. However, it is true that some people might even not be physically fit to participate into social parties and other gatherings. So, we are thinking of a system which will increase their social interaction with little active involvement from them. Our system aims to provide a software solution to this problem. The application will be somewhat like a chat application with some advanced features. The application will be used from the cell phone, PDA of the user in co-operation with a server installed at the home. The ultimate goal of the application is to remove loneliness of the elderly people by providing them more close connection with their friends and relatives.

4.7   Ensuring Privacy Protection

Modern people are very much concerned of their privacy. Any system that has threat of privacy violation might not be expected to be used by a large number of people. Privacy preservation is considered with great importance in our system. There are various aspects of privacy which are managed differently in our approach. In one side we should make sure that sensitive user data is never accessed by unintended authorities. On other side our system also shows ways of preserving location privacy which is a novel aspect of privacy violation.

Now, we give a detail description of the above services which our ultimate system intends to provide. The hardware and software components we have developed support most of these facilities. While developing the entire system we followed a modular architecture where individual module is responsible for specific task and a central control unit supervises, synchronizes and integrates the different tasks. Below we discuss the components in detail with description of implementation and functionalities.

5   Major Components

The In this section, we discuss the components of H2N individually. H2N follows a modular architecture which facilitates addition of new modules as/when required.

5.1   Remote Home Monitoring Tool

Continuously monitoring the statuses of electrical devices and certain environmental parameters of the home is the basic task of this tool. A number of mote sensors are placed in the rooms to collect data regarding temperature, humidity, light, sound, smoke etc. There is a special purpose switch which works with a device selection unit to monitor and control on/off state or operating level of any electrical device. Data from the sensors and the switch are sent to a server connected to the internet. An authorized user can log on to the website at anytime, from any place and using a PC, laptop or PDA. The server module displays status of home appliances/devices, doors, windows and values of selected ambient parameters graphically. The system interacts with the user through an interface having iconic representations of appliances/devices, doors, windows, rooms etc. The multimodal interface is customizable based on user's preference. It requires minimal typed input from the user and is easy to learn and use. One of the major goals of this tool is to ensure universal access to home monitoring system. It is accessible from any phone, PDA or computer connected to the internet. There is no constraint on the software or hardware platform of the client. It can schedule reports on home status at periodic times with specified intervals. Besides, fixed thresholds can be set up to check for an emergency situation (according to gathered data) and generate an alarm. The authorized users can also be immediately notified and can take measures before it is too late.

The major steps of developing this tool start with creating an interface on the web that mobile devices can access at anytime from any place and to have a TMote sensor-based monitoring system that can control the flow of electricity to home electric appliances. Finally we enable the web interface to send signals to the TMote monitoring system, effectively allowing the user to monitor and control electric appliances at home while they are away. The entire system comprises a hardware unit and a software unit. Major part of the hardware unit is an analog control switch which controls the electronic device connected to it. There is a TMote which works as wireless data transceiver to transfer data to and from the server. The overall hardware interface will resemble the picture of Figure 2. As shown in this figure any other electronic device can be attached to the switch and using a device selection unit a specific device can easily be chosen.

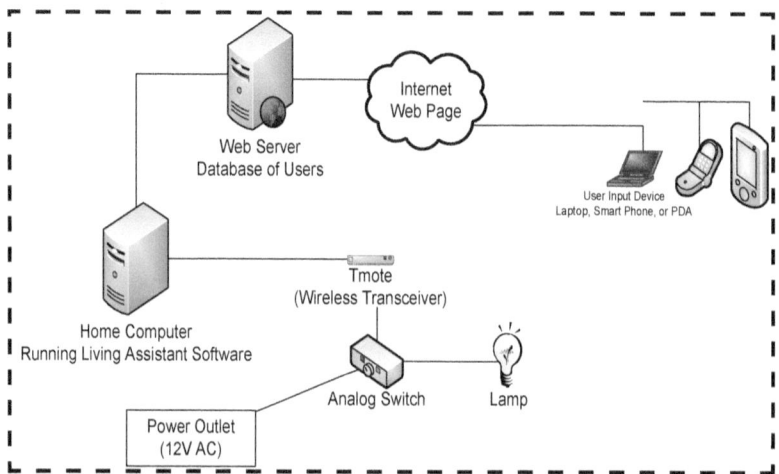

Fig. 2. Software Unit of Remote Home Monitoring Tool

The above figure presents the architecture of the software unit. Major components are TMote sensors, a home computer and a web server. Status of a device connected to the analog switch is stored in the home computer. A user accesses this data by logging on to the website through internet.

The prototype version of the tool is built using Visual Studio 2008, nesC, TinyOS [28] and JDK 1.6. Using HTML with JavaScript for our web architecture ensures that our system functions on most devices and still allows active interaction with the client monitoring and control software. We use switching relays and a single plug interface for our electrical hardware to promote easy and inexpensive prototype development and construction. The web page accessed by the user through a PDA, Smart Phone, or Computer with internet connection, is programmed using HTML and JavaScript.

The HTML acts as a wrapper to display the content to the user while the JavaScript is used to pull information from the user (input) as well as give output to the user. The user input is sent to an APACHE web server which hosts a database of customers as well as command information which is relayed to a Home Computer running the software module. The system sends information to a TMote sensor to carry out a user specified task. The diagram below shows the user interface of the system.

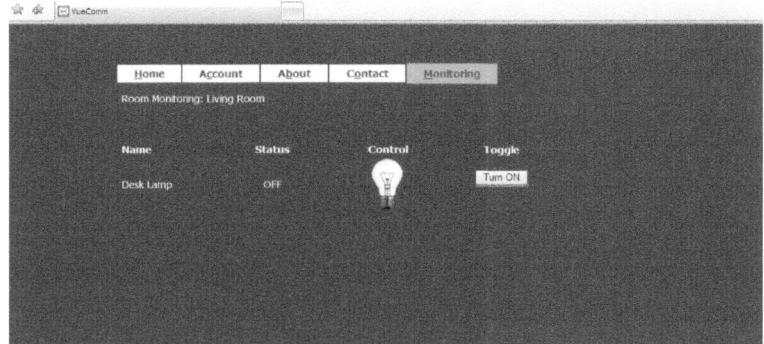

Fig. 3. Software Interface of the Remote Home Monitoring Application

5.2   Game Gloves

We have termed this unit as Wellness and Arm Rehabilitation (WeAR). WeAR functions just like any other existing joystick. But its actual purpose is different. WeAR intends to provide assistance to physically impaired people, especially elderly people with movement disorders, performing their regular physical exercises in more comfortable and enjoyable way as it seems to them that they are just playing computer games. The muscular movements carried on during the course of playing such games eventually serves as the required physical exercises.

At present a wired Game Glove system is built which is fully operating. Figure 4 presents the structure of the current Game Glove system and depicts how it actually looks and works.

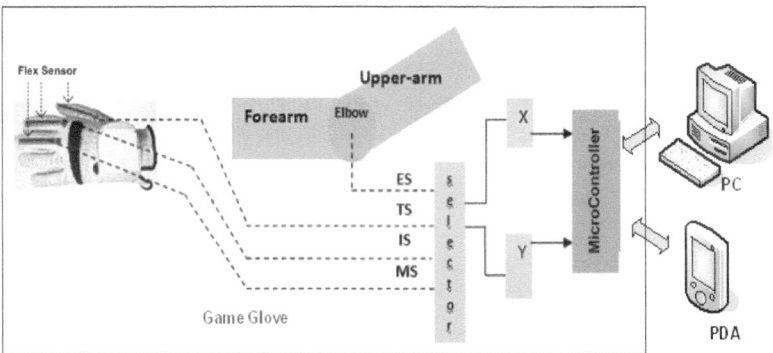

Fig. 4. Logical Diagram of Game Gloves system

The current system makes use of 3 flexible bend sensors to measure movement of the fingers. Signals coming from thumb, index finger and middle finger are denoted as TS, IS and MS respectively. Data from the potentiometer placed at elbow is termed as ES. The bi-directional flex sensor which we used is a unique component that changes resistance when bent. At the non-bent position the sensor has a nominal resistance of 10,000 ohms (10 K). As the flex sensor is bent in either direction the resistance gradually decreases. The system measures the rotation of elbow with the help of a potentiometer. All these 4 inputs come from the user and later pass through a selection unit where any two of those inputs are chosen which we term as X and Y. The μ-controller works with the X and Y inputs and performs the task of interfacing the whole external joystick unit with the PC unit which hosts any game software. The μ-controller is programmed in assembly language to deal with the registration process required to make the joystick identifiable by the native game controller.

5.3   Home Search Unit

This unit is supposed to consist of an iRobot, PDA, RFID tags and a server PC. A database of necessary household objects along with their current location is maintained at the server PC. At the initialization phase the database is populated with a list of objects and their locations. This list is periodically updated. Each object has an RFID tag attached with it and the RFID reader is carried by an iRobot. The iRobot moves throughout the home environment and visits every room periodically or on demand. For simplicity we assume the iRobot follows a fixed path for traveling from one room to another. While traveling it carries the RFID reader which transmits signal and as soon as it receives signal from a tag it recognizes that and updates the location of corresponding object.

5.4   Location Aware Fall Detection and Recovery Unit

This unit consists of a number of tmote sensors, RFID reader/tag, server, PDA etc. The iRobot is also used for finding the location where the patient has fallen. A group of accelerometer sensors are attached to the body of the user in order to continuously measure his physical activity level. During day time an extended period of time without any activity indicates toward an unusual situation which might have occurred due to fall down of the patient. The data collected by the tmote sensors are transmitted to the server which stores, analyzes them to compute duration of major inactivity and decides whether any mishap has happened. On the occasion the patient has fallen down, the server instructs the iRobot to find out exact location of the patient. The iRobot then starts traversing through the home carrying the RFID reader and as soon as it receives signal from RFID tag attached with the patient sends location information (in this case, room number) to the server. The server generates an alarm and sends to the PDAs of the relevant recipients. Immediately the recipients respond with their location and status based on which server program decides the nearest available person and notifies him.

5.5   Sleep Monitoring Unit

H2N includes a sleep monitoring unit. We focused on making this unit low cost, suitable for home use, and most importantly a continuous, long-term system. The sleep monitoring unit can be split into three major sections: nighttime data collection, daytime data collection, and analysis. Overall architecture of the sleep monitoring unit is depicted below.

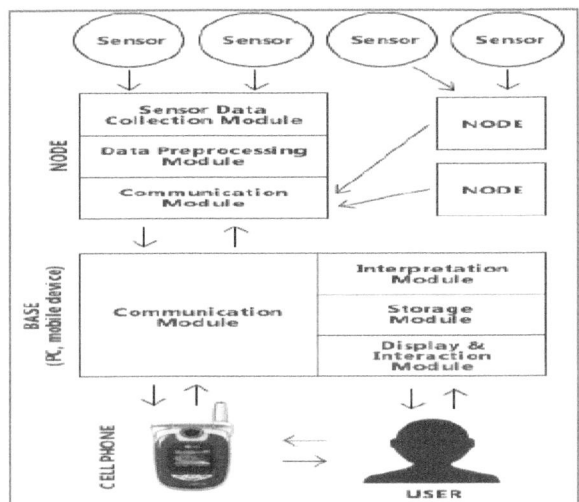

Fig. 5. Architecture of Sleep Monitoring Unit

Night-time Data Collection: We used a network of sensors and motes that communicate wirelessly using the Zigbee protocol and made a sensor-based system that is user friendly and not too obtrusive during sleep. Three of the sensors connect via wires to the main mote located on the person's arm. There are nasal and oral airflow sensors which are thermistors capable of measuring the patient's breathing, a characteristic especially important when diagnosing sleep apnea [20]. There is also a microphone placed near the base of the subject's neck to record sound such as snoring. The leg movement sensor, which is an accelerometer, is connected to its own mote and transmits data to the main mote wirelessly. We can add extra sensors to the network very easily. For instance, a simple passive infrared camera could be setup to record nighttime sleep movement patterns with more detail than the accelerometers do.

Day-time Data Collection: We seek to continuously monitor the person's lifestyle and habits that impact the condition of her sleep. Some of the factors that will be monitored throughout the day are: eating and drinking patterns (caffeine, alcohol, heavy/light meals, snacking, drinking before bed), exercise patterns (frequency, time of day, difficulty), and lifestyle (smoking, relaxing or stimulating activities before bedtime, sleeping schedule, amount of fatigue and stress level). This data could be entered in a variety of ways, but must be convenient for the user or it will not be entered at all. Therefore, the system will rely on everyday technology that the user already has access to. For instance, she could enter information through a text message or voice automated prompt on a cell phone. She could also go to a website and fill out a quick survey form. If none of the above is applicable, the user could keep track in a paper log and enter the data manually later in the day.

Data Analysis: All of the data collected throughout the day and night is relayed to a central location, which could be on the user's pc or at a central database accessed through the internet. The central database would allow access to the patient and other valid recipients only to ensure user privacy. Because data is stored in a computer or server, there is plenty of disk space for many weeks worth of data. Thus, instead of data from only three nights at a sleep center, a user could get a diagnosis from her last month of sleeping habits. This long-term solution is also viable because the technology is unobtrusive and would be practical for a patient to use every night for a month. Additionally, the system itself can give recommendations and customized reports based on the data it collects.

5.6   Situational Content Provider Unit

This is an enhanced chat application. Main objective of this application is to enhance social interaction of the user. In the background it analyzes the usage history to find out the preference, status of the user and then suggests or offers most suitable contents. The major functionalities of this special purpose application are listed below.

- It offers full featured chat facilities with most of the standard options.
- The application creates and maintains individual profile for each user. In the profile previous usage history is accumulated and based on that usage pattern is identified. Analysis of chat history also reveals the closest buddies of the user.
- There is a Frequency Calculation Unit which keeps track of how frequently the user is active in contacting with his buddies. Very low frequency indicates the user's reluctance to make social contacts. In that case the Recommendation Unit works on preparing a recommendation list which contains a number of advisory tasks to be accomplished.
- The application includes an Advisory Content Dispatcher Unit which can generate services automatically. It may remind the user to contact his closest friends/relatives or it may even create connection with his buddies automatically and encourage the user to continue chatting.
- Another module called Profile Guidance Unit can also be added to the application. This unit may track the upcoming social events happening at places nearest to the user and suggest him to participate in those events. This module may also perform some other additional tasks, for example, it may start playing some favorite music of the user.

All of the above services are intended to improve the social aspect of the life of elderly people by making them more involved in social activities. This will eventually help them remain sound both physically and mentally.

6   Evaluation

In this section, we present evaluation results of some of the modules which are fully functional. We have already built prototype version of game glove module. We tested the fully operating wired system (Game Glove) with handheld devices (PDA). The game glove was used for rehabilitation purpose for patients suffering from arm movement disability. An example of a prototype scheduler is shown in Figure 6b-d. The scheduler part of the Software interface on Handheld devices (PDAs and Cell phones) for Rehabilitation has been developed (Figure 6b and c), which illustrates only the reminder and data display features was developed to demonstrate monitoring capabilities.

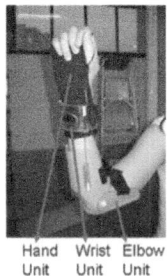 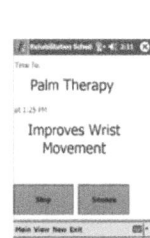 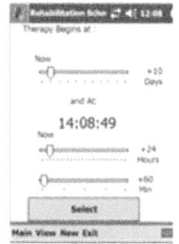 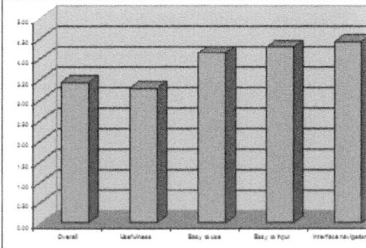

Fig. 6a. Game Glove

Fig. 6b. The Main Screen when there are scheduled events

Fig. 6c. To set date and time for scheduling the therapy

Fig. 6d. Overall rating by users of the Rehabilitation scheduler on a PDA/Cell phone

To show the user satisfaction about the initial the scheduler of Rehabilitation, a survey has been conducted and a graph has been plotted the numeric values of 5 criteria (overall rating, usefulness, ease of use, ease of input, and ease of navigation) of 10 people (shown in Figure 6d) where 5 is the most satisfied and 1 being the lowest.

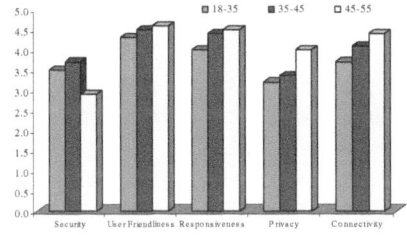 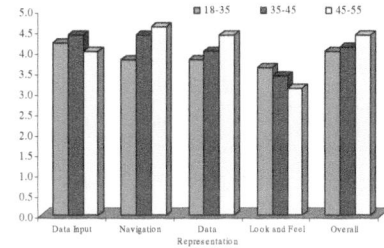

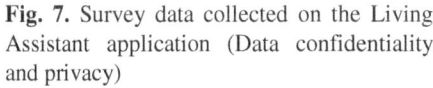

Fig. 7. Survey data collected on the Living Assistant application (Data confidentiality and privacy)

Fig. 8. Survey data collected on the Living Assistant application (Data representation and visual style)

Another module of H2N, the remote home monitoring unit, is also fully functional. We have collected user survey data on that module also. The user experience and opinion of the Remote Home Monitoring module has been examined by means of cognitive walkthrough among people from various age groups. The survey included 24 people of three different age groups with a questionnaire about the features of the application. The questionnaire contained questions about the usability of the prototype and the overall importance of certain concepts related to remote home monitoring system. Figure 6 exhibits the results of the survey. The category being considered in Figure 7 primarily covers data confidentiality and privacy issues along with the user friendliness and responsiveness of the application. From the graph it is evident that a user friendly interface is the most important and users seem to be less worried about security, especially in the higher age group. The usability category, as shown in Figure 8, reveals that the prototype requires enhancement in navigation, data representation and visual style.

7   Conclusion

In this paper, we propose H2N, a wireless sensor network based system for smart homecare that incorporates the essential elements of healthcare facilities. It extends healthcare from the traditional hospital or nursing home setting to the patient's home, enabling remote care-giving without the exorbitant costs of replacing existing home appliances. In H2N, a number of bio-sensors are able to collect data according to a physician's specifications without necessitating the patients to visit doctors at regular intervals. Besides the provision for regular monitoring, there are module like fall detection unit responsible for enabling immediate action. The entire system includes a home search tool to assist elderly people who are suffering from age-related memory decline. This tool along with other modules like remote device control, medicine reminders, sleep monitoring, object location and emergency communication make in-home tasks easier. We followed a multi-tiered architecture comprising both lightweight mobile components and more powerful stationary devices. Our system provides healthcare facilities without using any specialized medical tools and it requires very little fixed infrastructure which make it a viable solution for wide deployment. Besides providing conventional healthcare facilities, H2N proposes an intelligent software application with advanced features augmented with a basic chat application to assist people enhance their social involvement. Finally, we address this issue with great importance and propose techniques regarding how our system achieves privacy-awareness which is a major concern of modern people and such awareness is, in fact, motivating them towards home healthcare solutions in place of clinics or hospitals. Our future research is targeted towards finding out more robust privacy preserving techniques along with their practical deployment in real healthcare systems.

Acknowledgement. We thanks Michelle Johnson for her help with the game gloves.

References

1. Tapus, A., Mataric, M.J., Scassellati, B.: Socially Assistive Robotics. IEEE Robotics & Automation Magazine, 35–42 (2007)
2. Jovanov, E., Raskovic, D., Price, J., Chapman, J., Moore, A., Krishnamurthy, A.: Patient Monitoring Using Personal Area Networks of Wireless Intelligent Sensors. Biomedical Sciences Instrumentation, 373–378 (2001)
3. Dittmar, A., Axisa, F., Delhomme, G., Gehin, C.: New concepts and technologies in home care and ambulatory monitoring. Stud. Health Technol. Inform., 9–35 (2004)
4. Maki, H., Yonczawa, Y., Ogawa, H., Hahn, A.W., Caldwell, W.M.: A welfare facility resident care support system. Biomedical Sciences Instrumentation, 480–483 (2004)
5. MAYA Design, http://www.maya.com
6. Eaton Corporation, http://www.eaton.com
7. Gaddam, A., Mukhopadhyay, S.C., Gupta, G.S.: Development of a Bed Sensor for an Integrated Digital Home Monitoring System. In: IEEE Workshop on Medical Measurements and Applications, pp. 33–38 (2008)
8. Wu, C.L., Fu, L.C.: A Human-System Interaction Framework and Algorithm for Ubi-Comp-Based Smart Home. In: HSI 2008, Poland (2008)
9. Ahamed, S.I., Haque, M.M., Stamm, K., Khan, A.J.: Wellness Assiatant: A Virtual Wellness Assistant using Pervasive Computing. In: SAC 2007, Seoul, Korea (2007)
10. Islam, R., Ahamed, S.I., Talukder, N., Obermiller, I.: Usability of Mobile Computing Technologies to Assist Cancer Patients. In: Holzinger, A. (ed.) USAB 2007. LNCS, vol. 4799, pp. 227–240. Springer, Heidelberg (2007)
11. Ahmed, S., Sharmin, M., Ahamed, S.I.: GETS (Generic, Efficient, Transparent, and Secured) Self-healing Service for Pervasive Computing Applications. International Journal of Network Security 4(3), 271–281 (2007)
12. Ahamed, S.I., Sharmin, M., Ahmed, S., Haque, M.M., Khan, A.J.: Design and Implementation of A Virtual Assistant for Healthcare Professionals Using Pervasive Computing Technologies. Journal Springer e&i 123(4), 112–120 (2006)
13. Ahmed, S., Sharmin, M., Ahamed, S.I.: Ubi-App: A Ubiquitous Application using Ubicomp Assistant (UA) Service of MARKS for Universal Access from Handheld Devices. In: UAIS, pp. 273-283 (2008)
14. Mileo, A., Merico, D., Bisiani, R.: Wireless sensor networks supporting context-aware reasoning in assisted living. In: Proceedings of the 1st International Conference on Pervasive Technologies Related to Assistive Environments, Greece (2008)
15. Ruyter, B.D., Pelgrim, E.: Ambient assisted-living research in carelab. In: ACM Interactions (Special issue on Designing for Seniors: Innovations for Graying Times) (2007)
16. Velentzas, R., Marsh, A., Min, G.: Wireless Connected Home with Integrated Secure Healthcare Services for Elderly People. In: PETRA 2008, Greece (2008)
17. Vergados, D., Alevizos, A., Caragiozidis, M.: Intelligent Services for Assisting Independent Living of Elderly People at Home. In: PETRA 2008, Greece (2008)
18. Rialle, V., Lamy, J.B., Noury, N., Bajolle, L.: Telemonitoring of patients at home: a software approach. Journal on Computer Methods and Programs in Biomedicine, 257–268 (2003)
19. Lee, R., Chen, H., Lin, C., Chang, K., Chen, J.: Home Telecare System using Cable Television Plants – An Experimental Field Trial. IEEE Transactions on Information Technology in Biomedicine, 37–43 (2000)
20. Obermiller, I., Ahamed, S.I.: PATHOS: Pervasive at Home Sleep Monitoring. International Journal of Telemedicine and Applications, article ID 290431 (2008)

21. Kleinberger, T., Becker, M., Ras, E., Holzinger, A., Müller, P.: Ambient Intelligence in Assisted Living: Enable Elderly People to Handle Future Interfaces. In: Stephanidis, C. (ed.) UAHCI 2007 (Part II). LNCS, vol. 4555, pp. 103–112. Springer, Heidelberg (2007)
22. Holzinger, A., Searle, G., Wernbacher, M.: The effect of previous exposure to technology on acceptance and its importance in usability and accessibility engineering. Universal Access in the Information Society 10(3), 245–260 (2011)
23. Holzinger, A., Schaupp, K., Eder-Halbedl, W.: An Investigation on Acceptance of Ubiquitous Devices for the Elderly in a Geriatric Hospital Environment: Using the Example of Person Tracking. In: Miesenberger, K., Klaus, J., Zagler, W.L., Karshmer, A.I. (eds.) ICCHP 2008. LNCS, vol. 5105, pp. 22–29. Springer, Heidelberg (2008)
24. Holzinger, A., Searle, G., Kleinberger, T., Seffah, A., Javahery, H.: Investigating Usability Metrics for the Design and Development of Applications for the Elderly. In: Miesenberger, K., Klaus, J., Zagler, W.L., Karshmer, A.I. (eds.) ICCHP 2008. LNCS, vol. 5105, pp. 98–105. Springer, Heidelberg (2008)

Healthcare IVRS for Non-Tech-Savvy Users

Prasad Girish Rashinkar[1], Anirudha Joshi[1], Mandar Rane[1], Shweta Sali[2],
Salil Badodekar[1], Nagraj Emmadi[1], Debjani Roy[1], Riyaj Sheikh[1],
and Abhishek Shrivastav[1]

[1] Indian Institute of Technology, Bombay, Mumbai
[2] iGatePatni
{prasad.rashinkar,swetz21,colour,nagrajmumba,debjani.r,
riyajsheikh,abhishek.nmd}@gmail.com,
{anirudha,mrane}@iitb.ac.in

Abstract. The rapid increase in mobile penetration has cut through the literacy barriers even in the developing countries. It has paved a way for technological interventions in healthcare domain, using the mobile platform such as Interactive Voice Response Systems (IVRS). Over the past few years, IVRS have been looked upon as an intervention in frequent and non-frequent but time-critical health support systems for chronic diseases. We present an IVRS-based solution for a low-resource setting, to ameliorate the problems of People living with HIV/AIDS (PLHA). We discuss the strategy to deal with frequently and non-frequently used menus. We describe a style of interface added especially to meet the problem of selection of multiple and overlapping options. We highlight the use of flat messages (like health tips) and IRV-based quiz to provide information and shape users' understanding of the disease. We describe and discuss comparative study of usability evaluations of our system conducted with low literate rural users (independent of their HIV/AIDS status) in two villages of Maharashtra (India) in Marathi, the local language. Training provided to the users overcomes the problem of inability of abstract thinking in low literate users.

Keywords: HIV/AIDS, healthcare, adherence, user study, IVRS for chronic diseases, IVRS for low resource-settings.

1   Introduction

The treatment of chronic diseases such as HIV has moved, at least in part, from the medical and pharmaceutical domains to information and communication domain [1]. At the same time, technology usage has become widespread. Today, it seems feasible to provide personalised healthcare information technology (HIT) services to 'almost everyone'. In this paper, we investigate the issues related to usability of HIT for supporting treatment of chronic diseases to low-tech-savvy users but exposed to mobile telephony.

The growth in mobile phones has been quite recent and dramatic, and has managed to cut through several layers of society in a manner that was quite unexpected. For example, Figure 1 shows the number of mobile phones from Telecom Regulatory

A. Holzinger and K.-M. Simonic (Eds.): USAB 2011, LNCS 7058, pp. 263–282, 2011.

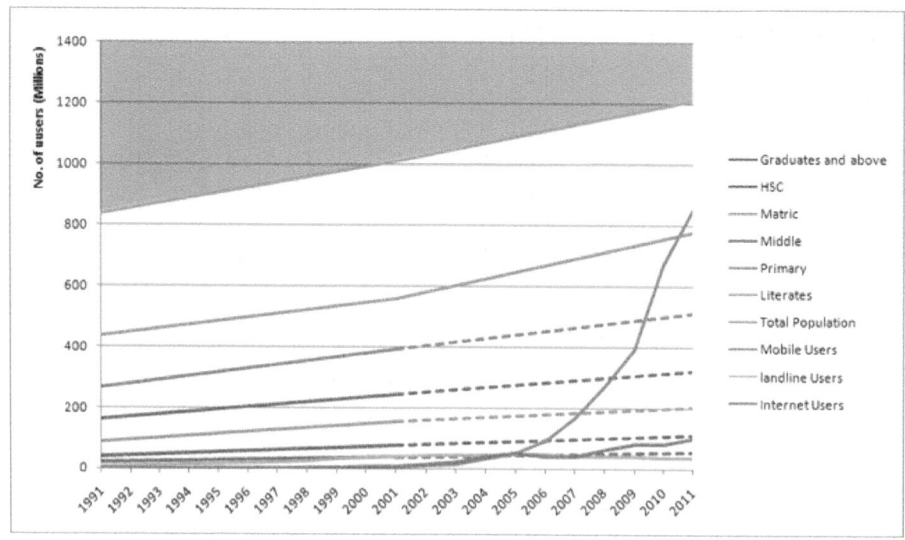

Fig. 1. Mobile, landline, and internet usage over the decade in India [3], [2], [4]

Authority of India (TRAI) [2] and the education figures from the Census in India over the past 20 years [3].

As of September 2011, there are 2.1 billion users of the internet [4] and 5 billion users of mobile phones in the world [5]. That means that there are 2.9 billion non-internet mobile users (NIMU), or about 45% of the world population. The proportion of NIMU is even greater in developing countries. For example, in India, there are 65% NIMU with the mobile phone penetration at 74% [2] and the internet penetration at less than 9% [4]. One implication of the increase in NIMU is that we can potentially provide services such as HIT to a large number of people over the phone. Unfortunately, several challenges have to be met before such services can be realised.

The growth of mobile telephony has been recent in developing countries, and several NIMU have limited abilities. They use mobile phones primarily for voice calls. Many NIMU still do not use features such as sending or reading SMS, adding a contact to the phonebook, or looking up missed calls [6], [1]. Many NIMU have limited exposure to other technologies. Many are from rural areas, with less exposure to urban amenities such as banking, public transportation, or entertainment. Many are either illiterate or have low levels of literacy.

A majority of NIMU phones do not support custom applications nor do they have a connection to the internet. Some lack colour displays or polyphonic audio capabilities. Interactive voice response systems (IVRS) are perhaps the only common technology that can be used to reach NIMU today. Yet, these too have many unsolved usability problems as we discuss below.

In this paper, we investigate several questions related to HIT based on an IVRS for NIMU. The next section discusses the prior work in the area of needs of People Living with HIV/AIDS (PLHA) and problems with IVRS. Section 3 describes the design of our system. Section 4 explains the method of our evaluation. Section 5 shows the results and the last section presents the discussion and conclusions.

2   Background

2.1   HIV and Technology Interventions

Though early on, opinions were mixed about whether HIT interventions would work for PLHA in the resource-limited settings of developing countries [7], later studies have shown promising results [8], [9], [10], [11].

Our recent study of the ecosystem of PLHA in private HIV clinics in India establishes that there is a need and an opportunity to make technology-based, user-centred interventions in management of antiretroviral therapy (ART) [1].

A few clear areas emerged where intervention was required: PLHA need support and reminders for daily pill-taking and they need help to track their adherence. During the initiation of antiretroviral therapy (ART), PLHA occasionally face symptoms such as side effects– systems could support PLHA to report symptoms and look up medical advice. It is important that the PLHA not only know the facts and procedures about HIV and ART, but also develop a conceptual understanding of the same.

Many PLHA need contextual repetition of information since much of it is new to them. We found that PLHA do not disclose their HIV status to their family, while some disclose only to the spouse or a sibling, or to a friend. The solution should support PLHA with different levels of disclosure, and should certainly not cause an accidental disclosure. We also found that PLHA socialise less because of stigma, but also can learn a lot from each other. There is an opportunity to enable anonymous socialisation amongst PLHA, where they can communicate securely, without the fear of any stigma.

We concluded that the solution should not be a stand-alone, independent activity; rather it should closely complement the ongoing efforts in the clinic. On the other side, the system can improve the efficiency of the clinic, secure health records, optimise the time of the PLHA in the clinic, and manage follow-ups.

The choice of a technology platform has significant implications in this ecosystem. Given the advances in mobile technology, in another context, it would be tempting to develop a solution for phones with a modern technology platform such as Android or iOS. However, this may not work in resource-limited settings for several reasons. Firstly, these platforms do not support languages in developing countries. Further, this would need additional expense for the PLHA to buy such a phone. Even if language support could be added and funding could be found to give away such phones, it could add to the stigma – the new mobile phone model may quickly become associated with HIV treatment. At the very least, it would be an intrusion in the life of a PLHA as he or she struggles to learn to use a new device. The solution should be grounded in the reality of a resource-limited setting and it should not add to the financial burden of the PLHA. We therefore decided to use the IVRS platform for our solution.

2.2   IVRS in Healthcare

Unlike applications on smart phones, which need internet connectivity and specific handsets, IVRS are relatively simple to realize. The users can access such a system with any mobile phone. IVRS applications can be used 'everywhere-whenever'. Further, users with lower levels of literacy can potentially use IVRS more effectively than applications that require the users to read text. This makes IVRS suitable for conveying health information to wide range of patients.

Researchers have been using IVRS as a simple and effective way of delivering healthcare information. IVRS were used to deliver recorded messages, instructions, reminders, or informational lectures [12], [13], [14], [15], [16]. Friedman reports a feasibility study of IVRS in the diagnosis and management of chronic diseases, improving adherence, promoting regular physical activity, modifying dietary behaviour, smoking cessation, and increasing mammography screening [17]. Results suggest a positive impact of IVRS on the patients. IVRS have been used to deliver counselling to patients cheaply [18], [19], [16]. Attempts have also been made to provide personalized health-related messages over the IVRS over a long period [13], [20]. In some studies, IVRS have been found to be more effective means of collecting sensitive personal data (such as sexual behaviour) than traditional interviews [21], [18], [22].

Though IVRS are often perceived to be associated with occasionally used applications such as travel, banking, or mobile services, in most studies, the users reacted positively to a frequently used IVRS for healthcare. However, privacy and security were a concern while providing personal information over the IVRS. To overcome this, a personal identification number (PIN) has been used to protect the data [22], [13].

Although the IVRS have been used in providing healthcare support, none of these studies was in resource-limited settings of developing countries or targeted to low-tech-savvy, low-literate users, which may have specific usability challenges.

Medhi et al. reports that low-literate users face difficulty in abstraction [23]. By nature, audio is ephemeral, and users cannot remember too many choices presented in an audio form. This often leads to a hierarchical menu system in IVRS, with choices of 3-5 items at a time. Users need to be capable of certain level of abstraction before they can start navigating such a hierarchy. It is not clear whether such users will be able to navigate hierarchical menus in IVRS.

Automated speech recognition (ASR) technologies have enhanced the user experience of IVR systems in many languages by reducing the need for hierarchical menus substantially by creating a dialogue. However, many of these users speak languages that do not yet have a robust ASR technology yet. While evaluating ASR against DTMF touch-tone in IVRS, touch-tone based IVRS were preferred by the low literate users [24], [25].

There could be specific problems associated with reporting symptoms and getting feedback in IVRS. Conventional menus in touch-tone IVRS could have the problem of overlapping choices for symptoms. For example, a menu could contain symptoms such as fever, rash, headache, and vomiting. If the patient is suffering from both rash and fever, it is not clear which option he should select.

Critical tasks in IVRS are often backed up by agents from a call centre. However, healthcare to chronic patients in developing countries is often provided by small clinics and nursing homes, which may not be able to afford such a call centre backup.

2.3   Objectives

While touch-tone IVRS present opportunities for helping chronic, low-tech-savvy patients in resource-limited settings to manage their treatment better, realising these opportunities may not be easy, given the usability problems and information-seeking behaviours of such users. Issues relate to low education, exposure to technology, behavioural aspects, and information overload.

In this paper, we investigate the issues related to usability of HIT for supporting treatment of chronic diseases for low-tech-savvy patients over IVRS. Can we make touch-tone IVRS usable enough by non-tech-savvy, low literate, rural users so that we can confidently provide HIT services to support treatment of chronic diseases in a resource-limited setting? Which strategies can be used to overcome the issues related to abstraction? How should frequent applications for such contexts be designed? How should infrequent, but critical applications be designed? What would be the extent of training required before these users can start using these applications confidently?

3   Design of the IVRS

An IVRS was designed to provide daily pill-time reminders and adherence feedback, relevant information, medical advice for common symptoms, and anonymous socialisation amongst PLHA. To solve the problem of overlapping menu items, two styles of menus were designed. The system is protected with a PIN to avoid accidental disclosure. The design was prototyped and evaluated through a formative pilot evaluation. In this section, we describe only the elements of the design relevant to the objectives described in the previous section.

3.1   Frequent Task – Pill-Time Reminders

The system provides daily reminders at the time when patients are supposed to take their dose. This scenario can happen in two ways. At the time of the dose, the patient can call the system. The system presents a menu, the first item of which is to report the dose. If the patient has taken the dose, he can select it immediately. In case the patient does not call the system, five minutes after the scheduled dose time, the system gives the patient a call and presents him a short menu. The system presents only three menu options – report that the dose was taken, report a delay in taking the dose, and report that the patient is going to miss the current dose. This input is also used to collect adherence information. In the other scenario, the options to report a delayed or missed dose is not provided, because it was assumed that probability of such an instance would be rare.

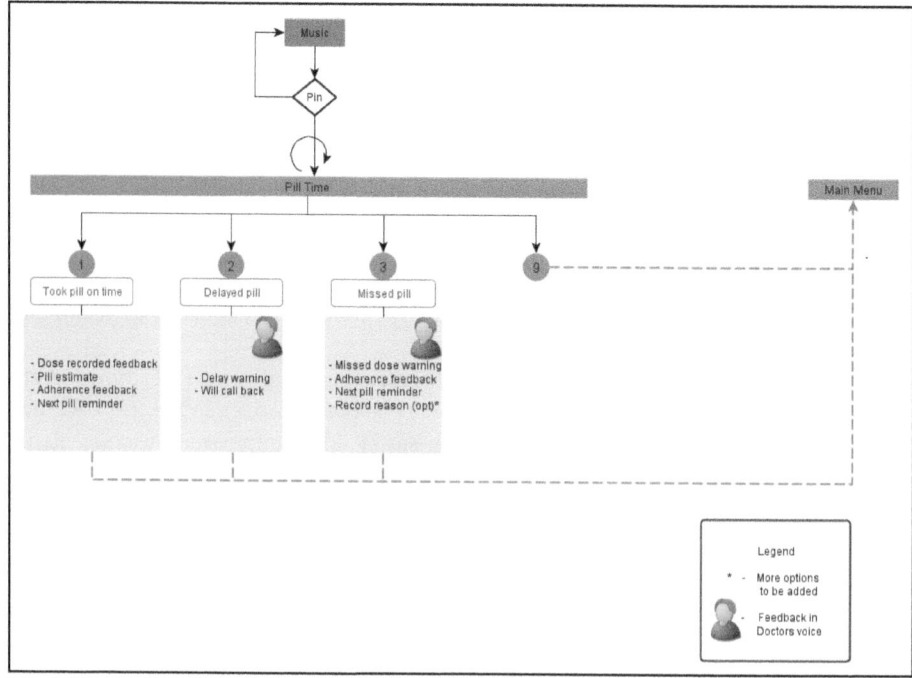

Fig. 2. Pill-time menu navigation

If the patient reports that he has taken the current dose, feedback about his or her current adherence is provided. Additional messages (such as appointment reminders or health tips) are provided after this. This task is a frequent activity, done several times a day (depending on the regimen). An important design consideration was that this task should be finished as quickly as possible. Therefore, all these messages are optional. The patient may listen to them, or may hang up immediately after reporting the adherence.

During an incoming call, the patient may report a delay in the dose. In such a case, the importance of taking pills on time is reiterated. The system calls back the patient after a period of 30 minutes. If the patient delays further, such calls are repeated until a 'pill time window'. In the last call, the patient is warned that his pill time window is over. The patient may also report a missed dose. In this case, the patient is given feedback about the missed dose in the voice of the treating doctor. This was used to leverage the trust of the patient in the doctor and to emphasise the importance of adherence. The feedback is titrated according to the adherence status. In the initial instances of missed doses, or if the adherence of the patient has been otherwise good, the feedback is gentle. On the other hand, if the adherence has been poor, the feedback gets gradually firmer, and warns the patient about potential negative consequences. If the adherence drops below a certain threshold, the doctor's voice advices the patient to meet him in the clinic. After the feedback, the patient is provided with an option to record a reason for the missed dose.

3.2   Infrequent but Critical Task – Looking up Medical Advice

During the early days of ART initiation, PLHA may experience symptoms and an apparent deterioration of health. It could be due to the side effects of the medicines, opportunistic infections, or an indication of a treatment failure. Some of these can be managed by over-the-counter medication or slight adjustments to lifestyles, while others may require urgent medical attention. The system provides first level of triage and immediate advice when the clinic may not be operational. The system also stores Information like user demographic, medical reports, ART regimen. Based on the information such as medical pre-disposing factors, ART regimen and current symptoms, doctors figure out the list of most likely occurring symptoms.

When the user calls the system, the system asks him if he is "*not feeling well*". The system presents the user with a list of likely symptoms. When the user chooses one or more symptoms, the system gives an appropriate, pre-recorded medical advice in the voice of the treating doctor.

While deciding the style of interface, it is important to understand that there are high chances of co-occurrence of more than one symptom. If two or more of such symptoms appear in a single menu, the user would get confused while reporting the symptom. Hence, there has to be a mechanism to select multiple symptoms from a menu.

3.3   Accessing Information Interactively – Quizzes

It is observed that most PLHA are unaware about the terminology such as ART, CD4 etc., conceptual knowledge about the disease, issues related to adherence, and the facts and procedures about the HIV/AIDS. To build the understanding about the disease, and to resolve misconceptions, it was decided to push information through personalized health tips and quiz.

Health tips are pushed as a part of a feedback in daily pill reminders. They were made contextual. In addition, the user can call the system and hear the relevant health tips. Quiz is the other medium to push the information. It encourages the user to try understand the question and guess the answer. It would be interesting to investigate which structure – a flat structure or the quiz - achieves a better retention of information by the users.

3.4   Overlapping Menu Items – Two Interface Styles

Like any IVRS, each option in the menu is assigned a distinct number on the keypad. To save the time of the user, the list of options is sorted in the decreasing order of likelihood of expected usage of an option. For IVRS navigation, we explored two styles of interfaces, namely, A and B.

Interface A

Interface A is the traditional IVRS style: In a menu, it presents all the options at once. The user is expected to listen to all the options and choose one of them. If the user chooses an option, the next menu (set of options) is presented. If the user does not give any input, the entire menu is repeated once again.

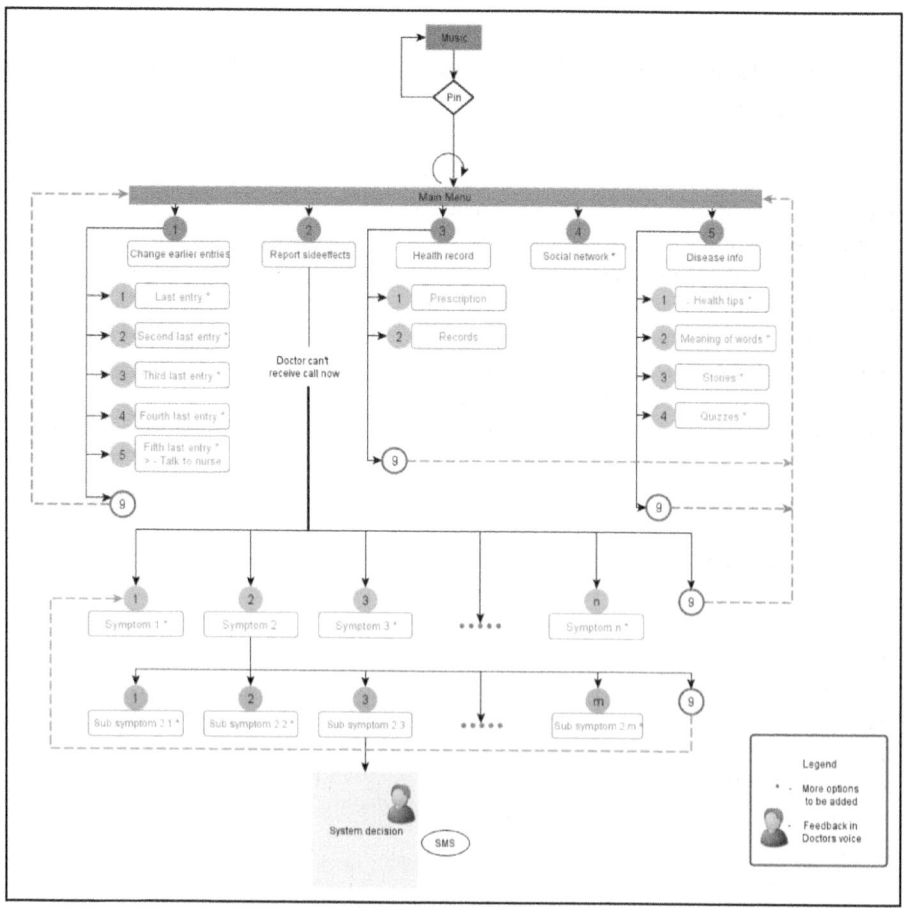

Fig. 3. Interface A

Interface B

Table 1. Mapping of keys to meanings in Interface B

Key	Meaning	Examples
1	Yes	"If you have taken your current dose, press 1", "If you have fever, press 1".
3	No	"If you have not taken your current dose, press 3", "If you have fever, press 1. Else, press 3".
2	Maybe	"If you have not taken your current dose yet but planning to take it later, press 2".
9	Go back	---

Interface B presents one option at a time. The user is supposed to answer the question with a 'Yes' or with a 'No'. Each input is processed at a new level of hierarchy in the menu structure. A 'No' is an explicit rejection of an option (unlike in interface A, where the selection of one option does not necessarily imply a rejection of another). This reduces the search space of possibilities and makes the search efficient. The implementation of interface B requires the user to use only four keys: 1, 2, 3, and 9.

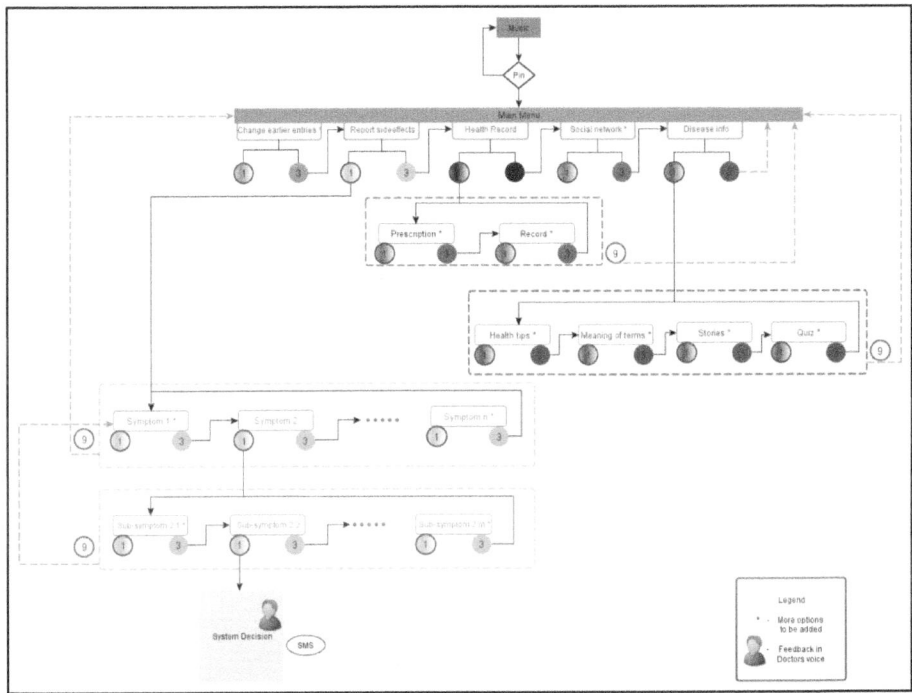

Fig. 4. Interface B

Comparison of the two interfaces

In case of interface A, user can listen to all the options in a menu, without having to give any input. He can decide his selection after considering all the options in the menu. While doing so the user has to remember all the options in the menu and has to keep a track of the input number associated with it. In interface B, the user does not have to remember any option and has to simply select or reject the current option. The input keys in interface B have the same meaning across all the menus as shown in fig. 4. This helps in habit formation, which in turn speeds up the process of user input and increases the performance.

All the options in a menu in interface A are available at the same point. The interface does not impose its bias or hierarchy, except for the sequence of the options in a menu. Interface B does impose a hierarchy.

Interface B overcomes the difficulty of selection of multiple options from a menu in which options overlap e.g., when it is possible to have both fever and rash independently or together. In such a case, interface A does not allow the selection of both the options.

A limit of 10 input options (keys 0-9) is imposed on interface A, while theoretically, interface B can have unlimited options in a menu.

Table 2. Comparison of Interfaces A and B

No.	Issue	Interface A	Interface B	Better
1	Memory load	High	Low	B
2	Cognitive load	Considerable	Little	B
3	Processing load	Considerable	Little	B
4	Freedom of selecting multiple options	Not allowed	Allowed	B
5	Input options	10	Unlimited	B
6	Introduction of bias	Little	Considerable	A
7	Description of all the options before selection	Allowed	Restricted	A

We expect interface B to take longer than interface A to navigate. To compensate this, we suggest the following two strategies:

1. Sort the options in each menu in the decreasing order of likelihood of expected usage of an option i.e. in the 'most-likely-first' order.
2. Present each menu in a short form, followed by a pause, expecting user input, and then the same menu in the full form e.g. "Headache? [Pause for user input] If you have headache, press 1. Else, press 3".

Both the interfaces provide the option to barge-in. In both the cases, sorting the menus according to the priority and context improves the performance.

3.5   Other Design Considerations

Prioritization of menu items: Decide the priority considering the usage, urgency, and the importance of the menu item in the context.

Consistency: Throughout the system, assign the same key to a menu item e.g. if 'A' is mapped to key '2', then each occurrence of 'A' should be mapped only to key '2'. It would lead to habit formation and better performance in the long term, on frequently used systems.

Forgivingness: Allow the users to correct the input they just gave e.g. provide the facility to undo the last selection and to go back to the previous menu.

Repetition of menu on no input: The usability evaluations revealed that until the users became acquainted with the system, a menu should be played at least five times consecutively on no input.

Context: In a web-based application, we have breadcrumbs to let the user know where he is in the interface. Giving the context is even more important in an IVRS since there is no visual support in an IVRS. To give the context, we give a feedback of the type: "You said <user's selection>". This is useful when user gives an incorrect input but does not realise it. This also helps users realise if they have landed on some unexpected menu on previous input.

3.6   Heuristic Evaluation

The goal of heuristic evaluation is to find the usability problems in the design so that they can be attended to as part of an iterative design process. Early evaluation helped in focusing on the key parts of the system and improving the system as a whole. Heuristic evaluation was conducted with a group consisting of 2 usability experts, 2 doctors and 1 Psychologist who is also a HIV counsellor. The experts were explained the basic functionality and purpose of the system and then were asked to perform the tasks that were considered crucial in terms of usability of the system. The first reactions on interface A were good as against interface B. They found interface B to be non-humanistic, difficult to understand, and most of the evaluators did miss the first word of every option due to frequent key inputs. Evaluators appreciated Interface A for considering IVR patterns with an explicit nature of options.

However once started, the doctors and usability professionals could navigate through interface B much faster as compared to A without errors. This means that though interface B introduces a new structure, it becomes easier as one starts using it.

The HIV counsellor liked the idea of quiz and considered it an indirect way to educate people.

To summarize, the feedback received is to consider the gradation in the adherence feedback given to the PLHA, only the serious problems needs to be escalated to the doctors, the system's voice should be sympathetic and the menus can be bilingual. Accordingly, the changes were made to the system.

4   Method

4.1   Protocol

Figure 1 shows that there is a large population falling within the category of illiterate and low literate (until primary school; fourth standard). In an attempt to target low tech savvy users within this band of 'illiterates' and 'low literates', following parameters were followed while selecting users for usability evaluation: age between 30 and 50, owner of a mobile phone, and educated up to a maximum of fourth standard. All the selected users were native Marathi-speakers. We assumed that if the solution could work for such a group of users, it should work very comprehensively with the highly educated and fairly tech-savvy users.

However, users participating in the usability evaluation were not PLHA as the current study is in collaboration with private clinics and these clinics usually have quite a few users matching the key demographics (age, education, and mobile usage) of the users targeted for the usability tests.

Users were carefully briefed about the purpose of the study and the activities involved. They were requested to provide an informed consent to participate in the study. Demographic information (age, gender, years of education, and years of mobile phone usage) pertaining to individual user was noted.

One of the interface types (A or B) was assigned to the users trying to keep user demographics relatively balanced on each style of interface. The experiment started with approximately 20 to 45 minutes training of IVRS, immediately followed by seven pre-designed tasks on the system. After each task, users were probed to get their reactions and perceptions. We used a post-test questionnaire to get user's feedback for further improvements and to estimate the usability of the system. The users were asked to rate their experience of using the system on a 5-point scale from 'very difficult' to 'very easy' at the completion of the test.

The training included some generic tasks, as well as a couple of infrequent and time-critical tasks taken from the designed system itself. All the usability tests were conducted at the choice of user's location but in a controlled environment.

A second round of evaluations was conducted with the same user, after a gap of 1 week from the first round. In round two, no training was provided to the users and the system was tested on the same tasks and the same interface that they had tested a week prior. The objective of second round was to check whether the speed of use and the error rates are inversely proportional to the frequency of usage.

The usability evaluation results of round one and two were assessed separately to find out whether the above stated objectives are met or not.

4.2   Pilot

Twelve pilot tests were conducted to finalise the protocol for the final usability evaluations. During the activity, the success rate was recorded at around 30%. A further analysis revealed the following reasons for failure:

1. Script and the language were not appropriate and thus needed an improvement.
2. User spent more time in completing the formalities viz. understanding his role and duties during the test, informed consent, demographics, etc. Hence, by the time training finishes, he was already exhausted.
3. Users tended to forget the task to be performed. This was not surprising since most of the users were exposed to an IVRS and a testing scenario for the first time.

The system was modified based on the findings of the pilot studies. To deal with the delay in the formalities before the usability test, it was decided to do the formalities at the time of user recruitment itself.

To reduce the cognitive load of remembering the task, a small booklet was created. It had the task description sheets. It was kept in front of the user so that the user could refer to it anytime during the tasks. In addition, the site maps were created to use during the training to give visual support to the users.

Apart from the above reasons, it was a concern whether the unique setting, which is under trial, needs more training. Since the pilot study did not point out the need of an extra training but to have a clear understanding about the amount of training required for such setting, training was considered a variable in usability testing. Hence, at this point we decided to conduct actual tests with two protocols: protocol 1 (P1): short training and protocol 2 (P2): long training.

4.3   Training

Users of the system often visit clinic for their regular checkups, the system helps doctors to diagnose the side effects, and upon the diagnosis, medical advice is given to the patients over the IVRS. These functionalities of the system can be life-critical at times. Therefore, it becomes very important for the user to give timely and correct input to the system and requires users to be well acquainted with the system right from day one. Hence, it was decided to train the users on a small number of frequent and critical aspects of the system. Half the sample size was trained on longer training and half on the shorter.

Short Training: We expect the most frequent activity on the system to be a user reporting that he has taken the current dose. He can do it either by calling the system proactively, or reporting when system gives a call. Therefore, this activity was included in one of the training tasks. The second activity chosen for the training is rare but time-critical and one in which accuracy matters the most. In this task, user has to report that he has some kind of illness (e.g. cold) and receive the prescription from the system (by listening to the system and by reading the SMS sent by the system).

Considering users' first interaction with the IVRS, the training had always been divided into three steps:

1.   Menu structure was explained verbally with a justification for every input.
2.   A demonstration was shown by putting moderator's phone on loudspeaker.
3.   The user was asked to perform the same task on his phone.

These steps were introduced to keep the traditional metaphor of learning: to begin with the theory, then the demonstration, and finally, the practical.

Long training: Half the users that were chosen were given long training. First, the users were given tasks that were not related to the system but demonstrated the functioning of IVRS. Things from user's day-to-day lifestyle were brought in to give a clearer conceptual understanding of the IVRS. The extended training includes following:

1. Introduction to the concept of IVRS:

The first training task was designed to acquaint the user with the mobile phone keypad and introduce him to the concept of listening to a machine and understanding the instructions properly. In this task, users were asked to input the digits spoken over the IVRS.

2. Teaching the concept of abstraction and hierarchical menu structure:

The concept was built slowly using three tasks. In the first task, the user has to select a '*Banana*', which is straightforward and appears as the second option. In the second task, the user is asked to select a '*fruit*' from a group of items and then '*Banana*'. The third task takes this learning a step ahead – it has two levels in the menu, i.e. selecting *Vegetable*, then *Brinjals*, and then answering the question '*how many?*'. After completing the tasks successfully, users were given the system-specific training that is the short training.

5   Users

All users had a very little exposure to the technology and to an urban environment. Most of the users had shared phones and a few were only acquainted with 'Red' and 'Green' buttons used to receive and disconnect the call. Though people had numeric literacy, when it came to punch in the keys to dial the number, people failed to do so. For example, one woman from Junnar could not locate the button '6'. It was observed that she used to count the numbers manually from left to right and then, from right to left. Therefore, she used to press '4' while trying to press '6', and vice versa.

Table 3. User demographics

# Users	Av. Age (y.)	Av. Mobile Usage (y.)	Education			Gender	
			0-2	**3-4**	**>4**	**M**	**F**
41	35.9	1.92	14	17	10	20	21

Legend: Av.: Average, y.: years, M: Male, F: Female

This group is a good representative of a section with the lowest level of education.

6   Findings

The 42 usability tests were conducted with seven predefined tasks. Users' responses were documented to analyze the usage, behavioural patterns, etc. For quantitative analysis, time taken for successful task completion, number of attempts, and errors during the task were recorded. User's statements, reactions were recorded which helped us to understand the issues and users' perception towards the system. This data helped us in judging the factors that affect the performance on the IVRS. Initially, we believed that the factors that affect the performance would only be the interface and the protocol. However, through the detailed analysis, it became clear that location (which implies the language) was the most critical factor that showed the significant diversity in the success rate.

As stated above, the two versions (short and long) of training lead to two distinct protocols for usability evaluations. The two protocols have been summarised below.

Table 4. Comparison of protocols

Protocol	Extended Training	Short Training	Site Maps	Average Time (in minutes)
P1	X	✓	X	20-25
P2	✓	✓	✓	40-45

Interfaces

The major reasons for failing to perform the tasks were inability to understand abstraction, length of menu, and the dialect (of the language of the IVRS) being different from one's own.

Interface A worked in most cases independent of location, gender, and protocol. Users of interface A learnt to barge in on their own, to speed up the task. However, it was observed that users found it difficult to answer the questions asked in interface B, even though they were supposed to answer to one question at a time. Reasons for this behaviour could be:

a. User is not sure whether .
b. End of the menu was not known. (i.e. "When would the menu end?")
c. It became stressful to keep taking decisions at every option.

Table 5. Data with respect to interfaces

Task	Interface					
	A			B		
	# Users	% Success	Time (m.)	# Users	% Success	Time (m.)
FT1	21	100.00	32.3	21	90.47	33.5
FT2	21	76.19	27.1	21	71.42	25.4
FT3	21	76.19	42.9	21	38.09	37.1
CT1	21	76.19	68.2	21	71.42	68.1
CT2	20	65.90	77.9	18	16.66	40.4
IT1	18	100.00	73.9	17	94.11	67.1

Legend: Av.: Average, m.: minutes, M: Male, F: Female, CT: Critical Tasks, FT: Frequent Tasks

Length of the menu: Although interface B has no visible constraint on the depth of the menu, it was observed during the usability testing that in interface B, users tended to lose their concentration and faith in the interface as they said 'No' to more and more options and their desired option did not appear in the menu. It was observed that people opted for an inappropriate option simply because the appropriate option was not presented and the user lost patience. Interface B is good if the desired option is found among the initial few in a menu.

Proximity of the buttons: We also observed that 4 users disconnected the phone by mistake at least once, while trying to press '3'. The combination of 1-3 was used to avoid unintentional input of 2, which would land the user on a wrong track.

Keystrokes and frequency of usage: Considering the number of keystrokes required to reach to the intended menu item, it is not advisable to use interface B style menu for routine and frequent tasks. Such a menu style cannot be used for the main menu, as the major functionalities of the system might remain hidden from most of the users if one does not reject the earlier options.

However, for the selection of multiple and potentially overlapping options from a menu, interface B should be used. Interface A does not facilitate this.

It is interesting to note that though the interface A has shown significantly higher success rates, interface B has been proved more efficient.

Protocol

The fundamental difference between the two protocols was the amount of training that was provided. The data does not show a significant difference between the success rates of the two protocols. The quantitative data shows that the extended training of 35-40 minutes is not required. Training users on TAMA tasks for 20 minutes is sufficient.However; it was clearly observable that the extended training had helped users in gaining confidence about the IVRS system. It helped the first-time IVRS users to understand the concept of listening to voice and answering the questions by pressing a number. It also helped them in being acquainted with the number pad. In addition, when put on protocol 1, the first-time users of IVRS were observed speaking to the system, acknowledging the system verbally (by saying 'hello', 'ok', 'no problem', etc.). During the process, they used to miss important words from the menu. This led them to listen to the menus multiple times.

Table 6. Data with respect to protocols

Task	Protocol					
	P1			**P2**		
	# Users	**% Success**	**Time (m.)**	**# Users**	**% Success**	**Time (m.)**
FT1	17	94.11	26.6	25	96.00	39.3
FT2	17	70.58	20.2	25	76.00	32.3
FT3	17	52.94	26.8	24	62.50	53.3
CT1	17	64.70	49.7	25	80.00	86.6
CT2	16	31.25	37.8	22	50.00	80.6
IT1	15	93.33	60.8	20	100.00	80.2

Another thing introduced in protocol 2 was the site map. Site map proved to be very useful in training, while explaining the interface details, and while explaining the abstraction used in the menus and the hierarchical navigation. Although users did not refer to site map while performing the tasks, it could be used as visual aid during the training.

Some issues regarding language were identified during pilot study as the reasons for a high failure rate. They were corrected before the actual usability evaluation started. The success rate in pilot studies was around 35%. With protocol 1 (keeping training the same), it went up to 87%.With protocol 2 and the extended training, it rose up to 90%.

Location

Table 7. Data with respect to location

| Task | % Success by Location and Interface | | | |
| | Junnar | | Pen | |
	A	B	A	B
FT1	100.00	88.88	100.00	91.66
FT2	90.00	88.88	63.63	58.33
FT3	90.00	62.50	63.63	25.00
CT1	80.00	88.88	72.72	58.33
CT2	77.77	16.66	54.54	16.66
IT1	100.00	100.00	100.00	87.50

Care was taken to include the regional diversities in the study. We selected the location Pen because it belongs to Konkan region, where Marathi is influenced by Konkani. Junnar is a small town in Pune district. Pune is known as a cultural capital of Maharashtra state and the Marathi spoken there is assumed the standard one. Table 7 shows the statistical analysis of the IVRS based on location. The success rate in Junnar was significantly higher than that in Pen ($p=0.01$). This difference was observed due to the difference in dialects of Marathi.

It was observed that the users got familiar with the IVRS concept and had no issues navigating through it. The users did remember the PIN correctly and also they remembered the music clue. The pill reminder tasks were executed successfully by the users although few of them could not comprehend the abstraction and menu hierarchy this time without training. The success rate of round two when compared with round one were higher though not significant.

User satisfaction ratings

Table 8. Analysis of SUS data

| | Interface | | Protocol | | Location | |
	A	B	P1	P2	Pen	Junnar
# of Users	19	20	17	22	23	16
Average SUS score	60.78	58.62	59.11	60.11	58.80	60.93

During SUS (the post-test questionnaire), users were probed for the need of PIN. As many as 17 users reported that PIN should be eliminated; 7 users were undecided, and the rest found that the PIN was an obstacle to access the information. We understand that the issues related to PIN would be better evaluated when the usability of the system is tested with the PLHA as the targeted audience had no stigma and hence they could not speculate the needs in such situations.

The experiment of using two voices - one as a system's voice (female voice) and the other for doctor's voice (male voice) was welcomed by the users and 39 out of 42 could recollect the two different voices. Some users associated the female voice with a nurse and the male voice with a doctor.

7   Conclusion and Discussion

The usability study confirms that the HIT services can be made usable to provide treatment support for chronic diseases to non-tech-savvy and low literate patients.

The resource-limited setting that has been chosen, deals with some of the inherent problems viz. navigation using the hierarchical menus, diversity in terms of culture, language and the geography. Hierarchical navigational problems associated with conventional IVRS designs can be minimized at the cost of brevity in the menu items. The low literate and non-tech-savvy users understand the expanded menu items better. For example, consider one of the menu items we had used, "*if you are going to take your dose later, press 2*". Such a prompt sounds very simple but during the pilot study, users could not comprehend it well and failed to report that they would be taking their dose later. We then expanded the menu to say, "*If you have not taken your dose yet, but plan to take it later, press 2*". This time the success rate was observed to be remarkably high. A similar observation was recorded while we transformed "*if you are not feeling well, press 2*" to "*if you are not feeling well or have any health related issues, press 2*".

The system designed needs users to be trained before they are exposed to the system. However the task success rates out of short-term training and long-term training are not significantly different, but SUS results show that the users who were given long-term training were more satisfied with the system and their individual performance relative to users who were imparted short-term training. We speculate that this perceived enhancement of satisfaction and performance in individual tasks completion is due to the nature of the long term training which is based on user's day-to-day lifestyle.

We thus believe that the issues related to the abstraction in case of IVRS, can be tackled by training users on the things from their day-to-day lifestyle and by making the hierarchical menus more expansive. Although which of the above two affects more is an unclear problem.

While designing IVRS for the patients of chronic diseases, one needs to segregate frequently used modules from non-frequently used modules by observing usage patterns. One need to consider that navigation should be reduced to minimise the time for frequent tasks. In our study, we have designed two distinct menus: pill time menu (frequent) and the symptoms menu (non-frequent). One option is one can customise menus based on time. For example, during the pill time, user is navigated to pill time menu if he has not reported the dose earlier. In case of infrequent but time-critical modules, one needs to follow the principles explained above such as expansivity and training. Whereas in frequently accessed modules, brevity is expected, as one would get habitual to the menu soon and at some stage, one might not listen to the options.

The usability tests showed that the first-time IVR users were comfortable using the system and could successfully complete their tasks in both types of interfaces. Users were found to be satisfied and this is reflected in their SUS scores. We found that for sensitive and critical health care systems utmost importance has to be given to content localisation as well as voice localization.

Menu repetition can be used to offer a better comprehension of the content. The time lost in repetition and expansivity can be minimised by incorporating a functionality to barge in. We found that even untrained users barge-in. In case of IVRS, usability of the system is correlated with the dialect of the users apart from other factors. The customization for dialect can be achieved through introducing redundancy and bilingualism in the menu items. For example *"aakadi or fit"*, where *aakadi* is a Marathi word for *fit*.

It is concluded that interface A can be effectively used for presenting a short list of menus. Interface B is especially useful in case of multiple selections. While diagnosing a patient's symptoms over the IVRS, doctors would want to know the complete set of symptoms. In order to obtain complete set of symptoms, one cannot use the traditional menu style of IVRS because it does not allow multiple selections from the same list. The interface B is seen to have worked in such situations where only one option is presented to the user at a time. Thus, this brings all the possible symptoms exhibited by the patient. We propose interface style B for dealing with overlapping symptoms where as interface A for all other menus. Evaluation of the combination of two interfaces is a beyond the scope of this study, although it will be interesting to see the results and user's reaction against the use the two interfaces together.

Acknowledgements. This project was funded through a grant from Johnson & Johnson Limited. We thank the doctors, counsellors, moderators, and the people living with HIV/AIDS for participating in this project and sharing their insights.

References

1. Joshi, A., Rane, M., Roy, D., Sali, S., Bharshankar, N., Kumarasamy, N., Pujari, S., Solomon, D., Diamond Sharma, H., Saple, D.G., Rutten, R., Ganju, A., Van Dam, J.: Design Opportunities for Supporting Treatment of People Living with HIV/AIDS in India. In: Campos, P., Graham, N., Jorge, J., Nunes, N., Palanque, P., Winckler, M. (eds.) INTERACT 2011, Part II. LNCS, vol. 6947, pp. 315–332. Springer, Heidelberg (2011)
2. TRAI: Telecom Subscription Data (July 31, 2011), http://www.trai.gov.in/WriteReadData/trai/upload/PressReleas es/837/Press_Release_July-11.pdf (accessed September 9, 2011)
3. Census of India, http://censusindia.gov.in/ (accessed 2011)
4. Internet World Statistics: Internet Users in the World, http://www.internetworldstats.com/stats.htm (accessed July 31, 2011)
5. Wikipedia, http://en.wikipedia.org/wiki/List_of_countries_by_number_of_ mobile_phones_in_use (accessed September 12, 2011)

6. Welankar, N., Joshi, A., Kanitkar, K.: Principles for Simplifying Translation of Marathi Terms in Mobile Phones. In: HCI, India, Mumbai (2010)
7. Kaplan, W.: Can the ubiquitous power of mobile phones be used to improve health outcomes in developing countries? (2006)
8. Chang, L., Kagaayi, J., Nakigozi, G., Packer, A., Serwadda, D., Quinn, T., Gray, R., Bollinger, R., Reynolds, S.: Responding to the Human Resource Crisis: Peer Health Workers, Mobile Phones, and HIV Care in Rakai, Uganda (2008)
9. Lester, R., Karanja, S.: Mobile phones: exceptional tools for HIV/AIDS, health, and crisis management (2008)
10. Fabricant, R.: Project Masiluleke. Interactions 16(6) (2009)
11. Benjamin, P.: Cellphones 4 HIV. In: mHealth potential in South Africa: The Experience of Cell-Life,
    `http://www.cell-life.org/images/downloads/Cell-Life_Organisation_Poster.pdf` (accessed 2010)
12. Leire, V.O., Morrow, D., Tanke, E., Pariante, G.: Elders' Nonadherence: Its Assessment and Medication Reminding by Voice Mail. The Cerontologist 31(4), 514–520 (1991)
13. Mundt, J.C.: Interactive voice response systems in clinical research and treatment. Psychi. Serv. 48(5), 611–612 (1997)
14. Lee, H., Friedman, M., Cukor, P., Ahern, D.: Interactive Voice Response System (IVRS) in Health Care Services. Nursing Outlook 51(6), 277–283 (2003)
15. Glanz, K., Shigaki, D., Ramesh, F., Bernardine, P., Bonnie, K., Friedman, R.: Participant reactions to a computerized telephone system for nutrition and exercise counseling. Pat. Edu. Counsel. 49(2), 157–163 (2003)
16. Mooney, K., Beck, S., Friedman, R., Farzanfar, R.: Telephone-linked care for cancer symptom monitoring: A pilot study. Ca. Pract. 10(3), 147–154 (2002)
17. Friedman, R.: Automated Telephone Conversations to Assess Health Behvior and Deliver Behaviorl Interventions. Journal of Medical Systems 22(2), 95–102 (1998)
18. Noell, J., Glasgow, R.E.: Interactive technology applications for behavioral counseling: issues and opportunities for health care settings. American Journal of Preventive Medicine 17(4), 269–274 (1999)
19. Glanz, K., Shigakia, D., Farzanfarb, R., Pintoc, B., Kapland, B., Friedman, R.: Participant reactions to a computerized telephone system for nutrition and exercise counseling. Patient Education and Counseling 49(2), 157–163 (2003)
20. Intille, S.: New Research Challenge: Persuasive Technology to Motivate Healthy Aging. IEEE Transactions on Information Technology in Biomedicine 8(3), 235–237 (2004)
21. Turner, C.F., Ku, L., Rogers, S.M., Lindberg, L.D., Pleck, J.H., Sonenstein, F.L.: Adolescent sexual behavior, drug use, and violence: increased reporting with computer survey technology. Science 280(5365), 847–848 (1998)
22. Schroder, K.E., Johnson, C.J., Wiebe, J.S.: Interactive Voice Response Technology applied to sexual behavior self-reports: a comparison of three methods. AIDS and Behavior 11(2), 313–323 (2006)
23. Medhi, I., Raghu Menon, S., Cutrell, E., Toyaman, K.: Beyond Strict Illiteracy:Abstracted Learning Among Low-Literate Users. In : ICTD, London (2010)
24. Sharma Grover, A., Stewart, O., Lubensky, D.: Designing Interactive Voice Response (IVR) Interfaces: Localization For Low Literacy Users. In: Computers and Advanced Technology in Education, St. Thomas (2009)
25. Sharma Grover, A., Plauche, M., Barnard, E., Kuun, C.: HIV health information access using spoken dialogue systems: Touchtone vs. Speech. In : 3rd Int. Conf. on ICTD, Doha, Qatar, pp. 95–107 (April 2007)

Experienced Barriers in Web Applications and Their Comparison to the WCAG Guidelines

Diana Ruth-Janneck

Technical University of Dresden, Private Lectureship Applied Computer Science,
01062 Dresden, Germany
diana.ruth-janneck@pdai.de

Abstract. A German organization established the study "Web 2.0 Accessible" in 2008 which asked Internet users with disabilities about the barriers they experience when using websites and web applications. This paper gives some interesting facts of the study which are useful for the design and implementation of accessible web applications. Therefore it raises classifications of barriers in various dimensions we have registered in the German study regarding the use of web applications by persons with disabilities and correlate these barriers with the WCAG 2.0 Guidelines and Principles to support the facts of the study. Furthermore the results will be supported by key results of other studies regarding web accessibility. The objective of this paper is to identify in practise experienced barriers for people with disabilities using websites and applications.

Keywords: Web Accessibility, Barriers, People with disabilities using the Internet, WCAG 2.0, Study Web2.0 Accessible.

1   Introduction

In our today's more and more digital world, it is necessary that web pages and web applications are accessible for all users and especially for users with disabilities. More than 8.6 million people with disabilities live in Germany. Their number represents about 10.5% of the German population [1]. The European Commission assumes that one fifth of the working age population have a disability and almost 60% of the population would be likely to benefit from web accessibility [2]. And this number does not include elderly people, which often experience similar problems to access web pages and their interactions. Thus, accessible web applications can be an important step to an inclusive web for all. But nowadays there are many problems and restrictions for users with disabilities. A German study was established in 2008 for the analysis of the actual state of the art regarding the Internet access by people with disabilities. The results provide important and practically relevant aspects for designers, developers and evaluators of accessible web applications. It outlines the most critical technical, design and editorial barriers for different user groups with disabilities. These results, in connection with the WCAG 2.0 Guidelines and the statements of the questioned users, are very useful to understand the needs and barriers of internet users with disabilities.

A. Holzinger and K.-M. Simonic (Eds.): USAB 2011, LNCS 7058, pp. 283–300, 2011.
© Springer-Verlag Berlin Heidelberg 2011

This paper gives an overview on the German study "Web2.0 Accessible" [3] at first. The most important applications for Internet users with disabilities and the applications showing the highest problem rates compiled in the study are especially interesting here. The second part of the paper consists of a comparison of the extracted most critical issues of web applications with the actual WCAG 2.0 Guidelines [4]. At the end of this paper, the most important aspects of accessible web applications are summarized.

1.1   Related Works

The facts about the barriers which are experienced in practice by people with disabilities are supported by the results of two other studies concerning web accessibility with user involvement. One important study was established by the Disability Rights Commission (DRC) in the UK [5] in 2004. It is a large-scale study which tested 1.000 popular British sites for technical compliance with the WCAG 1.0 Guidelines. Furthermore, 10% of these sites were tested with a group of 50 users with different impairments and by accessibility experts. The user statements and experienced key problems are the most interesting points for this work. Another helpful survey was a study on screen readers with 100 blind users in the US in 2007 by Lazar et.al. [6]. This study, whose findings have supported our results, recorded frustrations for blind users using the web. Several studies and research look for e.g. the compliance of government websites (e.g. MeAC [2] or Lopes et.al.[7]) or of popular websites with WCAG (e.g. Sullivan et.al. [8]) or with accessibility barriers for older people (e.g. Sayago et.al. [9]).

1.2   WCAG 2.0

The Web Content Accessibility Guidelines Working Group published the Web Content Accessibility Guidelines (WCAG) 2.0 as a W3C Recommendation in 2008. These guidelines cover "a wide range of recommendations for making Web content more accessible" [4]. In this way, the WCAG 2.0 want to consider people with various kinds of disabilities and make web content more usable to users in general. The WCAG 2.0 comprise the four principles of web accessibility: perceivable, operable, understandable and robust (POUR). Each of these principles implies one or more guidelines (12 in total) as a basis for the corresponding testable success criteria (60 in total) in different conformance levels. For each success criterion there is a number of sufficient and advisory techniques (incl. description, examples, resources, related techniques and tests) as well as failures. There are some documents which support the WCAG 2.0: "How to Meet WCAG 2.0" for developing and evaluating web content, "Understanding WCAG 2.0" for a better understanding of the guidelines and success criteria, and "Techniques for WCAG 2.0" with a collection of techniques and common failures. All these documents and layers of guidance (guidelines, success criteria, and techniques) "work together to provide guidance on how to make content more accessible [4]". Authors and developers have to consult all layers to make the web content as accessible as possible. The WCAG 2.0 provides three conformance levels: A, AA and AAA. Nevertheless the

WCAG 2.0 outline that even websites which conform to the highest level (AAA) will not be fully accessible to all users with a wide range of disabilities [4]. The WCAG 2.0 is a stable, referenceable technical standard which is designed to be widely applied to different web technologies. The supporting documents are based on the WCAG 2.0, but they can be updated and completed concerning new techniques, technologies or best practices. The guidelines and success criteria are written as testable statements that are not technology-specific. The document dealing with the techniques contains general techniques as well as technology-specific statements e.g. for HTML and XHTML, CSS, client- and sever-side Scripts, WAI-ARIA (WAI Accessible Rich Internet Applications Suite) and Flash.

1.3   Methodology

The following statements result from a qualitative analysis of the data from the online survey in connection with the transcription of the statements given in the interviews. The most important applications for Internet users with disabilities have been identified due to the highest usage frequencies in the different user groups. These applications have been compared with the recorded problem rates and with the interviewees' statements. These results have been the basis of developing the most important accessibility issues and critical aspects for the different user groups with disabilities and of connecting them with the corresponding WCAG Guidelines. The identified aspects are sorted in different tables according to the causing field like using techniques or editorial issues. Afterwards they are discussed in detail and compared with the other study results and user statements.

2   The German Study "Web 2.0 Accessible"

The German organization "Aktion Mensch" established the study "Opportunities and Risks of the Internet of the Future from the Perspective of People with Disabilities" [3] regarding the use of Web2.0 applications by disabled people in 2008 in whose evaluation the author significantly participated. This study offers reliable statistical data concerning the use of web applications by people with disabilities as well as which barriers and problems of use occur. It forms the statistical and qualitative basis for the statements and classifications made in this paper.

2.1   Methodology of the Study

The study involved three steps in order to collect both quantitative and qualitative data. On the one hand, experts from science and self-help organizations have been consulted to capture the current state of knowledge on Internet use by people with disabilities. Additionally, experienced Internet users with disabilities were questioned in group interviews about their experiences and habits with Web2.0 applications as well as about the barriers they experienced. The data from these steps about possible barriers in web applications were used for the concrete realization of the online survey which measured the scope of these barriers.

Disabled Internet users were questioned about habits of use and barriers with the help of an accessible online survey including mode of text, audio files and sign language videos. The online survey was organized in multiple areas to acquire several data [3, 10]:

- Demographic characteristics including kinds of disabilities and frequency of use of the web (participants without an impairment or with sporadic use were excluded here)
- Data on the use of assistive technologies and technical equipment
- Free text answers to "What is the best thing on the Internet for you?" and "What is the most annoying thing on the Internet for you?"
- Data on the behavior and intentions of use by selection from given lists ("I use websites for…" and "With the Internet I can …")
- Familiarity with different popular websites ("Which kinds of website do you know?" If the participant does not know the website, he will not get more questions about.)
- Questions about the prominence, the usage rate (from a list) and barriers experienced for the familiar websites; for every barrier noticed: free text answer for more explanation and a question about the kind of barrier (not operable, not perceivable, not understandable, no orientation)
- Graded compliance with regard to special advantages for disabled Internet users by using websites in a list of statements (e.g. "With the Internet I can communicate easier with others." on a scale from 0 to 100%).

The survey was supported with the help of special German websites for people with disabilities and self-help organizations in January and February 2008. A total of 671 people with disabilities have completed the questionnaire. This allows us to make precise statements on the test results from the perspective of the different kinds of disabilities, but not on all Internet users in general or all users with disabilities because of the non-representative basis [3].

2.2   Facts about the Study

People with different kinds of disabilities were interviewed during the study. In total, 10 people were interviewed as experts, 57 people were questioned in group-interviews and 671 people have completed the online-survey. Table 1 gives the total number of questioned people in the online survey with the different types of disabilities and the assistive technologies used most often in these groups [3] (also included in the survey: which assistive technologies do you use?).

The number of respondents in the groups Dyslexia and Learning and Cognitive Impairments was too small to make reliable statements about the barriers and strate-gies, but some tendencies could be deduced from the answers. We can make some statistical and qualitative statements about the experienced barriers and useful strate-gies concerning the other groups. The information is complemented by free text answers provided in the online survey and statements from the interviews. This has given us some interesting and concrete facts about the strategies developed and barriers experienced by Internet users with disabilities.

Table 1. Numbers of Questioned People and the Assistive Technologies Used Most Often

Type of Disability	Number of People Questioned[1]	Assistive Technologies Used Most Often
Visual Impairment	133	Screen magnifier (56%), Audio response software (22%), Screen reader (21%)
Blindness	124	Screen reader (91%), Braille Terminal (85%), Audio response software (70%)
Hardness of Hearing	96	Audio response software (16%), Screen magnifier (13%)
Deafness	260	Screen magnifier (7%), Audio response software (6%)
Motor and Dexterity Impairments	75	Special scroll wheels or trackball mouse (20%), Special keyboard/on-screen keyboard (17%), Voice recognition software (16%)
Dyslexia	41	Screen magnifier (32%), Audio response software (24%), Spell assist programs and voice-recognition facilities (20%)
Learning and Cognitive Impairments	35 and 13	Screen magnifier (22%), Audio response software (20%), Screen reader (13%)

These different kinds of disabilities are summarized for the following considerations into groups because the Internet is used with the help of similar assistive technologies (AT) or use strategies due to the respective disability-related restrictions. A definition and differentiation of the types of disabilities cannot be given at this point. All in all, it is remarkable that the magnification software was considered as of significant usage share by all surveyed user groups which is probably due to multiple restrictions or simplification of the perception of contents.

The people questioned distinguished themselves by a high technical standard of the Internet access so that it can be assumed that identified barriers are not caused by lacking technical equipment. The results of the study proved furthermore that the interviewees are very experienced in dealing with Internet applications, they show high usage frequency and have above-average experiences with Web2.0 applications

---

[1] As 82 participants have multiple impairments, the total number of questioned people is less then the sum over all user groups. These persons provide data for each affected user group with disabilities.

so that also factors like insecurity or low affinity to the Internet can be excluded [3]. A comparison with an annual German study (ARD/ZDF-Online-Study 2010) about the use of the Internet, which takes the whole German population into account, shows that Internet users with disabilities use the web about 6.5 days/week, internet users without disabilities use it only 5.1 days/week [1]. This fact underlines another result of the study "Web 2.0 Accessible": the Internet is one of the most important things in daily life for users with disabilities and it can help to live in a far more independent way. It is a tool for information and communication. For more than 40% of the questioned users with disabilities, Internet is a tool for the compensation of disability-related disadvantages [3].

Web accessibility is a very important fact for all questioned Internet users, particularly for blind users. 88% of them chose "accessibility is very important for me". Furthermore, 82% of the questioned people with blindness said that barriers disturb their access to the content. But web accessibility is also very important for 70% of the users with deafness and 70% of the users with cognitive impairments. The users with visual impairments have the smallest coincidence with 59% [3]. This is explainable with the circumstance that these users can manage accessibility problems in different ways. Accessibility problems are often invincible for users who are dependent on assistive technologies.

2.3   The Most Important Applications

The study inquired, among other things, prominence, use and problems in dealing with various Web2.0 applications and their functions. The most significant shares of utilization (more than 60% of use) and the highest problem rates (more than 20%) should indicate the value of certain application classes for the different user groups in the following comparison. Thus, it can be derived which applications are used very often and in which of them problems are frequently noticed.

Developers of applications with high usage and problem rates should increase the efforts with respect to accessibility. The usage rates given in the table were determined during the quantitative part of the study by the online survey. It indicates the proportion of those who have used or tried to use the application. The problem rate is calculated from the quotient of the problems and the use / attempt to use and provides a projection of the anticipated problems in the use of the application by the user groups [3].

Across all user groups, which have been questioned, the highest usage rates are to be observed concerning the reading of wikis. This kind of website causes least problems (problem rate between 6% and 13%) for most user groups. Deaf Internet users show the highest problem rate here (26%) because of problems in understanding the content[2]. The questioned participants mainly have problems with comprehensibility of the (user-generated) content (48% of all who have problems) and orientation on the website (39% of all who have problems) because of numerous links.

---

[2] The linguistic barrier concerning reading and writing, e.g. of wikis and comments, applies to deaf users because the German sign language differs substantially from the spoken and written language. Thus, deaf people experience a difficult access to the written language.

Table 2. Maximum Usage Rates and Rate of Problems[3]

	Visually Handicapped	Blind	Hard of Hearing	Deaf	Motor Disabilities
Usage Rate > 60%	Read wikis (79%), Make user registration (75%), View photos (70%), View videos (61%)	Read wikis (85%), Make user registration (80%), Write comments (60%), Listen to podcasts (60%)	Read wikis (68%), View photos (60%)	Read wikis (61%), View photos (60%)	Read wikis (84%), Make user registration (71%), View photos (65%)
Rate of Problems > 20%	Make user registration (41%), Edit user profile (30%), View videos (28%), Write comments (25%), Read weblogs (25%), View photos (23%), Listen to podcasts (21%)	Make user registration (69%), Edit user profile (58%), View videos (31%), Write comments (30%)	View videos (33%)	Read wikis (26%), View videos (23%), Write comments (21%)	Write comments (28%), Edit user profile (20%)
Problematic Aspects	Captchas, Completion of forms, Visual fields of applications	Captchas, Completion of forms, Visual fields of applications	Quality of media files, Audi-tory fields	Quality of media files, Linguistic problems, Auditory fields	Navigation, orientation and operability of web applications

---

[3] There are no reliable data about the groups Dyslexia, Learning disabilities and Cognitive Impairments given because the basis of results is too small (see table 1).

High shares of use are also mentioned for user registration in all groups. This is because a lot of web applications and services require a registration for full access. Problems here are based on inaccessible forms from the technical point of view and incomprehensibility of the explanations for the required data from the editorial point of view. Thus, 73% of those who have problems with a user registration chose "not perceivable" and 66% chose for "not operable" [3]. Visually impaired, blind and physically disabled persons are mostly confronted with these problems.

Much the same applies for editing user profiles and the use of forms. Forms and in particular Captchas limit the independent use here. Especially users with AT have problems with orientation on the website (53% of all who have problems), with operability of the form elements (50% of all who have problems) and with the perceptibility of the elements (47% of all who have problems). Similar problems are noticed on form-based and editor-based applications such as the writing in wikis or weblogs. The users show great interest in writing comments (e.g. 60% of blind users), but problems like those mentioned above limit the easy access and interaction [10].

Moreover, table 2 lists problems partially sighted and blind users with the use of primarily visual media like photos and videos notice. Disability-related restrictions and bad media quality are the main reason for it. Even hearing impaired and deaf Internet users stated problems with visual media which are caused by insufficient media quality as well as with the unlimited operability and availability of appropriate media players. Statements from free text answers [3] have given some more aspects: too small images, too small video windows or poor resolution, audio streams which are too noisy or added with background noise, unavailability of subtitles or sign language videos. Despite problems in access and use of media content, the high usage rates of visual and auditory content in all questioned user groups show big interests for these. This fact should emphasize the importance of making auditory, visual and other content as accessible as possible for all.

3   A Comparison of the Results with WCAG

Various areas of accountability and contributors in the development and operation process of a web application have to be identified for the prevention of barriers. They should be responsible for ensuring accessibility in their respective field of action. For the following comparison of the study results with WCAG 2.0 Guidelines (G), the facts have been organized in relation to the area of accountability. Different areas of accountability have been defined for this purpose which correlates to the different positions in the development process of web applications like developers, authors, designers and customers.

According to the description of the "Essential Components of Web Accessibility" from the W3C Web Accessibility Initiative (WAI) Group [12] which presents interdependencies between the components and roles, the four different areas of accountability are not independent at all. It is for this reason that some items in the tables are assigned to several areas. The four defined areas are: technical aspects, editorial aspects, design aspects and organizational aspects of web accessibility. A description of each can be found in the following paragraphs.

Furthermore, three tables concerning technical barriers, editorial barriers and design barriers have been developed. In the planning and development of a web application, a person in charge can consult the specific table to look up the most critical aspects and use cases compiled during the study und which WCAG Guideline correlates to them. In connection with the guidelines and technical documents of the W3C WAI Group, the responsible person can choose the relevant guidelines and select the corresponding success criteria and best practise.

For the comparison, the items of the classifications of barriers published in [11 and 13] were each collated with the WCAG 2.0 Guidelines. For better readability the results have been spread into one table for each area of accountability. Quantitative results concerning the aspects cannot be given in the tables because on the one hand the items are grouped according to the impairment groups, and on the other hand the different items are not exactly a part of the survey, but they were identified by the analysis of the study and the interviews. The items in the tables are based on the qualitative analysis of the survey, free text answers and the interviews, which figured out the most critical aspects in web applications today.

3.1   Technical Aspects

The area of technical aspects includes all critical aspects based on technical restrictions, conditions or implementations: e.g. techniques used (e.g AJAX, JavaScript), programming styles and restrictions in hard- and software because of assistive technologies (AT). Examples for these are Captchas, insufficient operability of flashplayers or missing semantics and markup in web forms. Web programmers, service providers and producers of utilities and AT are responsible for these aspects [13]. Guidelines for these groups are e.g. the documents from the W3C WAI: Web Content Accessibility Guidelines (WCAG), User Agent Accessibility Guidelines (UAAG) and Authoring Tool Accessibility Guidelines (ATAG) and evaluation tools like validators.

Table 3 shows the most important technical based accessibility issues of the different user groups, which have been extracted from the study, in connection with the corresponding WCAG Guidelines. All in all it is remarkable that technical barriers have a big influence on the operability of the applications with the AT used. So it is conspicuous that the user groups which are reliant on AT recognized most barriers. Visual impaired, blind and physically impaired Internet users have most problems resulting from technical problems with their AT. Most of the problems occur during the interaction with interactive elements and forms without a mouse. In some cases, these barriers hinder the independent use of the application by the affected user groups.

Table 3. The Most Important Technical Based Accessibility Issues for the Different User Groups in Connection with the Corresponding WCAG Guidelines

Type of Disability	Technical Aspects	WCAG Guidelines
General	Operability	2
	Semantics of web forms & buttons	1.3, 4.1
	Error messages	3.1, 3.3
	Semantics of media content	1.3, 4.1
	Operable & available player	1.1
Visual Impairments	Forms in PDF	3.3
	Captchas	1.1
	Operable forms & editors	2.1
	Operability with AT (e.g. JavaScript, flash, AJAX) & without mouse	2.1, 2.4, 4.1
Hearing Impairments	Download & control of podcasts	2.2
Motor and Dexterity Impairments	Operability of: web forms	2.1, 3.3, 4.1
	buttons	2.1, 2.4, 4.1
	drop-down-menus	2.4, 4.1
	players	2.1, 2.2, 2.4, 4.1
	activation of links	2.4, 4.1
	Operability without mouse	2.1, 4.1

Registration, Forms and Buttons. Forms and corresponding buttons, e.g. for user registration or buying processes, are relevant parts of a web page and have to work for all interested users. But there are problems with forms and buttons in a technical and in a cognitive way. This is also underlined by the rate of problems illustrated in table 2, which shows that e.g. 69% of blind users will probably have problems with user registration forms. But there are also high problem rates for this type of user interaction concerning the other user groups.

Problems in forms result from different aspects concerning different user groups, but the most important aspect for all user groups is language using in forms. Users have to understand what kind of input and in which format it is expected, why this data is needed etc. (G 3.3). Thus, explanations and labels are the most important aspects (see also par. 3.2). But if the explanation is too long, users with deafness and cognitive impairment for example, will not understand it [3]. The DRC-study[4] supports these results with significant figures, e.g. "complex terms/ language" is indicated as a key problem in the group of hearing impaired users [5].

Furthermore, access to forms with assistive technologies is the second big problem. This includes labels, input elements, selection elements, submit buttons, etc. Elements of forms which are not logically ordered (G 2.4) or which are not described with all necessary mark-ups (G 3.3) can cause problems for users which are dependent on the keyboard or on the special AT-functions of forms. They can have problems to reach the actual form element, to identify the label of the form element and to reach the submit button. Especially the tab order and focus behaviour (G 2.4 and 3.2) have to be taken into account when it comes to accessible forms. This fact is also supported by the study of Lazar et. al. [6], in which "poorly designed/unlabeled forms" is the third-highest point of frustrating points in web pages.

Some participants of the survey said that there are problems with comment functions when accessing with screen readers. The AT does not recognize the written text in the forms and they can not check their comments before submitting [3]. In large forms, e.g. for comments or for text in wikis, problems can occur with the reaction of the application to user controls. Unexpected processes can be the result. Another problem is the correct structuring and formatting of text in editor forms with AT. Participants said that they often do not format their comments or that they ask for help [3, 10].

The recorded problems underline that the design and implementation of accessible forms are very difficult. For this reason there is not only one guideline for forms but almost all guidelines are applicable for developing accessible forms because of the different dimensions that have to be considered in forms: operable, perceivable, understandable and robust. The last point is very difficult when implementing forms with new user-friendly techniques like AJAX. New technologies can help to prevent errors and support the user attention, but they can cause crashes for users with AT [14].

Moreover, the usability of forms in general is an important aspect which has to be well researched and realized. This includes e.g. the perceptibility of the elements and possibilities (e.g. in sliders or selection bars; G 1.1 and 1.4), the logic and programmed sequences of the elements (especially the keyboard access and focus; G 2.1 and 2.4) and the wording (G 3.3) as well. All programmers and editors have to think very carefully about forms and buttons to make them accessible in a perceptible, operable, understandable and robust way. Caspers [14] has established a good (German) tutorial for accessible forms, which includes design, error prevention and handling, HTML and CSS for forms, dynamics in forms (e.g. using AJAX), and methods for user tests.

Operability with Assistive Technologies. The operability of web pages and their compatibility with assistive technologies causes many problems for users who are dependent on AT. This key area is focused by two of four principles of the WCAG 2.0: Principle 2 Operable and Principle 4 Robustness. These principles affect to

---

[4] There is no direct comparison possible between the statistical results of the German study and the British study by the DRC or the American study by Lazar because they have different scopes. But the core results of the key problems are comparable.

keyboard navigation (G 2.1), navigation and orientation (G 2.4), and compatibility with current and future user agents including assistive technologies (G 4.1). The German study has ascertained that users often have problems with the operability of:

- Forms and buttons,
- Drop-down-menus,
- Players and editors and
- Multimedia components.

The central problem of all these aspects is lack of access without a mouse (G 2.1). This is particularly important for blind and physically impaired users. In the interviews and free text answers of the study, users said that they often can not operate players on multimedia sites and editors in wikis or weblogs when only using a keyboard. So they have no control of multimedia content. These problems are often expressed in interviews as well as in free text answer fields with regard to the application of wikis, weblogs, and media sharing websites [3]. The DRC-study confirmed this with significant figures concerning "incompatibility between accessibility software and web pages" for blind and partially sighted users [5]. In the US-Study of Lazar et al., "conflicts between screen reader and application" is indicated as the second-highest cause of frustration by blind Internet users [6].

Captchas. Captchas (G 1.1) pose a problem for 39% of the questioned blind people and for 5% of the visually impaired people. 50 persons said that this is the main barrier for an independent user registration because a screen reader can not recognize these figures. One way to solve this problem is the option to listen to an audio-file which represents the Captcha, but this is not the preferred way for most blind and visual impaired people [15]. Some of them use webvisum (www.webvisum.com/) which is a Firefox extension to solve graphical Captchas. The corresponding form element for the solution has to be accessible too.

Conclusion for Technical Barriers. Summarizing the technical aspects, we can see that the main problems occur in connection with AT. If programmers do not use all necessary mark-up, no logical structure of all elements and no alternative ways of access like audio-Captchas, some users with disabilities will have big problems to interact with the application. Another important aspect, programmers and utility producers have to take into account, is the ensurance of full access and interaction only with a keyboard as input device. Furthermore, developers have to ensure the accessibility of special features like applets in Java, PDF or flash. For these objects, the WCAG Guidelines are fully applicable, e.g. keyboard access (G 2.1), focus highlighting and order (G 2.4), alternative text (G 1.1), scalability (G 1.4) etc. Central importance should also be admitted to the accessibility of web forms. These measures are beneficial to all user groups because the readability, usability and accessibility of form elements are crucial for the independent participation e.g. in social networks.

3.2   Editorial Aspects

Editorial and content-related barriers contain insufficient editorial or structural content preparation for Internet requirements, e.g. difficult language, missing textual structures or missing semantics of media content [13]. Guidelines for web editors are e.g. "European standards for making information easy to read and understand" [16]. Table 4 shows main problems regarding the editorial aspects of a web application, which have been extracted from the study. This includes the understandability of the content in general, but also the understandability of all text elements of a webpage because these support the orientation, the user guidance and the content reception. One of the main points in the table, which is listed several times, is the issue of missing or unclear descriptions, semantics and mark-ups of media content. This implies for different user groups that they have no access to the content of media because there is no alternative text (G 1.1, 1,2, 1.3).

Table 4. Critical Editorial Aspects for Different User Groups in Connection with the Corresponding WCAG Guidelines

Type of Disability	Editorial Aspects	WCAG Guidelines
General	Understandability	3
	Orientation & clear arrangement	1.3, 1.4, 3.2
	Quality, size & contrasts of media content	1.4
	Descriptions of media content (alt text)	1.1, 1.2
Visual Impairments	Semantics of content	1.3, 4.1
	Descriptions of media content (alt text)	1.1, 1.2
	Numerous links	2.4
	Names of links	2.4
Hearing Impairments	Missing Videos in sign language & with subtitles	1.2, 1.4
	Quality of podcasts	1.4
Cognitive Impairments	Understandability	3.1
Motor & Dexterity Impairments	Semantics of content	1.3, 4.1

The most important critical point for all questioned user groups is language in the broadest sense. A large percentage of the Internet users have small or big problems in understanding the provided information. The problems result primarily from the use of difficult language and foreign words. In particular problematic are explanations, forms, and error messages as users often do not understand what they have to do or what is wrong.

Editors and programmers have to pay more attention to the wording and the explanations. It is an aspect which we can not check in an automatic way, only by creating more attention on readability. One solution to this is a very careful text editing and structuring of the web content. More attention to the content editors and their awareness of accessibility issues is needed.

This important fact underlined by its own principle in WCAG: Principle 3 Understandable. It emphasizes understandability of the information and the operation of user interfaces by users [4]. Guideline 3.1 addresses the content itself and requires to identify the language of text and mechanisms for abbreviations and pronunciations. According to guideline 3.2, the programmers have to make the web pages predictable in operation and appearance, which includes e.g. a consistent navigation and identification. This means that for example all buttons have the same wording for the same functions. The avoiding of errors and mistakes is in the focus of guideline 3.3. This includes the wording of labels, error messages and suggestions.

For almost all these criterions it can be checked automatically for whether they exist or not, e.g. if there is a label element or if there is an identifier for the language of the text. But only humans can check if the wording is understandable and formulated as easy as possible. Problems with the language are not only critical for interaction, but also for the user guidance of a website with regard to navigation and understandability of the provided information in general. The British DRC-study underlines these facts with its results. Language can pose an accessibility problem for all user groups which have been analyzed. The key problems for blind users are "incorrect or nonexistent labelling of links, form elements and frames". The central problem for dyslexic users arises from "complicated language or terminology". The survey has raised significant values in all groups concerning "confusing and disorienting navigation mechanisms" where the wording is a key factor for a predictable navigation [5]. This supports our findings concerning the problems with regard to orientation and navigation for all questioned user groups.

The German Study, the British DRC-Study and the study of Lazar et.al. have established another main problem: missing or unhelpful alt text for pictures and videos as it is required by G 1.1. This is a key issue particularly for blind users [3, 5, 6] in all studies. The lack of alternative media for audio-based information and missing subtitles or captures pose the key problems for hearing impaired users [3, 5]. A comparison of different accessibility studies published in McEwan et.al. [17] underlines this by showing that missing alternative text for images and objects is "the most fundamental accessibility problem in commercial website development".

In the evaluation of the interviews connected with the survey, it can be extracted that the different user groups with disabilities have different problems with language. Visual impaired and blind users often have problems if the wording of the navigation is not clear and easy and if headlines do not describe what the content represents (e.g. "Far too complicated! To get the overview is the main problem, then finding the entry ways and finally entering are just so complicated") [3, 6]. Users with hearing impairments, deafness and with cognitive impairments often have problems with understanding the content, especially in long text [3, 5]. Additionally, they have problems with writing texts like in comments or wikis, because they are often not very confident with the written language and that is why they are worried about the reaction of other users (e.g. "often there is somebody who says: you are stupid"). It is for this reason that these user groups use functions such as comments below average compared to the other questioned user groups (e.g. 60% usage rate in comments by blind people, but only 28% by deaf people) [3].

To sum up, the following list of issues concerns the language and understandability of text in websites [11]:

- Difficult language and foreign words,
- Content in general,
- Alt-Text and descriptions of media content,
- Names of links,
- Explanations and agreements,
- Error messages and suggestions,
- Expected input data,
- Names in navigation.

3.3   Design Aspects

In addition to technical and editorial barriers, design barriers can also have a considerable influence on the accessibility of websites and applications. These aspects affect the user guidance and perceptibility of functions and not least the aesthetic impression on the user. Design barriers are based on inadequate accessible design of user interfaces, e.g. insufficient contrast, background images or too small font sizes [13]. Table 5 links the most critical design based issues due to the accessibility of the web content and functionality, which have been extracted from the study, to the corresponding WCAG Guidelines.

Table 5. Critical Design Related Aspects for Different User Groups and the Corresponding WCAG Guidelines

Type of Disability	Design Aspects	WCAG Guidelines
General	Perceptibility	1
	Orientation & clear arrangement	1.3, 1.4, 3.2
	Perceptibility of functions	1.4, 2.4
	Quality, size & contrasts of media content	1.4
Visual Impairments	Quality of pictures	2.3
	Optimization for certain screen resolution	1.4
	Size of buttons & interactive elements	2.4
Cognitive Impairments	Orientation & clear arrangement	1.3, 1.4, 3.2
Motor and Dexterity Impairments	Arrangement of links	2.4

One of the most important and impressive facts of the study is that almost all Internet users have problems to access and interact with a web application because of deficient orientation and arrangement (G 1.3, 1.4, 3.2). The main problems are poor contrast and undersized fonts (G 1.4). The British DRC-study comes to similar results: all groups, except the blind users, have identified "graphics and text size too small" and "inappropriate use of colors and poor contrast between content and background" as key problems [5]. Furthermore, in our study as well as in the DRC-study almost all user groups outline problems with the layout and orientation on the website: "unclear and confusing layout of pages" and "confusing and disorienting navigation mechanisms" are the most referred key problems.

Another important aspect is the perceptibility of functions especially in editors and players (G 1.4, 2.4). The interviewees have formulated problems due to the non-perceptibility of functions with regard to almost all applications with media content. The effect is clear: if they can not detect or separate the functions, they can not use it.

Orientation, clear arrangement (G 1.3, 1.4, 3.2) and likewise problems with quality or size and contrast of media content (G 1.4) can be attributed to editorial and designer aspects. On the one hand, the design should intend suitable format templates and place holders and on the other hand the editorial staff has to process contents and media for the Internet and appropriately integrate it into the format templates. Navigation and contents must well identifiable structured (paragraphs, headings) and sufficient font size for the orientation and clarity of arrangements.

Table 6. Comparison of the Most Important Aspects of Accessible Web Sites as a Conclusion of the Regarded Studies

Aspect	Web 2.0 Accessible	DRC	Lazar	WCAG 2.0
Alt-text		X	X	1.1, 1.2
Links	X	X	X	2.1, 2.4
Forms	X	X	X	1.3, 2.1, 3.1, 3.3, 4.1
Plugins (PDF, Flash, …)	X		X	3.3
Navigation	X	X	X	1.3, 1.4, 3.2
Layout	X	X	X	1.3, 1.4, 3.2
Failures (screen reader problems)	X	X	X	2.1, 2.4, 4.1
Language	X	X		3.1
Media content	X	X		1.1, 1.2, 1.4, 2.2, 1.3, 4.1

4   Conclusions

Interestingly, the recorded results coincide very well with the four principles that characterize WCAG 2.0. Requests for perceptibility, operability and understandability have been articulated by the interviewed persons repeatedly. The principle of robustness is primarily reflected concerning the performance of web applications accessed with assistive technologies. The results presented here show the high practical relevance of both: the results of the study and WCAG 2.0 because the problems identified in the study reflect barriers which still occur and WCAG 2.0 documents can provide answers for their accessible implementation. Table 6 gives a summary of the most important aspects of accessible web sites and applications as a conclusion of the regarded studies.

The German study has identified wiki applications, registration and other forms, and media applications as the most important applications which are very interesting for people with disabilities although they are often faced with accessibility problems. The most important barriers for all user groups are understandability in the broadest sense, the use of forms and the operability of multimedia components, especially with assistive technologies.

Technical problems which are for the most part caused by insufficient operability of the applications with assistive technologies are especially noticed by visually impaired, blind and physically disabled persons. Hearing impaired and deaf Internet users particularly encounter problems of understanding due to insufficient or superficial treatment of content and media in formats they understand, e.g. videos in sign language or with subtitles. Therefore, primarily organizational and editorial aspects are perceived by this group. Even users with reading disabilities, such as dyslexia, as well as with learning and intellectual disabilities are affected by editorial aspects so that restrictions on account of the linguistic competence are experienced.

Therefore, there seems to be a need for more awareness not only of technical aspects of accessibility but particularly of editorial aspects. All elements of a web application such as links, labels, menus and the content itself have to be formulated very carefully and as easy as possible with different user groups in mind. To check the understandability of all contents, and in particular of elements for user interactions such as forms, web applications have to be evaluated by users with a variety of abilities because these in practice experienced problems will otherwise not be detected.

Acknowledgements. I give thanks to "Aktion Mensch" and to "Stiftung Digitale Chancen" for providing the study data and for the opportunity to evaluate it in detail.

References

1. von Eimeren, B., Frees, B.: Ergebnisse der ARD/ZDFOnlinestudie 2010: Fast 50 Millionen Deutsche sind online – Multimedia für alle? Media Perspektiven 7(8), 334–349 (2010), http://www.ard-zdf-onlinestudie.de/

2. European Commission: Assessment of the Status of eAccessibility in Europe. MeAC – Measuring Progress of eAccessibility in Europe. Bonn (2007)

3. Berger, A., Caspers, T., Croll, J., Hofmann, J., Kubicek, H., Peter, U., Ruth-Janneck, D., Trump, T.: Web 2.0/Barrierefrei. Eine Studie zur Nutzung von Web2.0 Anwendungen durch Menschen mit Behinderungen. Aktion Mensch e.V. Bonn (2010)

4. Caldwell, B., Cooper, M., Guarino Reis, L., Vanderheiden, G.: Web Content Accessibility Guidelines (WCAG) 2.0. W3C Recommendation. World Wide Web Consortium (W3C) (December 2008), http://www.w3.org/TR/WCAG20/

5. Disability Rights Commission (DRC): The Web. Access and Inclusion for Disabled People, London (2004)

6. Lazar, J., Allen, A., Kleinman, J., Malarkey, C.: What Frustrates Screen Reader Users on the Web: A Study of 100 Blind Users. International Journal of Human-Computer Interaction 22(3), 247–269 (2007)

7. Lopes, R., Gomes, D., Carriço, L.: Web Not For All: A Large Scale Study of Web Accessibility. In: Proceedings of the International Cross Disciplinary Conference on Web Accessibility 2010, pp. 10:1–10:4 (2010)

8. Sullivan, T., Matson, R.: Barriers to Use: Usability and Content Accessibility on the Web's Most Popular Sites. In: Proceedings of the ACM Conference on Universal Usability, pp. 139–144 (2000)

9. Sayago, S., Blat, J.: An Ethnographical Study of the Accessibility Barriers in the Everyday Interactions of Older People with the Web. In: Universal Access in the Information Society, pp. 1–13 (2011)

10. Cornelssen, I., Schmitz, C.: Presentation of Study Results "Opportunities and Risks of the Internet of the Future from the Perspective of People with Disabilities" (Vorstellung der Ergebnisse der Studie Chancen und Risiken des Internets der Zukunft aus Sicht von Menschen mit Behinderungen auf der Aktion Mensch-Fachtagung Einfach für Alle – Konzepte und Zukunftsbilder für ein Barrierefreies Internet) (2008), http://www.einfach-fuer-alle.de/studie/

11. Ruth-Janneck, D.: Multidimensionale Klassifizierung von Barrieren in Webanwendungen. Mensch & Computer, 13–22 (2009)

12. Henry, S.L.: Essential Components of Web Accessibility (2005),
http://www.w3.org/WAI/intro/components.php

13. Ruth-Janneck, D.: An Integrative Accessibility Engineering Approach Using Multidimensional Classifications of Barriers in the Web. In: Proceedings of the International Cross-Disciplinary Conference on Web Accessibility 2011, pp. 10:1–10:4 (2011)

14. Caspers, T.: Reine Formsache. Barrierefreie Formulare mit HTML, CSS & JavaScript (2011),
http://www.einfach-fuer-alle.de/artikel/barrierefreie-formulare/

15. Mayer, T.: 74,75 Points for Registration in Facebook (74,75 Punkte für die Facebook-Registrierung). BIK BITV-Test (2011),
http://www.bitvtest.de/infothek/artikel/lesen/facebook-1.html

16. Inclusion Europe: Information for all. European standards for making information easy to read and understand, Brussels (1999), http://www.inclusion-europe.org/LLL/documents/Information%20for%20all.pdf

17. McEwan, T., Weerts, B.: ALT Text and Basic Accessibility. In: Proceedings of the 21st British HCI Group Annual Conference on HCI 2008: People and Computers XXI: HCI...but not as we know it, pp. 71–74 (2007)

Visual Exploration of Time-Oriented Patient Data for Chronic Diseases: Design Study and Evaluation

Alexander Rind[1,3], Wolfgang Aigner[1,3], Silvia Miksch[1,3], Sylvia Wiltner[2],
Margit Pohl[2], Thomas Turic[3], and Felix Drexler[4]

[1] Institute of Software Technology & Interactive Systems,
Vienna University of Technology, Austria
{rind,aigner,miksch}@ifs.tuwien.ac.at
[2] Research Group Human Computer Interaction,
Vienna University of Technology, Austria
margit@igw.tuwien.ac.at, s.wiltner@aon.at
[3] Department of Information and Knowledge Engineering,
Danube University Krems, Austria
[4] Landesklinikum Krems, Austria

Abstract. Medical care, particularly for chronic diseases, accumulates a huge amount of patient data over extensive time periods that needs to be accessed and analyzed accordingly. Information Visualization methods hold great promises in turning data deluge into improved quality of medical care. Yet, patient data management systems mostly provide documents, form-based displays, or static visualizations. We present a design study of an interactive visualization system, called VisuExplore, to support long-term care and medical analysis of patients with chronic diseases. VisuExplore offers interaction techniques for effective exploration of time-oriented data and employs simple, but intuitive visualization techniques. It was developed in close cooperation with physicians. We conducted two user studies with nine physicians and 16 students, which indicate that our design is useful and appropriate for particular tasks.

Keywords: Information Visualization, time-oriented data, medical information systems, visual exploration, interaction techniques, user study.

1 Introduction

Modern medicine puts a huge amount of patient data at the attending physicians' disposal. Particularly in chronic disease care, data accumulates over extensive periods of time and physicians need to access and analyze it accordingly. Ongoing data integration efforts might bridge the technical gap between different data stores but not the gap between data stores and human expertise. In an effort to turn data deluge into improved quality of medical care, we present a design study of an Information Visualization (InfoVis) system to support physicians in exploring time-oriented health care data of patients with chronic diseases.

A. Holzinger and K.-M. Simonic (Eds.): USAB 2011, LNCS 7058, pp. 301–320, 2011.

Time and time-oriented data play an important role in health care, which is underlined by the definition of the electronic health record (EHR) as "the complete set of information that resides in electronic form and is related to the past, present and future health status or health care provided to a subject of care" [24]. In care for patients with chronic diseases and for analysis of such care, physicians often need to consult these records. While typical queries can be answered quickly, there are often situations that require deeper understanding of the recorded information (e.g., co-development of biometric variables, or how a change of therapy has affected patient status). In addition, physicians need to analyze multiple variables of different data types and irregular sampling. For such exploratory tasks, where they do not have a direct question but learn about the patient in their search, InfoVis holds great promise [10].

Current patient data management systems (PDMS), however, provide only a small part of what InfoVis has to offer for exploring time-oriented data. Often, patient data is available only in electronic documents or PDMS forms that show one examination at a time. This makes it hard to follow patient trends. Visualizations, if provided, are mostly static and do not allow powerful interactions. Furthermore, existing research for patient data visualization has engaged in different design studies that cannot be immediately transferred to our domain problem. These designs either focus on a single type of data (e.g., intervals) or special scenarios, like intensive care, which is mostly concerned with high-frequency, short-term data (cp. Sect. 2).

In close cooperation with physicians at a regional hospital, we have developed task-specific interaction and visualization methods for the diabetes outpatient clinic, called VisuExplore. Through our design, they can explore time-oriented data of a patient with chronic diseases in a coherent user interface. In order to represent variables of different structure, we visualize each variable or each group of homogeneously structured variables in a separate diagram. To provide a frame of reference, these diagrams are aligned to a common time axis. Tackling irregular and independent sampling, we draw items where they fit on the time axis. The use of simple and easy-to-understand visualization methods was requested by users and should make it easy for them to read and interpret the data. This is accompanied by an extensive set of interaction techniques that allows for flexible and effective exploration of the data. Providing a reasonable combination of simplicity and flexibility is a non-trivial achievement.

In general it is advisable to evaluate InfoVis systems with their target users. However, physicians at our partner hospitals have been very busy and we could recruit nine physicians for the usability investigation of VisuExplore. To complement this investigation, we repeated the user study with 16 students. With this combined approach we could back up the result and gain additional insights.

Contribution. This paper's primary contribution is a design study of InfoVis methods for medicine. Design studies have been characterized very well by Munzner [20], who also called for more work of this type. Following this, we describe the diabetes outpatient clinic as accompanying domain problem and the user requirements guiding our work (Sect. 3). Next, we present the visual encoding and interaction design of our approach (Sect 4).[1] In a case study we demonstrate the applicability of our approach (Sect. 5) and we report a user study with 16 students on its usability (Sect. 6). For a secondary contribution, we compare the results of this user study with a previous user study conducted with nine physicians [23]. Finally, we draw our conclusions and outline directions for future work (Sect. 7).

2   Related Work

There is growing interest in time-oriented data [2] with medical applications being tackled in some prominent design studies.

One group of designs works exclusively on quantitative patient data (e.g., heart rate). Typically, they encode each variable in a scatter plot or a line plot with time on the horizontal axis. The Time Line Browser [8] is a seminal work for the visual exploration of time-oriented patient data in general and this group of designs in special. It defines a solid theoretical foundation and powerful interaction techniques for time-oriented data but its design is generic and not aimed to be easy to use as the paper concentrates on underlying concepts. The Graphical Summary of Patient Status (GSPS) [25] used fine-tuned scatter plots for a high data–ink ratio and arranged them as small multiples. However, this design was intended for printing and is neither interactive nor flexible. The Medical Information Visualization Assistant (MIVA) [9] applies some features of GSPS' scatter plot and integrates them in an interactive design that allows flexible arrangement of medical variables. However, in contrast to our work it is limited to quantitative data and has scatter plots as its only visualization technique.

A second group of designs focuses on nominal patient data (e.g., period of hospitalization) and typically uses a visual representation similar to a Gantt chart, which shows items as bars parallel to a horizontal time axis. For this group, LifeLines [22] is a ground-laying design. Items are grouped to facets, which can be collapsed or expanded. The facets are comparable to our diagrams, but they cannot be rearranged and resized as flexibly. Patient History in Pocket (PHiP) [3] adapts this approach for a mobile device with limited display size and interaction capabilities. Zhang et al. [36] use vertical bars for the 'when' aspect in their design, which they structure based on the 5-W of journalistic reporting (who, what, where, when, why, and how).

There are other designs for patient data, which do not use a time axis. For example, VIE-VISU [15] provides a metaphor graphic of quantitative patient status over a time interval and repeats this graphic to show changes over time. Sundvall et al. [32] present a design that shows nominal data as placemarks on a zoomable map of the human body. They use animation to show development over time. The 5-W design of Zhang et al. [36] also contains a view of a stylized human body for its 'where' aspect. As a third view 5-W provides a directed graph

---

[1] This extends a short paper [28] written at an early stage of the project, which contained the overall concept and requirements analysis but no system design in detail and no user studies.

of events in the patient record for the 'why' aspect. These two views, however, show only the current patient status, but not development over time.

Comparing patient data to medical guidelines is a related domain problem and has yielded some designs that combine features from the groups of MIVA and LifeLines (e.g., CareCruiser [11], Midgaard [4]). However, these designs cater more to different tasks than open-ended exploration. In the surroundings of this work we also find the problem domains of querying patient databases (e.g., LifeLines2 [34], Similan [35]) and exploring patient cohorts (e.g., CareGiver [5], Dare [7], Gravi++ [14], TimeRider [27], VISITORS [16]).

Overall, VisuExplore stands out due to its flexibility and task-specific interactions for the exploration process. The exploration designs described above only work with either quantitative or nominal data and rely on a single visualization technique that shows development over time. Our design's interactions include most notably the flexible arrangement of variables, smooth zooming and resizing, measuring time spans, and keeping track of time and relevant items.

3   Domain Problem

In this section, we lay a foundation for our design study by describing the user requirements and a medical scenario that has accompanied our design process.

3.1   Methods for User-Centered Design

This work is embedded into a larger research project studying the application of InfoVis to medical care. We adopted a user-centered design approach [29] and involved potential users from the beginning. We conducted systematic requirements gathering through semi-structured interviews with five physicians at a regional hospital to assess how InfoVis could make their work easier and what kinds of mapping would be appropriate for their data. Furthermore, we chose a concrete medical scenario that would guide the design process and user studies. We used interviews and contextual observation of three patient encounters in the diabetes outpatient clinic to familiarize ourselves with the medical scenario.

We developed the design based on state-of-the-art InfoVis principles. The design underwent an iterative refinement process to gather expert reviews from InfoVis and human-computer interaction specialists in our team. In addition, we used prototypes, first on paper, then implemented in Java using prefuse [12], to test our approach informally with three physicians and a nurse, who are familiar with managing diabetes. These iterations culminated in a case study and a structured evaluation with nine physicians and 16 students, which we present later in this work.

3.2   Medical Requirements

Based on the interviews with the physicians we gathered the following user requirements:

- *Simple user interface:* The physicians need to gain quick and unambiguous insights. Thus, the interfaces and visualizations should be particularly clear and simple to use.
- *Flexible for various medical variables:* A single fixed configuration is not sufficient, because different patients or different medical disciplines require the analysis of different sets of variables.
- *Time-oriented data:* Various measurements of variables over time need to be followed. Development and co-development are of interest.
- *Interactivity:* A variety of interaction techniques such as (semantic) zooming, resizing of visualizations, grouping, opening medical documents from the visualization, and writing annotations should be included.
- *Multiple patients:* Some tasks require the comparison and filtering of data of patient cohorts, for example finding out whether some therapies are more effective than others.[2]

3.3   Medical Scenario

Diabetes mellitus is a chronic condition in which the human body is no longer capable of managing its glucose (blood sugar). To mitigate this, patients need to change their lifestyle, take oral medication, and/or inject insulin. Otherwise, they are at risk of many complications, e.g., cardiovascular disease, retinal damage, or diabetic coma. The choice of treatment depends on many factors including diabetes type, severity, comorbid diseases, and the patient's experience in keeping their glucose in the optimal range.

In this scenario, we take the point of view of a physician at the diabetes outpatient clinic. Examinations at the clinic are scheduled in intervals between six weeks to three months, depending on the patient's condition. The data set encompasses quantitative data (e.g., fasting blood glucose level, body mass index), nominal point data (e.g., concomitant medication to lower blood pressure), and nominal interval data (e.g., insulin therapy). However, some of the variables are optional and physicians only record them, if they expect relevant changes. In contrast, some other variables such as blood pressure or cholesterol level might also be recorded between two diabetes examinations by another department of the hospital. The data originates from two separate systems: a laboratory information system and a computerized physician order entry system. Together these factors make a good case for how relevant heterogeneous time-oriented data is in practice.

Physicians working for the diabetes outpatient clinic are interested in whether a patient's condition improves or worsens. They want to relate an improvement of some variables to the development of other variables, for example, losing weight and lower glucose. They need to know which types of therapy a patient already had and how these affected medical tests.

---

[2] In the following design process we came to the conclusion that we can support this requirement, analysing the development of multiple patients over time, better through a separate design study, which we present elsewhere [27].

4   Description of VisuExplore's Design

Next, we explain how our proposed interaction and visualization techniques (see Fig. 1) meet the domain problem presented above. For this, we set these techniques in context with state-of-the-art InfoVis research and use anonymized medical data as illustrative example.

4.1   General Layout

For efficient visualization of time-oriented data, research in InfoVis methods and human perception has yielded a considerable body of guidelines (e.g., [6,33]). However, there is no single visualization technique that can efficiently encode all types of time-oriented data needed for exploration of diabetes data (cp. [2]). Thus, we work with a collection of well-established visualization techniques, each of which can handle one class of time-oriented variables well. We combine diagrams of these techniques in a multiple-view visualization, where all views share the common time axis. Using the perceptually efficient encoding "position on a common scale" for the time aspects of all items of all variables allows the users to keep a common frame of reference. This makes it easy to find out about sequence, co-occurrence, and co-development of multiple, possibly heterogeneous variables. Thus, we accommodate for the important role time plays in fulfilling the tasks of this medical scenario (see Sect. 3.3). For the users, the time axis is visualized using the Gregorian calendar (see Fig. 1.v0). Vertical grid lines that extend from the time axis help users to look up time points of interest.

4.2   Visualization Techniques

VisuExplore provides four simple, but intuitive visualization techniques (see Fig. 1): A line plot and a bar chart for quantitative data as well as an event chart and a timeline chart for nominal variables.

Line plots and bar charts are well known and users can interpret them without training. Thus, we meet the design requirements for visualization that are simple to use and to interpret. The bar chart can be used, when individual values are of interest or should be compared. The line plot connects consecutive observations visually and, thus, can be used to spot and compare trends and patterns. The line plot uses a y-axis that scales automatically to a default value range, which is defined in the metadata. Alternatively, users can set it to scale fitting for the highest and lowest values in the patient's data. This allows users to follow changes that are small compared to the value and immediately determine the value range of a variable. However, this setting might lead to wrong insights as small fluctuations of a stable parameter may look like dramatic changes. Further, the y-axis may be set to extend to zero. This is particularly useful when ratios are important (e.g., body weight), but not for interval scaled variables (e.g., temperature). The bar chart uses the same y-axis but it will always extend to zero, because otherwise bar length would not be interpreted correctly.

For nominal data, we provide the *event chart*. It can visualize several variables in the same diagram. Each variable is positioned on a separate y-position.

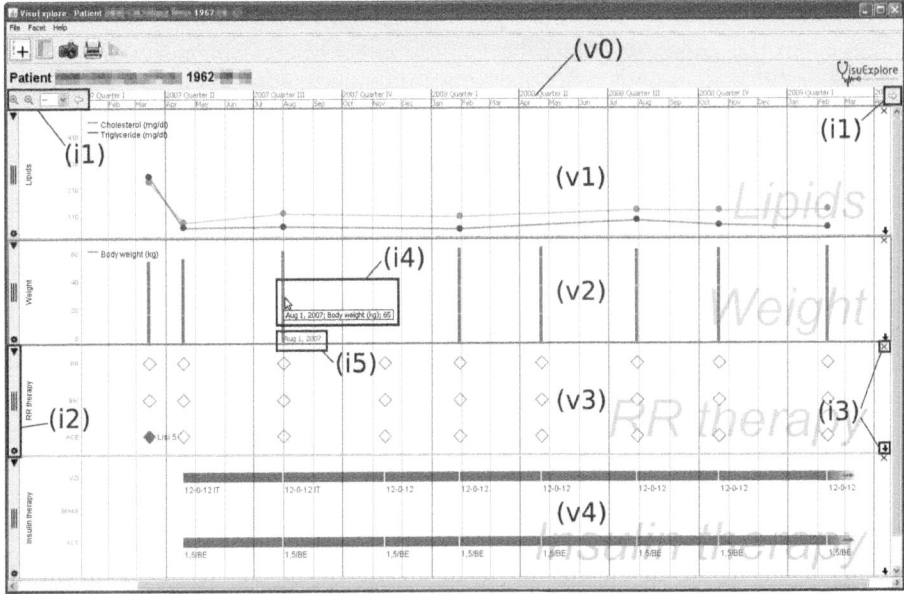

Fig. 1. Exploring medical data of a diabetes patient using the VisuExplore interface: Multiple groups of variables are visualized with different techniques in a multiple views display: Line plot (v1), bar chart (v2), event chart (v3), and timeline chart (v4). All visualizations share a common time axis (v0). Patient master data is printed above the time axis. Users can interact with the visualization through mouse actions inside each view, scrollbars, a toolbar for time (i1), two toolbars for views (i2, i3), and the menu. When hovering over an item, a tooltip (i4) prints the item's exact time and value. A mouse tracker (i5) marks the position of the mouse pointer with an orange line to keep users informed about items occurring together and their occurrence time.

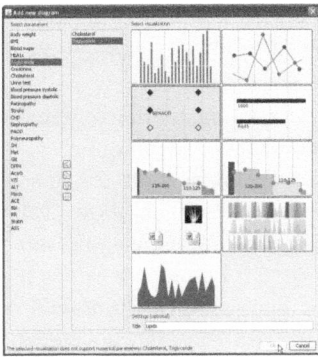

Fig. 2. Dialog to add a new diagram: Users select variables, a technique, and optionally a diagram title. The dialog will warn users, if they choose variables that are not supported by the selected technique. In the user study we used only bar chart, line plot, event chart, and timeline chart (top four options). The advanced visualization techniques were not visible in the user interface.

Basic shapes represent all variable observations and different nominal values are mapped to the shape or color. For example, in Fig. 1.v3 prescribed drugs are shown as filled diamonds whereas empty diamonds appear for drugs that are not prescribed. A short free text may go along with each of these shapes. In the figure they show an abbreviation of the brand name and the dosage.

So far, we presented visualization techniques for data that is valid for a point in time. When data of a nominal variable is valid for a time interval, we can use the *timeline chart* (see Fig. 1.v4). This chart type is a well-established technique and can be found in the group of designs around LifeLines [22]. We also devised a representation for intervals of which only the start time is known but not the end time (e.g., currently prescribed insulin therapy). We draw these intervals with the right edge fading out and an arrow should indicate that the timeline might extend longer than it is visible.

The collection of visualization techniques outlined above is not intended to be complete. Instead, we plan VisuExplore as a framework that is open for pluggable components as requested by Aigner et al. [2]. In fact, we have already integrated five advanced visualization techniques to demonstrate the extensibility of Visu-Explore (see Fig. 2): a semantic zoom chart (cp. [4]), a step chart, a silhouette graph, a horizon graph (cp. [26]), and a document browser. However, in the usability investigation we limited the prototype to simple techniques, because the introductory requirements analysis called explicitly for simple visualizations. In order not to overwhelm users we plan to evaluate advanced visualization technique one at a time.

4.3   Interaction Techniques

Above we discussed visualization techniques but much more is possible through interaction. Interaction is regarded as "at the heart" of InfoVis [31] and this might be even more true for exploration of time-oriented data.

A flexible and adaptable arrangement of variables was one primary requirement for VisuExplore (Sect. 3.2). Our design excels in allowing users interaction with variables. In this respect, it is more powerful than comparable approaches. Users can *add new diagrams* using a dialog window (see Fig. 2) where they choose variables and a visualization technique.

Each diagram is furnished with two toolbars, one on the left side (see Fig. 1.i2) and one on the right (see Fig. 1.i3), which allow users to adapt the diagram. The x icon in the top right corner *closes the view* and removes it from the display and the gearwheel icon in the bottom left corner opens a dialog window that *controls settings* of the chart (e.g., extending a numerical axis to zero). Furthermore, the toolbars allow users to *resize* the diagram depending on whether they want an overview by seeing many variables at once or analyze a few in details. They can collapse or expand the diagram to an outline with the triangle icon, which is used in multiple designs (e.g., LifeLines [22]). Alternatively, users can resize the diagram continuously by dragging the arrow icon or the bottom border of the diagram. The chart dynamically redraws during interaction and adapts to its height through optimized layout algorithms. By grabbing a diagram in the

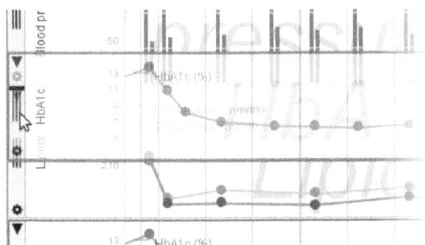

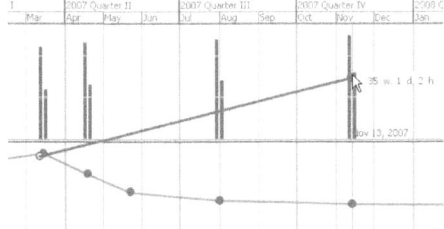

Fig. 3. Users can move a diagram by clicking and dragging the area indicated through three vertical lines in the left toolbar. While moving, the mouse drags a semi-transparent preview of the diagram and a blue bar marks the current insert location. Here the user moves "HbA1c" (green line plot) up, which will be inserted between "Blood pressure" and "Lipids".

Fig. 4. A measure tool allows users to determine the time interval between any two locations inside the visualization. Here the user finds out that a high blood pressure value comes about 35 weeks after a peak HbA1c reading.

middle of the left toolbar, users can *move* diagrams and thus rearrange the configurations (see Fig. 3).

For navigation in time, users can use the *pan* and *zoom* buttons in a dedicated toolbar next to the time axis (see Fig. 1.i1), shift the horizontal scrollbar, or drag the mouse in the visualization. There are also some predefined zoom steps, like one week or one year, which users can select in the toolbar. These replicated interactions make navigation usable for both beginners and more experienced users. During zoom, the time axis automatically adapts itself to use time units fitting the current temporal resolution, for example quarter of a year and month (see Fig. 1.v0). With the *mouse tracker* users can see, which observations occur together and at what time. This is implemented as an orange vertical line that follows the mouse inside the visualization (see Fig. 1.i5). A label accompanies the line and prints the time of its x-coordinate.

An important task when interacting with time-oriented data is to measure the duration of an item or the time difference between two items. Especially in exploring a medical record and in investigating possible cause-effect relationships, time differences between items of different variables need to be studied (e.g., does a change in insulin therapy result in a decrease of HbA1c within a certain amount of time). For this, we created the *measure tool* (see Fig. 4). Users can determine the time difference from a reference point to the current mouse location through a straight line and a label. The label is updated with every mouse movement and prints the time difference in reasonable time units. This works across multiple diagrams. Similar measure tools are common for spatial data (e.g., Google Maps), but we are not aware about such a functionality in other visualization approaches for time-oriented data.

Finally, users can interact directly with visual items representing entries in the data set. On mouse-over, an item is highlighted and a *tooltip* with its exact time and value pops up (see Fig. 1.i4). Users can also *mark one or more individual items as selected* by clicking on them. Further, users can open an additional window with a *table* containing the items of one diagram (see Fig. 5). Also in this table, users can select items – individually or block-wise. These items are then marked in the diagram and vice versa, which allows users to interact with one and watch the effects in the other. Users may also *sort* the items by their value or their occurrence time. Thus, it is possible to highlight, for example, the top five observations of a quantitative variable.

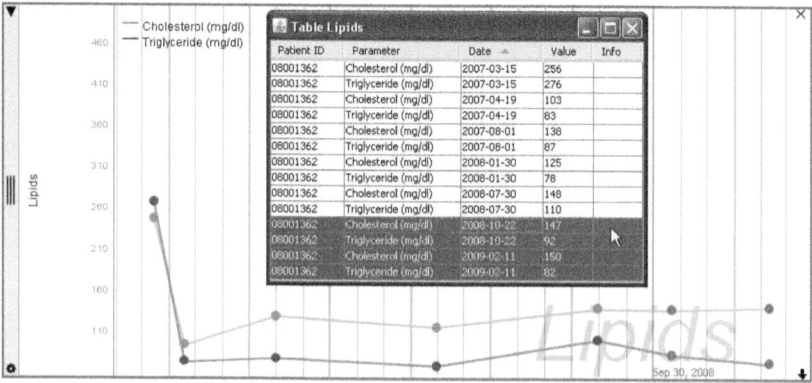

Fig. 5. The table window allows users to inspect all items in detail and sort them by each column. They can select items (color orange) by clicking. Diagram and table are linked, selecting an item in the table will select the corresponding item in the diagram. Here, the user has selected the four latest readings in "Lipids".

5   Case Study

In this section, we demonstrate our design in context of a concrete diabetes case that we obtained from our medical project partners. The insights reported here came up, while physicians tested our prototype.

5.1   Diagnosis of Latent Autoimmune Diabetes of Adults

In Fig. 6 we show a screenshot of our prototype applied to medical data of a diabetes patient. First, we have created eight diagrams and repeatedly rearranged them so that they provide a good overview of the patient's diabetes history: On top, there is an event chart of end organ damages that can be related to diabetes. Next, we added three line plots with body mass index (BMI), blood glucose, and HbA1c (an indicator for a patient's blood glucose condition over the previous several weeks). Below blood sugar values, we placed two timeline charts showing the insulin therapy and oral anti-diabetic drugs. Insulin is categorized into rapid-acting insulin ("ALT"), intermediate-acting insulin ("VZI"), and a mixture of these ("Misch"). Oral anti-diabetic drugs are grouped by five active ingredients/brands. Details about brand name or dosage in free text are shown in labels located under the timeline. The bottom two diagrams are related to

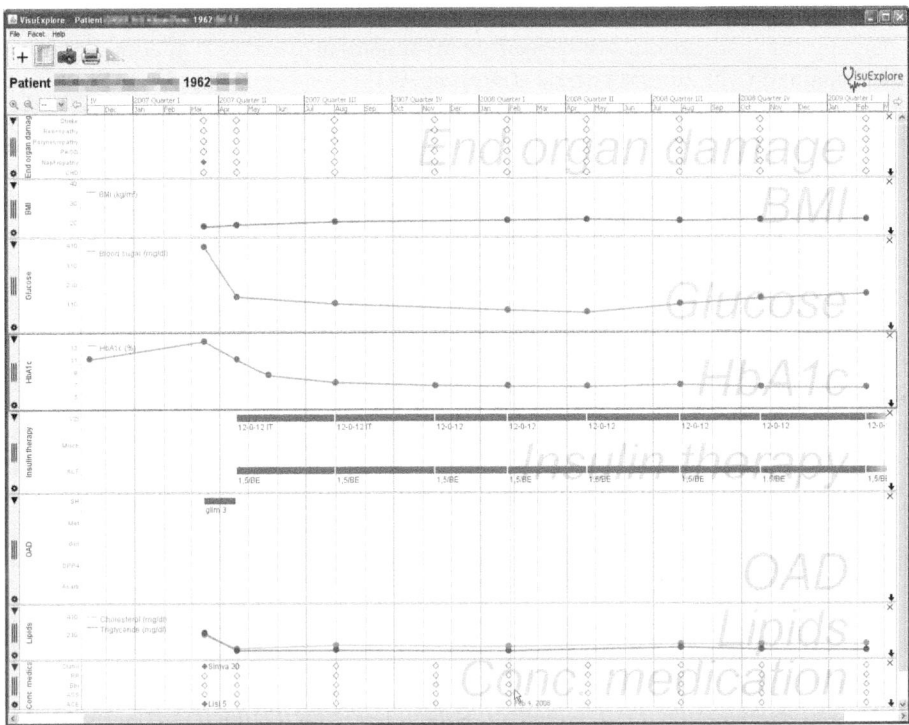

Fig. 6. Patient X (medical data extracted and anonymized in March 2009): Very high blood sugar values and a body mass index of 20.1 at admission are diagnosed as latent autoimmune diabetes of adults. First treatments are "SH glim 3", an oral anti-diabetic drug, with medication for elevated blood pressure and elevated blood lipids. After one month, blood sugar has improved and blood lipids have normalized. Patient switches to insulin therapy and continuously improves.

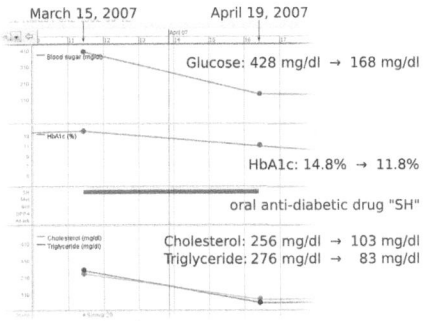

Fig. 7. First and second examination of Patient X show an improvement of blood sugar and blood lipid values

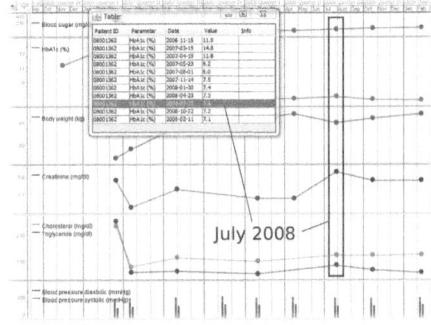

Fig. 8. Detecting local extrema of HbA1c, body weight, creatinine, cholesterol, and triglyceride in the July 2008 examination

blood lipids with a line plot of triglyceride and cholesterol and an event chart of concomitant medication. We chose this arrangement because it places diagrams with medical tests directly above diagrams of the related medical interventions. We reduced the height of some diagrams to fit them on a single screen. Then, we zoomed and panned to a period of two years and three months between November 2006 and February 2009, which shows all examinations.

This diabetes case (see Fig. 6) is a 44-year-old patient with initially very high blood sugar values. We can read the exact values 428 mg/dl glucose, 14.8% HbA1c from the tooltips. In addition, blood lipids values are high (256 mg/dl cholesterol, 276 mg/dl triglyceride). At the same time, the body mass index of 20.1 is rather low. Even though there is the suspicion of a nephropathy (damage to or disease of the kidney), these are also signs for latent autoimmune diabetes of adults, a special form of type 1 diabetes.

First treatments are "SH glim 3", an oral anti-diabetic drug, plus medication for elevated blood pressure ("ACE Lisi 5") and elevated blood lipids ("Statin Simiva 20"). After one month, blood sugar has improved (168 mg/dl glucose) and blood lipids have normalized (see Fig. 7). The patient switches to insulin therapy in a combination of rapid-acting insulin ("ALT") and intermediate-acting insulin ("VZI"). We use the measure tool with a reference point in April 2007 and move around to other examinations to get an impression of the time intervals relative to the start of insulin therapy.

Next, we open the tables for HbA1c and BMI because we are interested in exact values although we can see the trend from the visualization as well. We can see that the patient's condition almost continuously improves with a HbA1c value of 7.1% and a BMI of 23.5 on February 11, 2009. Only on July 30, 2008, we have a slightly higher HbA1c of 7.6% and a slightly lower BMI of 22.8. We want to find out more about July 2008 and add views of other variables: weight, creatinine, blood pressure (see Fig. 8). We notice that on July 30, 2008 also creatinine is higher than usually. A possible explanation for this is that the patient is dehydrated.

The suspicion of nephropathy has been wrong. Since April 2007, the insulin dosage stays stable and concomitant medication is no longer needed. The patient's overall condition has improved through blood sugar management.

In addition to nine examination dates with data on diabetes treatment, our system found two more HbA1c readings in November 2006 and May 2007. A physician involved in the case study wondered about the very high HbA1c value of 11.9% in November 2006 and why diabetes treatment had only started four months later. Furthermore, the examination in November 2007 lacks data about body mass index, glucose, and lipids.

6   Usability Investigation

6.1   Description of the Investigation

The main goal of the investigation was to assess whether VisuExplore was usable and the representations (mapping) of the variables understandable.

The subjects were 16 students. The results of this study are compared to another study with the same system and similar methodology (interviews) conducted with nine physicians (see [23]). An additional goal was to assess whether the results from the study with physicians and with students differed considerably. It is often criticized that evaluation studies are conducted with students, but we assume that at least some research questions, especially questions of usability, can also be answered using students as subjects.

The main research questions of the investigation were:

1. Which were the main advantages/disadvantages of the system?
2. Which forms of interaction are most useful?
3. Which of the proposed visualizations for the variables are appropriate?
4. Are the results of the study with students as subjects similar to the results of the study with physicians (experts)?

The subjects of the study were students. They were tested in two groups. One group (11 students studying computer science) participated in a lecture on Human-Computer Interaction and E-Learning. These students got an introduction of approximately two hours into the application domain and the system. They had to solve three tasks developed by a physician from a hospital participating in the project. They worked on their own with the system and had to fill in a questionnaire with open-ended questions more or less identical to the interview conducted with the physicians [23]. These students had ample time to work with the system – most took about 40 minutes to one hour – and were specifically asked to find usability problems. We decided that 11 students were not enough for the study; therefore we conducted an additional study with five students who studied languages or economics. This had the additional advantage that we did not only test computer science students. The second group received a short introduction into the application domain and system, worked with the system – also solving the three tasks – and then had to answer the same questions as the other students in an interview. The questions and tasks for both groups were the same. The only difference was that one group wrote down their answers and the others answered in an interview. The interview enables the researcher to check whether any misunderstandings occurred and to discuss the answers with the subjects. The results from both groups of students did not differ considerably, although the first one produced more usability problems because they worked longer with the system. The longer introduction and the extensive work with the system for the first group probably helped to overcome well-known problems occurring with questionnaires (subjects misunderstanding the questions, lack of contextualization) (see e.g., [1]).

Both groups got the same three tasks to solve. These tasks were identical to those for the physicians:

Task 1: Please look at the data of three patients (A, B, C), especially at blood sugar, cholesterol and body mass index. Can you see any relationships between the three parameters for these three patients?

Task 2: Look at patient D. Because of an illness, the patient has to take cortisone. What effects does this have on the patient's condition?

Task 3: Take a look at patient E. What can you say about his/her development? (Task 3 is a more general task for exploration).

We used qualitative methods for this investigation because they allow to get detailed information about usability problems in a very efficient manner. In addition, it is possible to analyze unanticipated or controversial usability problems more deeply. Furthermore, recruiting expert users is even harder for a controlled experimental approach. We also used qualitative methods for students because we wanted this study to be as similar to the study with the physicians as possible. In further research, we will also do a quantitative analysis of the log files and the thinking aloud protocols.

The main methods used in this study were a questionnaire with open-ended questions for one group and qualitative interviews for the other group. Questionnaire and interview consisted of the same questions. Sometimes the subjects uttered conflicting statements (e.g., that they appreciated a specific feature of the system, but nevertheless did not use it very often), therefore it is difficult to quantify statements.

6.2   Results

In this section, the results of the interviews/questionnaires are described in detail. The emphasis is on comments made by several subjects because we assume that these comments are more relevant for the assessment of the system than a comment made by just one subject. Quotations from the students are added in brackets.

Advantages of the system (research question 1). The answers concerning the main advantages of the system are fairly homogenous. Students noted that the system was easy to learn and intuitive. The interface was easy to handle. There were only a reduced number of features. This made the system easy to understand, but was seen as an advantage and a disadvantage by one subject. The visualization was seen as appropriate. It provides a fast and easy way to get an overview of rather complex data. Different variables can be compared at a glance.

The answers concerning the disadvantages are more heterogeneous, and most of the disadvantages are only noticed by a few subjects. Some of the subjects commented that the design was rather boring ("It looks like Excel."). They also complained that it is not possible to compare the data of two or more patients, which was not in the scope of VisuExplore's design aims. Many of them commented that scrolling in some cases was difficult. This was mainly due to the fact that the scrolling function by mouse wheel and automatic scrolling upwards/downwards when dragging a diagram were not implemented in that prototype. Some subjects also noticed that double-click did not work properly. Two of them also complained that there was lack of contrast concerning the colors which made it difficult to distinguish various variables.

In addition, the students found several different smaller usability problems.

Interaction (research question 2). Some of the interaction techniques were appreciated by the subjects while other techniques were criticized:

New Diagram/Delete Diagram: The method to create a new diagram was only appreciated by a few subjects. Several aspects of creating and deleting diagrams were criticized. Some of the subjects had difficulties to create new diagrams for different reasons. Several of the subjects complained that when a visualization technique was not available for a specific variable it was not disabled, but only after selecting the desired technique did an easy to overlook error message appear (cp. Fig. 2). This led to unnecessary user actions. Deleting diagrams also did not seem to be as intuitive as expected. One user, e.g., complained that it was not possible to select more than one diagram to make deletion more efficient.

Resizing Diagrams: Users liked this feature, and there were only a few complaints. It is an important possibility to change between overview and detail-view or to compare a larger number of diagrams.

Moving Diagrams: This feature was explicitly appreciated by eight subjects. They found it useful and well designed. Five subjects pointed out that scrolling and moving diagrams at the same time does not work, which makes this feature inefficient.

Select/Tooltip/Mouse-Over: The attitudes concerning these features were mixed. Six subjects found at least one of these features positive and useful. Four subjects complained that it was not possible to select more than one diagram. The subjects made several different suggestions on how to improve this feature.

Measure Tool: Ten subjects found this feature quite useful because it makes data easier to understand. They made several suggestions how to improve this feature ("rather click at start and end points instead of dragging the line from start to end point").

Pan/Zoom: Only one subject found this feature useful and well implemented. The other subjects criticized it quite heavily. They commented, e.g., that the zoom function does not give a detailed view of the region the subjects were interested in, but some other region. This led to some confusions and disorientation until some (not all) realized that the zoom function zooms into the middle of the time axis and not to the selected data item. Some subjects remarked that the zoom function is not necessary for the data presented in the test.

Visualization (research question 3). The system offered several visualization techniques (line plots, bar charts, etc.). The different possibilities to visualize the data were seen as very positive. Most of the visualization techniques are easy to understand. It is simple and intuitive to compare different variables over time. The subjects especially liked line plots and bar charts. The diamond shaped event charts were not understood intuitively and criticized by five subjects.

Most of the students appreciated the possibility to show several variables in one diagram because it makes the comparison of the variables easier ("ideal for up to three variables, more variables would be confusing"; "several lines in one diagram are easier to compare, they do not take up so much space"). No student explicitly criticized this feature.

Comparison to the study with physicians (research question 4). Basically, the results of the study with physicians and the study with students are fairly similar. It should be pointed out, however, that there are a few differences. The results for the question about the main advantages of the systems are more or less the same. Physicians as well as students found that the main advantages of the system are that it is easy to understand and to learn and that the visualization allows the interpretation of the data at a glance. The students found more usability problems, which is not surprising because many of them worked with the system for a longer period of time than the physicians and were specifically asked to identify such problems.

The attitude concerning the creation and deletion of diagrams was quite similar for physicians and students. For both groups we could identify mixed attitudes, some liked this features and some criticized it. Students as well as physicians liked the possibility to resize diagrams, although a few physicians argued that this features is not necessary or even misleading. Moving diagrams was also appreciated by physicians as well as students, although the students more often pointed out that there were technical problems concerning the implementation. Both physicians and students liked the select/tooltip/mouse-over functionality. Again, there are a few usability problems to solve which were noticed by both students and physicians. There are different attitudes concerning the measure tool for physicians and students. The students appreciated this tool much more than the physicians. Both physicians and students were critical concerning the zoom/pan functionality. This is probably due to some implementation problems and also to the fact that especially the zoom functionality is only necessary for large amounts of heterogeneous data. Several subjects (among physicians as well as students) pointed out that they did not really need to zoom to interpret the data provided during the test.

Concerning visualization techniques, physicians had a distinct appreciation for line plots. The students also preferred the line plots, but they also liked the bar charts. Both groups were skeptical about the diamond shaped event charts which they did not find intuitive and understandable. Physicians were more critical about combining several variables in one diagram because the scales of the variables are too different to represent them in one diagram.

In general, the results of the studies for physicians and students are quite similar. There are differences concerning the number of usability problems found because many of the students worked longer with the system than the physicians. Students also have a tendency to prefer more novel features (e.g., the measure tools), but it should be pointed out that they also found simple and well-known visualization forms much more useful than complex and new ones.

7   Conclusions and Future Work

Interactive InfoVis has the potential to help physicians exploring time-oriented patient data, which is of special relevance in patient-centric care for chronic diseases. We presented VisuExplore, a design study and a prototypical implementation of interactive InfoVis methods to support long-term care and medical analysis of patients with chronic diseases. Designing for such an exploration process, it is essential to consider the medical scenario and user requirements. During our iterative design and prototypical implementation phase, it became clear that our design needs to be flexible and adaptable as well as simple to use and to interpret in order to support the users in their exploration processes. Through combination of easy to understand and mostly well-established visualization techniques (e.g., line plot), powerful interaction techniques (e.g., rearrange diagrams, measure tool), and use of variable metadata we provide a design that meets these requirements.

We demonstrate VisuExplore's applicability using a case study to explore and analyze a patient with a non-typical type of diabetes. Furthermore, we conducted two usability studies, one with nine physicians (cp. [23]) and the other with 16 students, which we reported in this paper. These user studies indicate that our design is useful and appropriate for particular tasks. We have specifically analyzed usability problems connected to interaction techniques. As Lam [17] points out, less than a third of a large number of InfoVis papers she surveyed mentioned interaction explicitly. In doing so, we hope to contribute further to the development of a science of interaction [21]. Comparing the studies of physicians and students we found that the results were fairly similar. Therefore, we conclude that studies with students can be an adequate instrument for usability investigation. Though, for some questions, e.g., on the applicability of a feature, studies with domain experts are needed.

Starting from the work presented here, we see several directions for future research: First, results of the usability investigation point us at possibilities for improvement of VisuExplore. Specifically, we plan to improve the event chart visualization and interactions for panning, zooming, and scrolling. Second, we will do a quantitative analysis of the log files and the thinking aloud protocols. In future user studies, we will also investigate advanced visualization techniques in context of patients with chronic diseases. After adapting them for this concrete domain problem, we want to evaluate if they are more suitable than the simple visualization techniques described above. Third, to explore larger data sets quantitatively and qualitatively, we can apply temporal data abstractions. These visualizations of abstracted data (cp. [16,19]) can be integrated directly in our design and allow continuous exploration from overview to detail as we demonstrate with the semantic zoom chart. Furthermore, this should allow users to jointly explore variables of significantly different sampling frequency. Finally, our design can provide features to better support humans in an undirected exploration process. For example, users may wish to undo an interaction (e.g., closing a diagram), return to a previous state in their exploration history, or open a predefined set of diagrams (cp. [30]). Other features may afford to externalize hypotheses, which physicians have found during visual exploration, so they can discuss them with colleagues or analyze them statistically (cp. [13,18]).

Acknowledgments. This work was supported by the Bridge program of the Austrian Research Promotion Agency (project no. 814316) and the Centre for Visual Analytics Science and Technology CVAST (funded by the Austrian Federal

Ministry of Economy, Family and Youth in the exceptional Laura Bassi Centres of Excellence initiative). We wish to thank our partners: NÖ Gesundheits- und Sozialfonds, NÖ Landeskliniken-Holding, Landesklinikum Krems, systema Human Information Systems.

References

1. Adams, A., Cox, A.L.: Questionnaires, in-depth interviews and focus groups. In: Cairns, P., Cox, A.L. (eds.) Research Methods for Human-Computer Interaction, pp. 17–34. Cambridge University Press, Cambridge (2008)
2. Aigner, W., Miksch, S., Müller, W., Schumann, H., Tominski, C.: Visualizing time-oriented data—a systematic view. Computers & Graphics 31(3), 401–409 (2007)
3. Ardito, C., Buono, P., Costabile, M.F., Lanzilotti, R.: Two different interfaces to visualize patient histories on a PDA. In: Proc. 8th Conf. Human-Computer Interaction with Mobile Devices and Services, pp. 37–40. ACM (2006)
4. Bade, R., Schlechtweg, S., Miksch, S.: Connecting time-oriented data and information to a coherent interactive visualization. In: Proc. ACM SIGCHI Conf. Human Factors in Computing Systems (CHI), pp. 105–112 (2004)
5. Brodbeck, D., Gasser, R., Degen, M., Reichlin, S., Luthiger, J.: Enabling large-scale telemedical disease management through interactive visualization. In: Connecting Medical Informatics and Bio-Informatics, Proc. Int. Congress Eur. Fed. Med. Inform. (MIE), pp. 1172–1177 (2005)
6. Card, S.K., Mackinlay, J.D., Shneiderman, B. (eds.): Readings in Information Visualization: Using Vision to Think. Morgan Kaufmann, San Francisco (1999)
7. Catarci, T., Santucci, G., Silva, S.F.: An interactive visual exploration of medical data for evaluating health centres. Journal of Research and Practice in Information Technology 35(2), 99–119 (2003)
8. Cousins, S.B., Kahn, M.G.: The visual display of temporal information. Artificial Intelligence in Medicine 3(6), 341–357 (1991)
9. Faiola, A., Newlon, C.: Advancing Critical Care in the ICU: A Human-Centered Biomedical Data Visualization Systems. In: Robertson, M.M. (ed.) EHAWC 2011 and HCII 2011. LNCS, vol. 6779, pp. 119–128. Springer, Heidelberg (2011)
10. Fekete, J.D., van Wijk, J., Stasko, J.T., North, C.: The Value of Information Visualization. In: Kerren, A., Stasko, J.T., Fekete, J.-D., North, C. (eds.) Information Visualization. LNCS, vol. 4950, pp. 1–18. Springer, Heidelberg (2008)
11. Gschwandtner, T., Aigner, W., Kaiser, K., Miksch, S., Seyfang, A.: CareCruiser: exploring and visualizing plans, events, and effects interactively. In: Proc. IEEE Pacific Visualization Symp. (PacificVis), pp. 43–50 (2011)
12. Heer, J., Card, S.K., Landay, J.A.: prefuse: A toolkit for interactive information visualization. In: Proc. ACM SIGCHI Conf. Human Factors in Computing Systems (CHI), pp. 421–430 (2005)
13. Heer, J., Vigas, F.B., Wattenberg, M.: Voyagers and voyeurs: Supporting asynchronous collaborative visualization. Communications of the ACM 52(1), 87–97 (2009)
14. Hinum, K., Miksch, S., Aigner, W., Ohmann, S., Popow, C., Pohl, M., Rester, M.: Gravi++: Interactive information visualization to explore highly structured temporal data. Journal of Universal Computer Science 11(11), 1792–1805 (2005)
15. Horn, W., Popow, C., Unterasinger, L.: Support for fast comprehension of ICU data: Visualization using metaphor graphics. Methods of Information in Medicine 40(5), 421–424 (2001)

16. Klimov, D., Shahar, Y., Taieb-Maimon, M.: Intelligent visualization and exploration of time-oriented data of multiple patients. Artificial Intelligence in Medicine 49(1), 11–31 (2010)
17. Lam, H.: A framework of interaction costs in information visualization. IEEE Trans. Visualization and Computer Graphics 14(6), 1149–1156 (2008)
18. Lammarsch, T., Aigner, W., Bertone, A., Miksch, S., Rind, A.: Towards a concept how the structure of time can support the visual analytics process. In: Miksch, S., Santucci, G. (eds.) Proc. Int. Workshop Visual Analytics (EuroVA 2011) in conjunction with EuroVis 2011, Eurographics, Goslar, Germany, pp. 9–12 (2011)
19. Martins, S.B., Shahar, Y., Goren-Bar, D., Galperin, M., Kaizer, H., Basso, L.V., McNaughton, D., Goldstein, M.K.: Evaluation of an architecture for intelligent query and exploration of time-oriented clinical data. Artificial Intelligence in Medicine 43(1), 17–34 (2008)
20. Munzner, T.: Process and Pitfalls in Writing Information Visualization Research Papers. In: Kerren, A., Stasko, J.T., Fekete, J.-D., North, C. (eds.) Information Visualization. LNCS, vol. 4950, pp. 134–153. Springer, Heidelberg (2008)
21. Pike, W.A., Stasko, J., Chang, R., O'Connell, T.A.: The science of interaction. Information Visualization 8(4), 263–274 (2009)
22. Plaisant, C., Mushlin, R., Snyder, A., Li, J., Heller, D., Shneiderman, B.: LifeLines: using visualization to enhance navigation and analysis of patient records. In: Proc. AMIA Symp., pp. 76–80 (1998)
23. Pohl, M., Wiltner, S., Rind, A., Aigner, W., Miksch, S., Turic, T., Drexler, F.: Patient Development at a Glance: An Evaluation of a Medical Data Visualization. In: Campos, P., Graham, N., Jorge, J., Nunes, N., Palanque, P., Winckler, M. (eds.) INTERACT 2011, Part IV. LNCS, vol. 6949, pp. 292–299. Springer, Heidelberg (2011)
24. Potamias, G.: State of the art on systems for data analysis, information retrieval and decision support. Deliverable D13, INFOBIOMED project (2006), http://www.infobiomed.org/paginas_en/INFOBIOMED_D13_final.pdf (access July 14, 2010)
25. Powsner, S.M., Tufte, E.R.: Graphical summary of patient status. Lancet 344(8919), 386–389 (1994)
26. Reijner, H.: The development of the horizon graph. In: Bartram, L., Stone, M., Gromala, D. (eds.) Proc. Vis 2008 Workshop From Theory to Practice: Design, Vision and Visualization (2008)
27. Rind, A., Aigner, W., Miksch, S., Wiltner, S., Pohl, M., Drexler, F., Neubauer, B., Suchy, N.: Visually Exploring Multivariate Trends in Patient Cohorts Using Animated Scatter Plots. In: Robertson, M.M. (ed.) EHAWC 2011 and HCII 2011. LNCS, vol. 6779, pp. 139–148. Springer, Heidelberg (2011)
28. Rind, A., Miksch, S., Aigner, W., Turic, T., Pohl, M.: VisuExplore: gaining new medical insights from visual exploration. In: Hayes, G.R., Tan, D.S. (eds.) Proc. Int. Workshop on Interactive Systems in Healthcare (WISH@CHI2010), pp. 149–152. SIGCHI (2010)
29. Sharp, H., Rogers, Y., Preece, J.: Interaction Design: Beyond Human-Computer Interaction, 2nd edn. Wiley & Sons, Chichester (2007)
30. Shrinivasan, Y.B., van Wijk, J.J.: Supporting the analytical reasoning process in information visualization. In: Proc. ACM SIGCHI Conf. Human Factors in Computing Systems (CHI), pp. 1237–1246 (2008)
31. Spence, R.: Information Visualization: Design for Interaction., 2nd edn. Prentice Hall, Upper Saddle River (2007)

32. Sundvall, E., Nystrom, M., Forss, M., Chen, R., Petersson, H., Ahlfeldt, H.: Graphical overview and navigation of electronic health records in a prototyping environment using google earth and openEHR archetypes. In: Kuhn, K.A., Warren, J.R., Leong, T. (eds.) Proc. 12th World Congr. Health (Medical) Informatics (Medinfo 2007), pp. 1043–1047. IOS, Amsterdam (2007)
33. Tufte, E.R.: The Visual Display of Quantitative Information. Graphics Press, Cheshire, CT (1983)
34. Wang, T.D., Plaisant, C., Shneiderman, B., Spring, N., Roseman, D., Marchand, G., Mukherjee, V., Smith, M.: Temporal summaries: Supporting temporal categorical searching, aggregation and comparison. IEEE Trans. Visualization and Computer Graphics 15(6), 1049–1056 (2009)
35. Wongsuphasawat, K., Shneiderman, B.: Finding comparable temporal categorical records: A similarity measure with an interactive visualization. In: Proc. IEEE Symp. Visual Analytics Science and Technology (VAST), pp. 27–34 (2009)
36. Zhang, Z., Mittal, A., Garg, S., Dimitriyadi, A.E., Ramakrishnan, I.V., Zhao, R., Viccellio, A., Mueller, K.: A visual analytics framework for emergency room clinical encounters. In: IEEE Workshop on Visual Analytics in Health Care (2010), http://research.ihost.com/vahc2010/ (access May 5, 2011)

It's All about the Medium:
Identifying Patients' Medial Preferences
for Telemedical Consultations

Shirley Beul[1,2], Martina Ziefle[1], and Eva-Maria Jakobs[2]

[1] Communication Science/ eHealth: Enhancing Mobility with Aging,
Human Technology Centre, RWTH Aachen University,
Theaterplatz 14, 52062 Aachen, Germany
[2] Textlinguistics and Technical Communication,
Institute of Linguistics and Communication Studies,
RWTH Aachen University, Templergraben 83, 52062 Aachen, Germany
{beul,ziefle}@humtec.rwth-aachen.de
{s.beul,e.m.jakobs}@tk.rwth-aachen.de

Abstract. Coping with the consequences of the demographic change, industrialized countries have to adapt their health care systems to the increasing medical need of older persons despite the threatening shortage of physicians. In this context, telemedical services for communication between doctors and patients come into fore. However, it is unclear in how far users accept these new care concepts. Crucial for the success of telemedical services is the choice of the medium and its perceived appropriateness in different using situations. In this paper, an exploratory approach was undertaken to examine the users' acceptance of four electronic communication media (telephone, videophone, videoconference, interactive wall) in three different usage situations (additional service, urgency situation, exclusively telemedical consultation). 200 participants volunteered to take part. Findings show that the acceptance strongly depends on the specific situation and the type of communication media. User diversity, in contrast, did not show a major role for the acceptance of telemedical consultation.

Keywords: ehealth, telemedical consultation, teleconsultation, consultation medium, doctor-patient communicaton, user acceptance, interactive wall.

1   Introduction

The public eye focuses increasingly problems, which can be ascribed to the demographic change. Because of the postwar baby booms the demography of western countries became off-balance, and so demographic disequilibria were created. In comparison to previous generations, the post war generation comprises a very large cohort of people [1]. Taking improvements in healthcare, longevity among the elderly, and the delineated demographic imbalance into account, an increasing number of frail and old people hast to be provided with healthcare services in the close future [1]

A. Holzinger and K.-M. Simonic (Eds.): USAB 2011, LNCS 7058, pp. 321–336, 2011.

[2]. Problems like a higher demand for medical personnel [3] [4], or rising healthcare expenditures [5] are issues aging societies have to deal with urgently.

Accordingly, healthcare systems of industrialized countries currently change to cope with these upcoming consequences. In particular, the maintenance of area-wide supply of medical care despite the threatening shortage of doctors has been identified as a very serious challenge. One possible and also promising solution for the short-comings is the implementation of information and communication technology into the healthcare system [6]. In this context, telemedical services for the purpose of doctor-patient-communication gain in importance. First, they can facilitate an optimal allocation of physicians' human resources [7], second, they bridge the geographical separation between doctor and patient without wasting the patient's time and without causing transportation costs [8], and third, they give patients the possibility of having a doctoral consultation remotely, independent of time and location [9].

1.1   Telemedical Consultation

For launching a successful telemedical consultation service, the medium through which the consultation occurs, has to be chosen carefully [10]. Consequently, the used information and communication technologies (ICT) must be appropriate for this special purpose of use and, finally, accepted by its users [11]. For conceptualizing such a service, which is accepted and actually used by the target group, it is necessary to understand its prospective user group. Particularly, patients' demands for, require-ments on and preferences for media must be identified and carefully integrated in future electronic designs. Moreover, it is important if patients' preferences depend on certain demographic user characteristics (age, gender, state of health). Apart from these factors, the impact of the usage situation is also relevant, in particular, differ-ences between standard case and emergency case as well as different versions of the standard case. Many projects, which deal with electronic health services, currently investigate potential and pitfalls of telemedical consultations services and the nature of this special doctor-patient communication, which is altered by the use of electronic media. They deal with effects of oral and written communication; likewise real time and time-shifted communication is investigated.

Unfortunately, most of the recent studies regard a consultation medium exclusively in isolation [12] [13] [14], which impedes to compare the acceptance for those devic-es under study because the settings vary. Hence, it is unclear, which medium users prefer for an ICT-based medical encounter, if they would have the choice. Also, it is not understood so far, to which extent the choice for an electronic medium mediating the doctor-patient communication is influenced by the user scenario, in which patients communicate with doctors. To bridge this informational gap, acceptance motives of four devices for real time communication (telephone, videophone, videoconference, interactive wall) geared to three user scenarios (variations of the medical standard case) are examined.

1.2   Technology Acceptance of Assisted Medical Care Systems

Technology acceptance is a well-examined topic for quite a long time. Since the 1980ies, in which the boom of acceptance studies reacted to the area-wide introduction of PCs in offices, technology acceptance has become a key interest field of human computer interaction [15]. Even though the core interest of technology acceptance - understanding und predicting technology adoption behaviors of humans working or living with technology – has not changed since then, the topics, the implementation concepts of technology, and the fields, in which technology enters our personal environments, has changed considerably over time. In contrast to the altered technology domains and application areas, the understanding of technology acceptance underachieves the new requirements of innovative technology. This especially regards novel implementation of medical technology at home, which seems to be still more complex than in other technical systems: On the one hand, medical technologies are predominantly addressing the elderly, which is increasingly prone to diseases with increasing age. Ageing, dependency and illness have negative connotations in our culture, which is assumed to impact the acceptance of medical technology. On the other hand, as medical technology is increasingly incorporated in smart homes, it is often perceived as breaking into personal spheres, and touching intimacy and privacy issues. Furthermore, it should be considered that the health states and resulting feelings of (in)dependency on technology could also impact the willingness to accept electronic health applications and services.

Especially when focusing on telemedical consultation hours, any technology could be perceived as disturbing the established relationship between doctor and patient. However, the electronically mediated consultation hour and its acceptance could be also impacted by the type of the medium, which is used in the consultation as well as the type of the using situation, in which patients are seeking doctors' advice. This has not been addressed in research so far.

1.3   Questions Addressed and Logic of Empirical Design

In this paper, we examine if the acceptance of telemedical consultation hours is impacted by (1) the type of the medium (phone, videophone, videoconference, and interactive wall), (2) by the kind of using situation (additional service, case of urgency, exclusively telemedical consultation), and (3) user diversity (age, gender, health status). Several research questions were addressed: What role do user characteristics play for the acceptance for telemedicine? In which situations are telemedical services accepted? Are there conditions, which 'force' people to accept them? And more generally: Should telemedical services be designed under consideration of concrete user scenarios? How can telemedical services be introduced successfully within existing health systems? Should they be installed as additional services in a first step in order to reduce users' barriers?

2   Methodology

In the following section, the applied methodology of this study is delineated with particular attention in participants' characteristics, the structure and content of the questionnaire, and the considered research variables.

2.1   The Sample

200 participants took part in this study. They were aged between 17 and 83 years (M = 40.84, SD = 17.10). The gender distribution was almost balanced: the sample consisted of 51.5% female and 48.0% male respondents (0.5% is unknown).

For exploring participants' medial preferences under consideration of their age, the sample was split in three age groups. Their classification referred briefly to stages of life course geared to working life: The first group is aged between 17 and 29 years (M = 24.83, SD = 2.76, 66.2% female/ 33.8% male) and is regarded as 'career entrants', who have finished their education and have recently entered the job market. Group two encompasses participants between 30 and 59 years (M = 41.73, SD = 9.98, 44.6% female/ 55.4% male), who are referred to as 'settlers'. They are 'settling down' in several categories, e.g. job, social relations, and consequently, location. Moreover, this age group starts to deal with reduced health, sometimes also chronically-illness. The third group, the 'retirees', is aged between 61 and 83 years (M = 67.14, SD = 6.00, 43.9% female/ 56.1% male). In this period of life, people usually leave the job market sooner or later, (hopefully) enjoy their post-working life stage, and are confronted with senescence phenomena, and increasingly with diseases.

Apart from age, the respondents' health status was of special interest in order to find out if being healthy or chronically ill impacts the acceptance for the telemedical services under study. Although people of all age groups were addressed, older people (60+) were particularly encouraged to take part in this study because the prevalence for chronic diseases increases with rising age [16]. Consequently, addressing the elderly means to address the chronically ill, which was conducted to achieve a critical mass in order to be able to provide statistically significant information about the medial preferences of this group. The recruiting of respondents was carried out in relevant online forums, self-help groups for chronically ill patients (prevailing cardiacs), and senior online communities as well as in the authors' social networks. In the end, 30.0% of all participants (n = 60) indicated to be chronically ill, which requires seeing one or more doctors regularly. This group is aged between 21 and 82 years, (M = 49.30, SD = 18.00, 58.3% female/ 41.7% male). N = 106 (53.0%) affirmed being healthy. The age range in the healthy group is 17 - 83 years (M = 38.84, SD = 16.42). Among the chronically ill persons, 44.8% are female, 55.2% male. Unfortunately, 17.0% (n = 34), mainly females, did not give any information about their health status.

2.2   The Questionnaire

In this study, the questionnaire method (web- and paper-based) was applied because it allows reaching a large number of participants.

The questionnaire consisted of five different sections: Part one comprises a query of demographic and health data with respect to respondents' gender, age and health status. The following four sections were devoted to four telemedical services for remote doctor-patient communication. Each of them focused another consultation medium: a telephone, a videoconference on a computer monitor, a videophone, and a new ICT, a so-called interactive wall, which refers to a wall-sized multi-touch display and which was lately introduced in telemedical scenarios [17] [18]. The devices were delineated with respect to the presentation of the interlocutor, especially, if, how and which part of the interlocutor is visualized depending on the device. Furthermore, it was particularly emphasized that the presentation was reciprocal: One interlocutor is similarly presented for the other, as the other receives him/her verbally, and, depending on the device, also visually. In order to illustrate the functionality of the devices, each of them was depicted (Fig. 1).

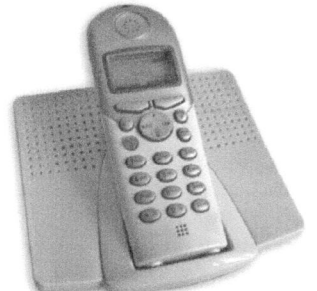

Telephone

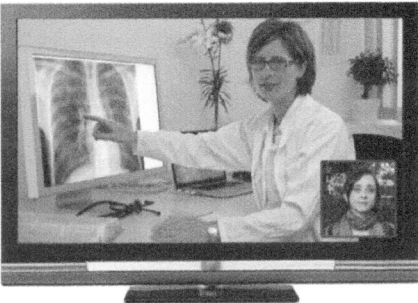

**Video Conference
on a Computer Monitor**

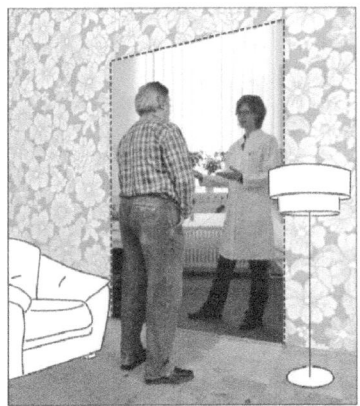

Interactive Wall

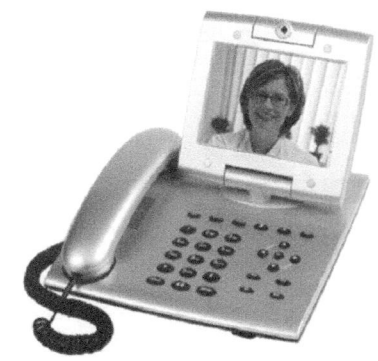

Videophone

Fig. 1. Visualization of consultation media in the questionnaire

Within these four sections, three different user scenarios were introduced. Every user scenario was gone through with every device. To support the participants in understanding the delineated situations (emotionally), all scenarios are based on one precondition: the respondents would know the doctor. They should think of their physician, who is familiar to them and they have a history with. For this reason, all scenarios are about 'your doctor'.

The first scenario outlines a situation, in which a telemedical consultation hour is implemented as an additional service to regular office hours (Tab. 1).

Table 1. User scenario 1: Telemedicine as an additional service

Your doctor offers in addition to his/her regular office hours a [*telemedical consultation hour*]. Would you use this service?
Yes, I would use this service inherently.
Yes, but only, if I cannot get an appropriate appointment with my doctor.
Yes, but only in cases of emergency.
No, I would never use this service.

The second scenario is about an urgent case, seen from the perspective of the patient. S/he needs to see his/her doctor, but s/he is busy with a lot of other patients. Therefore, the physician offers a consultation via telemedical service (Tab. 2).

Table 2. User scenario 2: Telemedicine in case of urgency

Your doctor is in high demand. You cannot get an appointment with him/her in the near future, but you are having an urgent matter of concern. S/he offers you alternatively [*telemedical consultation hours*]. Would you use this service?
Yes, I would use this service inherently.
Yes, but only in case of emergency.
No, I would not use this service. I would see another doctor (surgery, hospital).

Scenario three deals with an exclusive access to the doctor, who moved relatively far away for any reason. The patient wishes to stay under the physician's medical treatment, but, unfortunately, cannot travel so often. The doctor provides a telemedical consultation hour as a compromise (Tab. 3).

Table 3. User scenario 3: Telemedicine as exclusive access to a doctor

Your doctor has moved to another far off place. You would like to stay under his/her medical treatment, but you cannot travel permanently. S/he offers you a consultation via [*telemedical service*]. Would you use this service?
Yes, I would stay under my doctor's medical treatment and use this offer if needed.
Yes, but only in cases of dire emergency.
Yes, I would use this offer if needed. But I would look for another doctor who I can meet in person.
No, I would never use this service. I would directly look for another doctor.

By means of these scenarios we analyzed respondents' willingness to use certain devices for a telemedical consultation, which helped to explore a device's impact on user acceptance.

2.3   Research Variables

There were five independent variables. Two of them are related to the specific user scenario (additional service, urgency, exclusivity) in combination with different media (phone, videophone, video conference, interactive wall). Three variables refer to user diversity: One is users' age (<29 years: 'career entrants'; 30-59 years: 'settlers', 60+: 'retirees'). The second relates to the health states according to participants self-categorization into 'healthy' or 'chronically-ill' and the third addresses gender effects (96 males, 103 females). Dependent variables were preference data for telemedical applications in different user scenarios.

3   Results

Data were analyzed by multivariate analysis for variance, (M)ANOVA procedures, for repeated measurements if necessary. User variables (age, health status, and gender) were treated as 'between subject variables'. The level of significance was set at $p < 0.05$. Results, which reveal to be significant on the less restrictive 10%-level are referred to as marginal significant. First, we report on the outcomes with respect to the different user scenarios and media. Second, we look for effects of user diversity and potential interacting effects between variables.

3.1   Effects of Consultation Media

A first analysis referred to the different media, comprising participants' ratings, irrespectively of the using scenarios and user diversity. The ANOVA for repeated measurements revealed a significant effect ($F (3,174) = 8.7$; $p < 0.00$, Figure 2).

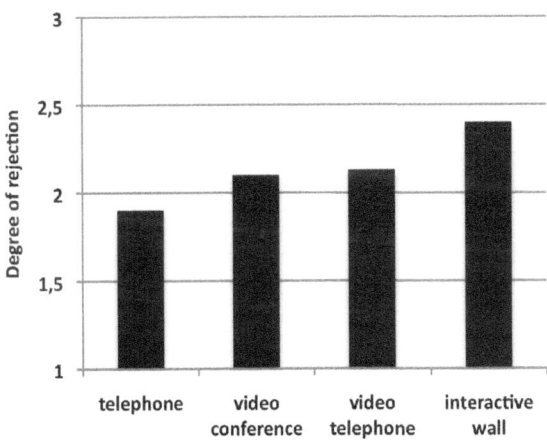

Fig. 2. Acceptance ratings regarding the four different consultation media (high values represent high degree of rejection)

As can be seen from Figure 2, the telephone (M = 1.9; SD = 0.78) is the most accepted medium. The interactive wall as the medium with which participants are mostly unfamiliar, represents the one with the strongest rejection (M = 2.1; SD = 0.75).
The PC mediated videoconference (M = 2.13; SD = .76) and the videophone (M =
2.4; SD = .84) range in between. No interaction effects of age, gender and health status were observed, showing a quite universal answering pattern.

3.2   Effects of Using Scenario

Three different user scenarios were presented to participants. First, participants had to
envisage that an additional telemedical service would be available at home. In the
second scenario, the urgency of the request for medical care was increased. Third,
participants were told that the doctor offers only telemedical consultation hours. Statistical analysis revealed a significant main effect of the using situation F (2.175) =
128.4; p < 0.00) regarding the acceptance of telemedical consultations (Figure 3).

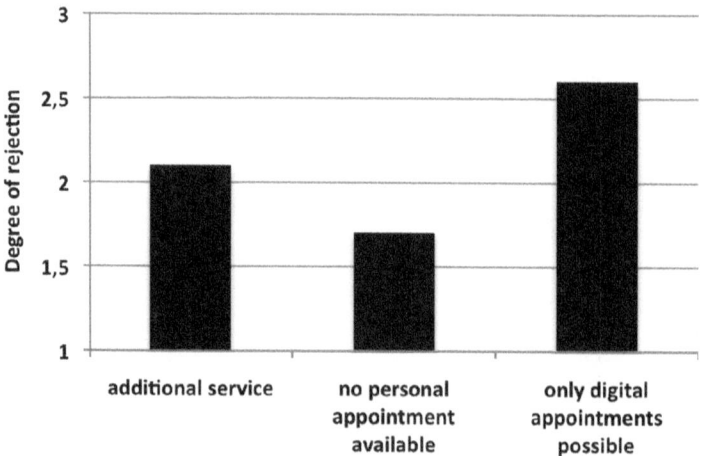

Fig. 3. Acceptance ratings regarding the three using situations (separated by the consultation
media). High values represent high degree of rejection.

Whenever only digital appointments with the physician would be possible leads to
the strongest rejection values (M = 2.6; SE = 0.7), followed by the offer that telemedical hours would be an additional service, which can be combined to the standard
procedure to have face-to face consultations with the doctor (M = 2.1; SE = 0.7). The
highest acceptance for the telemedical consultation hour received the scenario, in
which – temporarily – no personal appointment with the doctor is possible, but urgency for medical advice is high (M = 1.7; SE = 0.5).

3.3   Interacting Effect of Communication Medium and Using Scenario

In addition, a significant interaction effect of the type of the medium and the using scenario was detected ($F(6.171) = 6.3$; $p < 0.00$, see Fig. 4). As can be taken from Figure 4, the telephone is quite accepted whenever it is used as an addendum in addition to the conventional face-to face consultation as well as in a situation in which the doctor can not offer a personal consultation hour, but offers telemedical consultation in case of medical urgency. Though, the telephone is declined as the communication medium for only telemedical consultations. In case that temporarily no personal appointment with the doctor is possible, the video phone as well as the video conference would be the first choice, however both, the video phone and the video conference are to a much lesser extent accepted for additional electronic healthcare and both are also strongly rejected for completely telemedical consultation procedures with the doctor. The interactive wall at home is accepted in case for tele-consultations in case the doctor has no time to meet personally. As an additional service, the wall would be less accepted and for exclusive communication with the doctor, the wall is also no accepted communication medium.

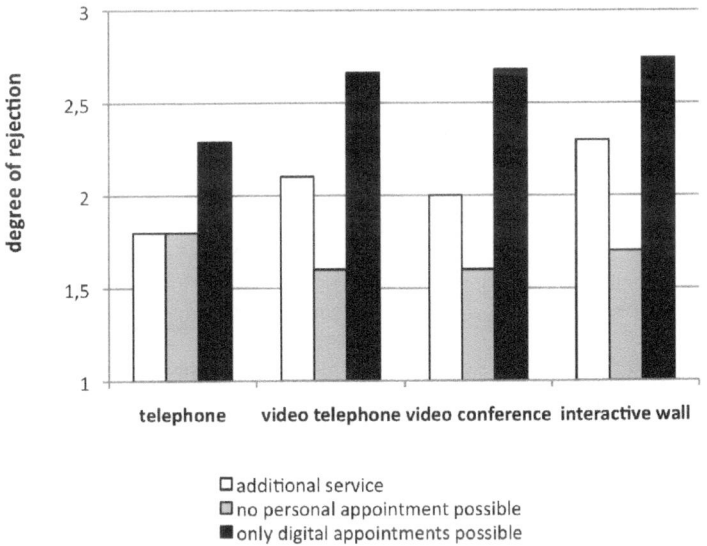

Fig. 4. Acceptance ratings regarding the three using situations (separated by the consultation media). High values represent high degree of rejection.

3.4   Effects of User Diversity

Three user characteristics have been analyzed in this research. First of all, we look for age effects, comparing younger, middle-aged and older users regarding their acceptance for telemedical services (differentiating user scenarios and the choice of communication media). Then, gender effects (n = 88 women, n = 88 men) are addressed followed by the effects of health states, comparing acceptance ratings of healthy (n = 97) vs. chronically ill (n = 58) persons.

While the age groups did not show significant differences regarding their choice of communication medium with the doctor (no interacting effect of age x media), there was a marginally significant interaction between age and the acceptance of tele-medical services depending on the using scenario $(F(4.12) = 2.3; p = 0.06)$. In Figure 5, descriptive outcomes of age groups are visualized.

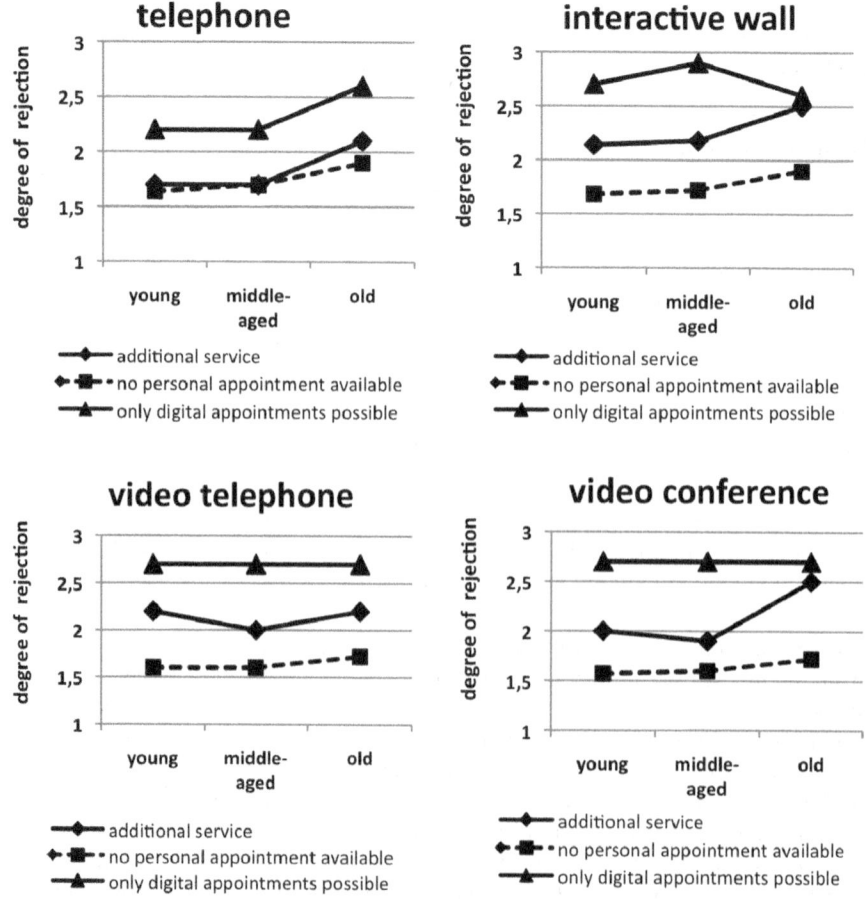

Fig. 5. Age effects in the four different media (separated by the using situations). High values represent high degree of rejection.

The oldest group – more than the middle-aged and the young group – rejects the telephone in all three using situations, but most strongly whenever only digital appointments are available.

Regarding gender effects, no interacting effects could be revealed, neither with respect to the choice of the appropriate communication medium nor with respect to the different using scenarios. Apparently, the acceptance for telemedical services is not gendered or affected by gender roles, but shows – overall – a similar acceptance pattern between men and women.

Finally, effects of health states are described. There was a marginal significant interacting effect of persons' health condition and the using scenario $F(2.6) = 2.9$; $p = 0.05$). Figure 6 depicts the descriptive findings. As can be seen there, the chronically ill persons show a higher acceptance of telemedical services when only digital consulting hours are available (due to their need of medical care) in comparison to healthy people. But – overall – they show lower acceptance levels for the additional electronic service and for the situation in which temporarily no personal consultation hour is available.

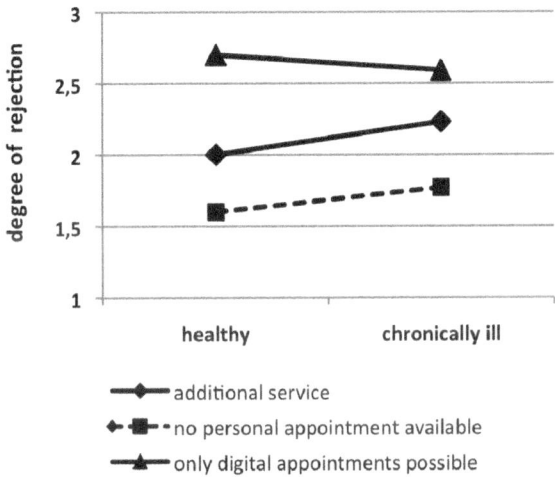

Fig. 6. Effects of health states on the acceptance of telemedical services depending on the different using scenarios. High values represent high degree of rejection.

3.5   Qualitative Findings

Any quantification of acceptance of telemedical services and a report on tolerated electronic communication media between doctors and patients are incomplete, as long as it is not understood which underlying cognitions or affects determine the extent of acceptance or rejection of communication media in the different using situations. Therefore, respondents had been given the possibility to comment on possible reasons in the questionnaire. Overall, participants frequently used this possibility. In the following, some of the comments of participants are detailed, as it allows a fruitful qualitative insight into possible objections people have.

The majority of concerns did not differ between the different using situations and communication media, but represent a generic attitude of a person towards telemedical consultations in general.

When classifying the kind of comments and their contribution to the discussion about telemedical services, we could identify five different types of argumentation lines. A first argumentation category refers to normative claims, a second regards concerns about the validity of the medical communication, a third category regards assumed technical concerns, but, as a forth type, also concerns regarding data and privacy protection. A fifth – less frequently reported – concern regards to feelings of discomfort when technology enters the living room.

Normative claims: First and foremost, normative claims were made, indicating persons' generic attitudes of how a good doctor-patient communication has to be. In most cases only the claim was raised, without having a practical or experience-based reasoning behind.

- *"If a doctor is serious, s/he must want to see me personally"*
- *"Physical examinations can only be done personally"*
- *"The doctor is not able to make a carful examination through the telephone"*
- *"A doctor must offer a personal consultation hour"*
- *"I do not want to wait for an electronic consultation hour, I want to see my doctor whenever I need it"*
- *"If a doctor has time for a videoconference, s/he then also should have time for a personal consultation hour"*
- *"I would have the feeling that the doctor does not take the appropriate time for my consultation"*
- *"I do not have the time to wait until the doctor invites me for an electronic consultation. I want to have the possibility to see the doctor whenever I need it"*

Concerns about the validity of the medical communication: many respondents also expressed their uncertainty whether diagnoses or medical advice delivered by the doctor via electronic medium is valid.

- *"Whenever I only have an electronic consultation, I would visit another doctor to get a second opinion"*
- *"I do not think that the doctor can have the same accuracy compared to the personal consultation. For example, s/he cannot use other instruments or devices s/he has in his/her doctors' office.*
- *"I do not trust the reliability and validity of the doctors' advice if s/he cannot see me personally- gestures and facial expressions as important communication channels are missing.*
- *"To my perspective, medical quality suffers in any case whenever mediated by electronic communication media, independently which"*
- *"I doubt that I can express exactly enough on the phone what I have"*

Technical concerns: Frequently, technical concerns were reported which could disturb a proper telemedical video consultation. As the video conference-scenario had been related to a computer, participants obviously transferred their negative experience when handling the computer to the ease of using the video conference.

- *"Anybody who has experienced break downs of the PC at home and who knows how long it takes until the PC works again properly can imagine how complicated the situation would be if the PC is the medium for the telemedical consultation"*

- *"I do not think that the display quality is high enough that the doctor can sharply recognize me or body parts"*

Concerns about data and privacy protection communication: Of course, respondents were also concerned about data protection.

- *"I do not trust the security of the internet and computers"*
- *"I would very much dislike that these sensitive data are stored on hard discs or are even connected to the internet*
- *"I do not think that the doctor can have the same accuracy in her/his medical advice than in the personal consultation. For example, s/he cannot use other instruments or devices s/he has in his/her doctors' office"*

Feelings of discomfort when technology enters private environments: The interactive wall but also the video conference (mediated by patients' PC) were assumed to cause discomfort at home and the feeling "that technology disfigures the cozy living environment".

- *"I do not think that the doctor and the patient can meet on an eye level, because the patient is at home, while the doctor acts on a business level"*
- *"I think such technology would be disproportionate"*
- *"I would not like such an abstruse installation at home"*
- *"I would feel restricted within my own home"*
- *"This is impersonal and unreal"*

4   Discussion

In this research, we focused on the user acceptance of telemedical services and users' medial preferences in order to identify acceptance patterns regarding the specificity of media for different using situations. As the perceived usefulness and the overall acceptance might be different depending on specific situations, three different using scenarios had to be evaluated. In the first, users had to envisage that the doctor would offer an electronic consultation hour in addition to the conventional consultation hour. The second scenario focuses on the situation, in which the patient has an urgent medical issue and the doctor is not able to offer a personal consultation. Instead, a telemedical consultation is available. In the third scenario, an exclusively telemedical consultation procedure is offered.

Regarding the media, the telephone as the most conventional medium received the highest acceptance, and the interactive wall the lowest, what surely is due to the different experience and familiarity level. When focusing on the scenarios, the majority of participants, independently from user characteristics, rejects the situation, in which only telemedical consultations are possible. The highest acceptance was given in the urgency condition, thus when the doctor has no time and instead offers a telemedical consultation hour. It is an interesting finding that user diversity does not play a role in the acceptance and preference rating, thus, showing that the overall attitude towards electronic assisted care systems do not vary with the social or gender role and not with the different perspectives of older compared to younger users. Solely, the health state revealed to be impacting acceptance. Chronically ill persons would more likely accept telemedical care in comparison to healthy people.

From the qualitative findings we saw a very clear picture. Generally, the attitudes towards telemedicine are quite reluctant if not negatively biased, independently of respondents' diversity. The reasons, which were noted as underlying cognitions, are mostly normative by nature. People seem to assume as a matter of fact that responsible doctors must see her patients personally, whenever patients need this. Also, medical care is assumed to decrease considerably when the consultation is electronically assisted or mediated. In light of the factual decrease in the availability of medical doctors [19] [10] and the shortcomings in the medical supply chain these attitudes seem precarious, if not alarming. It not only shows that there is a high personal claim regarding a certain quality of care and the undisputed naturalness with which persons take this doctor resource for granted. It also reveals the low awareness for the societal change and future shortcomings, which reflects a low public knowledge and an insufficient communication and information policy. Given the enormous move in modern and innovative technologies for medical home care and the increasing awareness for consideration of the human factor [21] [22], especially for the older user group [23], we need a transparent communication regarding the coming changes, the societal necessities in the context of telemedical care as well as an open discussion about benefits and barriers, which touches the general fear of privacy concerns and the high motivation of intimacy and face-keeping [25]. Moreover, not only the older user group is a sensible target group, but also the future seniors [26].

5   Limitations and Future Research Duties

Even though insights won by this study were informative, there are some final limitations to be considered which should be pursued in future studies. The first point in this context refers to the different familiarity status of the communication media under study. Of course, we all know the telephone and have a very detailed experience with the pros and the cons when using this technology. Also, our conceivability for the videophone and videoconference is quite high, as we are confronted with these media in the daily newscast. However, the interaction wall is quite unreal for most of the participants. The acceptance rating therefore is highly confounded with unfamiliarity, a global insecurity of how these systems work and an uncertainty whether these systems bring more negative effects than benefits. From a methodological point of view it can thus not be excluded that the unfamiliarity with the smart wall approach lead to a higher rejection than it would have been if participants would had the chance to see, feel and interact with such a wall [27]. Therefore, in future studies we will replicate the study, taking real technical devices and doctor-patient communication to learn if acceptance for telemedical services changes whenever patients can look and feel how such technologies might work and thus in how far they could really benefit from the technology.

Another major issue is the cultural dependency of the results presented here. Especially from the qualitative findings we saw an extremely normative view on "what doctors must do" and what people expect from the health care systems they are conversant with. It became evident that participants, used to a high economic standard in medical care, as industrialized countries are able to afford it, show a quite low acceptance for telemedical services in general, without having any hands-on experiences with telemedical consultation hours. However, it is clear that people used to other health care systems in other countries might have a completely different picture [28]. Future research will have to validate the findings using a cultural view and learning from other countries about the acceptance for telemedical systems.

Acknowledgments. We express our gratitude to our respondents for spending their time on filling in our questionnaire so patiently and sharing their perspectives on a sensitive topic with us. We also thank the anonymous reviewers for their helpful feedback on an earlier version of this manuscript.

This research was funded by the Excellence Initiative of the German federal and state governments.

References

1. Bloom, D.E., Canning, D.: Global Demographic Change: Dimensions and Economic Significance. In: Symposium on Global Demographic Change: Economic Impacts and Policy Challenges, pp. 9–56. Federal Reserve Bank of Kansas City, Kansas City (2004)
2. Leonhardt, S., Hexamer, M., Simanski, O.: Smart Life Support: model-based design and control of life-supporting systems. J. Biomed. Tech (Berl.) 54(5), 229–231 (2009)
3. Blum, K, Löffert, F.: Ärztemangel im Krankenhaus – Ausmaß, Ursachen, Gegenmaßnahmen. Deutsches Krankenhaus Institut, Düsseldorf (2009)
4. Beul, S., Mennicken, S., Ziefle, M., Jakobs, E.-M.: What happens after calling the ambulance: information, communication, and acceptance issues in a telemedical workflow. In: International Conference on Information Society, pp. 111–116 (2010)
5. Seshamani, M., Gray, A.: Time to death and expenditure: an improved model for the impact of demographic change on health care. J. Age and Ageing 33(6), 556–561 (2004)
6. Ziefle, M.: Potential and pitfalls of age-sensitive technologies in the e-health field. In: 1st European Conference on Ergonomics. Ergonomics in and for Europe. Quality of Life: Social, Economic and Ergonomic Challenges for Ageing People at Work (2010)
7. Yusof, K., Neoh, K.H.B., bin Hashim, M.A., Inbrahim, I.: Role of Teleconsultation in Moving the Healthcare System Forward. Asia Pac. J. Public Health 14(1), 29–34 (2002)
8. Miller, E.A.: The technical and interpersonal aspects of telemedicine: effects on doctor-patient communication. J. Telemed. Telecare 9, 1–7 (2003)
9. Bashshur, R.L.: On the Definition and Evaluation of Telemedicine. J. Telemedicine 1(1), 19–30 (1995)
10. Miller, E.A.: Telemedicine and doctor-patient-communication: a theoretical framework for evaluation. J. Telemed. Telecare 8, 311–318 (2002)
11. Buck, S.: Nine human factors contributing to the user acceptance of telemedicine applications: a cognitive-emotional approach. J. Telemed. Telecare 15, 55–58 (2009)

12. Parker, D.R., Demiris, G., Porock, D.: The usability of videophones for seniors and hospice providers: a brief report of two studies. J. Comput. Biol. Med. 35, 782–790 (2005)
13. LeRouge, C., Garfield, M.J., Hevner, A.R.: Quality Attributes in Telemedicine Video Conferencing. In: 35th Hawaii International Conference on System Sciences (2002)
14. Izqueirdo, R.E., Knudson, P.E., Meyer, S., Kearns, J., Ploutz-Snyder, R., Weinstock, R.S.: A Comparison of Diabetes Education Administered Through Telemedicine Versus in Person. J. Diabetes Care 26(4), 1002–1007 (2003)
15. Davis, F.D.: Perceived Usefulness, Perceived Ease of Use, and User Acceptance of Information Technology. MIS Quarterly 13, 319–340 (1989)
16. Ho, K.K.L., Pinsky, J.L., Kannel, W.B., Levy, D.: The Epidemiology of Heart Failure: The Framingham Study. J. American College of Cardiology 22(4), 6A–13A (1993)
17. Ziefle, M., Röcker, C., Wilkowska, W., Kasugai, K., Klack, L., Möllering, C., Beul, S.: A Multi-Disciplinary Approach to Ambient Assisted Living. In: Röcker, C., Ziefle, M. (eds.) E-Health, Assistive Technologies and Applications for Assisted Living: Challenges and Solutions, pp. 76–93. IGI Global, Hershey (2011)
18. Ziefle, M., Röcker, C., Kasugai, K., Klack, L., Jakobs, E.-M., Schmitz- Rode, T., Russell, P., Borchers, J.: eHealth – Enhancing Mobility with Aging. In: Tscheligi, M., de Ruyter, B., Soldatos, J., Meschtscherjakov, A., Buiza, C., Reitberger, W., Streitz, N., Mirlacher, T. (eds.) Roots for the Future of Ambient Intelligence. Adjunct Proceedings of the Third European Conference on Ambient Intelligence (AmI 2009), pp. 25–28 (2009)
19. Necheles, T.: Standards of Medical Care: How Does an Innovative Medical Procedure Become Accepted. Medicine & Health Care 10(1), 15–18 (1982)
20. Schmitt, J.M.: Innovative medical technologies help ensure improved patient care and cost-effectiveness. International Journal of Medical Marketing 2(2), 174–178 (2002)
21. Stronge, A.J., Rogers, W.A., Fisk, A.D.: Human factors considerations in implementing telemedicine systems to accommodate older adults. Telemedicine & Telecare 13, 1–3 (2007)
22. Warren, S., Craft, R.L.: Designing smart health care technology into the home of the future. Engineering in Medicine and Biology 2, 677 (1999), http://www.hctr.be.cua.edu/HCTworkshop/HCT-pos_SW-FutureHome.htm
23. Melenhorst, A.-S., Rogers, W.A., Bouwhuis, D.G.: Older adults' motivated choice for technological innovation: Evidence for benefit-driven selectivity. Psychology and Aging 21(1), 190–195 (2006)
24. Lalou, S.: Identity, Social Status, Privacy and Face-keeping in the Digital Society. Journal of Social Science Information 47(3), 299–330 (2008)
25. Ziefle, M., Röcker, C., Holzinger, A.: Medical Technology in Smart Homes: Exploring the User's Perspective on Privacy, Intimacy and Trust. In: The 3rd IEEE International Workshop on Security Aspects of Process and Services Engineering (SAPSE 2011). 35th Annual IEEE Computer Software and Applications Conference (2011)
26. Holzinger, A., Dorner, S., Födinger, M., Valdez, A.C., Ziefle, M.: Chances of Increasing Youth Health Awareness through Mobile Wellness Applications. In: Leitner, G., Hitz, M., Holzinger, A. (eds.) USAB 2010. LNCS, vol. 6389, pp. 71–81. Springer, Heidelberg (2010)
27. Cvrcek, D., Kumpost, M., Matyas, V., Danezis, G.: A Study on the Value of Location Privacy. In: Proceedings of the ACM Workshop on Privacy in the Electronic Society, pp. 109–118. ACM, New York (2006)
28. Alagöz, F., Ziefle, M., Wilkowska, W., Calero Valdez, A.: Openness to accept medical technology – a cultural view. Full paper submitted to the 7th Conference of the Austrian Computer Society Group: Human-Computer Interaction: Information Quality in eHealth. Springer, Berlin (under review)

Knowledge Discovery and Expert Knowledge for Creating a Chart-Model of a Biological Network - Introductory to Research in Chronic Diseases and Comorbidity

Ljiljana Trtica-Majnarić

School of Medicine, University J.J. Strossmayer Osijek, 31 000 Osijek, Croatia
ljiljana.majnaric@hi.t-com.hr

Abstract. By using an example of low antibody response to influenza vaccination, a new methodology approach is presented here, which can be introductory to research in chronic aging diseases, typically characterized with comorbidity. Starting with poor theory, this approach includes systematic health data record and approximate learning based on using data mining methods. By subsequent data mining, applied on already selected parameters, and supported by expert knowledge, selected health parameters can further be transformed, into functional pathophisiologic units. Graphical presentation of identified health disorders and their integration into a comprehensive visual model of the common biological network, provides additional information and improves our understanding of the topic, and can serve as a starting position for further research. In terms of Human-Computer Interaction, this approach seems challenging, by enabling computer automatic methods to be supported by human`s cognitive processes, which might be a solution when managing massive biomedical data, usually weakly structured.

Keywords: chronic aging diseases, comorbidity, systematic health data record, approximate learning, expert knowledge, visual modeling.

1 Introduction

Modern societies are marked by a domination of chronic aging diseases in morbidity and mortality causes. This takes on public health services a demand for protecting the public against these diseases through effective preventive measures [1]. The success of preventive strategies would be improved and economically justified if relied on the possibility of identifying factors responsible for prediction of the outcomes and/or definition of the target groups [2]. The problem is that, for many preventive tasks, risk and prediction factors have not yet been identified. In addition, it is not possible to select subjects into the target groups simple according to the diagnosis of a certain disease, or a medical condition, but it is rather based on using multiple factors [3]. This is due to the characteristics of chronic aging diseases, such as: 1) gradually changing continuum from health to a disease, 2) frequent subclinical disorders,

A. Holzinger and K.-M. Simonic (Eds.): USAB 2011, LNCS 7058, pp. 337–348, 2011.
© Springer-Verlag Berlin Heidelberg 2011

3) overlapping in genetic and environmental risk factors, and 4) shared clinical expression among related disorders. The consequences, on the population level, are: 1) the occurence of several diseases and medical conditions in one person (co- and multi-morbidity) and 2) the great interindividual diversity (including the number, combination and stages of disorders) [2,4,5]. In the context of clinical studies, the problem is a large heterogeneity of studied groups. These are also the reasons why Evidence-Based-Medicine (EBM) is not able to provide answers on many questions related to chronic aging diseases. Namely, EBM relies on the research methods which are essentially reductionist, i.e. based on randomisation due to only a few variables, while other diversity within the sample is rather neglected [6].

2   A New, Protocol-Based Method, Supported by Expert Knowledge, for Creating a Chart-Model of a Biological Network

In this paper, a new, protocol-based method, supported by expert knowledge, for creating a Chart-Model of a biological network, is presented, as an approach by which many medical uncertainties are likely to get a chance of being solved (Figure 1).

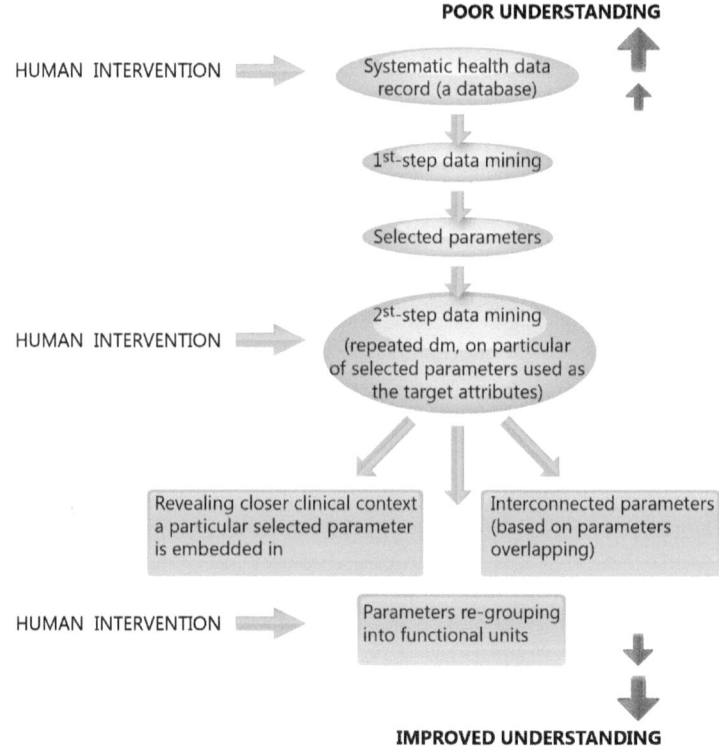

Fig. 1. The workflow of the protocol-based method for knowledge discovery supported by expert knowledge

As starting with poor theory, this concept includes systematic health data record and knowledge discovery for data approximation, based on using data-mining methods. In the second step-analysis, the same data mining procedure is repeated, for particular of the primarily selected health parameters, used as the target attributes, thus revealing closer clinical context a particular selected parameter is embedded in. Also, based on parameters overlapping, interconnected parameters are set apart, forming functional units. However, only by the support of expert knowledge, these interrelated parameters can be fully semantically transformed, into the recognisable pathophysiologic disorders. Finally, graphical presentation of the common functional network, by showing all identified medical conditions and pathophysiologic disorders, as well as the relationships among them, can be useful for subjects selection into the target groups, or - in the form of *an abstract relational model* - as the starting position for further research.

In terms of Human-Computer Interaction, this method can be the background for the early, exploratory learning phase, in software developing [7]. Involving an expert early in a task-analysis procedure, can provide answers on important questions such as the reliability and feasibility of the project.

This new concept is presented by using an example of low response to influenza vaccination.

3   Systematic Health Data Record

3.1   Theoretical Background

The classical methodology approach in biomedical science, such as a randomised controlled trial, or a case-control study, is strongly driven by the hypothesis. The results are expected to give an answer on the question if the proposed hypothesis is right, or not. Relatively well elaborated theories guide the choice of parameters used for analysis [6]. Even a decision on the choice of parameters for a multivariant linear analysis is based on yet well known background [8].

Differently, a methodology approach presented here, based on mapping the potentially relevant parameters in the poorly recognised input space, is useful for problems lacking in evidence, facilitating their further research. By tailoring the parameters from the large input space to the specifically defined outcome (a phenotype or a function) - this approach is likely to select components naturally interrelated within the common networks. This is similar to learning on co-morbidity (co-occurence, or clustering of diseases). In relation to this, it has been recognized that knowledge on causes of disease clustering can lead to better prevention strategies, by identifying yet unknown risk factors which can affect the outcomes [9].

Theoretical background of this sharing of diseases can be found in novel theories of aging, known as tending to reflect the complex and integrated nature of the human body [10]. An important assumption emerging from these theories is that, except for genetic and environmental factors, inner physiologic perturbations can also drive biological processes, thus implying self-sustaining (stochastic) nature of aging and developing chronic aging diseases. A step forward is a view that humans and their diseases are to be considered as the complex systems [11]. In complex systems, components respond to their environment by using internalised sets of rules that emerge from the action of biological networks. This behaviour is due to the highly integrated structure of the human body, from the molecular and cellular, to the systems levels [12]. Features arising from this structure include non-linearity, dependence on the starting position (in humans, this is the effect of the current health status) and fuzzy, rather than rigid boundaries between the biological networks. This is why it is not possible to predict the behaviour of the complex system with the certainty, just to make approximate conclusions on it, by mathematical modelling. In mathematical terms, that means that a complex system, to achieve its full description, should be determined by a range of numerical variables. The favourable fact is that a working mathematical model may not need to include all possible variables, as only a small number of them are likely to control the outcomes of the system. If we could identify these parameters, we would be able to reconstruct the biological network and to achieve better reasoning of the system.

Intensive literature search is necessary, to gain information on pathophysiologic mechanisms potentially associated with the problem of interest. In this way, also, the health status of subjects must be determined by many aspects, more systematically, than by using the classical methodology approach. Since a large amount of poorly proved data enter the analysis, knowledge approximation is necessary, to reduce the large dimension of the input space.

3.2   An Example: Low Response to Influenza Vaccination

The research question was: Which medical conditions and pathophysiologic changes do contribute to low antibody response to influenza vaccination?

The sample was consisted of 93 subjects, 35 males and 58 females, aged 50-89 years (median 69), characterized with multiple chronic medical conditions. The subjects were of the kind which are usually vaccinated against influenza in primary health care.

After taking a careful search across the literature (MEDLINE/PubMed and references screening), it could be realised that many disease-related factors and age-related pathogenetic changes, such as those indicating inflammation, nutritional, metabolic and neuro-endocrine status, chronic renal impairment, latent infections, and decreased humoral immune reaction, can alter the immune system functions of the importance for the response to influenza vaccine. Based on this information, a large number of 52 parameters in a total were collected, to systematically, by many aspects, determine the health-status of examined patients. Data included information on diagnoses of the main groups of chronic aging diseases, anthropometric measures and a wide range of laboratory and biochemical tests. Only those laboratory tests available in the real primary care system organization, were performed.

4   Knowledge Discovery - An Approximate Learning

Knowledge discovery corresponds to "making sense" of a large amount of data (a database). In other words, this is the process of *mapping low-level data (which are typically too voluminous to understand and digest easily) into other forms that might be more compact, more abstract, or more useful"* [13]. The key step in this process is the application of specific data mining methods, capable to extract information contents (patterns) from massive databases [14].

4.1   An Example: Low Response to Influenza Vaccination

On the prepared database, algorithms of the ILLM (Inductive Learning by Logic Minimization) system were applied, developed in the Laboratory for Information Systems, Institute Rudjer Bošković, Zagreb, to find meaningful patterns in the data. The main reasons for this choice were accessibility and good classification properties of this method [15,16]. In addition, this method seems to be appropriate for managing biomedical data because of its property to equally elaborate numerical and categorical data and to use a cut-off value for expression of the selected numerical parameters.

The result of application of ILLM algorithms on a database is a cluster of six parameters, best descriptors of the target outcome value, with the first parameter on the list ranking most important. Statistical measures "sensitivity" (the accuracy of the true positive results of the classification procedure) and "specificity" (the accuracy of the true negative results of the classification procedure) are used for expression of the statistically significant properties of the parameters selected in the cluster.

Since influenza vaccines are trivalent and factors related to past influenza viruses exposure also affect vaccination outcomes, it is not possible to establish the unique equation to link the health-status of patients with low antibody response to influenza vaccination (used as the target attribute value). For this reason, four reasonable definitions of the target outcome value were set up, leading to the selection, from the input database, of the four sets of health parameters. In making definitions, an intention was to maximally exclude the influence of factors related to past influenza viruses exposure, allowing health parameters to gain their full effect. In this way, a relatively large pool of 16 health parameters was selected from the initial input space, which is probably sufficient to deal with the heterogeneity of the target groups in different real-life situations of vaccination. That is, an initial number of 24 selected parameters (6 in each of four classifications) was reduced to 16, due to parameters overlapping between the clusters (Table 1).

Table 1. The starting number of 52 parameters in a database is reduced to 16

Classification	Nonoverlapping parameters	Overlapping parameters
No. 1	*homocisteine, creatinine clearance*	monocyte %, vitamin B_{12}, fT_4, tricep skinfold thickness
No. 2	*γ-globulins, IgA Helicobacter pylori, prolactin*	monocyte %, MCV (vitamin B_{12}), β-globulins
No. 3	*fasting glucose, albumin*	lymphocyte%, fT_4, β-globulins, monocyte %
No. 4	*age, TSH*	lymphocyte%, monocyte%, fT_4, triceps skinfold thickness

Selected parameters, found to overlap between two or more data mining classifications, are likely to indicate common intermediate mechanisms, linking chronic diseases with the immune system dysfunction (Table 1). Parameters specifically selected in particular classifications are likely to indicate specific, relatively well defined clinical conditions (clinical domains) associated with low response to influenza vaccination (Table 1). By comparing the results with the existing knowledge, following important clinical conditions were recognized: 1. impaired renal function, especially syndrome characterized with hyperhomocysteinemia [17,18], 2. chronic gastritis caused by *Helicobacter pylori* infection and accompanied by chronic humoral immunisation [19], 3. impaired glucose metabolism, accompanied by protein malnutrition [18], and 4. aging of the hypothalamus and pituitary gland, accompanied by the neuroendocrine system dysfunction [20].

These results also indicate towards the preferable selection of hematological and biochemical laboratory tests over the diagnoses of chronic diseases. We can speculate that a distinct set of laboratory tests should determine chronic health conditions, rather than the conventional, diagnosis-based disease classification.

5   Subsequent Data Mining, Supported by Expert Knowledge - Transforming Selected Parameters into Disorders

5.1   An Example. Low Response to Influenza Vaccination

We repeated the same data mining procedure, for most of selected health parameters, used as the target attributes. In this way, we could get closer insight into the clinical context a particular parameter is embedded in and in the way the selected parameters are interconnected forming functional units (Figure 2). By taking an additional search across the knowledge databases, for more information, and with the support of expert knowledge, meaningfull explanations could be joined to these newly formed groups of health parameters (Figure 2).

In this way, eight different recognisable disorders were identified, four of them representing well known clinical conditions, similar to those already defined by the first-step data mining selection procedure (Tables 1 and 2).

Based on this second-step analysis, four specific subgroups of patients, at higher risk for low response to influenza vaccination, could be identified, including: 1. patients with impaired renal function associated with hyperhomocysteinemia and impaired glucose metabolism, 2. patients with neurologic and mental disorders associated with hyperprolactinemia, 3. patients with chronic gastritis caused by *Helicobacter pylori* infection, and 4. patients with hypothyreoidism (Table 2, shaded).

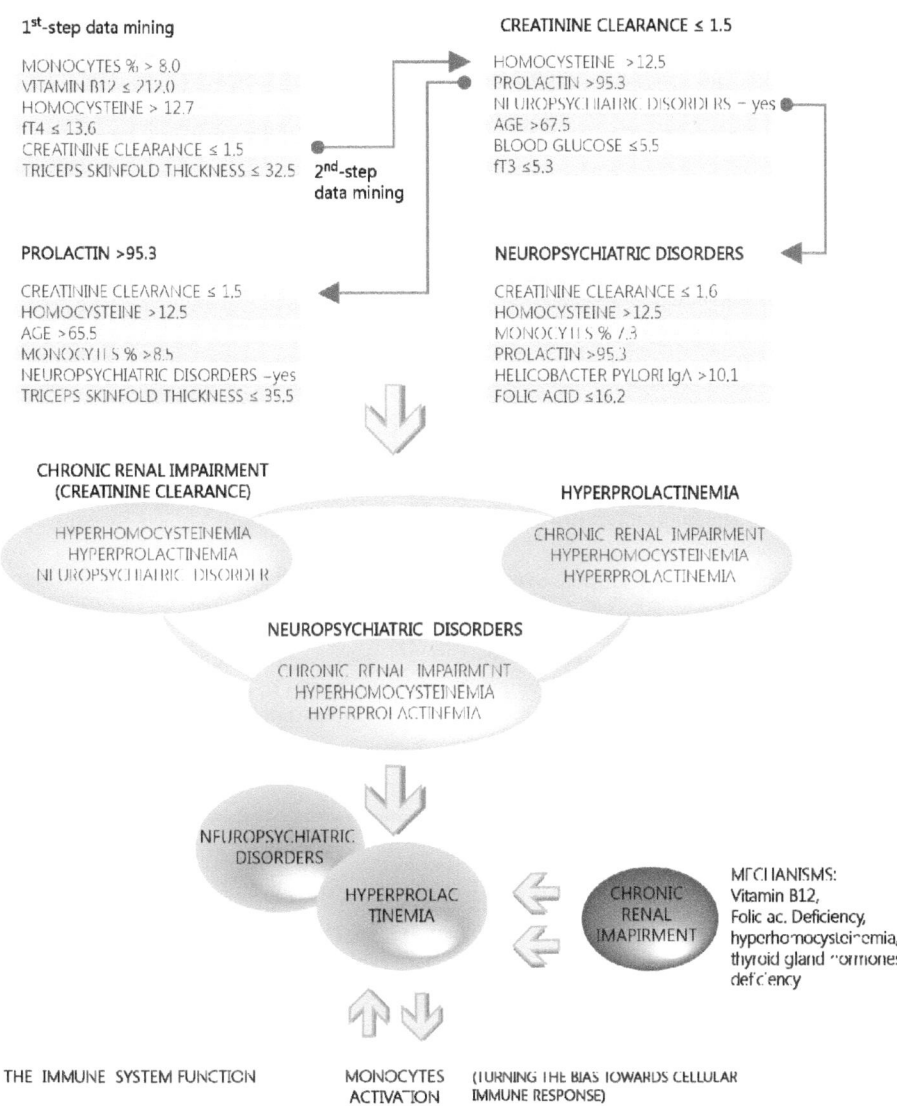

Fig. 2. A detail of the three-stage protocol. **Up:** subsequent data mining. **Middle:** interconnected parameters based on parameters overlapping. **Down:** a part of the biological network

Table 2. Recognisable disorders identified by subsequent data mining

	Identified pathogentic disorders	Clusters of parameters
1	Turning the bias of immune reaction from humoral and specific to cellular and nonspecific immune response	Decreased lymphocytes and eosinophils and increased monocytes and neutrophyls in WBC differential, low IgE
2	Vitamin B_{12} / folic acid deficiency/ hyperhomocysteinemia	Vitamin B_{12} / folic acid deficiency, hyperhomocysteinemia
3	Low-grade inflammation / protein malnutrition / chronic immunisation	Serum proteins electrophoresis (albumin, β, γ-globulins), increased triceps skinfold thickness
4	The thyroid gland hormones hypofunction	Decreased fT_4 and fT_3 and increased TSH
5	Impaired renal function / hyperhomocysteinemia / glucose metabolism impairment	Decreased creatinine clearance, increased homocysteine, normal (decreased) fasting blood glucose
6	Helicobacter pylori positive chronic gastritis	Increased Helicobacter pylori specific IgA and IgG
7	Neurodegenerative disorders, especially those connected with the changes in the hypothalamus and the pituitary gland	Increased prolactin and TSH, Diagnosis of the neuropsychiatric diseases
8	Older age	> 65 years

6   A Chart Model of the Biological Network — A Starting Position for Research in Comorbidity

At the final stage of the protocol, eight identified groups of interrelated parameters were graphically presented, allowing for better visual cognition of defined pathogenetic disorders (Figure 2).

By subsequent integration of these graphics, a comprehensive visual model of the common biological network, was built (Figure 3).

The constructed chart-model represents four, relatively independent, but interconnected clinical conditions, already mentioned above, which are likely to affect antibody response to influenza vaccination. These clinical conditions operate via common, partially shared mechanisms, including: the thyroid gland hormones hypofunction, vitamin B_{12} deficiency/hyperhomocysteinemia, inflammation, malnutrition and glucose metabolism impairment (insulin resistance). Although only simple, widely available hematological and biochemical laboratory tests were used in this study, several important immunologic disorders were identified, responsible for low

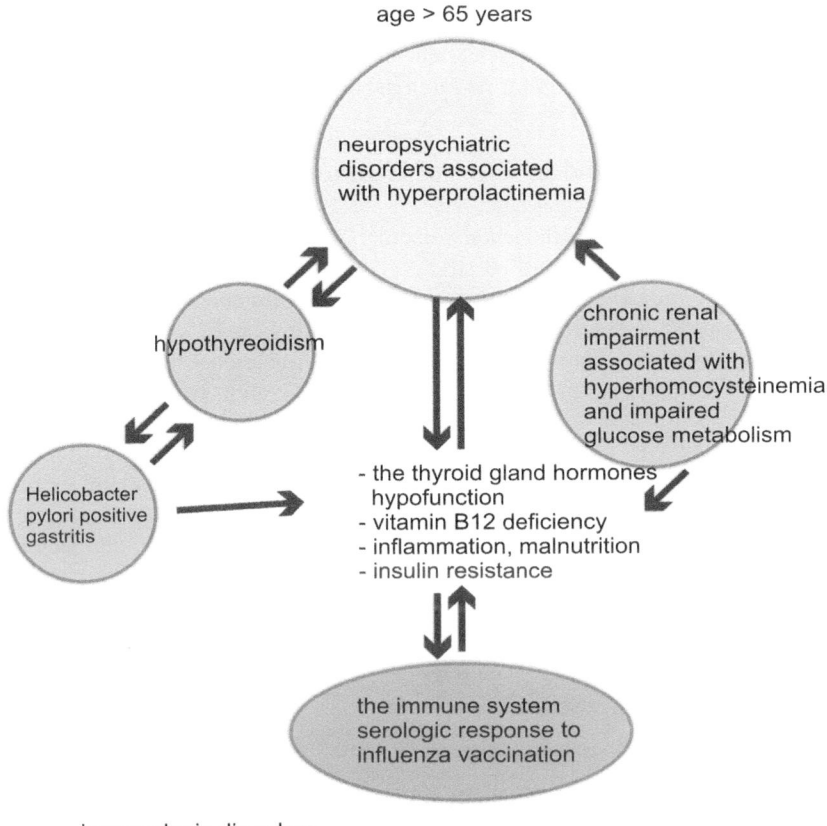

age > 65 years

neuropsychiatric disorders associated with hyperprolactinemia

hypothyreoidism

chronic renal impairment associated with hyperhomocysteinemia and impaired glucose metabolism

Helicobacter pylori positive gastritis

- the thyroid gland hormones hypofunction
- vitamin B12 deficiency
- inflammation, malnutrition
- insulin resistance

the immune system serologic response to influenza vaccination

immunologic disorders
- lymphopenia
- turning the bias of the immune reaction towards predominant nonspecific and cellular immune response
- decreased humoral immune response

Fig. 3. Visual presentation of the common biological network associated with low response to influenza vaccination

antibody response to influenza vaccination, including: general lymphopenia, turning the bias of the immune reaction from specific to nonspecific and cellular immune response, and decreased humoral immune response (Figure 3).

As the results also indicate, all of these disorders are concentrated in elderly population ($\geq$ 65 y), thus providing the mechanisms for the disability of elderly people to produce specific antibodies [21]. The fact that these identified clinical conditions are interconnected, means that several of them can occur in the same person. This correspondes with comorbidity, which is the characteristic of chronic aging diseases.

Construction of the chart-model provides more information, than it would have been by the simple extraction of health parameters from the prepared database. By mapping the relevant clinical conditions, relationships and mechanisms, within the common biological network, this visualised model can significantly improve our understanding of the health-status impact on the immune reaction. It can serve as the background for target groups selection when planning influenza vaccination protocols, or as a starting position for research in chronic aging diseases and comorbidity.

7   A New Method in View of Human-Computer Interaction

Clinical conditions and pathogenetic disorders, mentioned above as to be relevant for the issue, could not be identified strictly as the result of the automatic procedure of data mining application on the prepared database. Parameters linking into recognisable pathogenetic disorders were largely supported by expert knowledge (Figure 1). It is difficult to define what does this concept exactly mean, but it is likely to be close to the idea of an experienced and knowledgeable person engaged in research of the topic. In relation to this, some software developers has for a long time been trying to bring this matter to our attention. In general, there is an awareness that intelligent (automatic) processes for Knowledge Discovery may fail when data are weakly structured, leading to the modelling artefacts [22]. We suggest here the exact pathway of how to apply human cognitive resources to bridge this gap and to add meaning to the *"bare words"* (selected parameters). In addition, this approach is likely to be appropriate for the computer-based simulation purposes, since it is possible, by using this approach, to identify, in relatively easy and the short-time manner, health disorders with the potential relevance for the issue [23].

8   Conclusions

By using an example of low antibody response to influenza vaccination, we presented here an approach which can be introductory to research in comorbidity and medical problems lacking in evidence. As an indirect confirmation of the validity of this approach, there are evidence showing that human`s reasoning functions by considering temporally and spatially distributed information [24]. In this sense, graphical presentation of the selected parameters, by bringing topology to the rough data, is close to what we know is human`s mental model [22]. In terms of Human-Computer Interaction, this approach seems challenging, as it might become a preferable approach when managing massive biomedical data, usually weakly structured [22,23].

Acknowledgment. We would like to express our grateful thanks to Dr. Dragan Gamberger, Head of the Laboratory for Information Systems, Institute Ruđer Bošković, Zagreb, for his efforts and time spent in performing data mining models, necessary for data processing.

References

1. Pearce, N.: Traditional epidemiology, modern epidemiology and public health. American Journal of Health 86, 678–683 (1996)
2. Rockhill, B.: Theorizing about causes at the individual level while estimating effects at the population level. Implication for prevention. Epidemiology 16, 124–129 (2005)

3. Cooper, J.A., Miller, G.J., Humphries, S.E.: A comparison of the PROCAM and Framingham point-scoring systems for estimation of individual risk of coronary heart disease in the Second Northwick Park Heart Study. Atherosclerosis 181, 93–100 (2005)

4. Dawes, M.: Co-morbidity: we need a guideline for each patient not a guideline for each disease. Family Practice 27, 1–2 (2010)

5. Yang, Q., Khoury, M.J., Friedman, J.M., Little, J., Flanders, W.D.: How many genes underlie the occurence of common complex diseases in the population. International Journal of Epidemiology 34(5), 1129–1137 (2005)

6. Rosser, W.W.: Aplication of evidence from randomized controlled trials to general practice. The Lancet 353, 661–664 (1999)

7. Holzinger, A.: Interacting with Information: Challenges in Human-Computer Interaction and Information Retrieval (HCI-IR). In: IADIS Multiconference on Computer Science and Information Systems (MCCSIS), Interfaces and Human-Computer Interaction, pp. 13–17. IADIS, Rome (2011)

8. Campbell, M.J.: Statistics at square two, 2nd edn. Blackwell Publishing, Oxford (2006)

9. Gijsen, R., Hoeymans, N., Schellevis, F.G., Ruwaard, D., Satariano, W.A., van den Bos, G.A.M.: Causes and consequences of comorbidity: a review. Journal of Clinical Epidemiology 54, 661–674 (2001)

10. Kriete, A., Sokhansan, J., Bacoppock, D.L., West, G.B.: Systems approaches to the networks of aging. Ageing Research Reviews 5, 434–448 (2006)

11. Lipsitz, L.A.: Dynamics of stability: the physiologic basis of functional health and frailty. Journal of Gerontology 57(A), 115–125 (2002)

12. Plsek, P.E., Greenhalgh, T.: The challenge of complexity in health care. British Medical Journal 323, 625–628 (2001)

13. Fayyad, U., Piatetsky-Shapiro, G., Smyth, P.: From data mining to knowledge discovery in databases, `http://www.daedalus.es/fileadmin/daedalus/doc/MineriaDeDatos/fayyad96.pdf` (last access: July 20, 2011)

14. Witten, I.H., Frank, E.: Data mining. Practical machine learning tools and techniques, 2nd edn. Elsevier, Morgan Kaufmann Publishers, San Francisco (2005)

15. Gamberger, D., Šmuc, T.: Data Mining Server. Zagreb: Institute Rudjer Bošković. Laboratory for Information Systems, `http://dms.irb.hr` (last access: June 15, 2011)

16. Sonicki, Z., Gamberger, D., Šmuc, T., Sonicki, D., Kern, J.: Data Mining Server-On-line Knowledge Induction tool. Study in Health Technology and Informatics 90, 330–334 (2002)

17. Schroecksnadel, K., Frick, B., Wirleitner, B., Winkler, C., Schennach, H., Fuchs, D.: Moderate hyperhomocysteinemia and immune activation. Current Pharmaceutical Biotechnology 5, 107–118 (2004)

18. Pecoits-Filho, R., Lindholm, B., Stenvinkel, P.: The malnutrition, inflammation and atherosclerosis (MIA) syndrome - the heart of the matter. Nephrology Dialysis Transplantation 17(S11), 28–31 (2002)

19. Futagami, S., Takahashi, H., Norose, Y., Kobayashi, M.: Systemic and local immune responses against Helicobacter pylori urease in patients with chronic gastritis; distinct IgA and IgG productive sites. GUT 43, 168–175 (1998)

20. Magri, F., Cravello, L., Barili, L., Sarra, S., Cinchetti, W., Salmoiraghi, F., et al.: Stress and dementia: the role of the hypothalamopituitaryadrenal axis. Aging Clinical Experimental Research 18(2), 167–170 (2006)

21. Gross, P.A., Hermogenes, A.W., Sacks, H.S., Lau, J., Levandowski, R.A.: The efficacy of influenza vaccine in elderly persons. A meta-analysis and review of the literature. Annals in Internal Medicine 123, 518–527 (1995)

22. Holzinger, A.: Usability engineering methods for software developers. Communications of the ACM 48, 71–74 (2005)
23. Majnarić-Trtica, L., Vitale, B., Martinis, M., Reiner, Ž.: A view at the future - a dynamical, protocol-based and computationally intensive approach in cardiovascular risk assessment. Collegium Antropologicum 34(2), 437–445 (2010)
24. Piaget, J.: The psychology of intelligence, 5th edn. Routledge classics, London (2008)

Method to Improve Accessibility
of Rich Internet Applications

Junko Shirogane[1], Takayuki Kato[2], Yui Hashimoto[2],
Kenji Tachibana[3], Hajime Iwata[4], and Yoshiaki Fukazawa[2]

[1] Tokyo Woman's Christian University, 2-6-1, Zenpukuji, Suginami-ku, Tokyo,
167-8585 Japan
junko@lab.twcu.ac.jp

[2] Waseda University, 3-4-1 Okubo, Shinjuku-ku, Tokyo, 169-8555 Japan
{hosho0907,yui_hashimoto}@fuka.info.waseda.ac.jp, fukazawa@waseda.jp

[3] Oracle Information Systems Japan K.K., 11-1 Nagata-cho, chiyoda-ku, Tokyo,
100-6106 Japan
kenji.tachibana@oracle.com

[4] Kanagawa Institute of Technology, 1030, Shimo-ogino, Atsugi, Kanagawa,
243-0292, Japan
hajimei@nw.kanagawa-it.ac.jp

Abstract. Currently numerous websites contain dynamic content, but
it is difficult to create accessible websites with dynamic content compared
to those with static content. Because many platforms can realize Rich
Internet Applications (RIAs), it is important that this type of dynamic
content become accessible. We propose a method to improve accessibility
of RIAs. Our method consists of two phases. In the first phase, we develop
libraries to realize accessibility of RIAs. In the second phase, the libraries
are automatically applied to RIAs. As an example of platforms that
realize RIAs, our research focuses on JavaFX Script.

Keywords: Accessibility, RIA, Accessibility libraries, JavaFX Script.

1   Introduction

Although physically challenged and elderly users access many websites, there
are websites that usages by the users are not sufficiently considered. Often these
users cannot acquire sufficient information. To resolve this issue, web accessibility, which means that all users regardless of background (e.g. age, disability,
computer experience) can use websites without difficulty, is important.

To develop accessible websites, guidelines are prepared, such as WCAG (Web
Content Accessibility Guidelines) [2] and WAI-ARIA (Web Accessibility
Initiative-Accessible Rich Internet Applications) [1]. WCAG focuses on traditional static websites written by HTML (Hyper Text Markup Language).
Strategies of HTML for satisfying WCAG are described. WAI-ARIA focuses
on dynamic websites realized by RIAs (Rich Internet Applications). Strategies
of AJAX, HTML and JavaScript for satisfying WAI-ARIA are described.

A. Holzinger and K.-M. Simonic (Eds.): USAB 2011, LNCS 7058, pp. 349–365, 2011.

Currently many websites are intricately designed with RIAs. Flash [3] is one of popular platforms to realize RIA. For Flash, strategies to realize accessibility of Flash contents are prepared [4], and there are many researches of supporting to make Flash contents accessible [5][6].

As described above, there are many platforms realizing RIAs. Strategies to realize accessibility are introduced for some RIA platforms. However, there are RIA platforms that the strategies are insufficient. In these RIA platforms, it is necessary for web designers to develop websites along with accessibility guidelines, such as WCAG and WAI-ARIA. However, it is difficult to apply strategies for satisfying the guidelines like WAI-ARIA to the RIA platforms, because the language specifications of the RIA platforms are different from the RIA platforms in guidelines. Hence, it is difficult for web designers to implement accessible applications. As a result, challenged and elderly users have difficulty using websites with JavaFX Script applications.

Thus, our research focuses on improving the accessibility of RIAs to satisfy accessibility guidelines. As an example of RIA platforms, we focus on JavaFX Script. Specifically, we strive to prepare libraries to add accessibility functions to JavaFX components and provide a support system to apply these libraries to JavaFX Script applications.

2   Related Works

To realize accessibility of RIAs, a lot of methods are proposed. They can be classified into three types, such as development of accessibility strategies, evaluations of accessibility and realization of accessibility in user side.

Development of Accessibility Strategies

Gonzalez et al. have proposed accessibility APIs named Accessible Document Object Model (AccessibleDOM) [11]. Their work aims to resolve accessibility problems that occur in different platforms. Thus, AccessibleDOM is a platform independent API and complies the W3C DOM specifications. Using AccessibleDOM, some attributes, such as "name", "role" and "sate", can be attached to target applications, and improved accessibility can be realized.

Kawanaka et al. have proposed meta data of improving web accessibility, named Accessibility Commons [12]. Alternative text of images and headline tags for navigations are proposed. Accessibility Commons realize flexible diagrams for representing common meta data repository and a method of integrating different types of meta data. Web accessibility can be improved by Accessibility Commons.

However, these methods are not automatically applied to the target applications. In our method, a support to automatically apply JavaFX Accessibility Libraries to the target applications is available.

Evaluations of Accessibility

Fernandes et al. have developed "QualWeb" [13]. QualWeb evaluates web accessibility based on WCAG 2.0 [2] in both browser and command line environments. Also, QualWeb can evaluate accessibility of AJAX. In command line environments, HTML documents are evaluated. In browser environments, the transformed versions of HTML documents are evaluated. Using QualWeb, accessibility problems of not only HTML documents themselves but also representation of HTML documents in browsers can be extracted.

Sirithumgul et al. have proposed a method to evaluate web accessibility focusing on characteristics of disabilities [14]. In their method, first, barriers that challenged users use websites are extracted based on Walkthrough method, and the relevant checkpoints of WCAG to the barriers are selected. Then, the selected checkpoints are assessed. By this method, accessibility evaluations suitable for characteristics of challenged users can be performed.

Accessibility problems can be extracted by these methods, however, how to modify implementations is not often clear. Our method supports to automatically modify implementations along with accessibility problems.

Realization of Accessibility in User Side

H. Miyashita et al. proposed a browser called "aiBrowser (Accessibility Internet Browser for Multimedia)" [15]. Using aiBrowser, audio controls are provided to multimedia contents in websites. Due to these audio controls, users can adjust the volumes of multimedia contents and hear screen readers. Also, aiBrowser provides alternative user interfaces to operate inaccessible user interfaces for challenged users. Using aiBrowser, challenged users can easily operate multimedia contents.

D. Sato et al. proposed a strategy that resolutions are provided to users' requests [16]. In their strategy, there are two types of users, such as end users and support users. End users are challenged users that require to resolve accessibility problems, and support users are users that answer to end users. When end users find accessibility problems, they report the problems using the end user tool. Then, support users create meta data to resolve the problems or answer the problems using the supporter tool. In this strategy, challenged users can resolve accessibility problems without website owners' modifications.

However, to use these methods, it is necessary for users to obtain the specific tools for the methods and learn how to use the tools. In our method, because accessibility of RIAs are realized, users are not required to obtain any specific tools for our method.

3   Features

We strive to realize accessible JavaFX Script applications by preparing libraries for JavaFX Script applications and a system to apply these libraries. The features of our method are followings.

Realization of Accessibility of RIAs

When developing RIAs, it is difficult to realize enough accessibility, because web designers do not recognize enough how to realize accessibility of RIAs, and strategies of realizing accessibility are not enough provided for RIAs.

In our method, to make realization of accessibility of RIAs easy, libraries of adding accessibility functions to JavaFX Script applications are prepared. Using these libraries, strategies of realizing accessibility of JavaFX Script applications are provided. Also, using these libraries, RIAs satisfy accessibility guidelines. Thus, websites realized by RIAs become accessible for various types of challenged and elderly users.

Support of Applying Libraries of Accessibility

Even if libraries of adding accessibility functions to JavaFX Script applications are provided, it is necessary for web designers to learn how to apply these libraries to JavaFX Script applications. In addition, there are some libraries, and the usage of each library is different.

Thus, a support system for applying the libraries to JavaFX Script applications is provided. This system analyzes source programs of the applications and modifies the source programs for applying the libraries to the applications. Using this system, web designers can easily apply to the libraries to JavaFX applications.

4   Strategies

Our method consists of two phases to realize accessibility of JavaFX Script applications. Phase one prepares accessibility libraries, while phase two automatically applies these libraries to the appropriate applications.

4.1   Preparing Libraries of Accessibility

For JavaFX Script, strategies of realizing accessibility are not enough provided. So, to make JavaFX Script applications accessible for users, we have developed four accessibility libraries. These libraries are called "JavaFX Accessibility Libraries".

It is necessary to consider following backgrounds of users for accessible JavaFX Script applications. JavaFX Accessibility Libraries include support strategies for these users.

Visually impaired users. Visually impaired users cannot recognize the screen content with their own eyes, and often employ a screen reader, which is software that reads the text on a screen aloud. Thus, the reader library provides compatibility with screen readers. Thus, it is necessary to make screen readers available for JavaFX Script applications.

Also, it is difficult for these users to operate contents on JavaFX Script applications by a mouse, because a mouse is a device for pointing a content on a screen. In many cases, they perform all operations by a keyboard. Thus, it is necessary to make all operations of JavaFX Script applications available by a keyboard.

Users with weak eyesight. Users with weak eyesight have difficulty recognizing small content on a screen, and often increase the font size. Thus, the size library provides the ability to customize the content size of JavaFX Script applications.

Color impaired users. Color impaired users cannot recognize certain colors, which may limit their understanding of a screen. Thus, the color library allows the customization of the screen color.

Physically impaired users. Physically impaired users have trouble operating JavaFX Script content with a mouse, and they often employ the keyboard in lieu of a mouse. Thus, the keyboard library allows JavaFX Script applications to be operable with a keyboard as well as a mouse.

Elderly users. Elderly users often face one or more of the aforementioned issues. Thus, applications to support elderly users require similar support strategies.

4.2   Applying Libraries to JavaFX Script Applications

Even if JavaFX Accessibility Libraries are prepared, web designers must learn how to use the libraries, which imposes a financial and time burden on web designers. To aid web designers, we have prepared a system to apply the libraries to JavaFX Script applications. In our system, web designers input source programs, and code to apply the libraries is inserted into the source program.

Our method classifies the JavaFX Script components into two types: JavaFX Swing and custom components where the former is compatible with Java Swing components and the latter are developed by web designers. (Java Swing is a package to realize GUIs in the Java Programming Language.)

Java Swing components implement Java Accessibility APIs (Application Program Interfaces) [8], which are used to make Java applications accessible. Because JavaFX Swing components are compatible with Java Swing components, they can also be used to implement Java Accessibility APIs. JavaFX Accessibility Libraries are developed based on Java Accessibility APIs. Thus, these libraries can be applied to JavaFX Script applications.

However, specifications of custom components differ from JavaFX Script components and are often incompatible with Java Accessibility APIs. Thus, Java accessibility libraries cannot be automatically applied to custom components.

Currently JavaFX libraries are only automatically applied to JavaFX Swing components.

5   JavaFX Accessibility Libraries

In this paper, JavaFX Script components, which include both JavaFX Script and components developed by web designers, indicate the Graphical User Interface (GUI) components of JavaFX Script, such as button and text field components. Currently, the JavaFX Accessibility Libraries include the following.

5.1   Library to Adjust Component Size

GUIs are often too small for elderly users and those with weak eyesight. Thus, they are unable to understand the JavaFX Script components and text contained in them. Hence, the component size library (hereafter size library) allows the size of the GUIs to be adjusted. Specifically, the size of the window, components, and text can be simultaneously adjusted. Once a user selects from a font size list, their sizes are all altered.

Table 1 shows an example of the size library.

Table 1. Size library to adjust JavaFX Swing components

Component type	JavaFX Script component
button component	SwingButton
radio button component	SwingRadioButton
toggle button component	SwingToggleButton
label component	SwingLabel
text field component	SwingTextField
combo box component	SwingComboBox
check box component	SwingCheckBox

5.2   Library tp Adjust Component Color

In addition to those who are color impaired users, users with weak eyesight and elderly users often cannot recognize the color of GUIs. Thus, users need to be able to change the color. The color adjustment library (hereafter color library) allows users to change the colors of the foreground and background. The user selects a color combination from a list, and the JavaFX Script colors are automatically adjusted.

Table 2 is a list of background and foreground color combinations, which are defined based on Fujitsu ColorSelector [9], while Table 3 shows the components to apply the color library. All these colors are defined in CSS (Cascading Style Sheet) specifications [10].

5.3   Library of Implementing Keyboard Operations

Visually impaired and physically disabled users often have trouble operating a mouse, and they typically only use a keyboard to operate GUIs. When writing programs, web designers assign a shortcut keys to a specific JavaFX Script

Table 2. Color combinations for the background and foreground

Background color	Foreground color
#000000	#C0C0C0, #FFFFFF, #FFFF00, #00FF00, #00FFFF
#808080	#FFFFFF, #FFFF00
#FFFFFF	#000000, #808080, #800000, #FF0000, #008000, #008080,
	#000080, #0000FF, #800080, #808000
#FF0000	#FFFFFF, #FFFF00
#008080	#FFFFFF, #FFFF00, #00FFFF
#00FFFF	#000000, #800000, #008000

Table 3. Color library to adjust JavaFX Swing components

Component type	JavaFX Script component
button component	SwingButton
radio button component	SwingRadioButton
toggle button component	SwingToggleButton
label component	SwingLabel
text field component	SwingTextField
combo box component	SwingComboBox
check box component	SwingCheckBox

component. The keyboard operation library (hereafter keyboard library) groups JavaFX components. Different shortcut keys are assigned to components in a specific group. Buttons in different groups can be assigned the same short cut keys. When users use shortcut keys, they focus a specific group and users type a shortcut key. Then shortcut key event occurs on the component in the focused group. Due to this library, even if there are a lot of buttons, short cut keys can be assigned to all the buttons.

Table 4 shows the keyboard library applicable to JavaFX Script components.

Table 4. Library for keyboard operations of JavaFX Swing components

Component type	JavaFX Script component
button component	SwingButton
radio button component	SwingRadioButton
toggle button component	SwingToggleButton
text field component	SwingTextField
combo box component	SwingComboBox
check box component	SwingCheckBox

5.4 Library of Implementing Usage of Screen Readers

Because visually impaired users cannot view GUIs, they often employ screen readers. Consequently, it is important that they are able to hear the text. The screen reader library (hereafter reader library) allows screen readers to acquire text for JavaFX components, enabling users to employ screen readers. Specifically, web designers attach a name and description for each JavaFX component, and then the library places a transparent label component in JavaFX Swing, which is compatible with Java Swing. Finally, the screen reader speaks the name and description of the transparent label component.

Table 5 lists the JavaFX Script components the reader library is applicable to.

Table 5. Library to apply JavaFX Swing components to screen readers

Component type	JavaFX Script component
button component	SwingButton
radio button component	SwingRadioButton
toggle button component	SwingToggleButton
label component	SwingLabel
text field component	SwingTextField
combo box component	SwingComboBox
check box component	SwingCheckBox
slider component	SwingSlider

6   Generation of GUIs Realizing Accessibility

In our method, JavaFX Accessibility Libraries are automatically applied to JavaFX Script applications through individual JavaFX Script components. Figure 1 depicts a flowchart for our system operations. Source programs of a JavaFX Script application are analyzed, and accessibility problems are extracted. Then code to apply the accessibility libraries is generated. Finally, the problematic code is replaced with the generated code.

Hereafter we use a calculator program as an example. Figure 2 shows the GUI of the program, which includes label components to describe the application, text field to show a value, and button components to select numbers and operators. Figure 3 shows part of the source program for this calculator program.

6.1   Component Extraction

After source programs of a JavaFX Script application are entered, our system analyzes the source programs and extracts the JavaFX Script components. In this step, source programs are deconstructed into tokens, and components are extracted from the tokens. Then, the definitions of JavaFX Swing components are stored. The extraction stores the line number of each token. The target components of this extraction are followings.

- SwingButton
- SwingCheckBox
- SwingComboBox
- SwingLabel
- SwingList
- SwingRadioButton
- SwingSlider
- SwingTextField
- SwingToggleButton

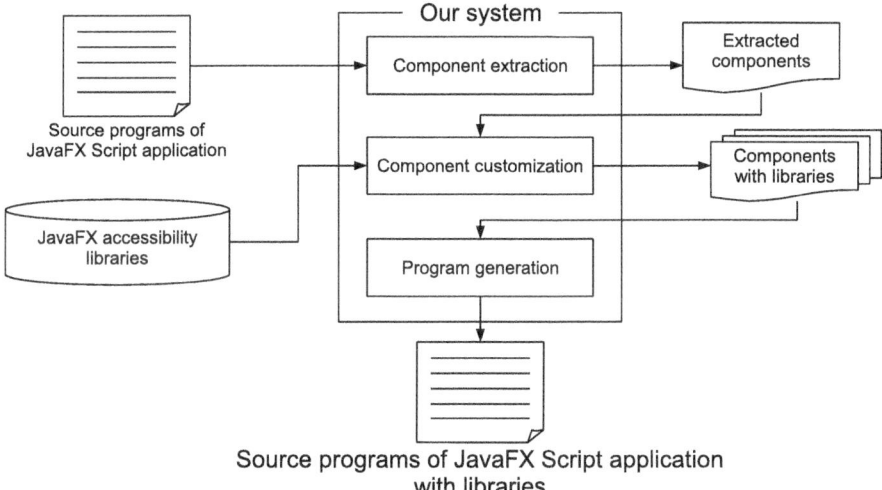

Fig. 1. System architecture

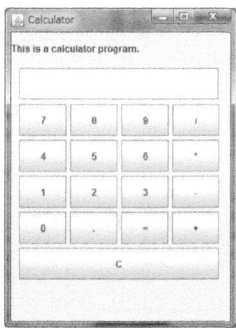

Fig. 2. Sample application (Calculator)

Figure 4 shows examples of the extracted tokens in a scenario with three types of JavaFX Script components: label component called SwingLabel, text component called SwingTextField, and button component called SwingButton.

6.2   Component Customization

Our system determines which JavaFX Accessibility Libraries are applicable to each component extracted in 6.1 and then generates the necessary code.

Adjustment of component size. To adjust the component size, our system evaluates each component separately to determine whether the size library should be applied. If the component is listed in Table 1, then our system generates code to apply the size library. Using the example in 6.1, this library is applicable to three types of components: SwingButton, SwingTextField, and

```
1    var myText = SwingLabel {
2         fill: bind Color.web(colorButton.accessibleForeColor);
3         text: "This is a calculator program."
4    }
5    var t = SwingTextField {
6         width: 100
7         height: 40
8         foreground: Color.BLACK
9    }
10   var b_0 = SwingButton {
11        text: "0"
12        foreground: Color.BLACK
13        width: 60
14        height: 40
15   }
```

Fig. 3. Source program of the sample application

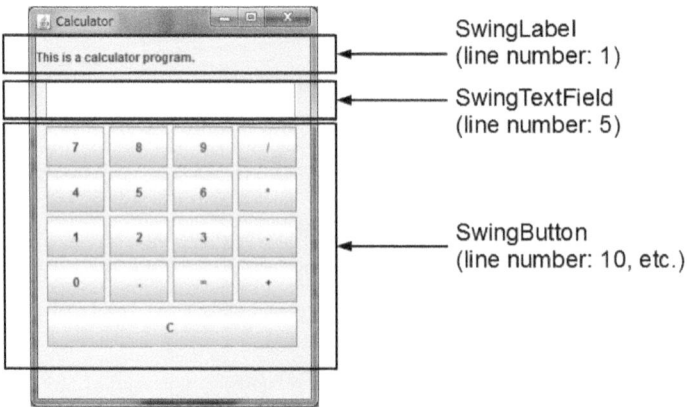

Fig. 4. Examples of extracted components

SwingLabel. Figure 5 shows an example of the code generated for the Swing-Button component.

```
width: AccessibleSize.AccessibleStage.width
height: AccessibleSize.AccessibleStage.height
```

Fig. 5. Example of code to apply the size library

Adjustment of component color. Similar to component size, our system determines whether the color library should be applied to each component. If the component is included in Table 3, then our system generates code for the color library. Figure 6 shows the generated code for this library using the example in 6.1. Specifically code is generated to adjust the foreground color of the SwingTextField component.

```
foreground: bind Color.web(AccessibleColor.accessibleForeColor)
```

Fig. 6. Example of code to apply the color library

Implementation of keyboard operations. To implement keyboard operations, our system evaluates each component individually. If the component is included in Table 4, then code is generated to apply the keyboard library. To use this library, a web designer must initially determine the assignment of concrete shortcut keys for each component. Using the example in 6.1, the keyboard library is applied to all SwingButton components. Figure 7 shows the generated code in the example.

```
var origScreen = MnemonicButtonScreen{};
var b_0 = MnemonicSwingComponent{
mnemonic1: KeyCode.VK_CONTROL
mnemonic2: KeyCode.VK_A
origScreen: origScreen

var MnemonicButtonGroup_g1 = MnemonicButtonGroup {
    GroupForcusKey1: KeyCode.VK_ALT
    GroupForcusKey2: KeyCode.VK_A
    }
var g1_A = MnemonicButton_g1_a.getMnemonicSwingButton();
MnemonicButtonGroup_g1.add(g1_A);
origScreen.add(MnemonicButtonGroup_g1);
origScreen.getAccessibleScreen(),
MnemonicButtonGroup_g1.get(),
origScreen.requestFocus();
```

Fig. 7. Example of code to implement keyboard operations

Implementation of usage of screen readers. To implement the reader library, our system assesses whether a screen reader is applicable to each component. If the component is listed in Table 5, then code is generated for the reader library. Web designers must initially determine an accessible name and description for the JavaFX Swing component where the former is a name and the latter is a description read aloud to indicate how to use the components. Using the example in 6.1, this library is applicable to all extracted components. Figure 8 shows the code for the SwingButton component called "9".

As described in 5.4, when executing the code in Figure 8, a transparent label, which includes a name and description, is placed on the target JavaFX Swing component. Screen readers speak the name and description of the transparent label. Figure 9 shows an image using the reader library and the example program shown in Figure 2.

```
var a = AccessibleContext.aButton {
    accessibleName:"Nine"
    accessibleDescription:"This button inputs nine."
    toolTipText:"Nine Button"
}
```

Fig. 8. Example of code to implement screen readers

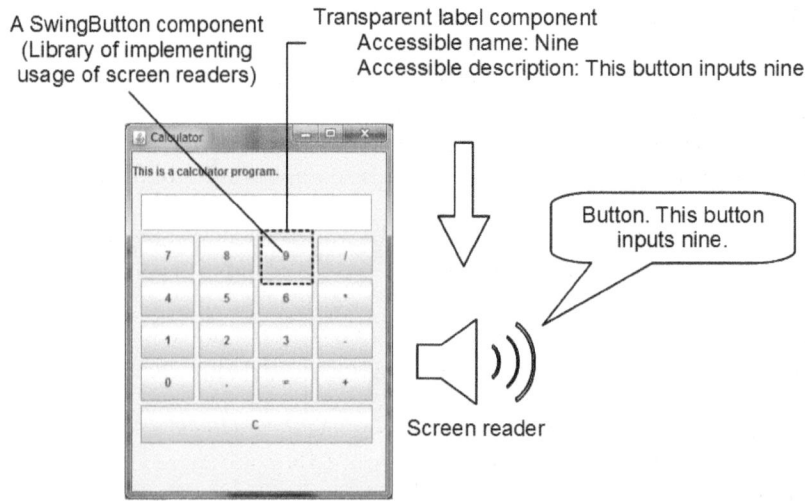

Fig. 9. Image of screen reader

6.3   Program Generation

After generating code to apply the JavaFX Accessibility Libraries, our system modifies the source programs of the JavaFX Script application. Based on the line number of each token extracted in 6.1, the target code is replaced with the generated code.

As shown in Figure 10, for size and color libraries, button components for adjusting are inserted. Using the "size" button allows users to select a font. Then the sizes of the text, component, and window are simultaneously adjusted, while the "color" button changes the combination of the foreground and background.

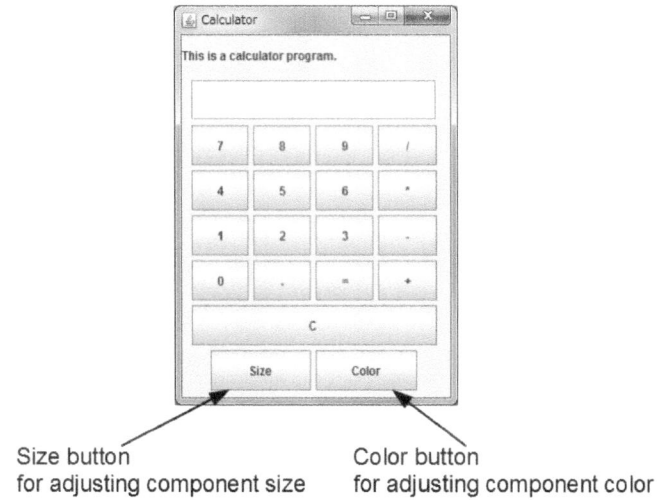

Size button
for adjusting component size

Color button
for adjusting component color

Fig. 10. Application after applying the libraries

7   Evaluation

We evaluated our method based on efficiency and appropriateness of the generated code.

7.1   Code Generation Efficiency

To confirm efficiency of our method, we compared the time required to realize accessibility and the amount of source programs. We assigned an evaluator, which determines accessibility to the sample program in following three scenarios.

Scenario 1. Realizing accessibility without JavaFX Accessibility Libraries
Scenario 2. Realizing accessibility with JavaFX Accessibility Libraries, but without our system
Scenario 3. Realizing accessibility with both JavaFX Accessibility Libraries and our system

Figure 11 shows the program, which has one window that includes a SwingLabel component, used in the evaluation.

Comparison of time. Table 6 shows the results where "scenario" indicates the different scenarios to realize accessibility of the program. "Size", "Color", "Keyboard" and "Screen reader" indicate size adjustment, color adjustment, keyboard operations, and usage of screen readers, respectively.

```
1 var label = SwingLabel {
2       fill: Color.WHITE
3       font : Font { size : 20 }
4       x: 20
5       y: 70
6       content: "Let's create accessible contents!"
7 }
8 Stage {
9       title: "Application title"
10      width:  380
11      height: 200
12      scene: Scene {
13          fill: Color.BLUE
14          content: [ label, ]
15      }
16 }
```

Fig. 11. Sample program for the evaluation

Table 6. Time to realize accessibility (minutes)

	Size	Color	Keyboard	Screen reader
Scenario 1	32.7	12.0	Impossible	Impossible
Scenario 2	5.0	1.2	5.9	1.5
Scenario 3	0.8	0.8	2.2	1.5

In scenario 1, because applying the "keyboard" and "screen reader" are time consuming, they are labeled as impossible. In scenario 2, "size" and "keyboard" require more time than "color" and "screen reader" because the evaluator is unfamiliar with "size" and "keyboard", they require more code modifications than "color" and "screen reader".

However, scenario 3 is the quickest. These observations indicate that our method to realize accessibility is time efficient, even if the evaluator is unfamiliar with the modifications in the evaluation.

Comparison of amount of source program. Table 7 compares the amount of source code required to realize accessibility. In this table, "size", "color", "keyboard" and "screen reader" are the same as in Table 6.

For the same reasons as Table 6, "keyboard" and "screen reader" are labeled as impossible as they required 497 and 174 lines, respectively. The amount of code for scenarios 2 and 3 with JavaFX Accessibility Libraries is less than "scenario 1". These results indicate that JavaFX Accessibility Libraries decrease the amount of code to be written, and web designers can effectively develop accessible JavaFX Script applications using our method.

Table 7. Amount of source program to realize accessibility (nubmer of lines)

	Size	Color	Keyboard	Screen reader
Scenario 1	73	63	Impossible	Impossible
Scenario 2	51	52	59	46
Scenario 3	51	52	59	46

7.2   Appropriateness of Code Generation

To confirm the appropriateness of the generated source programs, we executed the generated program of Figure 2 to confirm whether each library performed accordingly.

Library of adjusting component size. As described in 6.2, the size library added a button to adjust the size in the generated program. In our test, we verified that the text size is adjusted by pushing the button. The window and component sizes adjusted simultaneously and at the same rate.

Library of adjusting component color. Similarly, the color library added a button to change the color in the generated program. Upon clicking this button, the component colors changed accordingly where background and foreground colors were defined as one-to-one combinations based on the accessible combinations in ref. [9].

Library of implementing keyboard operations. To test the keyboard library, we assigned shortcut keys to each SwingButton component in Figure 2. Then we used these keys to assess their performance. All shortcut keys worked properly. For example, clicking SwingButton component "3" entered the number "3" in the SwingTextField component above the button. Thus, we assigned a shortcut key of "Ctrl+3" to enter the number "3" into the SwingTextField component.

Library of implementing usage of screen readers. Similarly, to test the reader library, we assigned accessible names and descriptions to the components in Figure 2. For example, we assigned an accessible name of "nine" and a descriptor of "this button enters the number nine" to the SwingButton called "9". Although the reader spoke the text, applying both the reader and keyboard libraries caused conflicts. Specifically, the reader library prevented implementation of the keyboard operations because the reader library places transparent labels on target components, and requires shortcut keys.

However, the above results confirm that the JavaFX Accessibility Libraries almost always perform appropriately. Thus, our system can effectively realize accessibility for JavaScript applications.

8   Conclusion

Herein we propose a method, which has two phases, to achieve accessibility of JavaFX Script applications. The first phase realizes accessibility libraries for JavaFX Script applications, while the second applies these libraries. Because our system automatically applies these libraries to JavaFX Script applications, the burden to web designers is small compared to other methods. Hence, our method effectively realized improved accessibility.

There are following some future works.

- Resolving conflicts between keyboard operations and screen readers
- Applying JavaFX Accessibility Libraries to components other than JavaFX Swing components
- Developing libraries of accessibility satisfying accessibility requirements, which JavaFX Script libraries do not include

References

1. Accessible Rich Internet Applications (WAI-ARIA) 1.0., http://www.w3.org/TR/wai-aria/
2. Web Content Accessibility Guidelines (WCAG) 2.0., http://www.w3.org/TR/WCAG20/
3. Adobe Flash Platform, http://www.adobe.com/jp/flashplatform/
4. Adobe Flash Professional CS5 accessibility, http://www.adobe.com/accessibility/products/flash/
5. Sato, D., Miyashita, H., Takagi, H., Asakawa, C.: Automatic accessibility transcoding for flash content. In: Proc. of the 9th international ACM SIGACCESS Conference on Computers and Accessibility (Assets 2007) (2007)
6. Cantón, P., González, Á.L., Mariscal, G., Ruiz, C.: Building Accessible Flash Applications: An XML-Based Toolkit. In: Miesenberger, K., Klaus, J., Zagler, W.L., Karshmer, A.I. (eds.) ICCHP 2008. LNCS, vol. 5105, pp. 370–377. Springer, Heidelberg (2008)
7. JavaFX Script - Overview, http://www.sun.com/software/javafx/script/
8. Java Accessibility: The Java Accessibility API, http://download.oracle.com/docs/cd/E17802_01/j2se/javase/technologies/accessibility/docs/jaccess-1.3/doc/core-api.html
9. Fujitsu ColorSelector, http://jp.fujitsu.com/about/design/ud/assistance/colorselector/
10. Cascading Style Sheets Level 2 Revision 1 (CSS 2.1) Specification, http://www.w3.org/TR/CSS21/
11. Gonzalez, A., Reid, L.G.: Platform-Independent Accessibility API: Accessible Document Object Model. In: Proc. of the 2005 International Cross-Disciplinary Workshop on Web Accessibility (W4A 2005) (2005)
12. Kawanaka, S., Borodin, Y., Bigham, J. P., Lunn, D., Takagi, H., Asakawa, C.: Accessibility Commons:A Metadata Infrastructure for Web Accessibility. In: Proc. of the 10th International ACM SIGACCESS Conference on Computers and Accessibility (2008)

13. Fernandes, N., Lopes, R., Carrico, L.: On web accessibility evaluation environments. In: Proc. of the International Cross-Disciplinary Conference on Web Accessibility (W4A 2011) (2011)
14. Sirithumgul, P., Suchato, A., Punyabukkana, P.: Quantitative evaluation for web accessibility with respect to disabled groups. In: Proc. of the 2009 International Cross-Disciplinary Conference on Web Accessibililty (W4A 2009) (2009)
15. Miyashita, H., Sato, D., Takagi, H., Asakawa, C.: Aibrowser for multimedia: introducing multimedia content accessibility for visually impaired users. In: Proc. of the 9th International ACM SIGACCESS Conference on Computers and Accessibility (Assets 2007) (2007)
16. Sato, D., Takagi, H., Kobayashi, M., Kawanaka, S., Asakawa, C.: Exploratory Analysis of Collaborative Web Accessibility Improvement. ACM Transactions on Accessible Computing (TACCESS) 3(2) (2010)

User-Centered Design of Accessible Web and Automation Systems

Helmut Vieritz[1], Farzan Yazdi[2], Daniel Schilberg[1],
Peter Göhner[2], and Sabina Jeschke[1]

[1] Institute of Information Management in Mechanical Engineering IMA, RWTH Aachen
University, Dennewartstraße 27, D-52068 Aachen, Germany
{helmut.vieritz,daniel.schilberg,
sabina.jeschke}@ima-zlw-ifu.rwth-aachen.de
[2] Institute of Industrial Automation and Software Engineering IAS, University of Stuttgart,
Pfaffenwaldring 47, D-70569 Stuttgart, Germany
{farzan.yazdi,peter.goehner}@ias.uni-stuttgart.de

Abstract. During the past decades, Web applications and industrial automation
systems – and their combination in e.g. pervasive computing – have gained
more and more importance in our daily life. However until now, user interface
accessibility remains as an important quality aspect and a challenge for implementation. The majority of accessibility requirements are shared between these
types of systems.

This paper presents a research on user-centered design and model-driven development of accessible user interfaces. The approach integrates the product
requirements of Web and industrial automation systems. The use of different interface models enables the description of particular UI aspects as structure or
behavior. User-centered design facilitates the integration of user-driven accessibility requirements.

The focus on the requirements of software development processes for Web
and automation systems shows that research on accessible user interfaces has to
consider the requirements of product analysis and design. Additionally, upcoming daily use in pervasive computing requires a comparison of requirements for
both system types.

Keywords: Accessibility, User-centered Design, User Interface Modeling,
Model-driven Design.

1   Introduction

During the past decades, Web applications and industrial automation systems[1] – and
their combination – have gained more and more importance in our daily life. Research
on Ambient Assisted Living (AAL) demonstrates new possibilities in daily life use of
all people. However until now, the usage of these applications is often restricted for

---

[1] With industrial automation systems we refer to products such as ticket vending machines,
washing machines or automated teller machines (ATM) systems.

A. Holzinger and K.-M. Simonic (Eds.): USAB 2011, LNCS 7058, pp. 367–378, 2011.

people with disabilities such as blind or deaf people since the User Interface (UI) design was not made with respect to their needs.

Existing accessibility recommendations as the Web Content Accessibility Guidelines (WCAG 2.0) [1] address mainly the run-time behavior. They are difficult to adapt to the requirements of early product development phases. Additionally, they are mainly created for Web applications.

Despite the importance of accessibility, it is still a big challenge integrating it to the industrial automation systems, due to reasons as the variety of user requirements for different groups or the difference between developer's mindset with that of the user. Additionally, restrictions may come from limited UI technology as smart phones with small screens or obstructive environment conditions as noise. Thus, accessible usage includes limited technology as mobile devices and restricting environments.

Both, industrial automation systems and Web applications share similar accessibility requirements. Here, the accessibility requirements are summarized in five criteria derived from the WCAG 2.0 [1], the WAI-Rich Internet Applications (WAI-ARIA) [2] and further research:

A. Metadata for documents describes author, title, document relations etc.
B. Navigation techniques as main or utility navigation, breadcrumbs or sitemap are supported.
C. Navigation through documents as skip links, access keys or short cuts can be given.
D. The UI model can describe user's workflow and serial order of UI components to assure that the order of interface components corresponds with user's workflow.
E. UI elements are described with role, state and state changing (behavior).

Often, User-centered Design (UCD) is recommended to ameliorate product accessibility [3, 4 and 5]. User-centered design is focused on user's needs and limitations during all the phases of the design process. Originally, UCD was intended to optimize the usability of products. Meanwhile, accessibility is seen as an essential part of usability and it is proposed to join users with disabilities in analysis, design and evaluation to enhance product accessibility [4]. The adaption of recommendations as well as the integration of users with disabilities in design requires expert knowledge. Additionally, systematic processes are lacking.

The focus of the presented research is the impact of product accessibility requirements on modern software development processes for Web software or automation systems. To overcome the mentioned problems, we propose user task analysis and modeling in early product design. Abstract task modeling allows describing user's workflow independent from the input and output technology. It is used in modeling multi-target and multimodality UIs [6].

Accessibility means that the products are usable for all users independent from their particular capabilities or age and without assistance by other persons [5] including free perception and control of all relevant information [1]. Relevant information refers to those being needed by the user to follow the intended workflow constituted by activities, actions and their relations. Therefore, the UI itself must assist the user to fulfill his or her working tasks and the usage must be easy to learn.

2   Related Research

Meanwhile, accessibility in product design is addressed by numerous international and national recommendations [e.g. 1, 2, and 3]. The WCAG [1] have the greatest impact on scientific research and discussion.

Accessibility in UCD is described by Henry [4] focusing on integration of users with disabilities in analysis and design and modeling is not included.

Approaches for Model-driven Design (MDD) in UI development can be classified in more practical or analytical concepts. Practical approaches are focused on usage in platform-independent development of UIs including development tools. Some examples are User Interface Markup Language (UIML) [8], User Interface Description Language (UIDL) [9], and Extensible Application Markup Language (XAML) [10]. Recent technologies as Microsoft Silverlight or Adobe Flex provide the separation of UI layout from UI behavior as well as from system core functionalities.

Analytical approaches are more abstract and include often a metamodel for all UI aspects, which describes UI structure, components, behavior, navigation, domain, and resources. Examples are User Interface Extensible Markup Language (UsiXML) [11], useML [12], Unified Modeling Language for Interactive Applications (UMLi) [13], Task Modeling Language (TaskML) [14] and Dialog Modeling Language (DiaMODL) [14]. However, analytical approaches are still under research and there is a lack of tool support for implementation.

Despite the promising potential, only few publications address the integration of accessibility in MDD of UIs. The Dante project [15] uses annotations in UI modeling to improve the navigation capabilities for visually impaired users. The authors have discussed particular aspects of UCD and MDD for accessible UIs in former publications [e.g. 16, 17]. The integration of different target platforms as the Web and mobile technologies is also addressed by the AEGIS EU-Project and the Raising the floor initiave.

3   Web Applications and Industrial Automation Systems

3.1   Accessibility Requirements

In this paper, Web applications and industrial automation systems are addressed. Their usage is more and more merged in pervasive computing e.g. navigation systems. Despite of obvious differences, many similarities form the ground for shared requirements and solutions in accessibility design. Some important similarities are:

- User disabilities, technological or environmental limitations lead to restrictions in Human-computer Interaction (HCI) e.g. acoustic interaction may be impossible.

- The combined use and limited interaction capabilities results in identical accessibility problems such as touchscreens require an alternative information representation for blind users.
- The spreading usage in daily life is associated with different user roles and characteristics.
- User and system workflow is automatized.
- Web technologies as HTML are used for UI implementation.

Regarding accessibility, important differences are:

- Industrial automation systems have often limited resources whereas Web applications are running on powerful clients and servers.
- Industrial automation systems have built-in UIs whereas interaction devices for Web applications e.g. browsers are running as separated clients allowing the usage of Assistive Technology (AT) for people with disabilities.
- Accessible Web content is typically a requirement of users with disabilities whereas for automation systems, accessibility is often driven by limited UI technologies or environment restrictions. Nevertheless, the requirements are similar and solutions can be adapted to the other field (see [7]).

We have used the WCAG to analyze and compare accessible HCI for Web and automation systems. A similar work was already done with the W3C Mobile Web Best Practices 1.0 [7]. More than 70% of the guidelines could be employed for the industrial automation system [7]. Hence, our concept uses WCAG as the basis to address the critical accessibility issues.

3.2   Model-Driven Design

A generic approach for accessible Web and automation systems needs a process model – User-centered Design process – and a structural model – the architecture model – for the development of the application. Model-driven design is very common in software engineering e.g. for automation systems. In Web development, MDD is already addressed by research activities. However, fast developing Web technologies and their diversity as well as the importance of creative aspects as layout impede the usage of MDD in Web engineering.

Model-driven design of UIs allows the abstract description of particular aspects of UI behavior or structure. Meanwhile, the Unified Modeling Language 2 (UML, [19]) is the lingua franca for modeling and graphical notation in software design. Here, UML diagrams are used to describe the different models of the UI. The abstract description of UI behavior provides a universal design making the usage of the UI independent from particular input and output devices.

Generic Architecture Model. A common architecture model is needed to merge the development processes for Web applications and industrial automation systems. The generic architecture of both is slightly different. Web applications are typically designed with layers for presentation, application logic and data persistence (three-tier architecture) e.g. the Model-View-Control (MVC) architecture pattern.

Otherwise, industrial automation systems are separated into the technical system which is automatized, the automation system itself and UI system [18]. The technical system includes all hard- and software which is needed to transform any kind of energy e.g. a heating system or matter e.g. a washing machine. The automation system controls the processes of the technical system e.g. to obtain a time-depending behavior or to communicate with other systems. The UI system is responsible for all aspects of HCI.

To bring Web and automation systems together, we have merged the layer architecture with the three main components and called them UI System, Computer System and Technical System. Figure 1 shows the generic application architecture which is applicable for Web and automation systems.

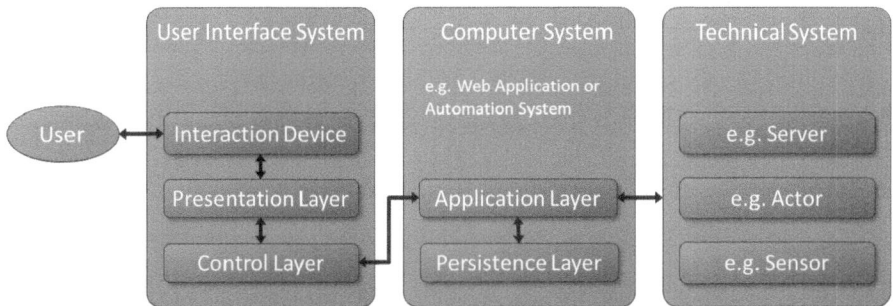

Fig. 1. Basic Architecture for Accessible Systems

The architecture combines common three-tier architecture with a separation of automation system and technical system. The UI system consists of an interaction device a presentation and a control layer. The interaction device may be a built-in UI as well as a client-based browser or screen reader. The presentation layer is responsible for HCI. Additionally, a control layer manages user control of the whole system and mediates between the UI and the computer system. The computer system compasses the application functionalities or the automation core and the persistence layer if data storing is needed. The technical system includes the complete hardware and software of the automatized system e.g. a ticket vending machine. The technical system of a Web application is the server operating system and the hardware.

User-centered Design for Human-computer Interaction. In this paper, we will focus on UI analysis and design for accessible UI systems. Regarding their UI, UCD is a promising approach for the UI development of Web and industrial automation systems, since both systems share similar accessibility requirements (see section 3.1).

Our modeling concept was developed in reference to the Cameleon Reference Model for UI modeling [6]. The reference model is designed to model UIs for multiple classes of users, platforms and environments (multi-target). It covers design and run-time phases of UIs. Figure 2 shows the four level model hierarchy for design.

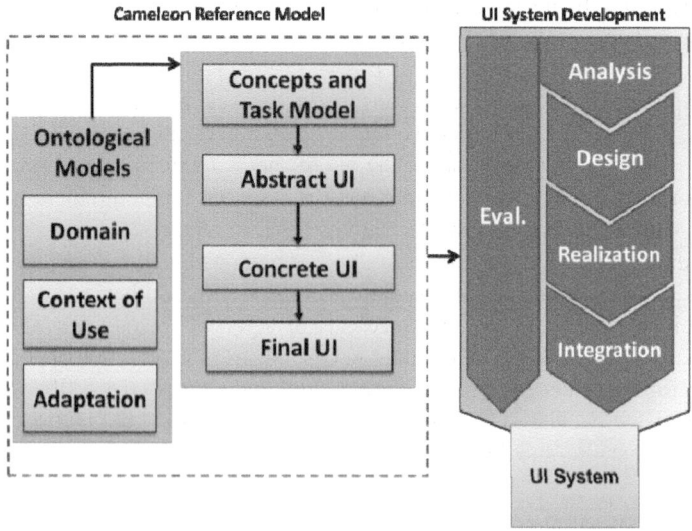

Fig. 2. Cameleon Reference Model [6] in UI Modeling

The highest level concepts and tasks allow the combination of design concepts with user tasks. The Abstract User Interface (AUI) model describes domain concepts independent from particular targets and input/output devices. It provides a semantical description of HCI with modes and dialogs. The Concrete User Interface (CUI) model gives an interactor-dependent description of the UI. Multimodal adaption of HCI can be integrated to support interaction modalities as visual, acoustical or haptic interaction. The Final User Interface (FUI) is the transformation of the CUI into source code as Java or HTML.

The Cameleon Reference Model is used as a master pattern for the design of essential UI models. Three types of models are essential [20] – the task (see section 3.3), the dialog (see section 3.4) and the presentation model (see section 3.5):

- The task model represents user's part of HCI. It comprises use cases, scenarios, activities, workflow etc.
- In the middle, the dialog model mediates between human and system activities. It describes HCI with modes, dialogs and basic interactions and transforms information from the active part of the user to the reactive behavior of the UI.
- The presentation model is a semantical description of the UI. It includes navigation, views, UI components, roles, behavior etc.

Additional models as the user model allow the design of more complex UI applications. Figure 3 gives an overview for the integration of essential modeling needs into the reference model.

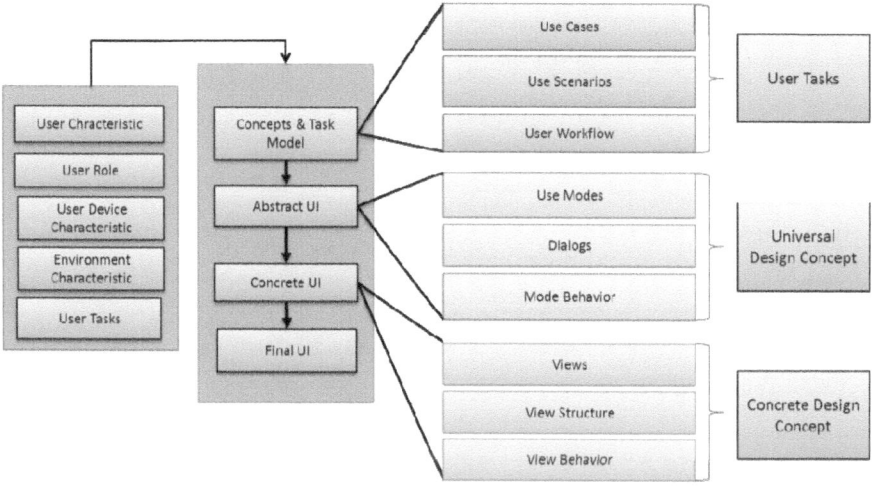

Fig. 3. Concept for UI Modeling

In a first step, requirement gathering helps to define design goals for user activities and system functionalities. Interaction concepts and user tasks are described by the task model with use cases, scenarios and activity diagrams (see section 3.3). Thereafter, the dialog model defines the abstract design of HCI with modes and interaction sequences (dialogs). A complete and abstract description of all essential HCI aspects provides the developer with a universal design concept for an accessible UI (see section 3.4). Finally, the presentation model allows the detailing of navigation, views and UI components regarding the visual, acoustic or haptic modality of HCI (see section 3.5).

3.3   Task Modeling

In the task model, activities as the main steps of user's workflow are described and detailed with user's workflow and basic actions. In UML, activities are sets of user actions. User-centered Design is often based on the analysis of user's tasks and workflow. Use cases and scenarios are detailed with activities and actions. The useML approach [12] provides a simple but powerful set of basic actions – so-called elementary use objects. Here, it is extended with graphical workflow description, constraints and UML notation. Figure 4 shows the structural classes of this task model.

The task model includes use cases, activities and basic actions (left side). Use cases are decomposed into activities and elementary actions further on. Not included are physical operations as mouse moving or key pressing since they are not independent from in-/output device. Thus, the description of user activities in task modeling remains independent from visual, acoustic or haptic interaction modality.

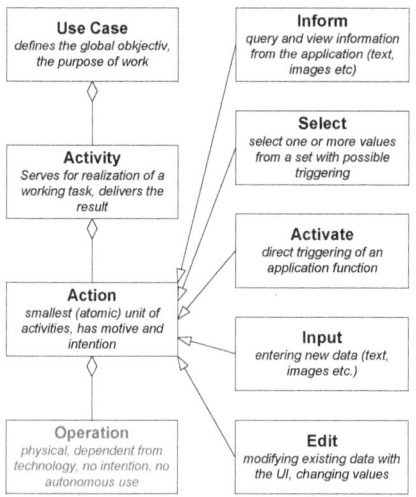

Fig. 4. Task hierarchy and elementary user actions

Atomic user actions represent the basic level of task modeling. A set of five predefined actions [12] (see Figure 4, right side) facilitates the modeling with UML activity
diagrams. They are named: Inform, Select, Activate, Input and Edit.

In UML 2, particular diagrams are well-suited for the graphical notation of models.
The active part of the user can be modeled with use case diagrams and activity diagrams. The reactive behavior of the UI is described in state chart diagrams. Structural
aspects are notated with class diagrams. Last but not least, sequence diagrams describe the sequential order of interaction.

Task modeling with UML allows not only the hierarchical decomposition of user
activities into basic actions but also the modeling of different workflow types as seria-
lized, parallelized, synchronized or competing. Even constraints and decisions are
supported.

Most aspects of task modeling are shared between Web and automation systems.
Typically, Web applications are dealing with complex information for the user whereas automation systems have decided sets of functionalities. The task model supports
both task characteristics.

3.4   Dialog Modeling

The AUI represents the dialog model. Human-computer interaction is described with
dialogs and modes of usage. Similar activities allow their combination within modes
of usage as an editor for different types of texts. A mode of interaction with the UI
provides a particular context for usage and only a certain set of user actions is allowed. Modes are sets of UI states [21] and possible user actions. A specific action
has a consistent effect within a given mode. Usability and accessibility requires an
elaborated mode design. Navigation in application can be modeled as the change of

mode. Finally, the AUI is focused on the semantic description of the UI and represents a universal design of the UI which can be used with different type of input/output devices as displays, screen readers, a mouse or keyboard.

Dialog modeling supports Web applications as well as industrial automation systems. Typically, a Web application has more dialogs or modes but is less restricted in the capabilities regarding visual, acoustic or haptic interaction modality. Thus, the universal design concept is better suited for Web applications than for automation systems.

3.5   Presentation Modeling

In the presentation model, the modes and dialogs are represented as views, the internal structure of views and UI components. A view is a single representation of the application UI at one time. Its UI components enable a particular set of user actions which correspond with context of mode and usage. A view is often but not necessarily assigned to a file as an HTML file or a Java object as a view controller. Navigation is provided with main and utility navigation, a sitemap, breadcrumbs or metadata about view relations.

Accessible main and utility navigation as well as a sitemap are additional accessibility requirements in modeling. They provide orientation, overview and navigation through the application interface. Navigation and sitemap facilitate the user access. User orientation (especially with AT) is easier if modes are mapped to single views.

For UI programming the object-oriented programming paradigm is extended with events to describe UI reactions and behavior on user activities. This programming paradigm is called event-driven programming. Therefore, UML class descriptions are extended with events (beside attributes and methods). To meet accessibility, only device-independent event handler as *OnFocus* or *OnActivate* are used. WAI-ARIA elements are used to describe the UI behavior during runtime.

The hierarchy of UI components is described with a class diagram and UI behavior with state chart diagrams. Even, the class model allows the description of component hierarchy or serial order of elements.

UI Components may be containers or single elements. UI containers as lists, table, articles, trees etc. consists of elements which are the basic components as buttons, headings, paragraphs, sliders, links etc. Here, the UI components for the presentation modeling are derived from recent UI development frameworks as Google Web Toolkit (GWT) [22], Microsoft Expression Blend (based on Silverlight and XAML) [23] or Java Server Faces (JSF) [24] implementations. These frameworks are focused one the design of interactive Web-based UIs and provide interactive components exceeding hypertext markup as HTML with e.g. color or date picker.

The MVC architecture pattern separates database design (model) from control and UI (view). The separation of UI and application design is well-suited to implement the user-driven models for the UI. Meanwhile, frameworks for Web application development support the usage of accessible UI components. Here, Web frameworks are evaluated. The evaluation has included the capabilities for UI development, tools for implementation, support for accessibility design with WCAG and WAI-ARIA etc.

The JSF-technology (e.g. Apache MyFaces (AMF) including Trinidad and Tobago subprojects) and the GWT provide generic accessibility support. The Web frameworks combine the MVC architecture pattern with libraries of UI components. MyFaces is an open source implementation of JSF. MyFaces Trinidad and GWT have built-in support for accessible UI elements. Google Web Toolkit implements more client-side functionality to obtain application behavior similar to desktop applications. WAI-ARIA is also supported in GWT. Now, prototypical implementation serves for detailed evaluation of model integration.

The mentioned technologies for implementation are typically Web-based. Thus, a good support is given for the integration of presentation modeling and implementation. Until now, automation systems with limited hardware resources may not support Web technologies for implementation. It is expected, that further development of technology will bring advances.

4   Conclusion and Outlook

The approach is focused on accessible Web applications and industrial automation systems. The majority of accessibility requirements are shared between these types of systems. Additionally, the usage of both systems is more and more merged in daily life use. Restrictions of user capabilities, technology or environment lead to similar requirements of product accessibility.

The approach examines the potential of UCD and MDD for accessible UIs. Model data describe much information which can be used to support AT with necessary data. Modeling includes static behaviors as site structure and navigation links. UML is used for graphical notation. Model-driven design supports the design of complex applications since particular aspects of structure and functionality are described in separate models. The integration of accessibility requirements in the process of development may help in future to integrate in and approach the knowledge of accessibility experts and software designers for the easier design of accessible UIs.

Until now, model data are translated manually into the runtime markup. Further work is necessary on accessibility-supporting model transformations as well as the design and implementation of a model compiler to support process automation.

Further on, the graphical UML-based notation of UI models is not naturally accessible. Text-based modeling notation e.g. Human-usable Textual Notation (HUTN) [25] can avoid this problem but still needs adaption to the UML metamodel.

The presented basic ideas are as well plausible for other platforms e.g. Desktop applications or for another user group e.g. elderly people. Further research may show that accessible Web and Desktop applications can be designed with one unifying approach and implemented with integrative technologies as Adobe Flex or Microsoft Silverlight.

Acknowledgement. We highly appreciate *"Deutsche Forschungsgemeinschaft"* (DFG) for funding the INAMOSYS project.

References

[1] World Wide Web Consortium. Web Content Accessibility Guidelines 2.0. (2008), http://www.w3.org/TR/WCAG20/ (last visited: July 21, 2011)

[2] World Wide Web Consortium (W3C): Accessible Rich Internet Applications (WAI-ARIA) 1.0. (2009), http://www.w3.org/WAI/intro/aria (last visited July 21, 2011)

[3] Swedish Administrative Development Agency (VERVA). Swedish National Guidelines for Public Sector Websites (2008), http://www.eutveckling.se/static/doc/swedish-guidelines-public-sector-websites.pdf (last visited: July 21, 2011)

[4] Henry, S.L.: Just Ask (2007), http://Lulu.com

[5] Deutsches Institut für Normung (DIN). Technical Report 124 – Products in Design for All (2002)

[6] Calvary, G., et al.: The CAMELEON Reference Framework. UJF, UCL, CNUCE (2002), http://giove.isti.cnr.it/projects/cameleon/pdf/CAMELEON%20D1.1RefFramework.pdf (last visited: July 13, 2011)

[7] W3C 2008. Mobile Web Best Practices 1 (2008), http://www.w3.org/TR/mobile-bp/ (last visited: July 21, 2011)

[8] UIML community 2009. User Interface Markup Language (UIML) (2009), http://uiml.org/ (last visited: July 21/2011)

[9] UIDL community 2008. User Interface Description Language (UIDL) (2008), http://www.uidl.net/ (last visited: July 21/2011)

[10] Microsoft Corp. 2010. Extensible Application Markup Language (XAML) (2010), http://msdn.microsoft.com/en-us/library/ms747122.aspx (last visited: July 21, 2011)

[11] UsiXML community 2010. User Interface Extensible Markup Language (UsiXML) (2010), http://itea.defimedia.be/ (last visited: July 21, 2011)

[12] Reuther, A.: Useml – Systematische Entwicklung von Maschinenbediensystemen mit XML. Technische Universität Kaiserslautern (2003)

[13] Da Silva, P.P.: Object Modelling of Interactive Systems: The UMLi Approach. University of Manchester (2002)

[14] Trætteberg, H.: Model-based User Interface Design. Norwegian University of Science and Technology, Trondheim (2002)

[15] Yesilada, Y., et al.: Dante – Annotation and Transformation of Web Pages for Visually Impaired Users. In: WWW Alt. 2004: Proceedings of the 13th International World Wide Web Conference on Alternate Track Papers & Posters, pp. 490–491. ACM Press, New York (2004)

[16] Göhner, P., et al.: Integrated Accessibility Models of User Interfaces for IT and Automation Systems. In: Proceedings of the 21st International Conference on Computer Applications in Industry and Engineering, Cary, NC 27511, USA (2008)

[17] Jeschke, S., Pfeiffer, O., Vieritz, H.: Developing Accessible Applications with User-centered Architecture. In: Seventh IEEE/ACIS International Conference on Computer and Information Science, ICIS 2008, pp. 684–689. IEEE Computer Society, Los Alamitos (2008)

[18] Lauber, R., Göhner, P.: Prozessautomatisierung. Springer, Berlin (1999)

[19] Object Management Group (OMG) 2010: Unified Modeling Language (Version 2.3) (2010), http://www.omg.org/spec/UML/2.3/ (last visited: July 21, 2011)

[20] Luyten, K.: Dynamic User Interface Generation for Mobile and Embedded Systems with Model-based User Interface Development. Transnational University Limburg (2004)

[21] Thimbleby, H.: Press on: Principles of Interaction Programming. MIT Press, Cambridge (2010)

[22] Google Inc. 2010. Google Web Toolkit (2010), http://code.google.com/intl/de-DE/webtoolkit/ (last visited: July 21, 2011)

[23] Microsoft Corp. 2010. Microsoft Expression (2010), http://www.microsoft.com/expression/ (last visited: July 21, 2011)

[24] Oracle Corp. 2010. JavaServer Faces 2, http://www.oracle.com/technetwork/java/javaee/javaserverfaces-139869.html (last visited: July 21, 2011)

[25] Object Management Group 2004. Human-usable Textual Notation (HUTN) (2004), http://www.omg.org/technology/documents/formal/hutn.htm (last visited: July 21, 2011)

Systematic Analysis of Mobile Diabetes Management Applications on Different Platforms

Eva Garcia[1], Clare Martin[2], Antonio Garcia[1],
Rachel Harrison[2], and Derek Flood[2]

[1] University of Alcalá, Spain
[2] Oxford Brookes University, UK
eva.garcial@uah.es, cemartin@brookes.ac.uk, a.garciac@uah.es,
rachel.harrison@brookes.ac.uk, derek.flood@brookes.ac.uk

Abstract. There are a number of mobile applications available to help patients suffering from Type 1 diabetes to manage their condition, but the quality of these applications varies greatly. This paper details the findings from a systematic analysis of these applications on three mobile platforms (Android, iOS, and Blackberry) that was conducted to establish the state of the art in mobile applications for diabetes management. The findings from this analysis will help to inform the future development of more effective mobile applications to help patients suffering from Type 1 diabetes who wish to manage their condition with a mobile application.

Keywords: usability, keystroke level modelling, mobile, heuristic evaluation.

1   Introduction

The development of usability evaluation methods for mobile devices and their applications is a growing area of research which has been fuelled by the rapid growth in the use of smart phones in recent years. Healthcare services in particular stand to benefit from the huge potential offered by the combined technologies of smart phones and cloud computing [1], particularly those associated with chronic conditions such as diabetes that require a high degree of self-management [2], but such interventions are likely to fail unless sufficient attention is paid to usability [3, 4]. Standard evaluation techniques [5] can be broadly applicable to mobile phone applications, but they often need to be adapted to consider additional factors such as context, connectivity and security [6].

This paper contains the results of a systematic evaluation of mobile applications for diabetes management. The study was conducted partly to discover the usability issues of existing applications in order to avoid repeating them in the design of a new application for diabetes management, and also to elicit functional requirements for this new application. In total, over 400 apps were examined in order to give a broad overview of the current status of smart phone based diabetes applications from a developer's perspective. This evaluation was conducted by usability experts, and consisted of a methodical survey based on efficiency, heuristics and functionality. A subsequent

A. Holzinger and K.-M. Simonic (Eds.): USAB 2011, LNCS 7058, pp. 379–396, 2011.
© Springer-Verlag Berlin Heidelberg 2011

evaluation is planned to investigate the potential problems that are experienced by patients while using some of these applications and to determine which interface components are most suitable for data input and output.

The methodology used here was devised in order to sift through the vast array of mobile applications that already exist for diabetes management, but it relies on general techniques that are equally applicable to other domains. This methodology has also been applied to spreadsheet packages [7]. The methodology comprises a series of steps that can be used to filter through a collection of applications by comparing functionality, efficiency and various other attributes that have been identified for use as mobile heuristics [6] such as personalization, ergonomics, flexibility, security and error management. In addition, the process was used to elicit functional requirements by collating a list of features offered by existing applications that will subsequently be ranked by potential users.

This paper is organized as follows. Section 2 introduces type 1 diabetes, Section 3 describes related work that has been conducted in this area. Section 4 explains the general steps of the protocol used to perform the analysis, and Section 5 presents the results obtained at each step of the protocol. Section 6 presents a discussion of these results and Section 7 discusses the threats to validity. The paper is then concluded in Section 8 with a summary of the work completed thus far and the work that will be performed in the future.

2   Type 1 Diabetes

Type 1 diabetes occurs when the insulin producing cells of the pancreas are destroyed leaving the body unable to control its blood glucose levels. People with this condition have to take insulin regularly to try to keep their glucose levels within a safe target range, and failure to do so can lead to short term complications such as heart palpitations or dizziness, and also longer term complications such as retinopathy and peripheral neuropathy.

Most medical professionals encourage patients to keep a diary containing their blood glucose levels before each meal, together with the corresponding carbohydrate intake and insulin dose, in order to help them stay within the target range. The insulin dose is usually calculated by the patient, according to the number of carbohydrates consumed and various other factors including exercise and hormones, but an increasing number of glucose monitors now offer a degree of decision support with such calculations. In addition, a vast number of mobile phone applications have been developed that help patients collect and maintain this information. These applications can now be distributed easily and quickly through locations such as the App store from Apple and the Android marketplace, making it easier for patients to experiment with them. Their usability varies greatly however, and it has been shown [8] that usability can be a determining factor in a users' choice of mobile application.

3   Related Work

Previous studies have been conducted to evaluate the effectiveness of mobile phones for assisting with diabetes self-management [2, 9], and some standards are emerging with regard to how to design mobile applications in general [10], as well as mobile medical applications in particular [11], but research about the usability evaluation of applications for mobile devices is still a relatively new area [12]. A comprehensive survey of the status and trends of 200 mobile-health applications was conducted in [13] but it differs from the work presented here in a number of ways: it considered a broader range of healthcare applications, it was based on the user perspective rather than that of experts and it was restricted solely to the iOS platform.

Some of the specific issues that affect the usability of mobile applications include the following [14]:

- *Mobile context*: this includes the location, identities of nearby people, objects and environmental elements that may distract the user's attention. In systems for diabetes management, the context is important as the need to measure blood glucose can arise at any time, in any place.

- *Connectivity*: network conditions (data transfer speed, reliability, strength of signals) may vary at different times and locations. Connectivity is significant for diabetes management systems, as the information collected by these apps may need to be synchronized with on-line repositories such as Microsoft© Health-Vault.

- *Small screen size*: the small screen size can significantly affect the usability of mobile applications. More specifically in systems for diabetes management, screen size affect the ability to visualize the stored data and graphics, which could be particularly problematic for patients with retinopathy, a common complication of diabetes.

- *Different display resolution*: different levels of display resolution on different mobile devices may cause different usability test results. As in the previous case, display resolution affects the ability to visualize data in graphics, and this could be a serious problem for patients with retinopathy.

- *Limited processing capability and power*: computational power and memory capacity of mobile devices are much less than those of desktop computers. Because of this, developers may have to disable some functions (e.g., high-resolution images and dynamic frame movement). In systems for diabetes management, the limited processing capability could affect the choice of dosing algorithm.

- *Data entry methods*: small buttons and labels limit users' effectiveness and efficiency in entering data, which may reduce the input speed and increase errors. The data entry method is crucial in diabetes management applications, since people must log data frequently, and they could be hindered by peripheral neuropathy, a common complication of diabetes.

4   The Evaluation Method

The methodology used here was devised as a way of filtering the large number of mobile applications that already exist for diabetes management to obtain a set that was small enough to evaluate in greater depth using relatively traditional techniques. The protocol used has been applied to other studies of mobile applications [7] and consists of the following steps:

1. *Identify all potentially relevant applications.* This step consists of searching the applications related to a particular keyword. Current online stores facilitate this task, such as the App Store from Apple, the Android Market from Google and the App World from BlackBerry.
2. *Remove light or old versions of each application.* The trial versions (those that offer a subset of the functionality offered by the corresponding full application or access to the full application for a limited period of time) should be removed as the corresponding full version will also be evaluated.
3. *Identify the main functional requirements and exclude all applications that do not offer this functionality.* Only the applications that meet all main requirements are carried forward to subsequent steps of the protocol.
4. *Identify all secondary requirements.* This step consists of identifying the secondary requirements that each application offers, i.e., the additional functionality that is not required in the step 3.
5. *Construct tasks to test the main functional requirements using each of the methods below:*
   a. *Keystroke level modelling (KLM)* [15] is used to provide a measure of efficiency for each application. New interaction methods provided by mobile devices have not been incorporated into KLM. Therefore it was not possible to predict the efficiency in terms of time, however it was possible to use the number of keystrokes as an indication of the efficiency of these applications.
   b. *Heuristic evaluation* [16] is used to identify some usability problems. Nielsen recommends performing the heuristic evaluation with between three and five evaluators. The heuristics used during this evaluation, shown in Table 1, were developed specifically for mobile applications in [6].

Table 1. Mobile usability heuristics

Heuristic	Description
A	Visibility of system status and losability/findability of the device
B	Match between system and the real world
C	Consistency and mapping
D	Good ergonomics and minimalist design
E	Ease of input, screen readability and glancability
F	Flexibility, efficiency of use and personalization
G	Aesthetic, privacy and social conventions
H	Realistic error management

5   The Results

The following section details the results obtained at each step of the protocol.

Step 1: Identify all potentially relevant applications.

To identify all potentially relevant applications a search of the online store of each platform was conducted using the keyword *"Diabetes"*. The results of the search on each platform are presented in Table 2. It can be seen that there are over 150 applications returned on both the iOS and Android platforms, but only 28 apps were found in the Blackberry App World.

Table 2. Number of apps returned by platform

iOS	Android	Blackberry
231	168	28

Step 2: Remove light or old versions of each application.

The next step of the protocol is to remove any light or old versions of applications already included in the results. As these applications are already represented, to evaluate both would require additional, unnecessary resources. The number of applications that were removed on each platform is presented in Table 3. It can be seen that only a small number, (less than 10%) of applications were removed, indicating that most applications are unique.

Table 3. Number of apps remaining after removing old and light versions

	iOS	Android	Blackberry
Number of Applications	231	168	28
Old or light versions	9	6	1
Apps remaining	222	162	27

Step 3: Identify the main functional requirements and exclude all applications that do not offer this functionality.

Recent studies have shown that users of healthcare apps prefer those that facilitate everyday tasks such as tracking blood glucose to those which are designed as reference tools [13]. The primary functionality was therefore chosen to model a daily diabetes management diary. The diary is only useful if the results can be visualized and transmitted to a backup computer however, and so tasks were developed to test these features as well. The functionality that was considered to be the minimum for any such application was mapped to the tasks shown in Table 4:

Table 4. Tasks to evaluate main functional requirements

Task	Functional requirements
1	Set measurement units
2	Log blood glucose level
3	Log carbohydrate intake
4	Log insulin dose
5	Display data graphically
6	Export data via email or similar

The reasons for choosing this functionality are outlined below:

- *Set measurement units*: some applications only permit units to be set to those used in a particular country, such as Mmol/L in Europe or Mg/dl in the United States. To be used internationally the app must allow the measurement units to be changed according to the users' preference.
- *Log blood glucose, insulin and carbohydrate*: Maintaining the blood glucose, insulin and carbohydrate levels over time can help patients with diabetes to better predict the onset of symptoms and take corrective action when necessary.
- *Display data graphically:* data in graphics can be easily understood and shows trends and patterns that can be used to indicate when patients are required to adjust the amount of insulin they are required to inject.
- *Export data via email or similar:* mobile devices have a very limited storing capacity, so there needs to be a facility to export data to an external source.

The descriptions and the developers' websites for each application were examined to exclude those that clearly did not offer the primary functionality shown in Table 4. After this, the remaining applications were downloaded and tested in order to determine if all six tasks could be completed and the results are summarized in Table 5. It can be seen that only a very small number of applications on each platform provided all of the necessary functionality.

Table 5. Number of apps on which all tasks can be performed

	iOS	Android	Blackberry
Number of apps	8	6	1

The applications that were excluded at this step were varied and included general medical information references to cookbooks offering recipes suitable for patients suffering from diabetes. Some of the applications did offer some of the desired functionality, but these applications were removed since the completion of all of the tasks was deemed to be essential for the effective management of diabetes.

Step 4: Identify all secondary functional requirements.

The purpose of this step was to elicit potential functional requirements that go beyond the minimum level identified in Step 3, which could subsequently be ranked by patients to obtain a measure of their usefulness. The requirements common to all the three platforms were as follows:

- *Log physical activity and other medication*: these factors, among others, can affect the insulin dose and are therefore logged by some applications.
- *Allow personal settings*: nearly all of the applications include a number of personal settings, such as the target blood glucose level. Some applications which featured a dosage calculator, for calculating the correct dosage, also allowed additional personal settings required for this calculation.

A number of additional features were found on only one or two platforms:

- *Decision support*: some applications offer basic support in calculating the insulin dose, but none offers any intelligent decision support.
- *Alcohol intake, illness, weight, blood pressure, allergies and hypoglycemia*: these factors, as well as physical activity and other medication, can affect the insulin dose and are therefore considered by some applications.
- *Carbohydrate database*: some applications include a database of nutritional information of certain types of food to facilitate calculations.
- *Discussion forums*: anonymous discussion forums can be a source of support for people with diabetes.
- *Export to online healthcare systems*: there is a growing demand for applications that store information securely in a way that can be shared with other selected users [17], including clinicians.
- *Ability to set reminders*: a number of applications have this facility, which is useful for long-acting insulin.
- *Backup and restore:* some applications have automatic backup and restore facilities over a wireless network. These facilities allow data to be recovered if the app is lost or damaged.
- *Add notes:* some applications allow users to enter a note with the logged data to record additional information about the data entered.
- *Insulin dose calculator*: some applications include a calculator for recommending insulin dosages.
- *Log pharmacies*: some applications have an option to log the information (phone, address, etc.) of pharmacies.
- *Log lab results*: there is an option to log the results of the laboratory analysis like sugar, A1C, HDL, LDL, cholesterol, triglycerides and creatinine.

A summary of the fulfillment of these requirements by applications on the three platforms is shown in Table 6.

Table 6. Additional requirements met by applications on each platform

Requirement	iPhone	Android	BlackBerry
Ability to set reminders	X	X	
Add notes		X	
Allow personal settings	X	X	X
Backup and restore		X	
Carbohydrate database	X		
Decision support	X		
Discussion forums	X		
Export to online health system	X		
Insulin dose calculator		X	
Log alcohol intake	X		
Log allergies			X
Log blood pressure		X	
Log hypoglycaemia	X		
Log illness	X		
Log lab results			X
Log other medication	X	X	X
Log pharmacies			X
Log physical activity	X	X	X
Log weight		X	

Step 5a: Perform keystroke level modelling analysis.

Each of the 15 apps that resulted from Step 3 were now subjected to a keystroke level modelling analysis, using the tasks listed in Table 4. The KLM was performed by counting the number of interactions required to complete each task.

Results for iOS

The results of the KLM analysis performed on the final 8 applications on the iOS platform are shown in Table 7.

Table 7. Results of KLM for iOS applications

Application Task:	1	2	3	4	5	6	Total
RapidCalc Insulin Dose Manager	10	2	1	3	2	1	19
GluCoMo	5	5	4	4	1	3	22
Diabetes Diary	5	3	3	2	3	6	22
Diabetes Personal Manager	3	7	4	3	3	6	26
DiabetesPlus	2	7	6	6	1	6	28
LogFrog DB	6	5	6	5	1	7	30
Diabetes Buddy Control your Blood Sugar	3	9	10	7	1	8	38
Diabetes Pilot	5	5	7	3	3	27	50

In Table 7 it can be seen that task 6 (export via email or similar) is far less efficient on the Diabetes Pilot app than any of the others. This is because it requires the user to type the entire address which can be difficult on a small keyboard rather than using default settings or the contact list.

Also task 1 (set measurement units) is less efficient on the RapidCalc app than the other applications because it is necessary to exit the application and enter the iPhone settings to carry out this task, but it is arguable that efficiency is less crucial here since the task is usually only carried out once.

The data logging occurs so frequently that it is essential for it to be as efficient as possible. The tasks that are concerned with data logging are 2 (log blood glucose), 3 (log carbohydrate) and 4 (log insulin), and the figures in Table 4 suggest the Rapid-Calc app and the Diabetes Diary app use the most efficient methods for this. Unfortunately this does not tell us anything conclusive about data entry methods, since RapidCalc uses sliders, whereas Diabetes Diary uses either a picker or a keyboard. The input methods used for each application are shown in Table 8.

Table 8. Data entry methods for iPhone applications

Application	Data Entry Method
RapidCalc Insulin Dose Manager	Sliders on same screen
GluCoMo	Pickers on separate screens
Diabetes Diary	Pickers or keyboard on same screen
Diabetes Personal Manager	Keyboard on same screen
DiabetesPlus	Pickers on separate screens
LogFrog DB	Dials on separate screens
Diabetes Buddy	Keyboard on separate screens
Diabetes Pilot	Keyboard on separate screens

Results for Android

The results of the KLM analysis performed on the final 6 applications on the Android platform are shown in Table 9. It can be seen that tasks 3 (log carbohydrate) and 4 (log insulin dose) are less efficient on the GlucoJournal app than on any of the others.

Focusing on data logging (tasks 2, 3 and 4), the most efficient application is Glucometro, and the least efficient is GlucoJournal. These data are consistent with the total scores, because the GlucoJournal and DiabetesBox apps score the worst in the KLM analysis, as they need 38 touches of the screen to fulfill all tasks, and the Glucometro app is the best, as it only needs only 29 interactions.

Table 9. Results of the KLM analysis for Android applications

Application Task:	1	2	3	4	5	6	Total
OnTrack Diabetes	4	7	8	9	2	5	35
Glucool	3	9	8	9	2	3	34
DiabetesBox	5	9	8	10	3	3	38
Glucometro	4	7	7	6	1	4	29
Track3 Diabetes Planner	5	9	9	6	2	4	35
GlucoJournal	3	5	10	13	2	5	38

The data entry methods of these applications shown in Table 10 do not really explain the differences in efficiency since all of the applications used a keyboard, and in general each number had to be input on a separate screen.

Table 10. Data entry methods for Android applications

Application	Data Entry Method
OnTrack Diabetes	Keyboard (on same or separate screen)
Glucool	Keyboard or "+" and "-" buttons (on separate screens)
DiabetesBox	Keyboard on separate screens
Glucometro	Keyboard on separate screens
Track3 Diabetes Planner	Keyboard on separate screens
GlucoJournal	Keyboard (on same or separate screen)

Results for Blackberry

The results of the KLM for the BlackBerry application are shown in Table 11.

Table 11. Results of KLM for the BlackBerry application

Application Task:	1	2	3	4	5	6	Total
iRecordit Diabetes Sugar Glucose and Health Tracker	20	57	16	13	2	11	119

As there is only one relevant application on the BlackBerry platform there is no comparison we can perform, but it is clear that task 5 is the easiest to accomplish (only 2 interactions) and task 2 is the most difficult to perform (57 interactions).

The data entry methods of this application is a picker for glucose and keyboard for carbohydrate and insulin, all on the same screen, as it is shown in Table 12. The picker for glucose is very small, and it contains only default values from which the user has to select one. The carbohydrates and the insulin can be entered through the keyboard.

Table 12. Data entry methods for the BlackBerry application

Application	Data Entry Method
iRecordit Diabetes Sugar Glucose and Health Tracker	Little picker (for glucose) and keyboard (for carbohydrate and insulin) on same screen

Summary of KLM Results

The process of conducting the KLM led to the following observations, all of which can affect the usability of mobile applications:

- Neither of the standard numeric keyboards offered by the iOS platform is ideal for the efficient input of decimal point numbers, since one is intended purely for integers and the other includes unnecessary symbols such as currency delimiters
- Pickers and sliders need to be designed carefully, since they are very difficult to use if they are too fine grained.
- If several numbers need to be input together then the screens should be designed so that they can all be input from the same screen.
- The haptic feedback offered by the keyboard on the Blackberry does not appear to offer increased efficiency but it may increase satisfaction.

Step 5b: Perform heuristic evaluation.

The applications that scored the best in the KLM analysis were then the subject of heuristic evaluation by three to five expert evaluators. For the purposes of this study, each mobile heuristic, defined in Table 1, was broken down into sub-divisions to be assessed by each evaluator using Nielsen's severity Ranking Scale as detailed in Table 13. Some of these sub-divisions were specific to the domain of diabetes management and are given in Table 14.

Table 13. Nielsen's Severity Ranking Scale (SRS)

Rating	Description
0	I don't agree that this is a usability problem at all
1	Cosmetic problem only. Need not be fixed unless extra time is available on project
2	Minor usability problem. Fixing this should be given low priority
3	Major usability problem. Important to fix, so should be given high Priority
4	Usability catastrophe. Imperative to fix this before product can be released

Table 14. Heuristic sub-divisions

A	A1 The battery status is visible
	A2 The network status is visible when transmitting data
	A3 The time is visible when entering data
	A4 The previously logged data and personal settings can be recovered if the device is lost
B	B1 The information appears in a natural and logical order
	B2 The information is presented clearly
	B3 You can see where everything is that you might need
C	C1 It is easy to see how to do tasks like entering blood glucose and carbohydrates
	C2 There are no objects on the interface that you would not expect to see
D	D1 The screens are well-designed and clear
	D2 The dialogues do not contain information that is irrelevant or rarely used
E	E1 It is easy to input the numbers
	E2 It is easy to see what the information on each screen means
	E3 You can easily navigate around the app
	E4 The screens have a 'back' button
	E5 The user can get crucial information 'at a glance'
F	F1 The user can personalise the system sufficiently
	F2 The system allows efficient input of data
G	G1 The design looks good
	G2 There are suitable provisions for security and privacy (eg Transmission of data is encrypted.)
H	H1 Users can recover from errors easily (If something goes wrong you can get back to where you were easily.)
	H2 If data is input incorrectly, it can be edited
	H3 There an Undo button, where appropriate

Each evaluator ranked each sub-division and provided evidence and comments for each ranking. This evaluation highlighted some problems that had not been identified by the KLM. For example, there are some applications that include unnecessary options or irrelevant information, which may confuse the user. Security was also identified as a problem of the evaluated applications, because none of these encrypt the data transfer, which would be appropriate for sending personal healthcare information over the Internet. Some applications show errors that are unrecoverable and cause the application to shutdown, which is disconcerting and annoying to the user. It is beyond the scope of this paper to give a full qualitative summary of the evaluation, which is presented in [18], but the summaries of the numerical rankings are included here.

Results for iOS

Five evaluators ranked the iOS applications, and a summary of the results is shown in Table 15.

Table 15. Average heuristic ranking for iOS applications

Heuristic:	A	B	C	D	E	F	G	H	Total
RapidCalc	1.1	0.9	0.4	0.4	0.8	1.3	1.3	2.0	8.2
GluCoMo	0.6	1.4	1.2	1.7	0.8	1.3	1.3	1.7	10
Diabetes Diary	0.5	0.8	0.9	0.5	0.9	0.7	1.4	0.8	6.5
Diabetes Personal Manager	0.6	0.8	0.9	1.1	1.1	0.9	1.6	2.3	9.3
Total	2.8	3.9	3.4	3.7	3.6	4.2	5.6	6.8	34

The application which produced the lowest score, and hence is deemed the most usable, was Diabetes Diary; and the least usable was GluCoMo, because it scored the most severe usability ranking. The heuristics that GluCoMo scored least well on were D and H, which were those concerned with minimalist design and error management, and this was probably because this application includes a lot of additional functionality beyond that specified by the tasks in Table 4.

The heuristics that had the highest total scores and were therefore the worst overall were G (Aesthetic, privacy and social conventions) and H (Realistic error management). This is because most applications did not offer any form of security when transmitting data, and because the iPhone does not include a 'Back' or 'Undo' button, unlike the other platforms considered here.

Results for Android

The four applications that were determined to be most efficient through the KLM analysis for the Android platform were also subject to heuristic evaluation, but this time by four expert evaluators. The average rankings for the Android applications are shown in Table 16.

Table 16. Average heuristic ranking for Android applications

Heuristic:	A	B	C	D	E	F	G	H	Total
OnTrack Diabetes	0.1	0.8	0.9	0.5	0.8	0.6	0.6	1.0	5.3
Glucool	0.3	0.3	0.4	0.4	0.3	0.6	0.6	0.3	3.2
Glucometro	0.5	1.0	1.4	0.8	0.9	1.1	0.6	1.7	8.0
Track3 Diabetes Planner	0.8	1.3	1.1	0.9	1.00	1.1	1.3	2.0	9.5
Total	1.7	3.4	3.8	2.6	3.0	3.4	3.1	5.0	26

The application which scored the lowest, and hence was most usable, was Glucool; and the least usable was Track3 Diabetes Planner. Some of the features that caused Glucool to score well were its good backup and restore options, its ability to log all data on a single screen and the clarity of its graphs. Track3 on the other hand was over-complicated with graphics that were difficult to interpret and no option to edit data. The heuristics that had the highest total scores and were therefore the worst overall were C (Consistency and mapping) and H (Realistic error management).

Results for Blackberry

Four expert evaluators performed the heuristic evaluation on the Blackberry application, and the averages of their evaluations are shown in Table 17.

Table 17. Average heuristic ranking for the BlackBerry application

Heuristic:	A	B	C	D	E	F	G	H	Total
iRecordit Diabetes Sugar Glucose and Health Tracker	2.44	1.58	1.38	1.88	1.5	1.5	1.75	0.42	12.4

The heuristic that was scored worst was A (Visibility of system status) because the battery status and the network status are never visible while using the application; the time is visible at the top of the screen but it is necessary to scroll down to add data which loses visibility of the status bar, including the time; and there is no option to backup up and restore the data leading to recovery problems. Heuristics D (Good ergonomics and minimalist design) and G (Aesthetic, privacy and social conventions) were found to be the next worst source of problems because some screens are too long and difficult to use; and the application does not have provisions for security and privacy as data is sent by unencrypted email.

6   Discussion of the Results

Perhaps the most striking observation is the sheer number of applications that are associated with diabetes management on each of the three platforms considered here. There were far more applications available for iOS and Android than Blackberry perhaps because the latter is aimed predominately at the business market. The quality of the applications was highly variable, with those written for the Android platform being particularly prone to crashing.

The keystroke level modelling highlighted some differences in the usability and efficiency of the apps on the various platforms. The number of keystrokes for finishing the tasks on average was 29 on the iPhone, 34 on the Android and 119 on the Black-Berry. The difference is evident especially between BlackBerry and the other platforms. This is due to the hard buttons that are on the BlackBerry devices, as opposed to the soft buttons and touch screens of the Android and iPhone devices. So with a Blackberry a key must be pressed several times to move the mouse or the cursor across the screen, but the other devices only need one click. The efficiency analysis has led us to suggest the following guidelines:

- Use default settings where possible (eg email addresses, dose calculation parameters)
- When using pickers and sliders, do not make them too fine grained, otherwise data entry is very inefficient
- When entering numeric data, display a numeric keyboard instead of an alphabetical keyboard, and only use the integer keyboard when appropriate.
- Do not use acronyms without explaining what they mean [19].
- Personalisation of settings should be adjusted within the app, rather than within the device settings

The heuristic evaluation exposed a different set of problems from the KLM, because it was guided by the mobile heuristics of [6], which are not related to efficiency. The most commonly breached heuristics were A, C, D, G and H, which lead us to the following associated guidelines

- The battery status and time should be visible while using the application. (A)
- The network status should be visible while sending data. (A)
- Provide options for backing up and restoring data. (A)
- Do not include unnecessary options or irrelevant information. (C)
- Do not overload a screen with too many elements [20]. (D)
- All data transmission should be encrypted.(G)
- Do not allow unrecoverable errors.(H)

The heuristic evaluation also showed that the most usable application was found on the Android platform. Glucool on the Android was found to contain the least usability issues across all platforms. The leading application on either of the other platforms was Diabetes Diary which was found to be less than half as usable as Glucool. The following shows how the best rated apps on each platform compare.

- The best application for the iPhone for the heuristic evaluation is the Diabetes Diary (rated 6.5), which was the second best rated (with 22 keystrokes) application in the KLM analysis of the iOS applications.
- The best application for the Android platform for the heuristic evaluation is Glucool (rated 3.2), which was also the second best rated (with 34 keystrokes) application in the KLM analysis.
- Finally, the best (and unique) application for the BlackBerry platform for the heuristic evaluation is iRecordIt (rated 12.4), which had 119 keystrokes in the KLM analysis.

The Diabetes Diary application has now been tested further on potential users in a subsequent experiment, which was restricted to the iOS platform for practical reasons.

The gathering of secondary functional requirements generated a wider range for the iOS platform than in the Android or Blackberry platforms, the latter of which was the most restricted, with only four additional functions. The full list of functionality gathered in Step 4 has also been presented to all of the participants in the user study for utility ranking. The most common functions are logging physical activity, logging other medication and allowing personal settings as they are included in applications of each of the three platforms, and so it is expected that these features will be rated highly by users.

7   Threats to Validity

This study had a number of limitations. First, it was restricted to applications running on the iOS, Android and Blackberry smart phone platforms. These were chosen because they have the highest market share in the UK [21], and jointly occupy 75.5% of the total market. It was also restricted to native applications, since such applications can take advantage of device-specific features which are particularly interesting to developers. The user perception of applications, as demonstrated by characteristics such as the popularity rating, was ignored because the goal was to assess each one solely according to the attributes listed above. Finally, recent studies have shown that users overwhelmingly prefer apps that use the unique features of mobile phones to facilitate tedious tasks such as tracking blood glucose to those which offer purely reference information [13]. Therefore, this survey was focused on apps that were designed for such purposes, and tasks were devised specifically to evaluate data entry methods, data visualisation and personalisation.

8   Conclusions and Future Work

This paper contains a summary of the results of a systematic survey of mobile applications for diabetes management across three smart phone platforms. The platforms operated on devices with different characteristics, with the iPhone being entirely touch screen, the Blackberry having no touch screen capability and the Android phone with touch screen capability, as well as the three standard keys (Home, Menu and Back).

This study concentrated on apps that were designed for frequent logging of data, but which also offered the capability for data visualisation, transmission and personalisation. The research has achieved its goal in terms of exposing problems with efficiency and various other attributes corresponding to mobile heuristics, as well as helping to elicit functional requirements, and this has resulted in a list of guidelines for development. It is hoped that the protocol followed here will therefore also prove useful to developers in other application domains, as it is a lightweight protocol which is not too time-consuming.

The study was restricted both in the choice of platforms, and in the choice of diabetes as a healthcare domain. Future work will include a survey of similar apps on other platforms, and research into self-management applications for other branches of healthcare. The work described here was restricted to expert evaluators rather than potential users, and utilised only two of the many existing techniques for evaluating user interfaces, namely KLM and heuristics. It might therefore be useful to consider incorporating other techniques in the future, such as cognitive walkthrough. Users are also being involved in a complementary user study, using the iOS app that scored best in this heuristic evaluation (Diabetes Diary). The purpose of the user study is to determine the nature and frequency of user errors, and to establish a comprehensive list of functional and non-functional requirements for the apps.

One of the shortcomings of this work was the KLM analysis, which involved counting the number of keystrokes to accomplish a task. This can be rather error-prone, since (for example) the number of finger swipes required to move a picker to a desired location can vary considerably, depending on the user. This is just one type of interaction introduced by mobile technologies that will be investigated in the future to determine how the KLM analysis technique can be adapted to provide a more accurate measurement of efficiency.

Acknowledgments. The authors would like to thank Oxford Brookes University and the University of Alcalá for generous support towards this research. They would also like to thank the expert usability evaluators who took part in the heuristic evaluation.

References

1. Alagöz, F., Calero Valdez, A., Wilkowska, W., Ziefle, M., Dorner, S., Holzinger, A.: From Cloud Computing to Mobile Internet, From User Focus to Culture and Hedonism: The Crucible of Mobile Health Care and Wellness Applications. In: IEEE 5th International Conference on Pervasive Computing and Applications, pp. 38–45 (2010)
2. Preuveneers, D., Berbers, Y.: Mobile phones assisting with health self-care: a diabetes case study. In: Proceedings MobileHCI 2008 Proceedings of the 10th International Conference on Human Computer Interaction with Mobile Devices and Services (2008).
3. Bellazzi, R.: Telemedicine and Diabetes Management: Current Challenges and Future Resarch Directions. Journal of Diabetes Science and Technology 2(1), 98–104 (2008)
4. Calero Valdez, A., Ziefle, M., Alagöz, F., Holzinger, A.: Mental Models of Menu Structures in Diabetes Assistants. In: Miesenberger, K., Klaus, J., Zagler, W., Karshmer, A. (eds.) ICCHP 2010. LNCS, vol. 6180, pp. 584–591. Springer, Heidelberg (2010) ISBN: 978-3-642-14099-0
5. Nielsen, J.: Usability Engineering. Morgan Kaufmann Publishers (1994)
6. Bertini, E., Catarci, T., Dix, A., Gabrielli, S., Kimani, S., Santucci, G.: Appropriating Heuristic Evaluation Methods for Mobile. International Journal of Mobile Human Computer Interaction 1(1), 20–41 (2009)
7. Martin, C., Flood, D., Harrison, R.: A Protocol for Evaluating Mobile Applications. In: Proceedings of the IADIS (2011)
8. Flood, D., Harrison, R., Duce, D.: Using Mobile Apps: Investigating the usability of mobile apps from the users perspective. International Journal of Mobile HCI (submitted)
9. Poropatich, R., Pavliscsak, H.H., Rasche, J., Barrigan, C., Vigersky, R.A., Fonda, S.J., et al.: Mobile Healthcare in the US army. Wireless Health, 184–187 (2010)
10. W3C. Mobile Web Application Best Practices, http://www.w3.org/TR/mwabp/
11. International Organization for Standardization. Medical devices – Application of usability engineering to medical devices. International standard ISO 62366: 2007, Switzerland (2007)

12. Kjeldskov, J., Stage, J.: New techniques for usability evaluation of mobile systems. International Journal of Human Computer Studies 60(5-6), 599–620 (2004)

13. Liu, C., Zhu, Q., Holroyd, K.A., Seng, E.K. Status and Trends of Mobile-Health Applications for iOS Devices: a Developer's Perspective. Journal of Systems and Software (July 2011)

14. Zhang, D., Adipat, B.: Challenges, Methodologies, and Issues in the Usability Testing of Mobile Applications. International Journal of Human-Computer Interaction 18(3), 293–308 (2005)

15. Card, S.K., Thomas, T.P., Newall, A.: The Psychology of Human-Computer Interaction. Lawrence Erbaum Associates, London (1983)

16. Nielsen, J., Molich, R.: Heuristic evaluation of user interfaces. In: The Conference on Human Factors in Computing Systems: CHI 1990 (1990)

17. Greenhalgh, T., Hinder, S., et al.: Adoption, non-adoption, and abandonment of a personal electronic health record: case study of HealthSpace. BMJ (Clinical Research Ed.) 341, c5814 (2010)

18. Martin, C. , Flood, D., Sutton, D., Aldea, A., Waite, M., Garcia, E., Garcia, A.: A System-atic Evaluation of Mobile Applications for Diabetes Management using Heuristics (submitted)

19. Nielsen, J., Tahir, M.: Homepage Usability: 50 Websites Deconstructed. New Riders Publishing (2001)

20. Rosenholtz, R., Li, Y., Mansfield, J., Jin, Z.: Feature Congestion: A Measure of Display Clutter. In: The Conference on Human Factors in Computing Systems: CHI 2005 (2005)

21. `http://www.onlinemarketing-trends.com/2011/04/smartphone-marketshare-2011-italyus-aus.html`

eHealth Service Discovery Framework: A Case Study in Ethiopia

Tesfa Tegegne and Theo van der Weide

Radboud University, Nijmegen, Netherlands
{tvdw,t.tegegne}@cs.ru.nl

Abstract. *eHealth* services just as general Health services mostly emphasize on patient record management systems. Unfortunately the information in these records is rarely used to provide quicker, personalized eHealth services and appropriate treatment especially in a low infrastructure context where health service providers are often overwhelmed by numbers leading to acute degradation in service delivery. Domain specific service discovery with personalization aims at providing user-aware services. This is very important in a low infrastructure context where most patient requirements particularly from rural areas are a consequence of low literacy levels. The focus of this paper is to describe a framework for eHealth service discovery in a low infrastructure context. To do this, we categorize the context of users and augment it with a user specific profile. Our framework provides ontology based, context-aware semantic and personalized services.

1 Introduction

Health services in a low infrastructure context are characterized by long queues, insufficient drugs, insufficient service providers and generally low literacy levels on the side of service consumers [22,19,18,6]. Services tend to be generic due to lack of specialized resources and a reasonable number of ailments can be avoided with appropriate education and advisory support. eHealth services are proliferating in countries with limited infrastructure (electricity, Internet) as a means of supporting the general health services. However, appropriate services need to be discovered first in order to support the provision of appropriate services to the right consumers. Moreover, customizing health services to different segments of patients can greatly save time while providing the available service to those that need it most.

In most developing countries, health services are provided by a combination of private and government centers, each with different capacity and competencies. As a result, health service providers are autonomous but rely on other centers for capabilities that they can not provide. To support this autonomous and dependence nature of health services, we consider the service-oriented architecture (SOA) (see [3,10]). The corresponding service-oriented computing (SOC) provides a system architecture in which a collection of loosely coupled services (components) directly communicate with each other using standard interfaces

A. Holzinger and K.-M. Simonic (Eds.): USAB 2011, LNCS 7058, pp. 397–416, 2011.

and message-exchanging protocols. Software services or simply services are self-contained, platform-agnostic computational elements that support rapid, low-cost and easy composition of loosely coupled distributed software applications. The functionality provided by a service can range from answering simple requests to executing sophisticated processes requiring peer to peer or client/server relationships between multiple layers of service consumers and providers [3,10].

Existing service oriented health care systems emphasize on patient record management, giving personalized health care assistance to patients, online consultation and advisory of patients. However, the communication among health professionals by modern technology has not yet been addressed. For example, Uganda implemented a wireless regional health care network to assist the rural health care workers in providing learning materials, email, and to enable outbreak reporting. Generally, this network is used for data collection systems. The eHealth systems developed so far does not provide professional assistance, for example when new cases or symptoms are encountered.

In this paper we first shortly describe some related work. In section 3 we elaborate on the application of Service Oriented Architecture in the health care domain. Then in section 4 we analyze the current situation of Ethiopia, derive next steps using a SWOT analysis and show how the architecture proposed is motivated from these next steps. In section 5 we describe service discovery in more detail and go into more detail about personalization and context awareness. We close in section 6 with some conclusions.

2   Related Work

Service discovery is one of the challenging activities of SOA. For example, Hasselmyer [10] describes the process of finding services. Most studies done sofar include service semantics, ontology based and context based service discovery. To the best of our knowledge, these three components have not been used together to discover services. In previous work service personalization or user profiling (user behavior and preferences) was given no attention. However, Hasselmyer [10] and Vu et al. [28] report that contextual information of services is available, complete and unambiguous. They ignore how to handle missing, redundant, or incomplete context information. In this paper we have divided context-awareness of services into service context and user context, which enables a richer handling of context.

In relation to health care service discovery very few research has been conducted [6,22]. For example, John et al. [22] mentioned eHealth projects under implementation in Uganda, South Africa and Nigeria (UHIN, Cell-Life and MindSet Health, LAMIS respectively), however as cited by Kehinde et al. and Drury [18,6], there are 12 million AIDS orphans in Africa. In line with this, Kehinde et al. [18] indicated that developing countries face challenges in providing accessible, efficient and equitable quality health services to their people.

3   SOA for Healthcare

The advancement of ICT and its application in different aspect have change the way we live, communicate and behave. Information Communication Technologies have gradually become part of our daily lives through Internet that allow computers and mobile phones to provide various remote services.

The application of ICT has become a worldwide trend. Impregnating Service-Oriented Architecture (SOA) to provide common activities and interests such as business, medicine, lifestyle, traffic, education, and entertainment has also become one of the popular methods in various industries.

The rapid rise of technology and its adoption into the healthcare field has caused healthcare organizations to collect an accumulation of non-interoperable systems that not only need to work together within the organization, but also are accessed from the outside. The burden of integration usually falls on the users of the system, who often are forced to access many different systems to complete one task. The use of a service oriented architecture (SOA), however, can improve the delivery of important information and make the sharing of data across a community of care practical in cost, security, and risk of deployment [14]. According to Peter [12] *SOA for healthcare is designed to give healthcare providers, healthcare benefit organizations, public health, and pharmaceutical companies the flexibility to leverage clinical and administrative business applications independently of the underlying computing platform.*

The ultimate purpose of integrating SOA for healthcare domain is to improve effectiveness, efficiency and service delivery. The application of SOA to healthcare service has the following objectives [12,14]:

- reduced stay
- improved patient outcomes/reduce risks
- revenue improvement
- staff efficiency
- improved patient and staff satisfaction
- reduced IT expenditure/maintainance costs
- improved information accuracy and availability
- exchange of medical information between care providers (hospitals, clinics, health posts) in order to get key information like patients' history, allergies, persistent medical problems, current medication (if any), and active treatments
- exchange of referrals between healthcare providers, labs and feedback of those referral visits
- a means to electronically order and monitor consumption of prescriptions

Effective and timely communication between patients, physicians, nurses, pharmacists, and other healthcare professionals is vital to good healthcare. Current communication mechanisms, based largely on paper records and prescriptions, are old-fashioned, inefficient, and unreliable. In the era of electronic record keeping and communication, the healthcare industry is still tied to paper documents that are easily mislaid, often illegible, and easy to forge [16]. When multiple healthcare professionals and facilities are involved in providing healthcare for a patient, the healthcare services provided are often not coordinated.

This section provides the application of Service Oriented Architecture (SOA) for healthcare domain in order to make health services accessible by anybody anywhere and anytime. Section 3.1 deals with the impact of SOA in healthcare. Section 3.2 addresses the use of mobile phones to improve healthcare services in low resources environment and a case study is presented in section 3.3.

3.1   The Impact of SOA in Healthcare for Developing Countries

A healthcare system based on a SOA has the potential to address many of the issues faced by health systems around the world by 1) extending the utilization of medical applications to different types of people including physicians, medical staff, personnel with limited training, and in some cases patients, 2) allowing for the coordination of various different types of multimedia inputs and outputs (text, images, and speech), and 3) creating a system that is flexible, nimble, and highly equipped for system changes [16]

Low level infrastructure development is one of the impediments of setting up a mobile health care system in a low-infrastructure country such as Ethiopia. Despite of its aggressively expanding ICT infrastructure a single state monopolized ETC (Ethiopian Telecommunication Corporation) hardly can meet the infrastructural demands for reaching the huge majority of the rural population.

Building a nationwide eHealth system on existing IT solutions would improve the efficiency of service delivery, enhance quality and enable cost savings for the health system- as well as for private health service providers. To establish such a system and reap its benefits, Ethiopia would need:

- establish centralized electronic health records (EHR) or customize the existing EHR;
- develop infrastructure utilizing already developed infrastructures (WoredaNet, SchoolNet, and mobile networks);
- enable migration from paper to electronic documents.

The ultimate purposes of developing electronic health system in Ethiopia are:

1. Information technologies are used to exchange medical information over a distance using audio, visual and data communication. The application comprises healthcare delivery and management such as diagnosis, treatment, consultation as well as education.
2. The doctor to population ratio is very low (1:37,000). To tackle this problem with mobile health is one of the options for the rural population. In addition, it gives an opportunity to share specialists' knowledge and experiences for remote hospitals, clinics and also for individual healthcare workers and patients, also at an international level.
3. The available health institutions can strengthen their network with referral and teaching hospitals. The existing few number of laboratories and research centers can disseminate their findings and laboratory results to other health

institutions. As an example, IIT Delhi and Tikur Anbesa hospital are working on TeleDermatology.

The existing 'digital divide' in communication technologies such as Internet is lessened by the mobile phone in the resource limited countries.

There is a significant growth of the number of mobile phone (12.2%) subscribers compared to fixed and Internet(1%) subscribers. Consequently, mHealth can play a pivotal role to provide health services for the rural population.

3.2   Anywhere Anytime mHealth

The application of mHealth carries the following promises [11]:

- quick and timely high quality affordable healthcare for all, everywhere, at anytime;
- overcoming healthcare shortage of staff and funding and optimization of patient care;
- enhancing preventive care;
- protecting human rights;
- educating and empowering citizens, etc.

No doubt the potential of mobile communications to radically improve healthcare services is enormous. The time has already proven this. Even in some of the most remote and resource-poor environments mobile health may drastically increased the quality and quantity of healthcare [11].

Mobile health is applicable for collecting clinical data and for quick exchange of information back and forth to medical staff, care givers and patients; for continuous education of healthcare professionals and providers. Many researchers suggest that mHealth is the top priority to alleviate chronic disease burden, scarce infrastructure and in general high level morbidity and mortality in the developing countries [11,6].

Mobile Health is no more an optional choice. The service is more and more advancing and acceptable both by citizens and medical professionals. It is already proven that remote care management service can enhance self-care, change health-related behaviors and improve outcomes in patients with a number of long-term conditions [1].

> *"Mobile Health is already a must, a fantastic challenge for the future but it requires cooperation and coordination at all possible levels, it requires networking and planning, readiness to learn from the others and no efforts to re-invent the wheel" [11].*

3.3   Case Study: Antiretroviral Treatment (ART)

Alexander is a farmer living in the village called Sana found in South Gondar zone in Amhara region. He lives with HIV viruses for the last two years. Two weeks ago he started taking antiretroviral viral drugs. However, recently, he experiences new symptoms such as nausea, diarrhea and headache. Alexander picks up his mobile phone dialling the special number he got for a consult. An automated dialogue system answers the call, asking Alexander the following information: name, age, address, when did he start antiretroviral treatment, when the new symptoms started and how severe they are, and also asks if he has any allergy. After obtaining the necessary information, the dialogue system sends the user request to the query interpreter, an agent that further analyzes the request. by adding personal profile information from the profile database and context information from the context repository. The enriched request is sent to the match making agent to look for the necessary consultation and treatment advises. As a result, the system responds to Alexander that such kind of additional symptoms are common for the couple of weeks after starting the antiretroviral treatment, therefore he has to continue the treatment for a couple of weeks and would the symptoms not disappear to consult a doctor face to face in the nearby health institution.

After 10 days Alexander's condition is getting worse so based on the recommendation of the system he travels to the health center. This story will be continued in section 5.1.

The above scenario depicts that mobile technology permits the venue of health control to shift from hospital systems to information systems deployed at the location where users live and move, promoting the evaluation from *facility-centered* services, mainly focussed on patient treatment within hospitals, to *patient-centered* services, providing anywhere anytime care support to patients while they are at home or on the move. Mobile aeromedicine, remote patient monitoring, location-based medical services, and emergency response represents examples of novel *patient-centered* services [27]. According to Toninelli et al. [27] security, interoperability and user and service mobility are some of the challenges in delivering mobile based healthcare enterprises. For example, Alexander needs to be provided with lists of treatments and precautions advices/consultations based on his physical conditions and his context.

Effective healthcare service discovery is a complex task in mobile healthcare environment and requires tackling several technical challenges at the state of the art, including security, mobility (user and device), interoperability, accessibility (availability), heterogeneity and reliability.

4   The SWOT Analysis

In this section we perform a SWOT analysis of the health care organization in Ethiopia as a motivation for the approach as presented in this paper. Typically a SWOT analysis is used to identify on the one hand the strengths and weaknesses (internal factors) of an organization and on the other hand the opportunities and threats (external factors) that come from its external environment. By confronting these internal and external factors in a so-called confrontation matrix, alternative best next steps may be obtained. A SWOT analysis is the base for developing a strategy for an organization that takes benefit from its strengths and the available opportunities, and is aware of the weaknesses of the organization and its external threats.

4.1   Background

Ethiopia is still ranking among the lowest income countries worldwide. The country also ranks high amongst the donor receiving countries worldwide. As a developing country, Ethiopia, has promising prospects with Figure 1 indicating one of the fast developing [7].

Table 1. Worlds top 5 fastest growing economies, taken from [7]

2001-2010		2011-2015	
1. Angola	11.1	1. China	9.5
2. China	10.5	2. India	8.2
3. Myanmar	10.3	3. **Ethiopia**	**8.1**
4. Nigeria	8.9	4. Mozambique	7.7
5. **Ethiopia**	**8.4**	5. Tanzania	7.2

Currently, Ethiopia still ranks among the worst countries in the world in terms of health service coverage and health outcomes. Per capita health expenditures are approximately 25$ PPP, which is significantly lower than the Sub-Sahara Africa average of 89$ PPP (World Bank 2004). The number of health workers per capita (11 nurses and 2 physicians per 100,000 inhabitants) remains extremely low even by African standards.

As in most low income countries, the Ethiopian health sector is dominated by the public sector: 73% of the nurses and 82% of the doctors work for the public sector. However, both the profit and non-profit sectors are growing. The governments' upcoming five years (2011- 2015) Growth and Transformational Plan (GTP) [21] looks promising for the health sector. In the year 2015, the primary health service coverage will reach 100%, maternal mortality rate will reduce to 267 per 100000 and number of mobile subscribers will be expected to reach 61.4 million.

Imbalance distribution of health professionals in the country: with only 36% of nurses and 17% doctors working in rural locations.The public sector remains by far the largest employer, with most doctors (74% working in public hospitals and the majority of nurses working in public hospitals (29%) or public health centers (27%). One-fifth of the doctors and a small proportion of nurses has secondary jobs in private and for-profit clinics in urban areas. Doctors in rural areas earn significantly more than those in urban areas, both in the public or private sector, whereas nurses earn slightly more in urban areas. Doctors working in urban public facilities receive more training and formal evaluation compared to their counterparts, whereas nurses in rural areas seem to work more hours and have more access to training compared with nurses in urban settings [23].

4.2   Strengths and Weaknesses

In this section we discuss the intrinsic (internal) factors of the Ethiopian health care system to consider their strengths and weaknesses.

Information and Communication Technology (ICT) developments in developing countries are still in their infant stage compared to developed countries. In most developing countries ICT is incorporated in governmental policy to solve societal problems. A strong point in the case of Ethiopia is that in the last five years every governmental organization has been involved in business process re-engineering (BPR), using ICT as a tool for improvement. We will refer to this strong point as S_1.

Also the Ethiopian government has improved connectivity by launching (1) an administrative network (WoredaNet) to connect all Ethiopian districts using VSAT technology and (2) a network for high schools (SchoolNet). We will refer to this strong point as strength S_2. However, these networks are provided by the Ethiopian Telecommunication Corporation (ETC) only, leading to a lack of competition in this market. Ethiopia is the last country in Africa monopolizing the telecom services including fixed, mobile, Internet and data communications. This monopolistic control has stifled innovation and retarded expansion. This is referred to as weakness W_1.

Mobile penetration is not huge yet but there is a lot of improvement from year to year. For example the number of mobile subscribers has grown from 500,000 in 2003 to 10.5 million in 2011. There are huge expansion programs, for instance the program to introduce fiber optic cables across the whole country. For example in Amhara region the mobile network coverage reaches about 90%, which provides the rural village to use mobile phones. This will be strength S_3.

The number of health facilities in the country has increased by 55% during 1997 to 2002. This increase rate is greater than the population growth rate in the same period, leading to an improved population-facility ratio. We also see a huge boost up of health professionals. Ethiopia's National Health Accounts show that total health expenditure had grown significantly from $230 million in 1996 to $1.2 billion in 2008. The country's per capita health expenditure has also increased over the last decade, from $4.09 in 1996 to $16.1 in 2008. The increase of health expenditure has been: 1996: $4.09, 2000: $5.6, 2005: $7.13, and 2008: $16.1. The strong point (referred to as S_4) is that we see growth, the weak point is that the actual levels still are very low (weak point W_2).

ICT as means of facilitating a solution to social problems has not yet been fully considered neither by government nor by society. Another problem to make a break through in the usage and development of ICT in healthcare and other sectors are low level education and less priorities given by the government for the advancement of the information and communication technology. This is referred to as weak point W_3. Creating awareness of ICT as an enabler of daily business processes needs to exert some extra efforts. ICT is delivered in schools only in the higher grades (11th and 12th). In most private schools, an ICT course is incorporated in the curricula contrary to governmental or public schools.

4.3   Opportunities and Threats

In this section we focus on the opportunities and threats (external factors) for the Ethiopian health care system that come from the external environment.

After years of international expansion of the Internet, in many areas we see new developments in developing global networks for cooperation and knowledge sharing internationally on the Internet. Around specific topics there are emerging worldwide communities that cooperate to develop such applications. Also for health care we see such developments. Examples are: Health Level 7 (HL7), European Telecommunications Standards Institute (ETSI). In the context of mobile applications we see mHealth Ecosystems and mHealth Initiatives. Most countries have established their eHealth and mHealth systems (Australia, Finland, USA, etc). These new developments offer interesting opportunities to improve facilities in Ethiopia taking advantage of international cooperation. This opportunity is referred to as O_1.

Opening up a society also has some well-known threats, mostly related to brain drain effects. For example, when people see new opportunities they want to make profit of them. This may cause a move of people from rural areas to cities, and from cities to international positions (outside Ethiopia). Migration of health professionals is one of the threats. For example Serra et al [23] say more than 50% of health professionals plan to migrate abroad in the next two years, expecting to earn higher salaries abroad. Also voice-online [30] reported that about 80% of doctors migrate to USA, Botswana , South Africa and middle est countries for better pay and conditions. Accordingly, the number of doctors working in US is more than the doctors working in Ethiopia. They also report that the satisfaction of health professionals with their career choice, economic situation and life in general, has deteriorated between 2004 to 2007. This threat is referred to as T_1.

Exponential growth both is an opportunity and a threat. We have seen many new developments to start following an exponential growth process. For example the introduction of the mobile phone. Exponential growth makes it possible to formulate strategies in a more ambitious way. Note that growth processes in society/nature usually follow the plateau model. The expected growth rate for Ethiopia (see Figure 1) for the coming years may indicate the start of exponential growth. This opportunity is referred to as O_2.

Exponential growth also poses some threats. Introducing new technology too fast will make the country too dependent from external sources. Especially when capacity building at a managerial level is not going hand-in-hand with the new introduction. This threat is referred to as T_2. This requires students to be trained at the international academic levels (bachelor, master and PhD) to manage actual technological processes, to find creative solutions for new problems, and to develop new policies.

Another opportunity is the continuing willingness of donor countries to support Ethiopia in their development process via special programs. This will be opportunity O_3.

Lower level education, lower level/no digital skill, and lower income may be some of the barriers to diffuse eHealth is a major threat to access ICT related services and equipments. This threat is referred as T_3. Inadequate technical infrastructure, knowledge and financial resources have an impact on the expansion of eHealth services.

4.4   The Proposed Strategy

The confrontation matrix combines internal factors (strengths and weaknesses) with external factors (opportunities and threats). In Table 2 we present the confrontation matrix for our case; + indicates a positive effect and − indicates a negative effect. For example a good infrastructure will help to fight brain drain, but monopoly will have a bad influence on taking advantage of opportunity O_1. From the confrontation matrix we see that the strong infrastructure and mobile phone both have a positive influence on the Internet. So using Internet opportunities to improve the health system seems a good option.

Table 2. Confrontation matrix

		Opportunities			Threats		
		O_1 Inter net	O_2 exp growth	O_3 funding	T_1 brain drain	T_2 exp growth	T_3 low educ
Strengths	S_1: global awareness	+	+	+	+	+	-+
	S_2: infrastructure	++	+	+	++	+	+
	S_3: mobile phone	++	++	+	+	+	+
	S_4: fast increase	+	+	+	+	+	-+
Weak nesses	W_1: monopoly	-	-+	-	- -	-	-
	W_2: low level	-	-	-	- -	-	- -
	W_3: ICT facilitator	-+	-+	-	-	-	-

4.5   Analysis of the Confrontation Matrix

The confrontation matrix relates the internal factors of an organization (strengths and weaknesses) with its external factors (opportunities and threats). A high correlation between an internal and external factor (++) suggests a candidate for a next step. In case of an strength, the next step tries to use this strength to take advantage of the related opportunity, or to protect from the related threat. In case of a weakness the next step is to avoid the weakness hindering in taking advantage of the opportunity, or in materializing the threat. We first focus on the most promising next steps and then discuss the main weaknesses to overcome.

First we focus on the strengths that are most helpful for the identified opportunities or most helpful to overcome threats.

S_2 **Infrastructure - O_1 Internet.** As we discussed in the previous subsection, the expansion of networking, electricity, telecommunication boosts up the number of internet users and increases the accessibility of the internet all over the country. The expanding infrastructure is a strong enabler for an efficient introduction of Internet technology.[1]

S_2 **Infrastructure - T_1 Brain drain.** The strongly emerging infrastructure can also help to overcome the brain drain threat in 2 ways. First, it might encourage educated people to find challenges by staying in their country, and it may make them a member of the international community without the need to actually move there. Second, those who still leave the country will more naturally and easily stay a member of their root community.

S_3 **Mobile phone - O_1 Internet.** As we discussed, the Internet is an excellent opportunity for Ethiopia to overcome infrastructural disadvantages. Since Ethiopia has a strongly developing mobile phone coverage, using the mobile phone is a good choice to benefit from the Internet opportunity. One of the specific opportunities we found in the SWOT analysis is the provision of internet services using mobile phones. Without any extra payment or charge, a user can access internet with the cost rate of air time. Its most simple format, the SMS messaging system, already provides such an access.

S_3 **Mobile phone - O_2 Exponential growth.** The effectiveness of the mobile phone strength is especially emphasized by the exponential growth that is to be expected from the introduction of this new technology.

Next we consider the weaknesses that are most threatening for the identified opportunities, or may be considered as negatively influence the threats identified. First we see from the confrontation matrix that there seem to be no major threats for the opportunities identified. With respect to the threats we have:

W_1 **Monopoly - T_1 Brain drain.** Monopoly may prevent newly educated people from being able to identify an effective way to define their contribution. Next steps can really hurt from a market situation that is too inflexible when it comes to adapting to a new technology.

W_2 **Low level - T_1 Brain drain.** Low level is seen as a major cause of brain drain.

W_2 **Low level - T_3 Low education.** Low education level is the major cause for low level.

In the next section we further explore on the role that the Service Oriented Architecture (SOA) can play for healthcare, and then we present a framework that conforms to the findings of the confrontation matrix as described above, and leads to the next steps as suggested by this matrix.

---

[1] For example, the number of mobile sites in Amhara region is about 501 which almost cover all the rural villages/kebeles of the region. Among this mobile stations 95% of them are functional and 5% will be start functioning in a few months. In 2010 the government of Ethiopia bought hundreds of VSAT from Gilat Satellite Networks Ltd company based in Israel. The satellite provides high quality voice, broadband data and video services for school-net and WoredaNet projects.

4.6 The Main Architecture

A health worker is performing medical tasks. At some moments, the health worker needs specific information, and will start a seeking task. As a part of this task concrete information units have to be matched with the actual information need as described in a query. This scheme of working has been described by Jarvelin and Ingwersen ([15]) and is displayed in Figure 1.

According to these authors, interactive IR comprises the work task, information seeking behavior of the user and context of retrieval. The figure considers different contextual factors in the process of service discovery, each contextual factor specifies its own information need/ information request in different perspectives, and its effect is independent from another contextual factors. The advantage of having these contexts helps to identify the appropriate services for the user request by considering current environment constraints, medical status and information seeking behavior of the user besides to personal profile and personal context.

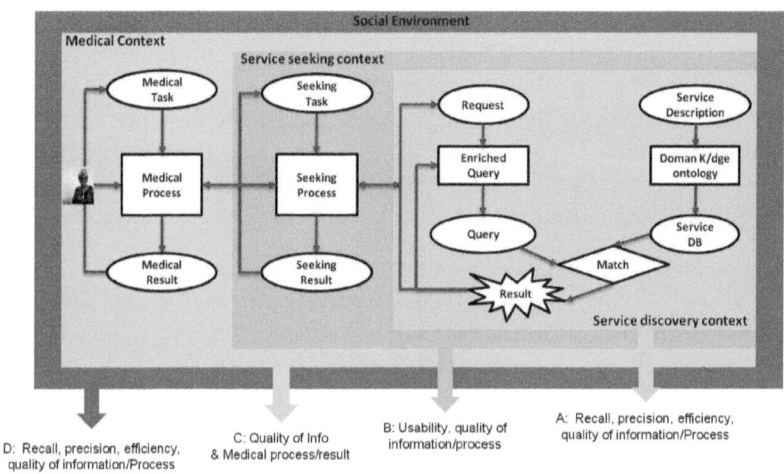

Fig. 1. Service Seeking frameworks and criteria adopted from [15]

In our architecture we focus on the seeking task, and how this can be supported by a service oriented architecture. The agents as described in our case in section 3.3 are presented in the architecture in Figure 2. The medical context is the dominating context, where technical support is obtained from modern technology. Figure 2 described the seeking process from a technical point of view. The dialogue system negotiates with the health worker to obtain a (completed) information or service request. Then the query interpreter further elaborates on the request by adding contextual and personal information to the request. Finally the match maker matches the request with the available services, and tries to find the best treatment (defined as a composition of services) for this request. When the match maker can not resolve the request, a human expert may be asked for advice. From the architecture we see how mobile technology is helping to empower the implemented knowledge distribution, and how experts can be involved with minor dependencies to the location.

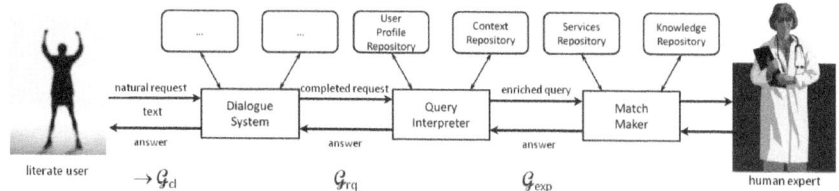

Fig. 2. The main architecture

5 Service Discovery

Typical eHealth setups in low infrastructure context involve Health Extension Workers (HEW) whose main role is to link the largely uneducated masses with Health centers. The proposed framework is presented in Figure 3 in detail. The figure consists of five components: *service Consumer, service provider, spoken dialogue system, service discovery engine, and service repository.* Service providers advertise services. Service consumer as denoted by its name requests services using either voice or text. In this framework our focus lies on voice/spoken based service request using mobile phone. The spoken dialogue performs speech recognition and converts the speech into text and vice versa (for detail see figure 4). The intention of using spoken based service query is to allow semi-literate and illiterate people to use the system. The service discovery engine performs query reformulation by incorporating additional information about users: user profile and user context. After formulating the user query, it processes the matchmaking, ranking and selection of services with respect to the user request. The service repository stores the advertised services.

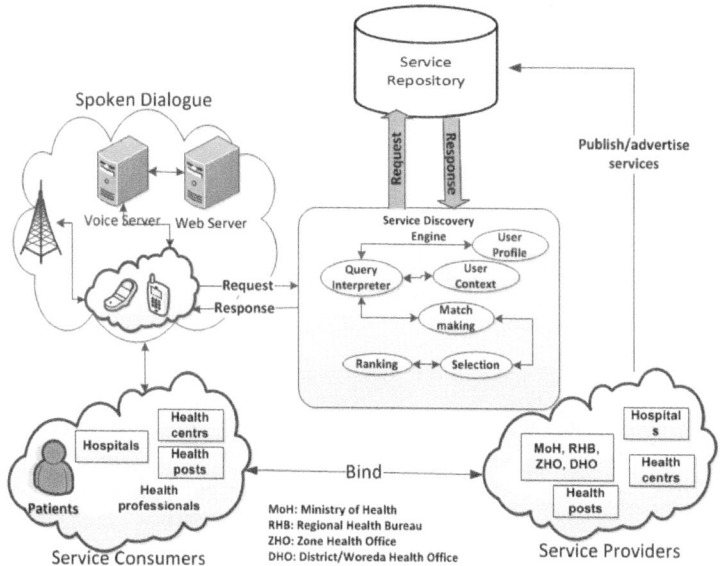

Fig. 3. Service discovery framework/architecture

5.1   Sample Session

In this part we present a sample session within our framework, continuing the case from section 3.3.

After 10 days Alexander's condition has gotten worse so based on the recommendation of the system he travels to the health center. The health center measures his CD4 finding no difference with the previous measurement. The nurse doesn't know what brought the additional symptoms therefore she uses her mobile to contact the eHealth System. Since the nurse is recognized as a health worker, she will get a higher access level into the system. She informs the health system about the symptoms, the lab results, the number of CD4 counted and when the treatment started. The system then asks the nurse to take additional tests and to send the results to the system. The match making agent matches the new patient request with the advertised services. Suitable (combinations of) service(s) found in the repository, are ranked based on user preferences, QoS, and semantics of services. If no matching (combinations of) services are found, then the match maker agent sends the request to the specialist team associated with the eHealth system. The specialist team forwards the services to the requester and to the service repository.

As a result, the nurse will receive the most promising alternative for treatment and reference materials. However HIV is a complex disease that requires specially trained physicians to deliver the complex care necessary for a healthy life. Complicated drug regimens with multiple side effects and long-term complications make treating the HIV disease a challenge. Hence, the system forwards Alexander's data to the HIV specialist. After accessing Alexander's health record, the HIV specialist will follow Alexander's dossier, and may for example contact the the nurse with the request to take an additional test.

The above scenario depicts how the working of the proposed framework. This framework can run on a mobile phone since the communication with the healthcare worker is based on relatively text or voice.

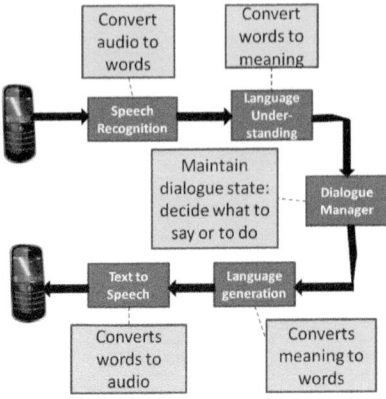

Fig. 4. Spoken dialogue system

5.2   Ontology Based Semantic Service

Service Ontology for Discovery. Ontology from the philosophical perspective is the science of study of being. Philosophical ontology handles the precise utilization of words as a descriptions of entities, it gives an account for those words that belongs to entities, and those do not [17]. In computing and information sciences an ontology represents the set of relevant concepts within a domain of interest and their relationships [17]. The ontology is a formal, explicit specification of a shared conceptualization of a domain, expressing the common understanding of the structure of descriptive information. The ontology makes explicit assumptions thereby separating domain knowledge from operational knowledge. A most important advantage is that an ontology is the basis for logic inference, giving a formal reasoning system for the underlying application domain. By mapping concepts in different ontologies, structured information can be shared. Hence, ontology is a good candidate for expressing context and domain knowledge.

According to D'Mello and Ananthanarayana [5], domain ontology (service ontology) plays a major role in matching service requests with web-based service functionality. Matchmaking algorithms make use of functional elements of web services and semantic relationships of concepts provided by the domain ontology.

The goal of domain ontology is (1) to capture the knowledge of related domains, (2) to provide common understanding of domain knowledge, (3) to determine terms commonly recognized by domain experts, and (4) to well-define these terms and their relationship from formalized patterns of various levels. Domain ontology provides (1) the definition of the domain concepts and their relationships, (2) the actions that may occur in this domain, and (3) the basic principles of this domain [13,5].

Describing Web services using ontology will enhance service discovery. The quality of that discovery depends on the used algorithms and techniques.

Semantic Service Discovery. The semantic matching based discovery mechanism retrieves meanings (semantics) from service descriptions through various means. Depending on the type of information obtained for match making, they are classified as information retrieval based methods, ontology driven methods, context information based methods, goal based methods and functional semantics based methods.

eSDF [25] deals with semantic matching discovery and the quality of service based matching. The former deals with the meaning of the services and the latter with QoS, usability, and personalization (preferences and interests). These two methods of service discovery will facilitate the selection and ranking of services with respect to the advertised and requested services.

The process of semantic service discovery consists of two steps: matching of functionality service aspects (the functional requirement) and service selection based on non functionality aspects of the services. Service selection involves semantic matching and ranking to select a single most relevant service to be invoked, starting from a given set of available services. Semantic service matching is the pairwise comparison of an advertised service with a required service (query) to determine the degree of their semantic match [5]. This process can be non-logic-based, logic-based or hybrid, depending on the nature of the reasoning style used by the matchmaker to compute partially or totally ordered matching degrees for the representations of service semantics. Subsequent ranking of services determines the order of their individual degrees of semantic matching with the given query.

The semantic based web service discovery explores all relevant web services based on the semantics of service functionality, service context, service usability, quality of service QoS) and service goals [3,5].

5.3   User Profile (Consumer Profile)

When a user wishes service behavior to be personalized based on the request a profile will be required. A user profile is a set of information, preferences, rules and settings recorded for that user [8]. In our framework we use personalization of service discovery as important element to discover eHealth services that better suit the user needs. Profiles may contain many individual data items (information, preference and rules) coming from various sources [8,25,26]. The profile will change by its usage or may be changed by a special profile updater agent.

User Profile Acquisition. To acquire user profile, the required information can be obtained explicitly, that is provided directly by the user, or implicitly through the observation of user actions/behaviors.

- **Explicit information.** The simplest way of obtaining information about users is through the data they input via filling forms or question answering techniques or from the user interfaces provided. Generally, the information gathered in this way is demographic data such as user's name, age, gender, job, marital status, and hobbies. Besides, user interests and preferences can be obtained explicitly. In this study we use spoken dialog systems to obtain user's information explicitly.
- **Implicit information.** User profile are often obtained based on implicitly collected information form user behavior or from user feedback. The main advantage of this technique is that it does not require any additional intervention by the user during the process of constructing profiles. Gauch et al. [9] give an overview of the most popular techniques used to collect implicit feedback, and the type of information about the user that can be inferred from the users behavior. User's browsing history, browsing activity, and search logs are some of the techniques used for implicit acquisition of user profile.

User profile Representation. According to Gauch [9] user profiles are generally represented as a set of key words, semantic networks and concept-based profiles. User profiles represented as weighted keywords are extracted and updated from the user request. The semantic network profile representation deals with the semantic relationship of keywords in the network. The bigger the weight, the more relevant the connected nodes. In concept based profiles, the user profile is compared with the whole concept of the user request rather than specific keywords. However, recently ontologies are used to represent user profile.

5.4 Context-aware Service Discovery

Context is defined by Dey and Abowd [4] as: *Any information that can be used to characterize the situation of entities (i.e. whether a person, place or object) that are considered relevant to the interaction between a user and an application, including the user and the application themselves. Context is typically the location identity and state of people, groups and computational and physical object.* Thus, context is used in three main cases: (i) presentation of information and services to a user, (ii) execution of a service and (iii) tagging of context to information for later retrieval.

In our framework we include characteristics as location, time and activity in the context. Furthermore, Dey and Abowd [4] says that context answers questions as: what, where, when and who. We therefore categorize context into service context and user context. The above information defines the context of the user whereas the service context includes: service price, service location, etc.

The context updater agent provides additional information about a service and a user, for example location. For that purpose, the context update is equipped with special agents. For instance a GPS agent that can track the user position, with the added benefit of being able to utilize location-related information. This extra information will improve service discovery.

The context can vary in time, therefore the context update may also involve a tracking function to signal context changes when they occur. The context updater might be a human, a system, or an digital agent on the Internet.

During service discovery the user context is matched against the service context in order to retrieve relevant services with respect to context-awareness. Context is very important for service discovery in an infrastructure-less and infrastructure based networks, since it can retrieve services that conform to the user's current context and service context. Healthcare services are very sensitive since the services are related to prevent human beings from death. Hence the context of the patient (such as blood pressure, temperature and other symptoms) should be accurate to provide remotely appropriate prescription, consultancy and support. Otherwise it would be cumbersome to treat the patient and to provide assistance to the health worker at a distance.

5.5 Personalized and Context Based Matchmaker

The process of service matching is to implement difference operation between service advertisements(S_A) and service requests(S_Q). Such an operation enables to extract from a subset of web service descriptions the part that is semantically common with a given service request and the part that is different.

The match maker ensures that the user will receive the service that is pertinent with user preferences, interests and user contexts. To do so, it receives the user profile, preferences and context from the request interpreter and it combines with service ontology in service repository/registry. After that the match maker matches the requested services with advertised services. The extracted services will be forwarded to reasoning to verify the services with respect to users profile, service description and contextualization. Later the ranking module ranks the extracted services (matched services) based on user preferences, user context and non functional properties of services. Finally, the services with maximal rank will be presented to the requestor. The match maker will further perform consistency check and validity of the user profile and quality of service [2].

5.6 eHealth Service

Internet-based health care is the application of information and communication technology in the whole range of health care functions. It covers everything from electronic prescriptions and computerized medical records to the use of new systems and services. This will cut down waiting times and reduce data errors [19,26]. Obviously the use of Internet, alike other sectors (e-business, e-learning), has facilitated the health care industry with access to information anywhere and anytime. Different challenges of eHealth have been identified (see [22]), for example process of design, implementation, delivery of services, identity management, infrastructure (wired/wireless), and security of information. However, most existing systems are in an experimental or infant stage [22]. In developing countries eHealth is an almost non-addressed issue. The emergence of e-Health has been shown to reduce the cost of health care and to increase efficiency through better retention and retrieval of records, better management of chronic diseases, shared health professional staffing, reduced travel times, and fewer or shorter hospital stays [20,29].

According to Tan [24], there is an eHealth paradigm shift: hospitals have been downsizing, reducing staff and closing hospital beds, new form of health providers alliance and new modalities of health service delivery is emerged in the introduction of the eHealth system. Thus the evolving eHealth system is a dynamic entity that is being continually shaped by economic, political, technological, and social forces.

Email, phone, PDA, cellular phones enhance long distance communication among health workers, patients, and other professionals. Besides, the eHealth empower the health workers and patients through e-learning, e-consultations, teleconferencing, etc. Moreover, eHealth system can help attract and retain health professionals in rural areas by providing professional development training and by creating a collaborative environment among the health professionals [6,24].

6   Conclusion

The emergence of Internet is changing the way people live. Service orientation is being applied to all sectors of human life, such as health care. Most developing countries have little coverage of society's health even though the spread of disease is high. In order to reduce this problem electronic health is an option. As eHealth has impacted on developed countries, it will bring a change also in developing countries such as Ethiopia that suffer from high migration of medical doctors inside and outside the country. In this paper we propose an eHealth service discovery framework which can facilitate the effectiveness of eHealth. The framework provides various facilities to create, specify, discover and select health care services. Especially, the framework covers the ignored part of service orientation to customize services based on user/consumer requirements. Our framework will serve for both wired and wireless networks.

References

1. Satisfaction: the effect of a telephone based care management service on patient outcomes in the uk. In: Jordanova, M., Lievens, F. (eds.) Med-e-Tel: The International Educational and Networking Forum for eHealth, Telemedicine and Health ICT, Electronic Proceedings, Luxexpo, Luxembourg
2. Alam, S., Iqbal, Z., Noll, J., Chowdury, M.M.R.: Semantic personalization framework for connected set top box environment. In: Second International Conference on Advances in Human-Oriented and Personalized Mechanisms, Technologies, and Services, CENTRIC, pp. 97–102 (2009)
3. Bianchini, D., De Antonellis, V., Pernici, B., Plebani, P.: Ontology-based methodology for e-service discovery. Information Systems 31(4), 361–380 (2006)
4. Dey, A.K., Abowd, G.D.: Towards a better understanding of context and context-awareness. In: The Workshop on The What, Who, Where, When, and How of Context-Awareness (CHI 2000), The Netherlands, April 3. The Hague (2000)
5. D'Mello, A.D., Ananthanarayana, V.S.: A review of dynamic web service description and discovery techniques (2010)
6. Drury, P.: ehealth: A model for developing countries. eHelath International 2(2), 19–26 (2005)
7. The Economist. A more hopeful continent. the lion kings? africa is now one of the world's fastest-growing regions, January 6 (2011)
8. ETSI. Etsi eg 202 325: human factors (hf); user profile management (2005)
9. Gauch, S., Speretta, M., Chandramouli, A., Micarelli, A.: User Profiles for Personalized Information Access. In: Brusilovsky, P., Kobsa, A., Nejdl, W. (eds.) Adaptive Web 2007. LNCS, vol. 4321, pp. 54–89. Springer, Heidelberg (2007)
10. Hasselmyer, P.: On service discovery process types (December 2005)
11. ITU. Question 14-2/2: Mobile ehealth solutions for developing countries (2009)
12. Peter, M.J.: e-health is the way via soa (March 1, 2007),
    http://www.allbusiness.com/technology/
    software-services-applications-information/10559505-1.html
    (visited September 06, 2011)
13. Ji, X.: Research on web service discovery based on domain ontology. In: 2nd IEEE International Conference on Computer Science and Information Technology, pp. 65–68. IEEE (2009)
14. Juneja, G., Dournaee, B., Natoli, J., Birkel, S.: Improving performance of healthcare systems with service oriented architecture, March 07 (2008),
    http://www.infoq.com/articles/
    soa-healthcare;jsessionid=A66D6FE007C7B77C311C7326F9D467F2
    (visited September 06, 2011)

15. Ingwersen, P., Järvelin, K.: Information seeking research needs extension towards tasks and technology. Information Research 10(1) (October 2004), http://informationr.net/ir/10-1/paper212.html

16. Kart, F., Moser, L.E., Melliar-Smith, P.M.: Building a distributed e-healthcare system using soa. IT Professional 10(2), 24–30 (2008)

17. Kayed, A., Nizar, M., Alfayoumi, M.: Ontology concepts for requirements engineering process in e-government applications (2010)

18. Kehinde, A., Nyongesa, H., Adesina, A.: ICT and information security perspectives in e-health systems. Jou. of Mobile Com. 4(1), 17–22 (2010)

19. Malindi, P., Kahn, T.M.: Providing qos for ip-based rural telemedicine systems (2008)

20. McClure, P.D.: e-health and america's broadband networks an examination of how broadband services enhance health care in america (2007)

21. MOFED. Performance evaluation of the first five years development plan (2006-2010) and the growth and transformation planning (gtp) for the next five years (2011-2015) (July 2010)

22. Oladosu, J., Emuoyinbofarhe, J.O., Ojo, S.O., Adigun, A.O.: Framework for a context-aware mobile e-health service discovery infrastructure for rural/suburban health care. Journal of Theortical and Applied Information Technology, 338–351 (2009)

23. Serra, D., Serneels, P., Lindelow, M., Montalvo, J.G.: Discovering the Real World Health Workers' Early Work Experience and Career Preferences in Ethiopia. The World Bank (May 2010)

24. Tan, J.: E-Health care Information Systems: An Intro. for Students and Professionals. Ebook (April 2005)

25. Tegegne, T., Kanagwa, B., van der Weide, T.P.: An ehealth service discovery framework for a low infrastructure context. In: 2nd Int. Conf. on Computer Technology and Development, Cairo, Egypt, November 2-4, pp. 606–610 (2010)

26. Tegegne, T., Kanagwa, B., van der Weide, T.P.: Service discovery framework for personalized ehealth. In: Int. Conf. on Services Science, Management and Engineering, SSME 2010, Tainjin, China, December 26-28 (2010) (in press)

27. Toninelli, A., Montanari, R., Corradi, A.: Enabling secure service discovery in mobile healthcare enterprise networks. IEE Wireless Commmunication, 24–32 (June 2009)

28. Vu, L., Hauswirth, M., Aberer, K.: Towards p2p-based semantic web service discovery with qos support (2005)

29. Weerasinghe, D., Elmufti, K., Rajarajan, M., Rakocevic, V.: Xml security based access control for health care information in mobile environment (2006)

30. Weitzman, Y.: Doctors fleeing in record numbers, September 24 (2007), http://archive.voice-online.co.uk/content.php?show=12043 (visited September 06, 2011)

PROP – A Medical Expert System for Preoperative Testing

Karl Entacher[1], Gerhard Fritsch[2], Vinzenz Huber[3], and Sabine Klausner[1]

[1] Salzburg University of Applied Sciences, Urstein Süd 1, 5412 Puch / Salzburg, Austria
{karl.entacher,sabine.klausner}@fh-salzburg.ac.at
[2] Paracelsus Medical University, Department of Anesthesiology, Perioperative Medicine and Intensive Care Medicine, Müllner Hauptstrasse 48, 5020 Salzburg, Austria
[3] Versicherungsanstalt öffentlicher Bediensteter, Faberstraße 2A, 5020 Salzburg, Austria

Abstract. Preoperative evaluation is carried out in an inhospital and outpatient way and may easily cause double examinations. This paper deals with the initiation of a medical application, named "Präoperative Befundung" (PROP) which is applied by clinicians, internists, family doctors and pediatricians since the year 2008 within the framework of an Austrian Reformpoolproject. The aims of the project are the standardization of preoperative evaluation, the prevention of double examinations and unnecessary tests, by a unique Patient-Anamnesis-Matrix. Moreover knowledge discovery about the preoperative process in general and economical optimization for public health insurance companies was focus of the project. How the system exactly works and how it was possible to make medical professionals using it will be explained in the paper. Empirical results from a two year application of PROP within a Reformpoolprojekt in the state of Salzburg, Austria will be demonstrated.

Keywords: Preoperative evaluation, preoperative diagnostic guideline, data analyses.

1 History and Motivation

Patients undergoing surgical procedures have to be evaluated preoperatively. In most of the involved institutions stringent guidelines for preoperative testing are missing. Thus local algorithms based on expert opinion are widely spread. The current process of preoperative evaluation may easily cause double examinations. One reason therefore is a communication gap between inhospital and outpatient medical professionals. To prevent such double examinations and to standardize preoperative evaluation was the main reason to initiate the development of a user-friendly web based preoperative diagnostic guideline (PROP) focusing on the improvement of the preoperative process [1, 2, 3, 4].

The main goals of the project were:

— Standardization and optimization of the preoperative processes
— Economization by reducing the quantity of tests

A. Holzinger and K.-M. Simonic (Eds.): USAB 2011, LNCS 7058, pp. 417–428, 2011.

— Forcing the medical quality in the special sphere of risks
— Efficient usage of resources in the hospital by using outpatient structures
— Optimization of the preoperative procedures: shorter ways for patients, physical and mental stress of older patients and children and
— Knowledge discovery for the preoperative evaluation process in general.

During the start-up period of the project (from 2006 to middle of 2008) a prototype of PROP was implemented and applied by test users. Later, the PROP project team decided to adapt the "ÖGARI guideline" [5] in order implement a unique Patient-Anamnesis-Matrix within PROP for standardization purposes of the preoperative diagnosis. This guideline has been created by a team named "Präoperative Evaluierung" and defines the standardization and harmonization of preoperative patient evaluation for interior departments in anesthesiology and extra mural institutions. PROP is applied by clinicians, internists, family doctors and pediatricians since the year 2008 within the framework of an Austrian Reformpoolprojekt in the state of Salzburg. The execution of this project and the achievement of its objectives have been evaluated by the Paracelsus Medical University in Salzburg [7, 8].

The following chapters contain a general description of the functionality of the software, special software features and technical information, application details within the Reformpoolprojekt and empirical results during a constant two year application period of PROP.

2   General Functionality of the Software

The web-based preoperative diagnostic application PROP (http://prop.fh-salzburg. ac.at) is a "self-explanatory" expert system where medical professionals may input anonymous, patient-related information in order to get a standardized preoperative indication.

A number of 32 parameters classified in 13 categories (type of surgical procedure, ASA-Classifications, lung, metabolism, liver, kidney, coagulation, neurology, oncology, gynecology, drugs, dyspnoea, hematology, heart) of the patients, the patients' history, and some general information such as demographic measurements, type of public health insurance company and related parameters are requested. For outpatient users, the hospital of referral is also stored. Via a standardized Patient-Anamnesis-Matrix the system generates a preoperative indication based on the input data. As mentioned above, the matrix is based on the 13 categories. The first category, namely types of surgical procedure is itself defined by 5 parameters: minor-, heavy-, adipositas-, major orthopedic- and pulmonary surgery. The other groups except of the group heart which has three different types of cardial risc factors with 5 subgroups have between 1 and 3 subgroups. Every parameter accords to defined examinations.

The PROP user is able to see a preview list of his activated information and the proposed preoperative tests. After activation of the "finalization" button the data is stored and a print out of the diagnosis is provided containing an anonymous Patient Identification (Pat_ID). The printout is the basis for the preoperative examination and is handed out to the patient. More details about the functionality and features will be explained in the following section.

2.1   Special Software Features and Further Details

The software PROP provides a platform for inhospital and outpatient health professionals, for special users like insurance companies and the PROP administrator. The different users receive selected views and special roles within the system. Medical professionals generate their preoperative tests slightly differently for the inhospital or outpatient application.

PROP Administrator

The PROP administrator is able to automatically perform certain statistical evaluations, like user statistics or details about the diagnosis combinations which were carried out and further descriptive statistics.

Additionally, the administrator is able to generate user identifications and permissions (username, password), certain user group assignments and may define a clear assignment of the symptoms to the necessary examination within the Patient-Anamnesis-Matrix. Via the administrator, the diagnosis guideline changes are entered and can be applied immediately by the users. Thus the users have access to the most recent version of the algorithm.

Patient-Anamnesis-Matrix

The Patient-Anamnesis-Matrix is the basis for the generation of the standardized preoperative evaluation via PROP. It is based on currently 32 parameters which result in the necessary examinations from the derived symptoms which are certain combinations of these parameters (see the introduction in Chapter 2). The matrix was fixed in the year 2008 in the "ÖGARI guideline" [5].

Public Health Insurance Company User

Every medical professional need to provide the insurance company with the PROP generated Pat_ID to be able to get the corresponding medical fee. For quality management purpose of their service and the ability to countercheck the diagnosis results according to a certain Pat_ID, it is possible for public health insurance company users to insert this ID into a defined interface in the PROP system and to verify the results.

Anonymity and Login of Users/Patients

One of the main requirements of the project was to provide anonymity protection of medical professionals and patients. No user/patient details are stored in the current system. As already mentioned above, the patient is identified via the anonymous Patient Identifier. The medical professionals get their user name and password after the execution of a PROP-workshop at the medical council of Salzburg. From the system it would hardly be possible to find out which of the users applied which patient, only if the finalization date and timestamp is known exactly.

2.2   Procedures for PROP Users

If a user wants to generate a preoperative evaluation using PROP, someone opens a browser with the current URL http://prop.fh-salzburg.ac.at. The first page of the application is opened which shows some general information about team members in charge and other participants of PROP. It is then possible to continue the process by signing in. Therefore, it is important that cookies are activated in the browser. After the login, a general page is opened with information for new users about PROP and about the philosophy of the project.

For being able to fill in the anamneses form, the "Start" button in the text or the "Anamneses" link on the left hand side has to be activated. The first part of the questionnaire is opened where general patient information like sex, age, referral to the hospital (only for outpatient area) and to which public health insurance company the patient belongs is queried. Then the user can switch to the next page where information about the "Type of surgical intervention" is asked. It is necessary to choose one selection of the radio button list. As an example, this page from the PROP System is shown in Fig. 1. The continuative pages described in the following are generally structured in the same way. At the next page the "Anamneses" based on the "ASA-Classifications" [5] is asked. The "Explanation" pages which may also be activated from the left menu answer how the classification is defined. If a user inserts incorrect data it is possible to return to the previous page via a special button in order to correct the input. Hereby it should be mentioned that the "Back" button offered from browsers is not the correct way to return, because information could be stored wrongly.

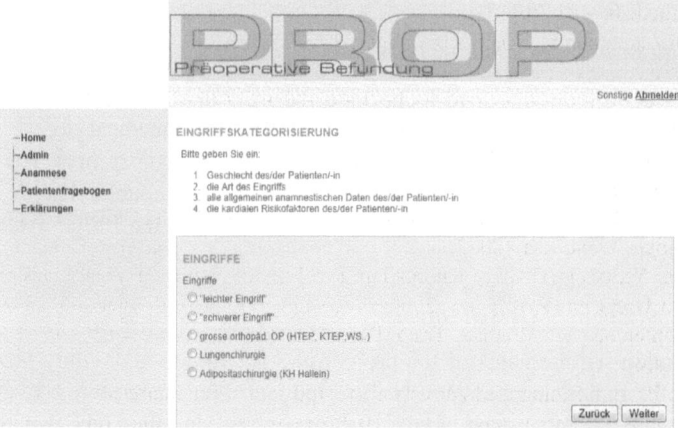

Fig. 1. Example-page from PROP where a user can choose the "Type of surgical intervention"

The next page of the form shows the "Cardial Risk factors" which are categorized in three areas, namely low, intermediary and heavy risk factors. In future versions of PROP this section will be abandoned as guidelines [6] do not use this grading anymore. The "Show Diagnosis" button which can be activated on this last page completes the anamneses process. The user gets a preview list of all his activated buttons and the resulting preoperative tests which are recommended. The evaluation process may be finished via the "Cancel", the "Fill in a new form" or the "Finalize" buttons. Only the "Finalize" button generates the Patient Identifier and forces the process to store the date in the system. From this moment the user is not able to change information of the current patient any-more.

As a final step the preoperative evaluation result may be stored or printed out by activating the "Printout" button. Then, a print version of the result will be generated containing the Patient Identifier. Additionally, the referral to the corresponding hospital is given. In the current preoperative process in the state of Salzburg, the medical professional provides the printout to the patient who takes it to the hospital where the preoperative testing is carried out. The medical professional saves the Patient Identifier and provides it to the public health insurance company. The saving process of the results and the corresponding ID can be easily carried out locally on every computer with HTML, but cannot be opened again by the user via the PROP system. Otherwise, data security and transparency of the user could be violated.

2.3   Technology and Infrastructure

The software is written in the programming language C#[1]. As development platform Microsoft Visual Studio 2008[1], Microsoft SQL Server 2008[1] as database is used. The current PROP system is running on a Windows 2008 Server[1]. The backup has a size of 2 Gigabytes which currently contains about 40 000 patient results and user information.

The server is located at the Salzburg University of Applied Sciences and provides online access for the PROP users. Additionally a virtual private network (VPN) connection via a Cisco[2] PIX firewall is provided in order to allow outpatient medical professionals to apply PROP using their e-Card system[3]. It has to be mentioned that the main part the PROP users connect to the application via the Internet. Fig. 2 exhibits the current architecture of the system.

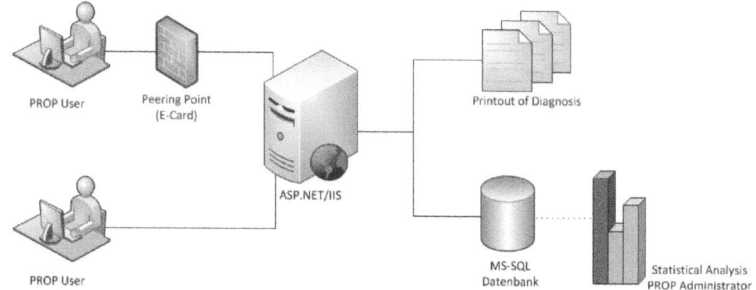

Fig. 2. Architecture of the PROP system during the period of the Reformpoolprojekt

---

[1] http://www.microsoft.com/ (Jul. 2011)
[2] http://www.cisco.com/ (Jul. 2011)
[3] http://www.peeringpoint.at/ (Jul. 2011)

Consortium and license holder of PROP

Currently, the owner of the PROP license is the SAGES KV - a union of the Salzburger Gesundheitsfonds (SAGES http://www.salzburg.gv.at/sages) and the public health insurance organization, i.e. the Krankenversicherungsträger (KV) in Salzburg.

Until the end of the year 2011 the project will be applied as an extended form of the Reformpoolprojekt in Salzburg. The Austrian countries Burgenland, Lower Austria and Upper Austria are also testing the software since the beginning of this year. Further members of the PROP project are:

- the Austrian Medical Chamber (http://www.aerztekammer.at/) as a part of the development team and provider for the training workshops for medical professionals;
- the Paracelsus Medical University (http://www.pmu.ac.at) where the external evaluation [7] of the Reformpoolprojekt was carried out;
- the Medical Center of Salzburg (SALK http://www.salk.at/) with the Department of Anesthesiology, Perioperative Medicine and Intensive Care Medicine as a part of the development team;
- the Austrian Society of Anesthesiology, Resuscitation and Intensive Care Medicine (ÖGARI http://www.oegari.at/);
- the National Health-Insurance of Austria (http://www.sozialversicherung.at/);
- the Salzburg University of Applied Sciences (http://www.fh-salzburg.ac.at/) where the software was developed and hosted during the project phase.

3   Empirical Results

This section contains first results from an empirical analysis of a constant two year application of PROP during the final period within the Reformpoolprojekt in Salzburg, from March 2009 to March 2011.

Currently, 403 users are employing the application and are assigned to certain roles (compare Table 1). In Salzburg seven inhospital, 362 outpatient members and five users for public health insurance companies have access to the role-adapted system. Other users like the PROP administrator, four test users for Lower Austria and eight for Burgenland are implemented as well. Sixteen other test users are installed in order to provide temporary accesses for interested organizations.

Table 1. Current number of users listed in roles

Number	Role names
1	PROP administrator
5	Health insurance company users
7	Inhospital users Salzburg
28	Test users for Burgenland (8) and Lower Austria (4) and others
362	Outpatient users in Salzburg

The following statistical analyses are carried out using the software SPSS 18.0.0[4]. In Table 2, the patient quantities and frequencies applied by PROP are shown per quarter. Within the two year period a total number of 22 646 preoperative evaluations are stored. The first quarters contain between 2 400 and about 3 900 patients. In last year's 2nd and 3rd quarter the number of evaluations is significantly lower, since inhospital and outpatient users applied a smaller number of patients. The reason therefore is that the external evaluation period of the Reformpoolprojekt finished at this time and therefore inhospital users stopped their trial execution of PROP. At the beginning of 2011 these users started the application of PROP again. Table 3 below shows the amount of applied patients for the inhospital and outpatient case.

Table 2. PROP application frequencies during a two year period

Quarterly Division	Year	Period	Absolute frequency	Relative frequency
2nd Mar. – 31st May	09	Q1_1	3 853	17,0%
1st Jun. – 31st Aug.	09	Q2_1	3 266	14,4%
1st Sept. – 30th Nov.	09	Q3_1	3 887	17,2%
1st Dec. – 28th Feb.	09/10	Q4_1	2 856	12,6%
1st Mar. – 31st May	10	Q1_2	2 367	10,5%
1st Jun.– 31st Aug.	10	Q2_2	1 737	7,7%
1st Sept. – 30th Nov.	10	Q3_2	2 163	9,6%
1st Dec. – 2nd Mar.	10/11	Q4_2	2 517	11,1%
Total			22 646	100,0%

Table 3. Frequencies of patients in the outpatient and inhospital area for the two year period

Grouping	Frequency	Percentage
outpatient	14 689	64,9%
inhospital	7 957	35,1%
Total	22 646	100,0%

In Fig. 3 an error bar plot (99% confidence interval) of the user access times in minutes (time between login and preoperative evaluation result in the database) divided into the number of patients in the outpatient and inhospital area is shown. In the outpatient area the users need less than 5 minutes for finalizing one patient and the estimation of the average access times is very accurate. A slightly decreasing trend is visible during the observation period. Because of the fact that outpatient users apply trainings before getting their PROP access, the time for preoperative evaluation via PROP is continuously low. In comparison, the inhospital users need time to learn how to apply the system. Furthermore, the login session of inhospital users is longer than in the outpatient case in general.

---

[4] http://www.ibm.com/software/analytics/spss/ (Jul. 2011)

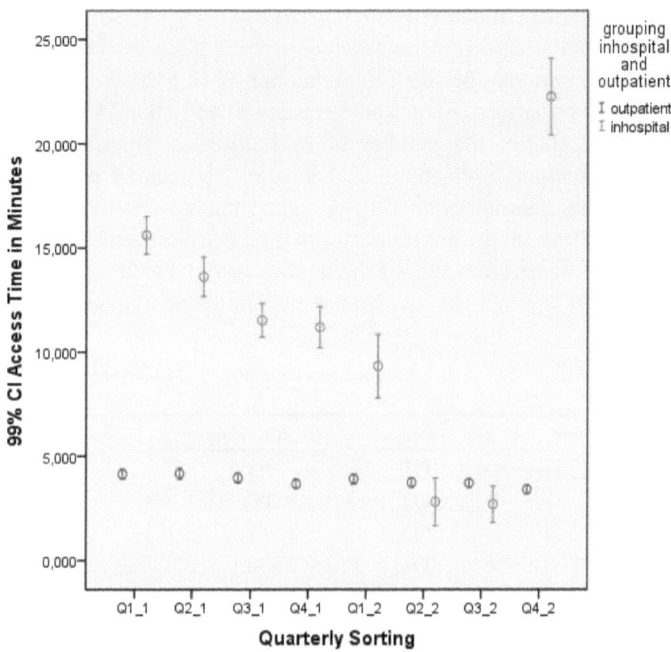

Fig. 3. Access times for inhospital and outpatient PROP users (99% confidence intervals)

In the inhospital case there seems to be more time provided for the evaluation process in general. In the first five quarterly periods there is a continuous decrease of the access time which demonstrates how the users learned to deal with the system. In the 6th and 7th quarter the access time is very low whereas in the 8th quarter the average time increased rapidly from about 5 minutes up to over 20 minutes. As already mentioned above, this is due to the fact that the period for external evaluation of the PROP project finished at this time and therefore inhospital users stopped the trial execution of PROP. At the beginning of 2011 the usage of PROP was started again by new inhospital users and therefore the access times obviously increased.

In Fig. 4 the frequencies for the type of surgical intervention for the whole observation period are shown as bar chart. Table 4 contains the corresponding absolute quantities. As can be seen from the chart, the number of female patients is significantly higher than those of male patients except in the case of "lung surgery". Minor surgeries are carried out for female patients about 10% more often than for male patients. The reason therefore may be that women take part in preventive medical examinations to a greater extent. In relation to the other type of surgical interventions, the "adipositas surgery" is carried out rarely, but for female patients 50% more often than for masculine ones. This surgical intervention is in the state of Salzburg only offered in the hospital of Hallein.

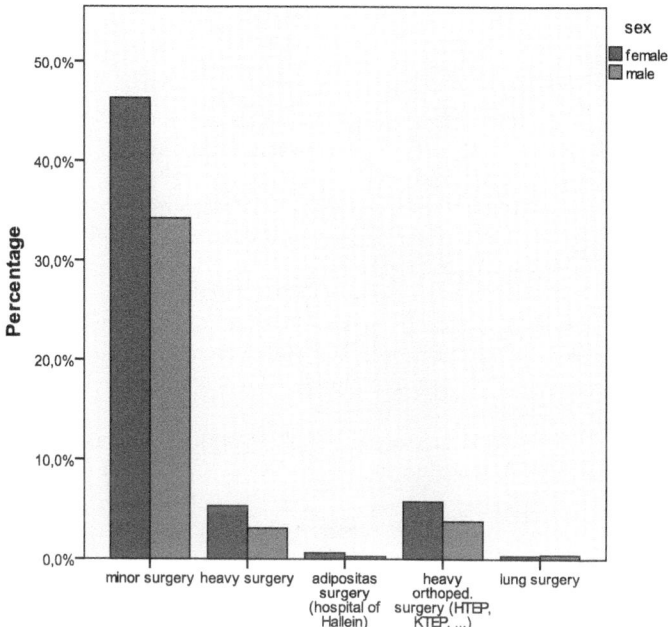

Type of Medical Intervention

Fig. 4. Type of medical intervention for female and male patients for the period of two years

Table 4. Type of operation in absolute and relative frequency for male/female patients

Type of Operation	Frequency	Percent	Men	Women
minor surgery	18 217	80,4%	7 738	10 479
heavy surgery	1 892	8,4%	698	1 194
adipositas surgery (hospital of Hallein)	195	0,9%	56	139
major orthoped. surgery (HTEP, KTEP, …)	2 149	9,5%	851	1 298
pulmonary resection	164	0,7%	92	72
Total	22 617	100,0%	9 435	13 182

Fig. 5 shows an overview of the number of PROP patients belonging to a certain public health insurance company. The corresponding numerical values are given in Table 5. In the latter table the English denominations with German abbreviations in brackets are given. The abbreviations stand for Versicherungsanstalt öffentlich Bediensteter (BVA), Salzburger Gebietskrankenkasse (SGKK), Sozial-versicherungsanstalt der gewerblichen Wirtschaft (SVA), Sozialversicherungsanstalt der Bauern (SVB) and Versicherungsanstalt für Eisenbahnen und Bergbau (VAEB).

Most of the patients (82%) in Salzburg are members of the SGKK, of which 32% are male and 50% female patients. A number of 8.5% of all patients in PROP are members of the BVA and the remaining 9.2% are members of SVA, SVB or VAEB.

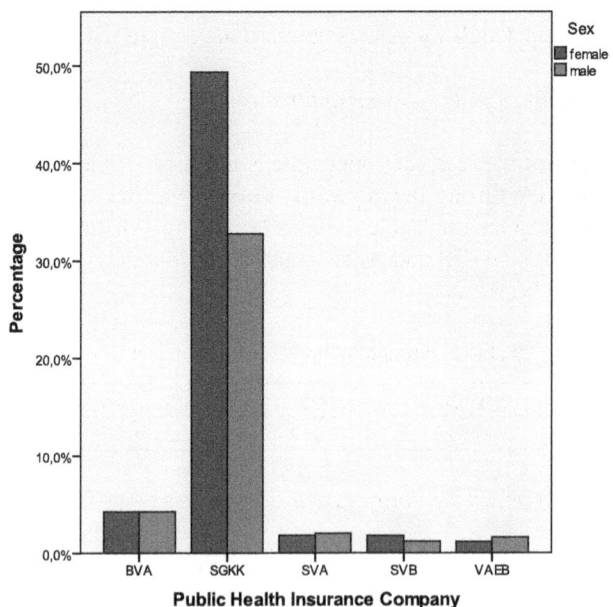

Fig. 5. Number of female and male patients per public health insurance company

Table 5. A list of public health insurance companies and their patient frequencies

Public Health Insurance Company	Frequency	Percentage	Men	Women
Insurance institution of public servants (BVA)	1 917	8,5%	958	959
Regional medical insurance of Salzburg (SGKK)	18 581	82,0%	7 411	11 170
Social Security institution of the industrial economy (SVA)	860	3,8%	451	409
Social Security Institution of the farmers (SVB)	668	2,9%	266	402
Insurance institution of railway and mining (VAEB)	620	2,7%	361	259
Total	22 646	100,0%	9 447	13 199

4   Summary and Future Perspective

From the project start up to now, about 40 000 patients have been preoperatively evaluated using the web application PROP which was applied within a Reformpoolprojekt in the state of Salzburg, Austria from 2008 to 2011. The evaluation algorithm of PROP is based on the "ÖGARI guideline" for preoperative testing [5]. Application experience and evaluation of the project have demonstrated the economic potential of this standardized preoperative procedure and the prevention of double examinations was verified [1, 2, 3, 7, 8].

Since then, the usage of the software is well accepted by the PROP users and the usage is reported to be very easy. The acceptance of the application was constantly improved due to the introduction and information process by the PROP consortium (Sect. 2.3) and the training workshops organized by the Austrian Medical Chamber. The team at the Salzburg University of Applied Sciences had to deal with requests from the outpatient medical professionals via telephone but mainly with very easy duties such as password resets, login support and general questions on the IT infrastructure of their medical practice, such as support for printout from a web browser, i.e. questions which are not directly related to with PROP. Therefore, the system was provided with small services for user support in order to answer general technical questions like "How and where can I print out the diagnosis?", "How may I reset username and password?", "How is it possible to save the password permanently in the browser?" and so on.

The goal of the present paper is to provide a technical description of the PROP system and to demonstrate empirical results from a constant application PROP during a two year period within the Reformpoolprojekt. These results contain general patient frequencies, types of medical interventions, insurance classifications and important differences between female and male patient behavior. The user access times (time between login and preoperative evaluation result) demonstrate the learning effect of the application of PROP in the inhospital and outpatient case.

The application of PROP during the Reformpoolprojekt phase also showed some suggestions for possible future adaptions. In Fig. 6 recommended further extensions for an improved PROP system are visualized. In order to provide a connection to medical information systems, a universal interface which allows a standardized data transfer is necessary. The export of the diagnoses may be realized in the format HL7 (Health Level 7) which is a standard medical protocol. The diagnosis itself could be stored in in the system in form of Extensible Markup Language (=XML) files which offer a standardized data format and well defined options for data exchange and - processing.

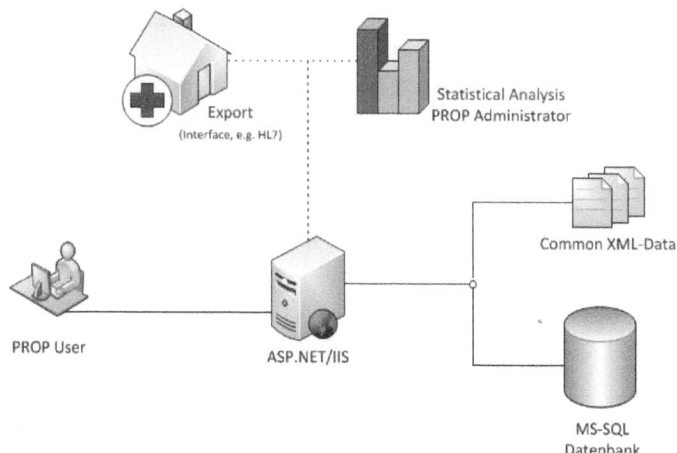

Fig. 6. Recommended architecture for a future PROP system

Acknowledgment. The authors would like to thank all colleagues from the organizations involved in the execution and development of the project (see Sect. 2.3) especially Dr. Beate Stolzlechner from SAGES for her support. The first author is supported by the FWF project L526-B05.

References

1. Huber, V.: ÖKZ: Ohne Blutbild in den OP? Das Österreichische Gesundheitswesen 51(6) (2010)
2. Fritsch, G.: ÖGAM-News: Reformpoolprojekt, Präoperative Befunde" – Vision, Performance und Realität. Ärzte Krone, no. 15/16 (2010), http://www.oegam.at/
3. Huber, V., Gerner, H.: Reformpoolprojekt, Präoperative Befundung im Bundesland Salzburg, Soziale Sicherheit – Fachzeitschrift der Österreichischen Sozialversicherungen (December 2009), http://www.hauptverband.at
4. Reform im Spital bringt Millionen Euro, Salzburger Nachrichten, October 30 (2010), http://www.salzburg.com
5. ÖGARI - Österreichischen Gesellschaft für Anästhesiologie, Reanimation und Intensivmedizin, ÖGARI-Leitlinie, Präoperative Evaluierung (2008), http://www.oegari.at/web_files/dateiarchiv/205/Quellleitlinie %20Präoperative%20PatientInnenevaluierung%20Juni%202011.pdf
6. Fleisher, L.A., Beckman, J.A., Brown, K.A., Calkins, H., Chaikof, E., Fleischmann, K.E., Freeman, W.K., Froehlich, J.B., Kasper, E.K., Kersten, J.R., Riegel, B., Robb, J.F., Smith Jr., S.C., Jacobs, A.K., Adams, C.D., Anderson, J.L., Antman, E.M., Buller, C.E., Creager, M.A., Ettinger, S.M., Faxon, D.P., Fuster, V., Halperin, J.L., Hiratzka, L.F., Hunt, S.A., Lytle, B.W., Md, R.N., Ornato, J.P., Page, R.L., Tarkington, L.G., Yancy, C.W.: ACC/AHA 2007 Guidelines on Perioperative Cardiovascular Evaluation and Care for Noncardiac Surgery: Executive Summary: A Report of the American College of Cardiology/American Heart Association Task Force on Practice Guidelines (Writing Committee to Revise the 2002 Guidelines on Perioperative Cardiovascular Evaluation for Noncardiac Surgery): Developed in Collaboration With the American Society of Echocardiography, American Society of Nuclear Cardiology, Heart Rhythm Society, Society of Cardiovascular Anaesthesiologists, Society for Cardiovascular Angiography and Interventions, Society for Vascular Medicine and Biology, and Society for Vascular Surgery. Circulation 116, 1971–1996 (2007)
7. Flamm, M., Sönnichsen, A.: Reformpoolprojekt Präoperative Diagnostik PROP – Evaluationsbericht. Paracelsus Medizinische Privatuniversität, Institut für Allgemein-, Familien- und Präventivmedizin, Salzburg (2010)
8. Fritsch, G., Flamm, M., Seer, J., Soennichsen, A.: Economic Aspects of Preoperative Testing. Abstract 9, Cleveland Clinic Journal of Medicine 77 (2010)

Utilizing Acquired Healthcare Knowledge, Based on Using Electronic Health Records

Sara Nasiri[1], Mohammad Mehdi Sepehri[1], and Marjan Khobreh[2]

[1] Department of Industrial Engineering, Tarbiat Modares University (TMU), Tehran, Iran
[2] Institute of Knowledge Based Systems & Knowledge Management, University of Siegen
sara.nasiri62@gmail.com,
mehdi.sepehri@modares.ac.ir,
khobreh@informatik.uni-siegen.de

Abstract. In today's healthcare systems; health records are the bases to exchange information and knowledge among healthcare professionals. Thus Electronic Health Record (EHR) is considered as one of the main elements of Knowledge Management (KM) in healthcare organizations. Despite all advantages of EHR, the vast amount of data, information and knowledge leads to difficulties for defining a practical-oriented framework. Thus simplification of the analysis, presentation and usage of information and knowledge acquired from EHR is significantly important. In this paper a new Dashboard-Oriented EHR Model (DOEM) is proposed for the KM in healthcare, based on using EHRs for gathering health records from health organizations and KM techniques for processing and analyzing the acquired data and information. DOEM is designed for customizing different healthcare stakeholders' requirements, for effective transforming of data and information into actionable information (knowledge), and for efficient sharing of experiences and creativities of healthcare knowledge contributors.

Keywords: Knowledge Management, Electronic Health Record, Knowledge Discovery, Knowledge Sharing, Dashboard.

1 Introduction

Over the past decade, with the rapid advance in Information Technology (IT), the healthcare industry has increasingly embraced new IT and web based applications in the search for opportunities for higher-quality care [1]. Recently, a growing interest in the electronic health (E-health) concept is causing significant changes in the healthcare environment [1], [2]. As healthcare industry moves into the e-health era, healthcare organizations are becoming knowledge-based communities connected to hospitals, clinics, pharmacies, and customers for sharing knowledge, reducing costs, and improving the quality of care. Thus, the success of e-health depends critically on the collection, analysis and seamless exchange of clinical and medical information or knowledge within and across the above organizational boundaries [1], [3]. 'Electronic

A. Holzinger and K.-M. Simonic (Eds.): USAB 2011, LNCS 7058, pp. 429–439, 2011.

Health Record(EHR) is an important e-health concept for shared medical documentation, where data objects of care providers' local Electronic Medical Records(EMRs) can be conditioned to communicate with other care providers in order to maintain, review or share medical data objects' [4]. 'Although EHR can provide legal support, or allow the development of population studies that constitute another type of knowledge with a purpose like, for example, resource allocation, the basic objective of EHR is to integrate knowledge on the health of patients. Therefore, the contexts of healthcare in which EHR for Knowledge Management (KM) can have an outstanding interest include healthcare planning (i.e., Public Healthcare Systems), management (i.e., healthcare services, hospitals or primary care areas) and to support the professionals (i.e., medical, surgical and nursing services)' [5]. As mentioned in World Health Organization KM strategy (WHO KM strategy), translating knowledge into policy and action, sharing and reapplying experiential knowledge, and leveraging E-health in countries are strongly required to fill the gap between "what is known" and "what is done in practice"[6]. Due to the vast amount of data, information and knowledge in EHR the technical issues of practical implementation has its own challenges. Even though ample research is done on tracking, logging and authenticating data access, little research is done on: (i) how valuable was the accessed data to the healthcare professional, (ii) how this data was utilized by the healthcare professional and (iii) what data would this healthcare professional have actually been exposed to if this data was not present at the time of search [7]. The emergence of such questions is because of the complex nature of the issue and the need for a better model to properly address the related problems. Based on studying of prior efforts indicated either as research projects or empirical studies, prior proposed models are quite complex to be practically applicable and most of healthcare organizations are not motivated to use complex systems because of time, resource and cost-intensive issues. Also, while proposed models tend to be comprehensive and globally utilizable, they are suffering the lack of simplicity for easy implementation, maintenance and development. Thus simplification of the analysis, presentation and usage of information and knowledge acquired from EHR is significantly important.

In this paper first an introduction is given on EHR, its contents and where it stands in the healthcare environment. Further, the role of KM in healthcare is described by reviewing the available literature. Finally a new dashboard-oriented model is proposed for the KM in healthcare, based on using EHRs for gathering health records from health organizations like hospitals, clinics, health insurance, etc., and KM techniques for processing and analyzing the acquired data and information. This dashboard is also designed for customizing different healthcare stakeholders' requirements, for effective transforming of data and information into actionable information (knowledge), and for efficient sharing of experiences and creativities of healthcare knowledge contributors. Basically this paper is the outcome of literature study and analysis of existing EHR approaches for integration of KM methods and techniques in healthcare practices particularly for healthcare initiatives and contributors.

2   EHR Data Management

'An EHR is a collection of data and information gathered or generated to record clinical care rendered to an individual. It is a comprehensive, structured set of clinical, demographic, environmental, social and financial data and information in electronic form, documenting the health care given to an individual. Considerable effort is spent in standardization of EHR in different regions. Different standards -CDA, CCR, HL7 and DICOM- exist but most of the countries suffer from lack of using these standards' [8], [9]. EHR as defined by ISO is a bank of a comprehensive and longitudinal (long term from cradle to grave) patient-centered health-related information to support efficiency and integration of healthcare quality of care by also providing plans, goals and evaluations of patient care [10], [11]. By definition, EHRs are distributed medical patient electronic data and, in due time, will partially (if not fully) replace paper-based medical records to improve the quality of healthcare for patients. EHRs are distributed in order to get assistance from multiple healthcare professionals. Authenticated healthcare professionals are able to gather data in an EHR, in or out of a healthcare environment, from multiple locations [10].

The primary purpose of an EHR is for continued care of the patient. The EHR should be comprehensive with all significant clinical and administrative information pertaining to a given patient, enabling the attending clinician to provide effective continuing care and to determine the patient's condition at any given time. EHRs should enable all activities that physicians perform with paper records. The EHRs should also enable healthcare providers other than the attending clinician to review the patient and render his/her expert opinion or continue the patient's care at any time. Secondary purposes are research/historical, epidemiology/public health, statistics, education, peer review, utilization studies, quality assurance, legal document (used as evidence) and healthcare policy development [8].

The content of an EHR consists of administrative and clinical data. This content should be comprehensive and expressive, addressing all aspects of the healthcare process for all related disciplines and authorities. There should be no restrictions on the type of data that can be entered into the EHR. The administrative content includes:

- Identification/demographic data - patient unique identifier or medical record number, address, next of kin/guardian, sex, ethnic origin, complete name, date of birth, place of birth, marital status, religion, mother's maiden name, etc.
- Financial data - Employer, health insurance, type of coverage.
- Social data - Race, family status, etc.

Clinical data includes medical history, physical examination, clinical orders, progress notes, pathology reports, radiology reports, ECG, EEG, EMG, consultations, operative data, anesthesia, medication data, monitoring data and observations.

Ideally, the EHR includes all available patient data, irrespective of its source and provides medical professionals with meaningful views on these data [8].

It can be seen that there is a large amount of data for every person and effective management of this data is a very challenging task. The use of EHRs offers significant benefits in healthcare. Direct access to patient history, lab tests and imaging from the point of care eliminates the delay required for the medical attendants to dispatch and retrieve physical records from distant physical locations. Loss and misplacement of patient records x-ray films, which frequently happen with physical paper folders, can be considerably alleviated [12]. 'The system supports better decision making in patient treatments with ability to countercheck interaction between drugs, allergies, as well as abnormal result of investigation to lessen life threatening situations' [13]. With respect to the mentioned benefits of EHR in healthcare, as healthcare organizations are drowning in information overload, KM is believed to be the current savior of organizations [14].

3   Healthcare Knowledge Assets

Data is a series of facts that has not been processed for use i.e. no specific effort has been made to interpret or understand the data. Information is data given context, with meaning and significance. Knowledge is created by transforming information through reasoning and reflection into beliefs, concepts, and mental models [15], [16]. A KM cycle process can turn data into information and form information into knowledge involving various activities [1], [17]. The Healthcare Information and Management System Society (HIMSS) broadly defined e-health as IT-enabled healthcare system that improves the access, efficiency, effectiveness and quality of clinical and business processes utilized by healthcare organizations, practitioners, and patients in an effort to accomplish some combination of the following objectives: cut costs, increase revenues, streamline operations, improve patient satisfaction, and contribute to the enhancement of medical care. As healthcare organizations are drowning in information overload, KM is believed to be the current savior of organizations [14]. Currently, IT allows for supporting a knowledge-centric view so the e-health solutions must begin to take advantage of these new capabilities. The health care industry has increasingly tried to embrace the KM–enabled technologies and applications to improve the access and transfer of e-health information and knowledge at all levels (physicians, nurses, therapists, diagnosticians, and pharmacists) [1], [3]. The KM-enabled healthcare system is becoming the new trend in e-health. In the context of healthcare processing data and generating information is crucially vital to support healthcare services e.g. clinical decision making [5]. Healthcare data sources are administrative, basic healthcare or clinical complexes (e.g., diagnoses, procedures, evolutions, comparatives, assessments, etc.)[5]. However in healthcare organizations, applying KM is only fulfilled on the basis of well structured and managed information. 'When referring the concepts of information and knowledge in the scope of health, there are differences between explicit, tacit, and implicit information, according to the source from where they come' [5].

Thus, *explicit information* is the result of scientific research in the biomedical sector, but also of the assessment of healthcare services and assistance. *Tacit information* is the result of healthcare professionals experience in their clinical practice, and *implicit information* is contained in clinical files. Similarly, *explicit knowledge* is acquired by means of documentary sources, both internal and external.

Tacit knowledge is the one present in people as a result of their experience and *Implicit knowledge* results from the working practice of healthcare professionals. The main knowledge sources in the area of health are healthcare professionals who *own the tacit knowledge intrinsically.* This sort of knowledge is the one with a greatest value in the KM process [5]. The process can be subdivided, for example, into creating internal knowledge, acquiring external knowledge, storing knowledge in documents versus storing in routines, as well as updating the knowledge and sharing knowledge internally and externally [1], [18]. In light of the extant literature [17], [19], the KM process can be generically represented as four cyclic activities: knowledge acquisition, knowledge codification, knowledge transfer, and knowledge application as shown in Fig 1. Knowledge acquisition includes all activities involved in the acquisition and development of knowledge. Knowledge codification involves the conversion of knowledge into accessible and applicable content. Knowledge transfer includes the sharing of knowledge from its point of creation or codified to the point of use. Knowledge application includes retrieving and applying codified knowledge in support of actions, decisions or problem-solving. Ideally, these activities do not represent a monolithic set of activities, but an interconnected and intertwined set of activities.

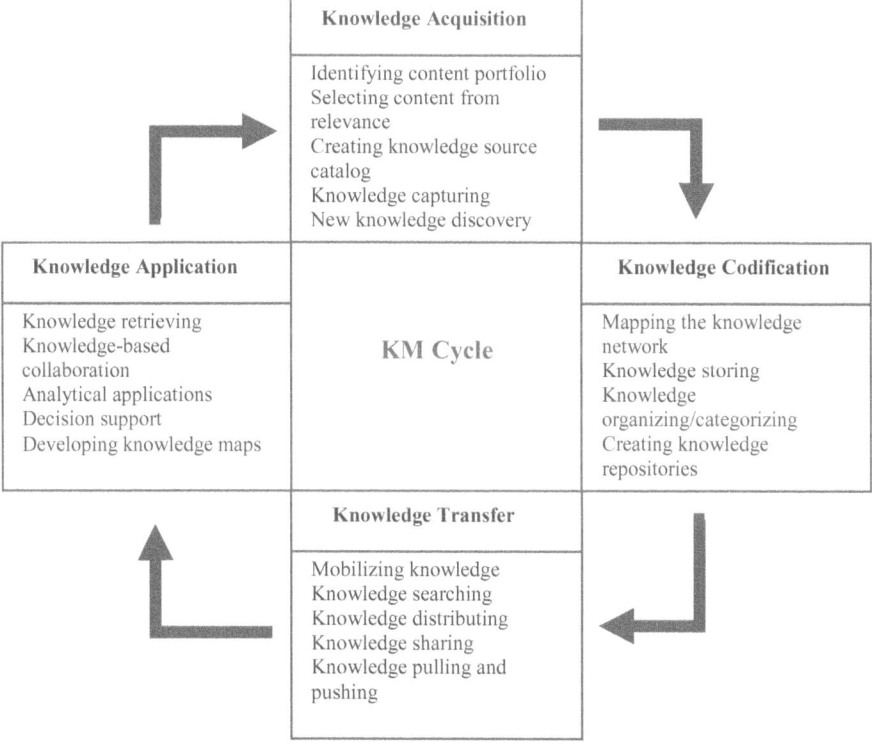

Fig. 1. KM Cycle, [17], [19]

Data and text mining is often used during the knowledge discovery process and is one of the most important subfields in knowledge management. Data mining aims to analyze a set of given data or information in order to identify novel and potentially useful patterns [20]. These techniques, such as Bayesian models, decision trees, artificial neural networks, associate rule mining, and genetic algorithms, are often used to discover patterns or knowledge that are previously unknown to the system and the users [21] . Because of their predictive power, data mining techniques have been widely used in diagnostic and healthcare applications. Data mining algorithms can learn from past examples in clinical data and model the oftentimes non-linear relationships between the independent and dependent variables. The resulting model represents formalized knowledge, which can often provide a good diagnostic opinion. Data mining is also used to extract rules from healthcare data. For example, it has been used to extract diagnostic rules from breast cancer data [22]. Text mining aims to extract useful knowledge from textual data or documents [23], [24]. Although text mining is often considered a subfield of data mining, some text mining techniques have originated from other disciplines, such as information retrieval, information visualization, computational linguistics, and information science.

Based on KM process steps and these techniques, a conceptual model to customize a dashboard for KM based on using EHR is proposed in the next section.

4   Dashboard-Oriented EHR Model (DOEM)

KM activities can supply healthcare industry with enhanced quality of care and is increasingly becoming a knowledge-based community [1]. Utilizing KM Systems (KMS) to manage medical information and healthcare knowledge to support the full spectrum of knowledge needs in the EHR has become an important issue for patients and professionals. Due to the vast amount of data and information in EHR, it is always a very complex task to find out the relations between different instances of data and information. It would be significantly convenient if data and/or information are presented to the target group according to their needs and demands. This would also help in sharing the knowledge more effectively. It is also important to devise a model that could satisfy every stakeholder in healthcare, from patients to physicians and etc. The proposed model can be seen in Fig.2 which includes different contents of EHR, customizable dashboards, knowledge types and the KM activities. As mentioned before EHR consists of different contents like administrative (identification, finance and social data) and clinical data (medical history, physical, examination, clinical orders and etc.).

In this context, KM has an important functionality to deploy strategies, techniques, methods and tools to capture, refine, organize, store, share and transfer *explicit/tacit/implicit knowledge* [25]. In fact, EHR can be used as a tool for KM to acquire data, information and knowledge. The knowledge cycle can also be seen in Fig 2. First, explicit knowledge can be acquired from data and information stored in

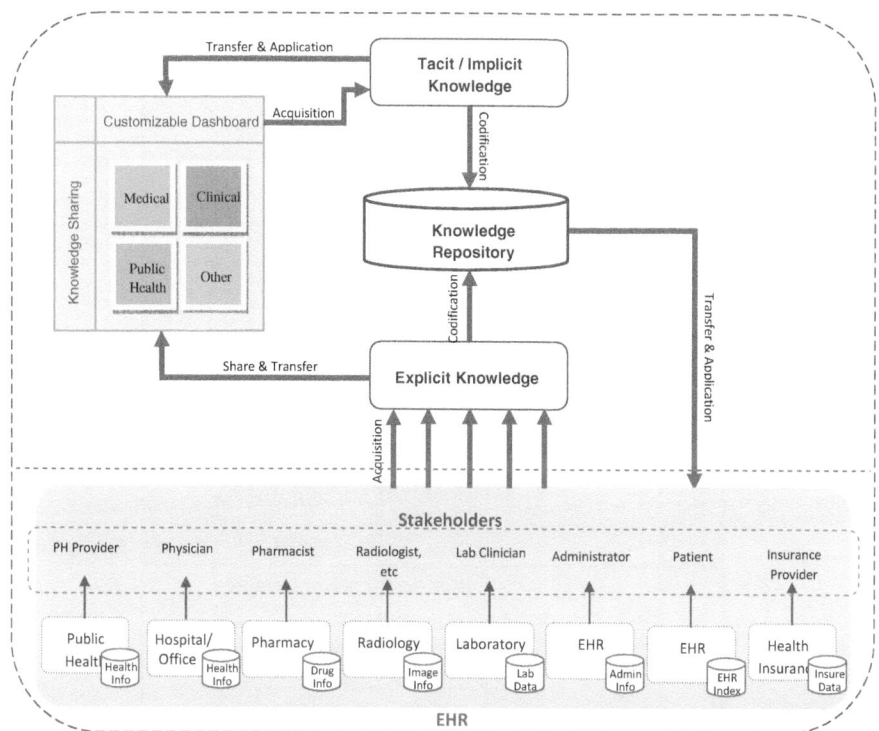

Fig. 2. DOEM Architecture

EHR using proper data and text mining methods. This knowledge will then be codified to be stored in the knowledge repository. It can also be transferred and shared by the use of dashboards to the users of each dashboard. On the other hand the stakeholders (shown in Fig.2) as the owners and contributors of knowledge, play the main role in KM and their tacit and implicit knowledge should be revealed by the means of dashboards. The acquired knowledge will also be codified to be stored in the knowledge repository. The gathered knowledge in knowledge repository is also transferred to be used and applied by the stakeholders of EHR. Each of these KM processes in knowledge cycle is powered by its own IT tools. A list of such tools can be seen in Table 1.

A customizable dashboard is proposed in our conceptual model in order to discover and gather the tacit and implicit knowledge of knowledge owners. The dashboard should be designed based on the related EHR content, knowledge stakeholders and their workplace culture. Customizable Dashboard is the means to help understanding the relations of different data acquired from EHR while giving the right information in the right time to the right person. It also provides each group of stakeholders with a selected set of knowledge and information based on their role in the healthcare.

Table 1. Selected IT tools to support certain KM activities, Adapted from [1]

ID	KM Process	IT Tools
1	Acquisition	Data mining Text mining Discussion forums Dashboards
2	Codification	Databases Data warehouse Knowledge repositories Operational knowledge store Electronic publishing
3	Transfer	Intranet and Extranet Workflow systems Groupware Dashboards
4	Application	Rule-based personalization Intelligent agent Knowledge-based systems Expert systems Case-based reasoning Clinic decision support systems

Different dashboards should be designed to fit the various requirements of the professionals of every healthcare domain. Some of the main features and attributes of dashboards are as follows.

- They should be designed according to the level of expertise and the needs of their users.
- They should only show what each user must know. Thus time is not wasted on unwanted information and no mistakes are made due to lack of information.
- Using IT enabled equipment; real-time feedback of the user can improve knowledge and information presentation. Such interactive interface can also be used to gather the information needed for knowledge discovery.

By using well-designed dashboards with the mentioned properties great advantages can be gained. These advantages are listed in Table 2.

The inclusion of the mentioned benefits depends on the type and the usage of the dashboard. For instance, in the domain of clinical healthcare, medical and clinical histories of patients grow larger and larger through time and it is important to only show the effective information and knowledge in the dashboard for healthcare

Table 2. Advantages for DOEM

ID	Benefit	Description
1	Collaboration and Knowledge Sharing	Dashboards provide a good framework for collaboration of healthcare stakeholders to share their ideas and experiences about different medical and clinical issues. It can also improve the culture of knowledge sharing in the healthcare society.
2	Interoperation	Dashboard can provide interoperation between different implementation of EHR and KMS.
3	Categorization	Data and information categorization in dashboards enables easy codification of the discovered knowledge.
4	Education	A dashboard can provide its users with up-to-date knowledge tailored to their needs, obtained from the knowledge repository. In long term, this can be seen as a tool for educational purposes.

professionals. This can be done by proper data/text mining which is the task of knowledge discovery in KM. When healthcare professionals have the right information and knowledge in the right time and are able to share their knowledge with each other, they will be able to make more accurate decisions. Moreover, with the help of KM these decisions can be used to acquire the tacit and implicit knowledge of healthcare professionals which can be stored in the knowledge repository and can be used by other persons. It should be noted that such knowledge should be verified by a certified group of experts before it can be used as a new source of knowledge. Using such dashboard not only decreases medical errors, but also increases the available knowledge in the healthcare society. The following items can be included in a dashboard designed for a physician: patient demographics, problems/diagnoses, medication, allergies, patient charts, documents, lab tests, confidential notes, images and other helpful data. Custom-designed forms and questionnaires can be present in the physicians' dashboard to acquire his/her diagnostics results and decisions. Another example could be the patient dashboard which can be used to inform the patient and his/her family about his/her circumstances and give him/her the proper advices according to the information in the EHR and knowledge about his/her clinical and medical issues. This will help to improve the awareness of the patients which is a very big challenge in today's healthcare. The patient dashboard can also be used by him/her to enter or correct his/her information in his/her records and also guide him/her through the medical and clinical process if needed. Accordingly, the following items can be included in a patient dashboard: allergies, vaccinations, medical family history, prior prescriptions, medical guidelines and other helpful data.

5   Conclusion and Outlook

Regarding the WHO KM strategy and the importance of e-health in today's world, reconsideration in implementation of EHR as one of the main elements of e-health seems inevitable. Also, effective usage of the huge amount of data in EHR is a challenging task and every stakeholder in the healthcare society should be satisfied. Furthermore, building a sharing culture and capacity to use and reapply scientific and experiential knowledge is of great importance [6]. Some of the interesting aspects of KM are knowledge sharing and knowledge transfer with great potential for innovation, time and cost savings [26]. Eventually, using KM techniques will help building the sharing culture and along with tacit and implicit knowledge discovery, paves the way for reapplying scientific and experiential knowledge. In this regard, a conceptual model for EHR with a KM approach is proposed in this paper. In this model, customizable dashboards are used to highlight the relations between the data from EHR, help in discovery of tacit and implicit knowledge of the knowledge owners and ease the knowledge sharing between stakeholders. Different dashboards should be designed for every domain to meet the requirements of the related stakeholders. While KM activities are done on the explicit knowledge derived from EHR, the knowledge stored in the knowledge repository can be reused and shared by the use of dashboards. Although some attributes of the mentioned dashboards are described in this paper, selecting a framework and defining the steps needed for real implementation of such dashboards can be the subject for more work. Moreover, adapting different clinical workflows and procedures into this model should be taken into account for any implementation.   Further work can also be done by extending different aspects of KM described in the model, for real implementations.

References

1. Hsia, T.L., Lin, L.M., Wu, J.H., Tsai, H.T.: A Framework for Designing a Nursing Knowledge Management Systems. Interdisciplinary Journal of Information, Knowledge and Management 1, 14–22 (2006)
2. Lin, B., Umoh, D.: E-healthcare: A vehicle of change. American Business Review 20(2), 27–32 (2002)
3. Bose, R.: Knowledge management-enabled health care management systems: Capabilities, infrastructure and decision-support. Expert Systems with Applications 24, 59–71 (2003)
4. Duennebeil, S., Sunyaev, A., Leimeister, J.M., Krcmar H.: Strategies for Development and Adoption of EHR in German Ambulatory Care. In: Pervasive Computing Technologies for Healthcare (PervasiveHealth) (2010)
5. Montero, M.A., Prado, S.: Electronic Health Record as a Knowledge Management Tool in the Scope of Health. In: Riaño, D. (ed.) K4HelP 2008. LNCS, vol. 5626, pp. 152–166. Springer, Heidelberg (2009)
6. World Health Organization: World Health Organization Knowledge Management Strategy. World Health Organization Geneva Switzerland. WHO/EPI/KMS/2005 1, 1–16 (2005)
7. Bakker, A.R.: The need to know the history of the use of digital patient data, in particular the EHR. International Journal of Medical Informatics 76(5-6), 438–441 (2007)

8. Koppar, A.R., Sridhar, V.: A workflow solution for electronic health records to improve healthcare delivery efficiency in rural India. In: eTELEMED, pp. 227–232 (2009)
9. Arnold, S., et al.: Electronic Health Records: A Global Perspective. In: A Work Product of Healthcare Information and Management Systems Society (HIMSS) (2008)
10. Razzaque, A., Jalal-Karim, A.: Conceptual Healthcare Knowledge Management model for adaptability and interoperability of EHR. In; European, Mediterranean & Middle Eastern Conference on Information Systems (2010)
11. Garde, S., Knaup, P., Hovenga, E.J.S., Heard, S.: Towards Semantic Interoperability for Electronic Health Records: Domain Knowledge Governance for openEHR Archetypes. Methods of Information in Medicine 11(1), 74–82 (2006)
12. Hameed, S., Mustapha, S., Mardhiyah, A., Miho, V.: Electronic Medical Record for Effective Patient Monitoring Database. In: Proceeding of the International Conference on Computer and Communication Engineering (2008)
13. Ghahramani, N., Lendel, I., Haque, R., Sawruk, K.: User satisfaction with Computerized order Entry System and its Effect on Workplace Stress. Journal of Medical Systems 33, 199–205 (2009)
14. King, W.R., Marks Jr., P.V., McCoy, S.: The most important issues in knowledge management (2002)
15. Kebede, G.: Knowledge Management: An information science perspective. International Journal of Information Management, 416–424 (2010)
16. Zins, C.: Conceptual approaches for defining data, information and knowledge. Journal of the American Society for Information Science and Technology 58(4), 479–493 (2007)
17. Nonaka, I.: The knowledge creating company. Harvard Business Review 69(6), 96–104 (1991)
18. Alavi, M., Leidner, D.E.: Knowledge management and knowledge management systems: Conceptual foundations and research issues. MIS Quarterly 25(1), 107–136 (2001)
19. Gover, V., Davenport, T.H.: General perspectives on knowledge management: Fostering a research agenda. Journal of Management Information Systems 18(1), 5–21 (2001)
20. Fayyad, U.M., Piatetsky-Shapiro, G., Smyth, P.: From Data Mining to Knowledge Discovery in Databases. AI Magazine 17(3), 37–54 (1996)
21. Chen, H., Chau, M.: Web Mining: Machine Learning for Web Applications. Annual Review of Information Science and Technology 38, 289–329 (2004)
22. Kovalerchuk, B., Vityaev, E., Ruiz, J.F.: Consistent and Complete Data and 'Expert' Mining in Medicine. In: Cios, K.J. (ed.) Medical Data Mining and Knowledge Discovery. Physica-Verlag, New York (2001)
23. Chen, H.: Knowledge Management Systems: A Text Mining Perspective. The University of Arizona, Tucson (2001)
24. Hearst, M.A.: Untangling Text Data Mining. In: Proceedings of ACL 1999: The 37th Annual Meeting of the Association for Computational Linguistics, Maryland, pp. 20–26 (June 1999)
25. Khobreh, M., Ansari, F., Nasiri, S.: Knowledge Management Approach for Enhancing of Urban Health Equity. In: Proceedings of ECKM 2010, pp. 554—565 (2010)
26. Ansari, F., Holland A., Fathi, M.: Advanced Knowledge Management Concept for Sustainable Environment Integration. In: Proceeding of the 2009 8th IEEE international Conference on Cybernetic Intelligent Systems UK, September 9-10, pp. 1–7 (2009)

Navigability of an Ontology-Based Web Site

Kyungsil Min, Sungkyu Chun, Hwansoo Kim,
Hyosook Jung, and Seongbin Park*

Computer Science Education Department,
Korea University, Seoul, Korea

Abstract. A web site should be designed carefully because if the structure of the site is complex, users can be disoriented. A navigable web site is one where users can find desired information as they freely move around at the site. It is important to construct a navigable web site because the navigability of a web site can indicate how accessible the information contents in the site might be. In this paper, we present a way by which a navigable web site might be created. Our method utilizes an ontology that specifies important concepts in the domain of interests and describes how they are related. A web site is modeled as a directed graph and navigability is measured by two quantities: time spent and the number of web pages visited by a user during an information retrieval task. Experimental results indicated that navigability increased as the degree of similarity between the structure of the site and that of ontology increased.

Keywords: ontology, navigability.

1 Introduction

Working with computers in the information society becomes necessary for most people regardless of age and profession. Thanks to the Internet which is often called the sea of information has developed, people can rapidly exchange information and communicate with others. While surfing the Internet, people can search the information they need to know or share the information with others. At that time, while they easily find the right information in some web sites, they cannot find out the desired information in other web sites even though it exists somewhere in the web site. In addition, when surfing the Internet, some people do not know why they have followed specific paths and have seen the wrong information which they do not need. This symptom is called 'lost in hyperspace' or 'disorientation' [2][5][6][9]. It means that people lose their contexts of searching and they do not know where they are located in the sea of information.

In this paper, we present a way by which a navigable web site could be created, where the navigability of the web site refers to how efficiently a user finds the information that the user wants when navigating through the site [1]. A navigable web site allows a user to find out information in the web site easily

---

* Corresponding author.

A. Holzinger and K.-M. Simonic (Eds.): USAB 2011, LNCS 7058, pp. 441–453, 2011.

and reduces the symptom of lost in hyperspace. Our method utilized an ontology that describes concepts and their relationships in a domain of interests [13]. More specifically, information that exists in the web site is connected using hyperlinks according to the structure specified by an ontology so that it can help users follow meaningful links in the web site.

To evaluate how ontology influences the navigability of a web site, we measured time spent and the number of web pages visited by users during information retrieval tasks in web sites that contained the same contents, but had different link structures.

We conducted two types of experimentations.

First, in order to test whether an ontology influences navigability at all, we created a web site that reflected the structure of an ontology completely (type A) and created a web site that reflected the structure of the ontology partially (type B). Both types of the sites had the same contents, but their linking structures were different. It turned out that users could navigate better in type A site than type B site.

Second, to evaluate how the degree of similarity between the structure of an ontology and the structure of a web site influences the navigability of the site, we created three web sites. The contents of the sites were the same, but they had different link structures. More specifically, one site reflected the structure of the ontology completely (100 %), another site reflected the ontology nearly completely (70 %), and the other site reflected the ontology partially (30 %). It turned out that the more the site reflected the structure of the ontology, the navigable the web site was.

So, the problem of designing a navigable web site reduces to the problem of designing a good ontology for the domain of interests that constitute the contents of the web site. In addition, since ontologies can be processable by machines [16], it becomes possible to measure the navigability of a web site by checking how much the linking structure of the site resembles the structure of an ontology for the site.

This paper is structured as follows. Section 2 describes related works to our research. Methodology of the current research is explained in section 3. Section 4 describes experimental results and the paper concludes in section 5.

2   Related Works

The success of a web site is influenced by how easily users can navigate the web site [10][17] and the design of a web site to minimize the symptom of 'lost in hyperspace' is an important issue for web based education, distance learning, and hypermedia-based learning environment such as VLE [17][14][20][21]. Especially, if the amount of information in the site is large, users can easily get lost in the sea of information [19]. However, the measure of navigability is not simple or easy to define [8].

There have been approaches to evaluate how navigable a web site is. Navigable web sites refer to ones where users can find desired information easily as they move around at the sites. Since navigability is a qualitative attribute of a web site, quantitative evaluation is not always easy and certain assumptions or approximations have been made.

Aaronson [1] presents a numerical index that measures how well-organized or easy to navigate a hypertext system is. A hypertext is modeled as a directed graph, where a node represents a web page and directed links exist between nodes if their contents are related. In order to specify how two nodes may be linked, three types of links are defined. A first type is a virtual link which is an ordered pair of web pages (p_a, p_b) meaning that p_a could conceivably contain a link to p_b based on the content of p_a and p_b. A second type is a mandatory link that is an ordered pair of web pages (p_a, p_b) that must exist because the contents of p_a and p_b are closely related. A mandatory link is included in the virtual links. The virtual and the mandatory links should be chosen by the hypertext designer or someone else who has knowledge about the hypertext's content and purpose. A third type is a real link that is an ordered pair of web pages (p_a, p_b) signifying that p_a actually links to p_b in the hypertext. The set of real links should contain mandatory links.

Figure 1 depicts two possible hypertexts that can be constructed given a specification about virtual links, mandatory links, and the number of maximum links.

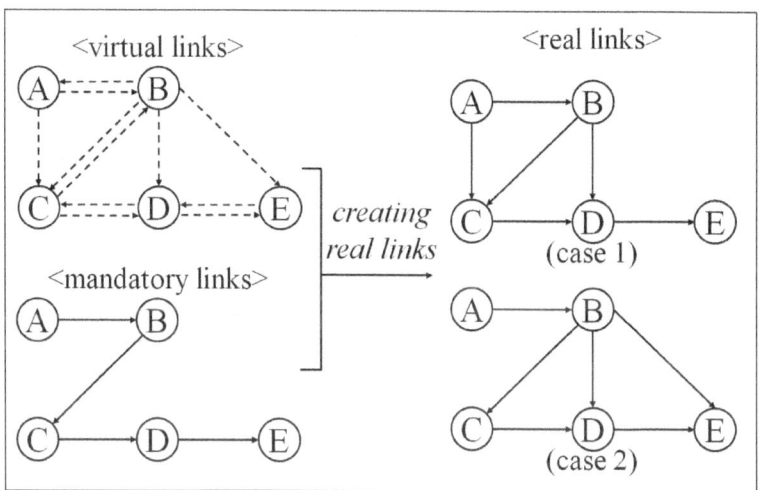

Fig. 1. Construction of a hypertext subject to the constraints (i.e., virtual links, mandatory links, and the maximum number of links that can exist in the hypertext)

Left part of the figure shows that there are five web pages (i.e., A, B, C, D, E), eleven virtual links (i.e., dashed links such as a link from A to B, B to A, etc), and four mandatory links (i.e., A to B, B to C, C to D, D to E). We assume that the maximum number of links that can exist is six. Since there are four mandatory links, it means that two more links need to be selected from the set of virtual links. Right part shows two possible hypertexts that can be constructed which satisfy the constraints; i.e., both of hypertexts include mandatory links and two additional links are selected from the set of virtual links.

The index reflects user demands for a page denoted as d_{p_a} which represents how important the hypertext designer judges to p_a. It also incorporates a factor α called attention span that represents the likelihood that users will follow a path through the hypertext without becoming sidetracked. The index is defined as follows:

$$\psi = \sum_{p_a,p_b \in P, p_a \neq p_b} d_{p_a} d_{p_b} \alpha^{r_{p_a,p_b} + \gamma_{p_a,p_b} - 2}$$

where r_{p_a,p_b} represents the length of the shortest real path from p_a to p_b and γ_{p_a,p_b} represents the length of the shortest virtual path from p_a to p_b, respectively. The experiment on actual hypertext systems shows that as the index value increases, the number of pages accessed to find information decreases and the speed of finding information increases.

Smith [2] defines various path measures such as indicators and ratings of user's lostness, efficiency and confidence while using a hypertext system. The measures of lostness are produced in terms of the path measurements. There are two lostness indicators. One considers the number of different nodes accessed while searching (N) compared with the total number of nodes accessed while searching (S). The other is a comparison of the number of nodes required to complete a task (R) and the number of different nodes visited while search (N). It also produces a lostness rating (L) compared to a user performing a 'perfect search' as follows:

$$L = \sqrt{(\tfrac{N}{S} - 1)^2 + (\tfrac{R}{N} - 1)^2}$$

It assumes that in a perfect search a user visits exactly the number of nodes accessed as being required to complete a task. It means that the value of N/S is 1 and the value of R/N is 1. The lostness rating increases as lostness increases. The lostness rating is 0 in a perfect search.

Gwizdka and Spence [3] used lostness measure based on counts of visited web pages such as revisits and lostness, and statistical properties of the web navigation graph such as compactness, stratum and similarity to the optimal path. These measures can be used to diagnose user navigational problems and identify problems in web site design. It is because users in hypermedia navigation have often experienced cognitive overload and lostness. They examine some structural and temporal measures to predict lostness and task success during the web navigation.

Metacognition can help users learn materials in hyperspace and Chiazzese et al.[18] presented results of a pilot study for an educational tool which improved students' awareness during surfing activities.

Recently, ontology has been used to help users navigate in a hyperspace. In general, ontology [11] defines a set of representational primitives to model a domain of knowledge. The representational primitives consist of classes, attributes and relationships and their definitions contain information about their meaning and constraints on their logically consistent application. The ontology is a specification of an abstract data model that is independent of its particular form.

Woukeu et al. [12] present ontological hypermedia which is the use of ontologies as conceptual models of knowledge to improve navigational capabilities in hypermedia systems. The resources are represented by using concepts and their relationships in a defined ontology are used to create conceptual links as well as classical links. The resulting hypermedia is more beneficial to the users and enables reasoning over the resources by queries.

Jung et al. [4] presents a system that automatically provides a user with links that are semantically related using an ontology.

3   Methodology

In this section, we describe the main ideas behind our approach.

There are two research problems that we address. First, we intend to construct a navigable web site. Second, we would like to measure how the navigability of a web site changes as the degree of similarity between the ontology and the web site increases.

For the first problem, we propose to use the information specified in an ontology. As we can see from figure 1 in section 2, in general there are different hypertexts that satisfy the constraints about virtual links, mandatory links, and the maximum number of links. When creating a hypertext, ontology is viewed as specification about virtual links and when real links are added, we refer to the ontology and select links until the number of links becomes the maximum number of links that can exist in the hypertext.

Figure 2 shows this idea.

Left part of the figure describes the information in an ontology which can be easily expressed using an ontology language such as OWL [16], where the concepts are represented as classes and the concept relations are represented as properties.

For example, the concepts are defined by <owl:Class> and the concept relations are defined by <owl:ObjectProperty> which describes relations between two classes. <owl:ObjectProperty> specifies the domain and range class and then relates the domain class to the range class. So, part of the above ontology can be expressed as follows:

```
<owl:Class rdf:ID="A">
  <owl:Class rdf:ID="B">
    <owl:ObjectProperty rdf:ID="fromAtoB">
      <rdfs:domain rdf:resource="#A" />
      <rdfs:range rdf:resource="#B" />
    </owl:ObjectProperty>
```

For the second problem, we evaluate how an ontology influences the navigability of a web site using two measures: time spent and the number of web pages visited by a user during an information retrieval task. To verify that an ontology-based

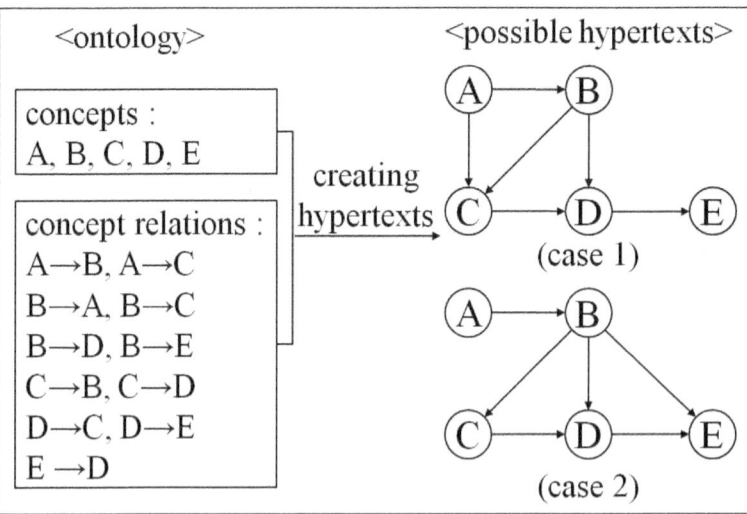

Fig. 2. Construction of a hypertext subject to the constraints specified in an ontology

site is more navigable than sites that do not reflect ontological information, we constructed sites that contained the same contents with different link structures. Then, we conducted information retrieval tasks against users, where each user was asked to find a web page that contained target information. When the information retrieval task ended, we checked how differently the users performed the navigational tasks by analyzing their navigational data. (i.e., we measured the number of web pages visited by a user and the total time spent on each question.). It turned out that as the degree of similarity between the structure of an ontology and the structure of a web site increased, the site became more navigable.

4 Experimental Results

In this section, we describe experimental results. We had two types of experiments. The first experiment was to check whether a web site that reflected the structure of an ontology completely (type A) was more navigable than a web site that was constructed by reflecting the same ontology partially (type B). The second experiment intended to evaluate how the degree of similarity between the structure of an ontology and the structure of a web site affected the navigability of the web site.

In the first experiment, we developed two types of web sites for learning Japanese; A-type site was designed based on an ontology, Japanese WordNet which is available up at http://nlpwww.nict.go.jp/wnja/index.en.html; B-type site was designed by modifying the structure of A-type site slightly.

Each page in both type of sites had one entry word and was connected to at least one other page. However, while all pages in A-type site were connected to other pages according to the semantic relation, some of the pages in B-type site were connected to other pages randomly. Each type of web sites contained 25 web pages and the number of different links between A-type and B-type was 10.

Figure 3 depicts the idea about constructing two types of the web sites. There are seven concepts (w_1, w_2, $\cdots$, w_7) in the J-WordNet which are connected each other. We need to construct a hypertext using seven web pages (n_1, n_2, $\cdots$, n_7) each of which corresponds to a concept in the J-WordNet. A-type site follows the structure of J-WordNet completey, but B-type site follows the structure partially.

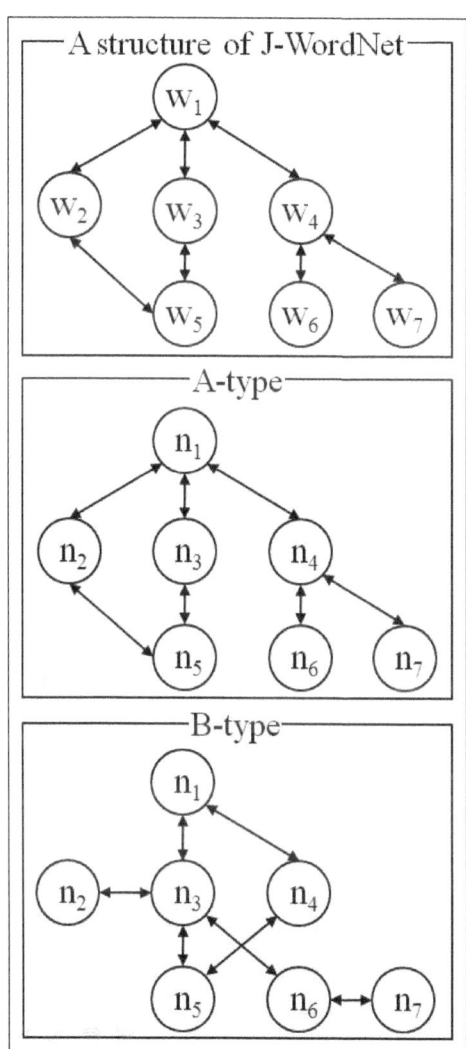

Fig. 3. Two types of Japanese language learning web sites

Specifically, A-type site was constructed as follows;

1. We chose an initial word. By using the word as a query, we searched the related words in Japanese WordNet.
2. In the words that were found, we selected some words that students at the intermediate level could understand. (This experimentation was conducted for Korean students who were taking intermediate level Japanese class.)
3. We created web pages whose entry words were either the initial word chosen at step 1 or its related words selected at step 2. Then, we made a hyperlink from the initial word to the selected words as its related words. (Note that each web page had one entry word.)
4. By using each entry word as a query, we repeated searching the related words in Japanese WordNet and made hyperlinks from the web page that had the entry word to web pages that had related words until the total number of the web pages became 25.

B-type web site was constructed as follows;

In the web pages created in A-type, we chose some pages randomly and made the pages link to other web pages that were not semantically related. We made sure that each web page had at least one incoming link to avoid a situation where some web pages existed as islands. In other words, all web pages were accessible from some other web pages.

We tested each web site against eight college students (ID 1 to ID 8) and calculated the navigability of each site using WebNavi program [7] that can record the web pages visited by the students and elapsed time for each of the visited pages. Students were asked to find specific information in the web sites. Four students performed the task in A-type first and then did the task in B-type, and the remaining four performed the task in B-type first and then did the task in A-type. At that time, they did not know which site was constructed based on Japanese WordNet. There was a time limitation (10 minutes for each site). After 10 minutes passed or students completed the answer sheet in one type, they were asked to move to the other type. When they completed the answer sheets in each type, the experiment ended.

The result of the experiment showed that A-type site was more navigable than B-type site. The students spent less time finding the target information in A-type site than in B-type site. While the students spent about 5 minutes on average in A-type site, they mostly spent more than 10 minutes in B-type site. In addition, the students in A-type site visited fewer web pages than in B-type site. The number of web pages visited in B-type site were approximately 4 or 5 times more than those in A-type site

We also found that the students performed the task faster in A-type site than in B-type site regardless of the order of experimentation (i.e., A-type → B-type or B-type → A-type). Especially, some students in B-type site did not complete the answer sheet. Except for one student whose log was erroneously recorded, the time spent in A-type site was less than that in B-type site and the number of web pages visited in A-type site was fewer than those in B-type site. As for the order of the experimentation, the students who moved from A-type site to

B-type site spent more time than those who moved from B-type site to A-type site. Our interpretation is that because the student felt the psychological anxiety when they did not complete the first answer sheet in B-type site, it might have affected their abilities to complete the second answer sheet in A-type site.

Table 1 shows the results of the first experiment.

Table 1. The experimental result about Japanese learning site

sequence of the performance	student ID	the spent time in A-type	the spent time in B-type	the number of web pages visited in A-type	the number of web pages visited in B-type
A-type → B-type	1	4' 24"	More than 10'	31	125
	2	4' 23"	More than 10'	31	151
	3	2' 3"	More than 10'	24	265
	4	5' 22"	More than 10'	69	218
B-type →A-type	5	5' 13"	5' 54"	33	27
	6	3' 22"	More than 10'	31	240
	7	7' 16"	More than 10'	64	89
	8	5' 35"	More than 10'	56	89

In the second experiment, we built an ontology about data structure and developed three types of web sites for studying data structure each of which reflected the structure of the ontology differently.

Figure 4 depicts the idea of constructing three types of hypertexts. There are eight concepts $(C_1, C_2, \cdots, C_8)$ in the ontology. We need to construct a hypertext with eight web pages $(n_1, n_2, \cdots, n_8)$ each of which corresponds to a concept in the ontology. The first site (fully corresponding site) reflects the structure of the ontology completely. The second and the third sites reflected the structure of the ontology nearly and partially, respectively. Specifically, each web site had 57 nodes and 80 links. The link structure of the first site fully corresponded with the structure of the ontology. In other words, the structure of the web site reflects the structure of the ontology completely. The link structure of the second site nearly corresponded with the structure of the ontology. The structure was 70 % similar to the structure of the ontology. The other links in the site were randomly rearranged, but each web page had at least one incoming link. The link structure of the third site partially corresponded with the structure of the ontology. The structure was 40 % similar to the structure of the ontology. The other links were randomly rearranged, but each web page had at least one incoming link.

We tested each of three sites against nine college students (ID 9 to ID 17). Each student was assigned to each site and given information retrieval tasks that consisted of 15 questions. They were asked to finish the task within 50 minutes. The results of the experiment showed that the students spent least time finding the target information in the site whose structure corresponded with the ontology 100 percent. The number of web pages visited by the students was the smallest in the site whose structure corresponded with the ontology

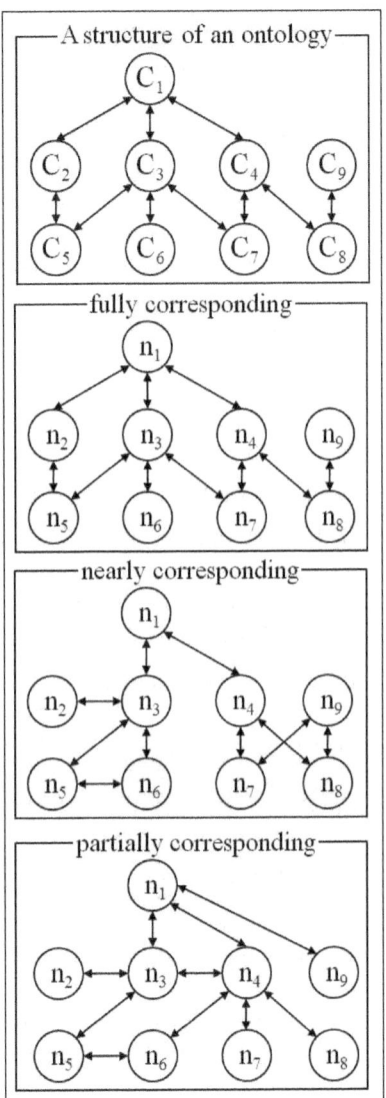

Fig. 4. Three types of web sites that reflect the structure of an ontology differently

100 percent. Students spent most time finding the target information in the site whose structure corresponded with the ontology 30 percent. The number of web pages visited by the students was the largest in the site whose structure corresponded with the ontology 100 percent.

Table 2 and table 3 show the experimental results about the second experiment.

Table 2. The experiment of Data structure learning site

the rate of the correspondence	student ID	the spent time	the number of visited web pages
40 percent	9	43' 7"	373
	10	50' 1"	318
	11	33' 10"	345
70 percent	12	31' 37"	113
	13	22' 31'	136
	14	45' 1"	183
100 percent	15	15' 59"	100
	16	16' 12"	139
	17	16' 46'	117

Table 3. The result of the experiments

the rate of the correspondence	the spent time on average	the number of web pages on average
40 %	42' 6"	345.3
70 %	33' 3"	144
100 %	16' 19"	118.7

5 Conclusions and Future Works

Navigability of a web site can affect the quality of the web site [15]. Even if a lot of information exist in a web site, if the site is not navigable, users can become easily disoriented. So, navigability of a web site can indicate how accessible the web site might be.

In this paper, we addressed two research problems that are relevant to accessibilty of information. First, we dealt with how a navigable web site could be constructed. To this end, we utilised an ontology that specified important concepts and their relationships in a domain of interests. Second, we evaluated how the navigability of a web site increased as the similarity between the structure of an ontology and the structure of a web site increased.

We conducted two types of experiments.

First, in order to test whether an ontology could influence the navigability of a web site at all, we created two types of web sites with the same contents (i.e., Japanese language learning materials) that had different link structures. In this experiment, we found that a web site that reflected the structure of an ontology completely was more navigable than the site that reflected the structure of the same ontology partially.

Second, in order to measure how the similarity between the structure of a web site and the structure of an ontology influences the navigability of a web site, we created three web sites with the same contents (i.e., data structure learning materials) that had different link structures. It turned out that as the similarity between the structure of a web site and the structure of an ontology increased, the navigability of the site increased.

Designing a navigable web site is an important and diffult problem that involves some issues.

First, we should start with a *right* ontology. Since there could exist different ontologies for the same domain of interest, we have to select reasonably good ontologies that can indicate what might be good virtual links.

Second, assuming that we have selected an ontology, we should also select mandatory links and real links from the set of virtual links specified in the ontology.

Third, once a web site is created according to this approach, the navigability of the site needs to be calculated realistically using a formula as well as pilot experimentation.

Currently, we are working on an ontology-based quantitative formula that can evaluate the navigability of a web site. The formula will still incorporate factors such as user demands and relevance of pages as in [1], but include a term that indicates the similarity between the structure of a web site and the structure of an ontology.

In the future, we plan to generalize the results of the current work. For example, quality of navigation can be determined by various aspects which were not reflected in the current work and browsing context of a user can contribute as well. These should be reflected when navigabilty of a web site is evaluated. We also plan to experiment with more realistic web sites and a set of ontologies rather than just one ontology. Finally, we plan to work on how the concept of navigability changes in the context of the Semantic Web [16]. We believe that in order to access the information on the Semantic Web, users still need to browse the Web site since the structure of the Semantic Web is hypertext [22]. In other words, even though information is represented in a way that computers can interpret directly on the Semantic Web, users still need to surf on the Semantic Web in order to access the information. But, the situation is different from the Web since some computations can be done by aoftware agents. So, the navigability of a Semantic Web site should be defined differently.

References

1. Aaronson, S.: Optimal Demand-oriented Topology for Hypertext Systems. In: Proceedings of 20th Annual International ACM SIGIR Conf. on Research and Development in Information Retrieval, pp. 168–177 (1997)
2. Smith, P.A.: Towards a practical measure of hypertext usability. Interacting with Computer 8(4), 365–381 (1996)

3. Gwizdka, J., Spence, I.: Implicit measures of lostness and success in web navigation. Interacting with Computers 19(3), 357–369 (2007)

4. Jung, H., Kim, H., Min, K., Park, S.: The Ontology-based Web Navigation Guidance System. Journal of Korean Association of Computer Education 12(5) (2009)

5. Yatim, N.: A Combination Measurement for Studying Disorientation. In: Proceedings of 35th Annual Hawaii International Conference on System Sciences, pp. 138–144. IEEE Computer Society (2002)

6. Otter, M., Johnson, H.: Lost in hyperspace: metric and mental models. Interacting with computers 13(1), 1–40 (2002)

7. Lee, S.H., Jung, H., Park, S.: A navigational guidance system for Web-based Education. In: Proceedings of sixth Conference on IASTED International Conference, Web-Based Education, vol. 2, pp. 206–209 (2007)

8. Zhang, Y., Zhu, H., Greenwood, S.: Website complexity metrics for measuring navigability. In: Proceedings of 4th International Conference on Quality Software, pp. 172–179 (2004)

9. Conklin, J.: Hypertext: An Introduction and Survey. Computer, 17–41 (1987)

10. Palmer, J.: Web Site Usability, Design, and Performance Metrics. Information Systems Research 13(2), 151–167 (2000)

11. Gruber, T. (2007),
http://tomgruber.org/writing/ontology-definition-2007.htm

12. Woukeu, A., Wills, G., Conole, G., Carr, L., Kampa, S., Hall, W.: Ontological Hypermedia in education: A framework for building web-based educational portals. In: Proceedings World Conference on Educational Multimedia, Hypermedia and Telecommunications, pp. 349–357 (2003)

13. Heflin, J., Volz, R., Dale, J.: Web Ontology Requirements, Proposed W3C Working Draft (2002), http://km.aifb.uni-karlsruhe.de/projects/owl/index.html

14. Herder, E.: Modeling user navigation. In: Brusilovsky, P., Corbett, A.T., de Rosis, F. (eds.) UM 2003. LNCS, vol. 2702, pp. 417–419. Springer, Heidelberg (2003)

15. Gonzalez, F., Palacios, M.: Quantitative evaluation of commercial web sites: an empirical study of Spanish firms. International Journal of Information Management 24(4), 313–328 (2004)

16. Antoniou, G., van Harmelen, F.: A Semantic Web Primer. The MIT Press (2004)

17. Zhou, Y., Leung, H., Winoto, P.: MNav: A Markov Model-Based Web Site Navigability Measure. IEEE Transaction on Software Engineering 33(12), 869–890 (2007)

18. Chiazzese, G., Ottaviano, S., Merlo, G., Chiari, A., Allegra, M.: Surfing Hypertexts with a Metacognition Tool. Informatica 30, 439–445 (2006)

19. Banciu, D.: e-Romania - A Citizens' Gateway towards Public Information. Studies In Informatics and Control 18(3), 205–210 (2009)

20. Glusac, D.: Dynamically Organization of Educational Contents for E-Learning. International Journal of Computers, Communications & Control 3, 316–321 (2008)

21. Page, T., Thorsteinsson, G., Niculescu, A.: Management of Knowledge in a Problem Based Learning Environment. Studies in Informatics and Control 18(3), 255–262 (2009)

22. Goble, C., Bechhofer, S., Carr, L., De Roure, D., Hall, W.: Conceptual Open Hypermedia = The Semantic Web? In: Semantic Web Workshop (2001)

Navigating through Very Large Sets of Medical Records: An Information Retrieval Evaluation Architecture for Non-standardized Text

Markus Kreuzthaler, Marcus Bloice,
Klaus-Martin Simonic, and Andreas Holzinger

Institute for Medical Informatics, Statistics and Documentation,
Auenbruggerplatz 2, 8036 Graz, Austria
{markus.kreuzthaler,marcus.bloice,klaus.simonic,
andreas.holzinger}@medunigraz.at

Abstract. Despite the prevalence of informatics and advanced information systems, there exists large amounts of unstructured text data. This is especially true in medicine and health care, where free text is an indispensable part of information representation. In this paper, the motivation behind developing information retrieval systems in medicine and health care is described. An overview of information retrieval evaluation is given, before describing the architecture and the development of an extendible information retrieval evaluation framework. This framework allows different information retrieval tools to be compared to a gold standard in order to test its effectiveness. The paper also gives a review of available gold standards which can be used for research purposes in the area of information retrieval of medical free texts.

Keywords: information retrieval, medicine, text mining, evaluation, gold standards.

1 Introduction and Motivation

Retrieving information from a large amount of medical free text is an important factor in clinical research, quality assurance, and medical accounting [1]. Also, with the introduction of large medical information systems, legacy texts are being processed by optical character recognition systems, digitized, and fed into archive systems. Medical professionals are often confronted with masses of free text and must deal with the task of finding the relevant information. Consequently, there is a need for smart information retrieval systems that can operate on this type of text, and the current systems in use are far from being infallible [2]. We believe that to make this data more accessible, usable, and useful, both the technological aspects, as well as human aspects, must be taken into consideration [3].

Although language understanding in general is still an unsolved problem, restricted domains such as medical notes and letters seem to be more tractable. This holds even more for the task of information retrieval where a thorough text understanding is not required and the identification of the concepts mentioned

A. Holzinger and K.-M. Simonic (Eds.): USAB 2011, LNCS 7058, pp. 455–470, 2011.

in a text together with the detection of their polarity suffices in most cases. However, the medical language used in our system poses a number of particular challenges:

- Abbreviations are frequent, often ambiguous or even ad hoc.
- There may be typos and optical character recognition (OCR) errors.
- A mixture of different languages (e.g. German, Latin, English) is used together with expressions of medical jargon.
- The same concept may be expressed in various ways using synonyms and linguistic variations.

As far as the context is concerned, homonyms are often only resolvable when knowing the context in which they belong. For a doctor, as long as the free text content is clear, correct spelling is not entirely important.

Meeting the information demand of medical professionals poses challenges that go beyond classical information retrieval. The first is robustness with respect to the mentioned *variability* and *noise* of the underlying texts. Another challenge is to take into account the semantic relations in the medical domain. These involve, in particular, taxonomic, functional, and anatomic relations. For instance, searching for reports of neoplasms in the gastrointestinal tract means having to match to all kinds of tumors and carcinomas in many parts of the body, such as the esophagus, stomach, intestines etc.

Of course, it must also be possible to evaluate a system's performance, in order to compare it with other solutions currently being used or systems that are under development. Furthermore, it is of importance to be able to compare any system's performance against a human expert who is executing the same task. Human experts possess knowledge about the typical idiosyncrasies that are contained within free texts, and are able to apply previous experience and knowledge to the search request to get high precision *and* high recall values from the information retrieval process. On the other hand they must use much longer expressions in their chosen query language to get the required information, which contrasts the way semantic information retrieval works; the input to the tool is in a human readable form.

This paper, besides providing a review of information retrieval testing and available gold standards that can be used for this purpose, concentrates on the description of a test environment for information retrieval systems working on medical free text copora. The test environment allows the comparison between the human expert's results and the retrieval tool's results according to an information need. The core elements of the evaluation framework that must exist were identified, and these components were grouped together as one graphical user interface (GUI) in order to provide a user-friendly front end to the system, following usability engineering methods [4]. The GUI supports the speedy evaluation of an information retrieval tool (IR Tool) and also aids the developer of the tool in further enhancing it.

The remainder of the paper is organized as follows: Section 2 motivates information retrieval in medicine and health care and gives a review regarding information retrieval evaluation. Furthermore, openly available gold standards that can be used for free text information retrieval testing are listed. Section 3 describes the entire evaluation architecture identifying the main components that the architecture consists of and logically groups them together. Section 4 depicts the results of the evaluation environment concentrating on the arrangement of components in the GUI. Finally, Section 5 concludes the paper and gives an outlook of open questions and future research directions in this area.

2 Theoretical Background and Related Work

In this section we are motivating information retrieval in the context of medical textual data. Afterwards, a short overview of information retrieval testing is given, concentrating on available gold standards which can be used for information retrieval research. This is an important aspect due to the fact that in order to test any information retrieval system's usefulness in the medical domain, data must be used which, by its nature, is *very sensitive*.

2.1 Information Retrieval in Medicine and Health Care

To enhance quality of patient care and to provide a better use of evidence, information retrieval systems are increasingly used by physicians [5]. Information retrieval system evaluation is an ongoing are of research [6,7,8] and advanced text mining techniques help to handle the information overload, for example in medical literature [8,9]. In contrast to this, text mining methods lack enhancement in the area of medical information and documentation systems [1,3,10]. Sophisticated medical information retrieval systems have to handle very large sets of medical documents, where typically *non-standardized* text makes up a significant amount of this patient data. This data, often called free text in literature, has been very long in the focus of research [11,12,13] and has not lost its importance [14]. The automatic analysis of text is still a challenging problem [15,16,17], which is in contrast to the effort which has to be made to produce text. Relevant relationships can stay completely undiscovered, because relevant data are scattered and no investigator has linked them together manually [18].

2.2 Information Retrieval Evaluation

According to [19] the standard procedure to measure information retrieval effectiveness comprises; a document collection, a test suite of information requests expressible as queries and a set of judgments for each query-document pair, which defines each pair as either relevant or not relevant. The result of this binary classification process to an information need is called a *ground truth judgment of relevance* or simply a *gold standard*. Another important fact is that the test collection should be a sample of the kinds of text that will be encountered in the operational setting of interest and particularly for testing information retrieval systems that work on medical free text data, it is hard to find utilizable corpora that can be used for information retrieval research [20]. In extension

to [20] we want give a review of openly available free text corpora which can
be used as gold standards for research purposes (Table 1). We therefore concentrate our review on copora containing text types which pose the challenges
mentioned in Section 1 which differ significantly from text corpora used in the
field of biomedical natural language processing (bioNLP) for example. Typically
in bioNLP most of the annotated texts are drawn from biology literature or from
abstracts of scientific literature (e.g. MEDLINE), so *not* reflecting the difficulties in computer based patient records. For the sake of completeness we want to
mention The National Centre for Text Mining (NaCTeM)[1] which is an excellent
resource finding corpora which can be used for bioNLP. Table 1 which is an
extension to [21] gives an overview of available test corpora for medical free text
information retrieval and extraction evaluation. An excellent overview to other
copora which can be used for natural language processing (NLP) can be found
at `http://nlp.stanford.edu/links/statnlp.html#Corpora`.

Table 1. Available free text gold standards in the medical domain

Corpus Name	Description
Computational Medicine Challenge	1954 reports are assigned with ICD-9-CM codes from a radiology department. The corpus was initially used for testing and evaluating different classifiers [22].
ImageCLEFMed	The data set comprises ca. 50 000 images with textual annotations. Even though made up for content based image retrieval, the textual content to each picture plus annotations can be used as a gold standard for text based information retrieval testing [23,24].
Ogren	The corpus contains 60 clinical notes annotated with functional disorders. [25].
CLEF Corpus	The set exits of 167 medical documents annotated with diseases, drugs, body regions etc. as well as their internal relations [26].
i2b2	The text corpus comprises 889 anonymized epicrises and contains annotation which can be used for evaluating algorithms for the task of de-identification of clinical records. A subset of the texts further on contains annotations about the smoking status of the patient [27,28].
BLULab	The BLULab NLP Repository contains a collection of ca. 100 000 de-identified clinical records from multiple U.S. hospitals during 2007. The reports are annotated with ICD-9 Codes. `http://nlp.dbmi.pitt.edu/nlprepository.html`

The Text REtrieval Conference (TREC, `http://trec.nist.gov/tracks
.html`) has recently started a track with the following aim: "The goal of the
Medical Records track is to foster research on providing content-based access
to the free-text fields of electronic medical records." The BLULab corpus will

---

[1] `http://www.nactem.ac.uk/`

be used for this purpose and judged information needs through pooling will be available soon.

Having chosen a collection of interest, a metric must be decided upon. Typically one differs between metrics for *ranked* (Precision, Recall, Fallout, F-Measure) and *unranked retrieval results* (R-Precision, Precision at k, Mean Average Precision (MAP), Normalized Discounted Cumulative Gain (NCDG)) [29,30]. Beside pure statistical evaluation metrics other levels of testing should be considered. [31] stated testing at the engineering level, the input level, the processing level, the output level, the use and user level, and the social level that should be accounted for. Furthermore the human factor and human information behavior [32], in the context of information retrieval systems, are important factors when developing such systems. The systems must be capable of satisfying user needs and therefore human factors play an important role [33] for the acceptance of the retrieval systems as a whole.

3   Methods and Materials

This section describes the generic architecture that was developed for information retrieval testing based on *medical* free text corpora. We start by specifying the objective target and requirements of the overall system. Based on these requirements main components are identified, which are described in Section 3.2. The next section concentrates on the human computer interface (HCI) aspects that were considered when developing the GUI for the test framework, by logically grouping together the mentioned components. At the end we depict the overall architecture, containing the different parts identified previously.

3.1   Objective Target and Requirements

The main objective was to evaluate an information retrieval system within an integrated test environment and to compare the performance achieved by the IR Tool to that of a human expert who searched for the same task. As a representation metric the precision, recall, fallout, and F-measure operating figures were chosen to gauge the performance of the IR Tool. A further requirement for the test environment was that different versions of one IR Tool and their corresponding evaluation values could be saved. As a consequence, different versions can be loaded and compared according to their performance values. Besides testing different versions of one IR Tool, the framework working in the background also supports the integration and test of different IR Tools. Therefore the main requirements for the system are:

- To support the developer in enhancing the IR Tool. Therefore, both a test set (3034 ICD-annotated pathology reports) and a training set (508 ICD-annotated pathology reports) were created. The test set allows the developers to only see the statistical evaluation. The training set, on the other hand, provides the developer with the chance to view details as to why a text was found or not found by the IR Tool.

– Evaluation results with preset information retrieval parameters can be saved and compared to evaluation results from previous test runs. For example two runs with different information retrieval parameters.
– A user friendly graphical interface, which logically groups together components in a consistent way. In particular, statistical evaluation values between different IR Tool versions, and between the training and test data, were arranged in a way that makes them easy to compare them at a first glance.
– To be easily extendable to accommodate new test or training sets of different text types. For example, pathology inflammation and radiology thorax.
– The framework should also support the integration of different IR Tools. This makes it possible not just to compare different versions of one tool but different versions of different IR Tools.
– To make it easy to navigate through the different result sets of the IR Tool (true positives, false positives, false negatives, true negatives and all found).
– To highlight texts that differ between different result sets of the expert and the IR Tool according to an information need, to gain quick access.
– To ensure that the evaluation environment is accessible online with different user rights for different developers.

3.2   Component Identification

Considering the requirements from the previous sections, we identified the core components that the evaluation architecture must consist of. These components are:

Data Base. A data base specifies a certain type of medical free text reports. The text's type in our case are pathology reports. It is the data that the IR Tool must perform actions on.

Training Data. The training data is an annotated set of medical reports which belong to a certain data base. All medical reports which belong to a certain training data type can be fully accessed, so all details belonging to this text are displayed. This means that it is possible to enhance the information retrieval system for this particular type of data.

Test Data. The test data is an annotated set of medical reports which belong to a certain data base. No medical reports that belong to a certain test data type can be accessed, and therefore no details belonging to this text are displayed.

Test Case. A test case defines a specific set of queries. For example, the test case "One Word" comprised the queries "Hepatitis", "Appendicitis", "Colitis", and "Gastritis".

Query. A query belongs to one or many test cases. A query on its own consists of three search requests.

Search Request. There are three types of search requests.
   – *Expert Search Request.* This is the human expert's search statement used to fulfill the information retrieval task.

- *Information Retrieval Search Request.* This is the statement that is used as an input for the IR Tool.
- *Gold Standard Search Request.* This is the statement that is used to get the truth out of the gold standard. That means that reports that correctly belong to the diagnosis 'hepatitis' are returned, for example.

Test Case Result. An evaluated test case returns a test case result. A test case result consists of one or many query results.

Query Result. An evaluated query returns a query result. The query result also contains the results of different evaluation metrics.

Information Retrieval Tool. This is the IR Tool, where benchmarks should be performed on.

Information Retrieval Parameters. The information retrieval can be enhanced by further tuning specific parameters which influence the results.

Evaluation Metric. To determine the quality of the information retrieval system an adequate metric has to be used.

3.3   Component Grouping

Concerning the requirement that a user-optimized GUI had to be created, this section describes the logical grouping of the components identified in the previous section which are finally associated to a view. This grouping resulted in the following three views and functionalities:

Search and Evaluate. Abstractly spoken, a test case is used in conjunction with specific information retrieval parameters on training data and/or test data that belong to a certain data base, with the aim of evaluating the performance of the IR Tool. Therefore, the data, test case, query, and information retrieval parameter selection process should be grouped together in their own section of the GUI. We refer to these elements as *Komponenten Pool I.*

The evaluation of a test case produces a test case result. To cater for this, there must be a section in the GUI where different views of the test case result can be selected. This result view selection comprises of:

- *Data Selection.* This is used to choose whether to show the evaluation results that belong to the training data or to the test data.
- *Query.* This is used to select a specific query result from the test case result.
- *Sub Set.* This is used to select the amount of true positives, false positives, true negatives, false negatives or all found.

We refer to these elements as *Komponenten Pool II.*

The result view is the third section of the GUI. It comprises of the following components:

- Training data based evaluation results from the expert and the IR Tool.
- Test data based evaluation results from the expert and the IR Tool.

- A section that comprises of a list of found reports along with their identifiers, how many were found, and the search request that lead to the
  result. Such a section has to be set up for the Expert, the IR Tool and
  the Gold Standard.
- A field where query results can be annotated with further information.
- A field where any save options can be selected. This is required as it is
  possible for test case results to be saved to a data medium.

We refer to these elements as *Komponenten Pool III*.

Load and Compare. As mentioned in Section 3.1, it is essential that evaluation values for previous versions of the information retrieval system can be
loaded and compared. To achieve this, the following elements are required:

- *Test Case Result Filter*. Because many different IR Tool versions will be
  tested using different test cases, it was deemed necessary to allow certain
  test case results to be filtered that match certain criteria.
- *Filtered Test Case Results*. If the filtering process results in different test
  case results, the user can choose to compare these.

Again we refer to these elements as *Komponenten Pool I*.

The comparison of two test case results should be feasible in a user friendly,
well-arranged way. The following menu items are necessary:

- *Data Selection I*. This menu item allows one to toggle whether the results
  belonging to the training- or test data should be shown. The selection is
  connected to the first loaded test case result.
- *Query*. This menu item allows one to toggle which query result of the test
  case result should be shown. The selection is connected to both loaded
  test case results.
- *Sub Set*. This menu item allows one to toggle what result set should be
  shown (true positives, false positives, false negatives, true negatives and
  all found). The selection is connected to both loaded test case results.
- *Data Selection II*. This menu item allows one to toggle whether the
  results belonging to the training- or test data should be shown. The
  selection is connected to the second loaded test case result.

We refer to these elements as *Komponenten Pool II*.

Two loaded test case results must be compared in a user-friendly way with
the following content:

- Evaluation results based on the selected data (either training data or
  test data) from the human expert and the IR Tool.
- A section that comprises of a list of found reports along with their identifiers, how many have been found, and what the search request was that
  led to the result.
- A field where query results can be annotated.

Both these fields must appear twice, so that it is possible for two case results
to be compared. Again, we refer to these elements as *Komponenten Pool III*.

Details. When developing the IR Tool, it is possible to not only get evaluation values but also to get detailed information as to why a certain report was found or not. Developers of the IR Tool are allowed to have a certain amount of insight into these details, but only for reports which belong to the training data. If required, they can get detailed feedback regarding each report in order for them to be able to enhance the retrieval performance. Conversely, developers have no insight into the details of the medical text corpora that belong to the test data. Performing a test run using test data only returns evaluation values according to the chosen metrics, as stated in Section 3.2. Any further access is disallowed. Aside from the aforementioned details, developers are also able to change the inspected report in this view in order to inspect how the information retrieval system deals with the altered text. Developers can then see if the changed text is found or not, according the details contained within that text. With the IR Tool Console the following functionality and content is mapped:

- The full content of the report is displayed.
- The IR Tool parameters which are responsible for this result are displayed and can be altered.
- Information about the scoring-process regarding the reports affiliation to the information need can be read.
- The report can be altered and the outcome of the retrieval process using the altered text can be checked.
- The semantic presentation of the report (Concept Graph) is displayed.

These elements are referred to as *Komponenten Pool Details*.

3.4   Architecture

This section describes the architecture and the components within this architecture as displayed in Fig. 1. The design is a typical three-tier architecture, which is specified in more detail in the next paragraph.

Client Tier. Contains the views as described in Section 3.3. The user is interacting with the environment via a web-browser.

Logic Tier. The communication with the server is realized with the Spring MVC paradigm. Important server side components are the corresponding controllers for the views (Search and Evaluate, Load and Compare, Details). The controllers are using the Java-based evaluation framework to handle the test logic. The framework consists of an evaluation logic, communicating with three main components: Data Bank Handler (DB Handler), the Metrics Module (Metrics) containing different statistical evaluation measures and IR Tool handler (IR Handler).

Data Tier. The data tier exists of three elements:

- Every data basis is stored in a data bank, containing medical reports split up into training- and test data. Further on test cases, queries and corresponding results are saved. A new data basis (e.g. radiology thorax) is saved in a new data bank.

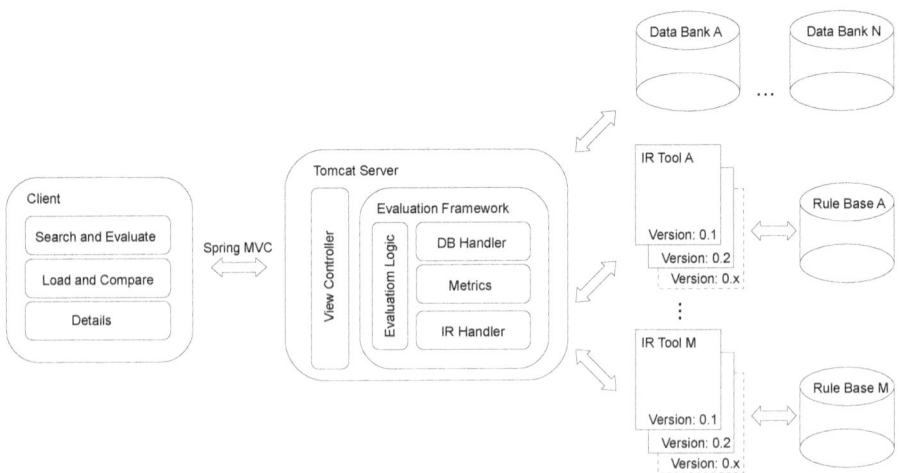

Fig. 1. Architecture of the evaluation environment

- The IR Tool under test. As well as the testing of different versions of *one* IR Tool is supported, *different* information retrievals tools can be integrated.
- Lots of information retrieval technologies communicate in the background with a rule base, which contains further logic that is needed for the retrieval process.

4   Results

This section describes the results of the GUI and provides some screen shots of the completed system. Therefore this section concentrates on the arrangement of the components of the developed information retrieval test environment. Statistical evaluation results and a detailed survey of the benchmark can be found in [34].

4.1   Hardware and Software Setup

The entire system was developed as an online, web application. The website itself runs on the Apache Tomcat web server, has a MySQL backend and was developed using the Spring Model-View-Controller paradigm in the Java programming language. The physical server runs the FreeBSD operating system on an Intel processor. The IR Tool under test was developed by ID Berlin (ID Information und Dokumentation im Gesundheitswesen GmbH & Co. KGaA ID) and uses the ID MACS® Server as rule base in the background. The IR Tool's retrieval process is based on a semantic text representation of the medical reports. This is achieved by applying a natural language processing technique to the texts, and the resulting concepts are parsed to a Wingert nomenclature [35,36,37].

4.2   Graphical User Interface

In Fig. 2 it is possible to see the arrangement of all important GUI components that were defined in Search and Evaluate. At the top of the web page all elements belonging to *Komponenten Pool I* are visible. Beneath these are the result view selection elements grouped into *Komponenten Pool II* - most of the page is dedicated to *Komponenten Pool III*. As mentioned in Section 3.1, one of the requirements was to compare the results achieved by an expert with the results achieved by the IR Tool's information retrieval process. Therefore, any different document identifiers are highlighted so that the user can see them at a glance. The evaluation results from the training data are placed next to the results from the test data, so that the user can quickly and directly compare the values achieved by the precision, recall, fallout, and F-measure algorithms. By clicking on any report, the user accesses the details of the text, assuming they have the sufficient access rights (Fig. 4).

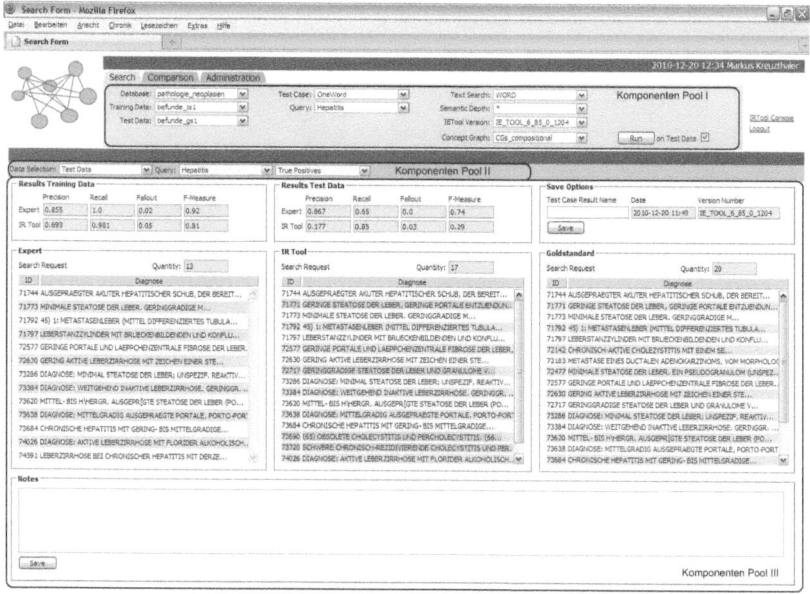

Fig. 2. Search and Evaluate View

The arrangement of the components we defined for the Load and Compare view is described in Fig. 3. Again, elements belonging to *Komponenten Pool I* are at the top of the screen where the user can select which test case results should be loaded. Beneath it is the result view section *Komponenten Pool II*, as well as *Komponenten Pool III*. As can been seen from Fig. 3, both loaded test case results are arranged in such a way as to allow the user to compare the different IR Tools easily.

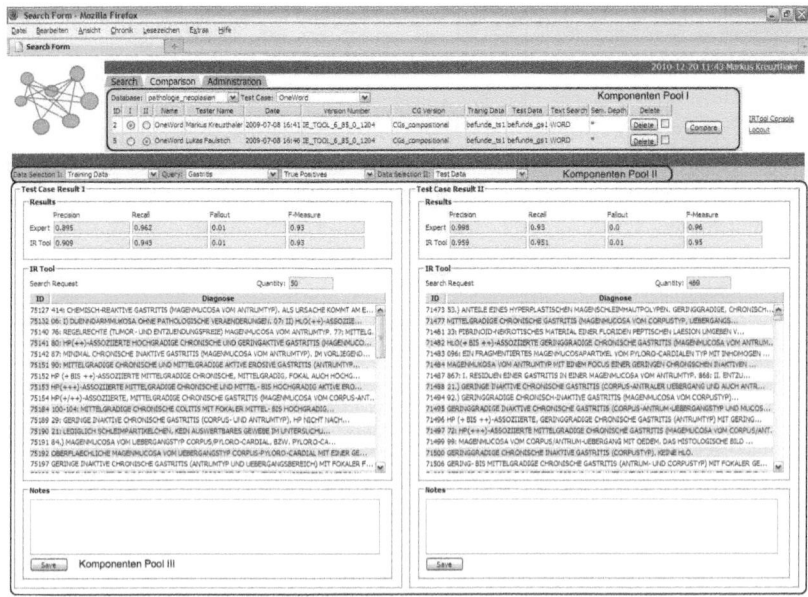

Fig. 3. Load and Compare View

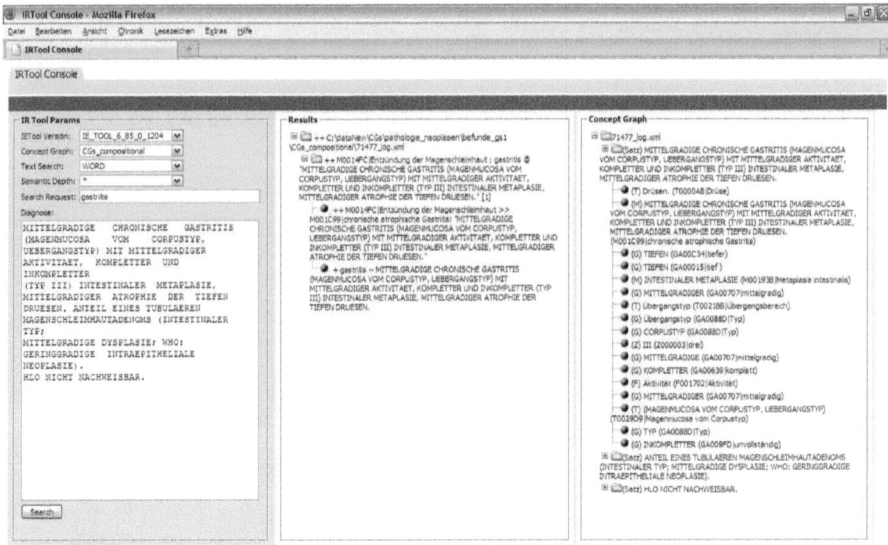

Fig. 4. Details View

By clicking on a report, the details view appears (Fig. 4). As can be seen from the image, the left side of the view shows the full report and all the IR Tool parameters. In the center of the view is the information regarding why the diagnosis was found or not. On the right hand side, the results of the report's natural language processing and its mapping to the Wingert nomenclature is shown. Further, you can directly alter the text and repeat the search on the updated text by clicking on "Search".

5   Conclusion and Outlook

In this paper, do our best knowledge we tried to expand the review on available medical free text gold standards which was made by [21]. In addition, we presented an information retrieval evaluation architecture, described its core components, and explained the development of a user friendly GUI that groups these components in a logical and consistent way.

Future work will concentrate on how to dynamically integrate other information retrieval tools so that they can be compared and contrasted to one another. In the German speaking community there are just a few companies that provide solutions or prototypes for medical free text retrieval or information extraction (e.g. SemFinder, ID Berlin, Averbis). Instantiating a challenge using our evaluation architecture would be of interest.

The development of new gold standards to address other fields of medicine is also of the utmost importance. Furthermore, there are some tools that claim to be applicable to general free text medical corpora, and these should be rigorously tested. The kernel of our system, namely the gold standard developed specifically for this project's needs, currently contains only German texts. Multi-lingual information retrieval in the medical domain is the subject of ongoing research.

During the development of the tool, it became apparent that there is no open source ground truth for German medical free texts in existence [20]. The development of such open source ground truths for medical reports, which span several medical fields, and are multi-lingual, are of special interest and warrant much effort in the future. It is clear that if such open source gold standards were to exist, it would certainly help the information retrieval tool community and would definitely encourage others to join this field.

To conclude, information retrieval in the field of medicine is becoming increasingly important and relied upon. This is especially reflected through the fact that a Medical Records Track has been started recently at the TREC so the information retrieval community will become aware of the challenges medical free text retrieval pose. We previously stated that this topic should be introduced as a track to the TREC in [34]. Semantic search seems the only possible way to search medical free text corpora and return meaningful results, while at the same time this area of research is being hampered by a number of factors, such as a lack of an open source gold standard initiative in the German speaking community. The evaluation environment presented here constitutes our contribution towards medical free text retrieval.

References

1. Holzinger, A., Geierhofer, R., Errath, M.: Semantic information in medical information systems-from data and information to knowledge: Facing information overload. In: Proc. of I-MEDIA, vol. 7, pp. 323–330 (2007)
2. Buckley, C.: Why current ir engines fail. In: Proceedings of the 27th Annual International ACM SIGIR Conference on Research and Development in Information Retrieval, pp. 584–585. ACM (2004)
3. Holzinger, A., Geierhofer, R., Mödritscher, F., Tatzl, R.: Semantic information in medical information systems: Utilization of text mining techniques to analyze medical diagnoses. Journal of Universal Computer Science 14(22), 3781–3795 (2008)
4. Holzinger, A.: Usability engineering methods for software developers. Communications of the ACM 48(1), 71–74 (2005)
5. Hersh, W.R., Hickam, D.H.: How well do physicians use electronic information retrieval systems? JAMA: The Journal of the American Medical Association 280(15), 1347 (1998)
6. Robertson, S.E., Hancock-Beaulieu, M.M.: On the evaluation of ir systems. Information Processing & Management 28(4), 457–466 (1992)
7. Tange, H.J., Schouten, H.C., Kester, A.D.M., Hasman, A.: The granularity of medical narratives and its effect on the speed and completeness of information retrieval. Journal of the American Medical Informatics Association 5(6), 571 (1998)
8. Brown, P.J.B., Sönksen, P.: Evaluation of the quality of information retrieval of clinical findings from a computerized patient database using a semantic terminological model. Journal of the American Medical Informatics Association 7(4), 392 (2000)
9. Sullivan, F., Gardner, M., Van Rijsbergen, K.: An information retrieval service to support clinical decision-making at the point of care. The British Journal of General Practice 49(449), 1003 (1999)
10. Noone, J., Warren, J., Brittain, M.: Information overload: opportunities and challenges for the gp's desktop. Studies in Health Technology and Informatics 52, 1287 (1998)
11. Gell, G., Oser, W., Schwarz, G.: Experiences with the aura free text system. Radiology 119, 105–109 (1976)
12. Gell, G.: Aura: routine documentation of medical texts. Methods Inf. Med. 22, 63–68 (1983)
13. Zingmond, D., Lenert, L.A.: Monitoring free-text data using medical language processing. Computers and Biomedical Research 26(5), 467–481 (1993)
14. Holzinger, A., Geierhofer, R., Errath, M.: Semantische informationsextraktion in medizinischen informationssystemen. Informatik-Spektrum 30(2), 69–78 (2007)
15. Gregory, J., Mattison, J.E., Linde, C.: Naming notes: transitions from free text to structured entry. Methods of Information in Medicine 34(1-2), 57 (1995)
16. Holzinger, A., Kainz, A., Gell, G., Brunold, M., Maurer, H.: Interactive computer assisted formulation of retrieval requests for a medical information system using an intelligent tutoring system. In: Proceedings of ED-MEDIA, pp. 431–436 (2000)
17. Lovis, C., Baud, R.H., Planche, P.: Power of expression in the electronic patient record: structured data or narrative text? International Journal of Medical Informatics 58, 101–110 (2000)
18. Smalheiser, N.R., Swanson, D.R.: Using arrowsmith: a computer-assisted approach to formulating and assessing scientific hypotheses. Computer Methods and Programs in Biomedicine 57(3), 149–153 (1998)

19. Harter, S.P., Hert, C.A.: Evaluation of Information Retrieval Systems: Approaches, Issues, and Methods. Annual Review of Information Science and Technology (ARIST) 32, 3–94 (1997)
20. Kreuzthaler, M., Bloice, M.D., Simonic, K.M., Holzinger, A.: On the Need for Open Source Ground Truths for Medical Information Retrieval Systems. In: International Conference on Knowledge Management and Knowledge Technologies, vol. 10, pp. 371–381 (September 2010)
21. Roberts, A., Gaizauskas, R., Hepple, M., Demetriou, G., Guo, Y., Setzer, A., Roberts, I.: Semantic Annotation of Clinical Text: The CLEF Corpus. In: Workshop Programme, p. 19 (2008)
22. Pestian, J.P., Brew, C., Matykiewicz, P., Hovermale, D.J., Johnson, N., Cohen, K.B., Duch, W.: A shared task involving multi-label classification of clinical free text. In: Proceedings of the Workshop on BioNLP 2007: Biological, Translational, and Clinical Language Processing, pp. 97–104. Association for Computational Linguistics (2007)
23. Hersh, W.R., Müller, H., Jensen, J.R., Yang, J., Gorman, P.N., Ruch, P.: Advancing biomedical image retrieval: development and analysis of a test collection. Journal of the American Medical Informatics Association 13(5), 488 (2006)
24. Müller, H., Deselaers, T., Deserno, T.M., Clough, P., Kim, E., Hersh, W.: Overview of the ImageCLEFmed 2006 Medical Retrieval and Medical Annotation Tasks. In: Peters, C., Clough, P., Gey, F.C., Karlgren, J., Magnini, B., Oard, D.W., de Rijke, M., Stempfhuber, M. (eds.) CLEF 2006. LNCS, vol. 4730, pp. 595–608. Springer, Heidelberg (2007)
25. Ogren, P.V., Savova, G., Buntrock, J.D., Chute, C.G.: Building and Evaluating Annotated Corpora for Medical NLP Systems. In: AMIA Annual Symposium Proceedings, p. 1050. American Medical Informatics Association (2006)
26. Roberts, A., Gaizauskas, R., Hepple, M., Davis, N., Demetriou, G., Guo, Y., Kola, J.S., Roberts, I., Setzer, A., Tapuria, A., et al.: The CLEF corpus: semantic annotation of clinical text. In: AMIA Annual Symposium Proceedings, p. 625. American Medical Informatics Association (2007)
27. Uzuner, Ö., Luo, Y., Szolovits, P.: Evaluating the State-of-the-Art in Automatic De-identification. Journal of the American Medical Informatics Association 14(5), 550 (2007)
28. Uzuner, Ö., Goldstein, I., Luo, Y., Kohane, I.: Identifying patient smoking status from medical discharge records. Journal of the American Medical Informatics Association 15(1), 14–24 (2008)
29. Baeza-Yates, R., Ribeiro-Neto, B., et al.: Modern information retrieval. Addison-Wesley, Reading (1999)
30. Manning, C.D., Raghavan, P., Schütze, H.: Introduction to information retrieval. Cambridge Univ. Pr. (2008)
31. Saracevic, T.: Evaluation of evaluation in information retrieval. In: Proceedings of the 18th Annual International ACM SIGIR Conference on Research and Development in Information Retrieval, pp. 138–146. ACM (1995)
32. Wilson, T.D.: Human information behavior. Informing Science 3(2), 49–56 (2000)
33. Lew, M.S., Sebe, N., Djeraba, C., Jain, R.: Content-based multimedia information retrieval: State of the art and challenges. ACM Transactions on Multimedia Computing, Communications, and Applications (TOMCCAP) 2(1), 1–19 (2006)

34. Kreuzthaler, M., Bloice, M.D., Faulstich, L., Simonic, K.-M., Holzinger, A.: A comparison of different retrieval strategies working on medical free texts. Journal of Universal Computer Science 17(7), 1109–1133 (2011)
35. Wingert, F.: Automated indexing based on SNOMED. Methods of Information in Medicine 24(1), 27–34 (1985)
36. Wingert, F.: Morphologic analysis of compound words. Methods of Information in Medicine 24(3), 155 (1985)
37. Wingert, F.: An indexing system for SNOMED. Methods of Information in Medicine 25(1), 22–30 (1986)

TagTree: Storing and Re-finding Files Using Tags

Karl Voit[1], Keith Andrews[2], and Wolfgang Slany[1]

[1] Institute for Software Technology (IST),
Graz University of Technology,
Inffeldgasse 16b/2, A-8010 Graz, Austria
`Karl.Voit@IST.TUGraz.at`, `Wolfgang.Slany@tugraz.at`
[2] Institute for Information Systems and Computer Media (IICM),
Graz University of Technology,
Inffeldgasse 16c/1, A-8010 Graz, Austria
`kandrews@iicm.edu`

Abstract. Although desktop search engines are now widely available on the computers of typical users, navigation through folder hierarchies is still the dominant mode of information access. Most users still prefer to store and search for their information within a strict hierarchy of folders.

This paper describes TagTree, a new concept for storing and retrieving files and folders using tagging and automatically maintained navigational hierarchies. TagTree is compatible with all currently prevalent software environments. A prototype implementation called *tagstore* provides a flexible framework for experimentation and a testbed for both usability studies and longer term field tests.

Preliminary test results show a very positive user acceptance rate of using TagTrees for storing and re-finding files.

Keywords: Tags, information re-finding, information architecture, folders.

1 Introduction

Users keep the vast majority of their personal files on local hard disk drives, even though network storage is becoming more popular. Successfully managing and accessing this data is crucial: finding the right information becomes increasingly difficult, as the sheer amount of information increases.

There are two kinds of information access methods: *navigation* (or *browsing*) methods, where the user typically steps through a hierarchy of folders, and *search* methods, where the user is magically transported to the item of interest. Much recent research has concentrated on search methods, in the form of desktop search engines and their query interfaces [1]. Navigational methods for local file retrieval have changed little from the principles described in the 1960s: files are placed into a hierarchy of folders. Cross-links to other destinations are hardly used by users, and operating systems make it hard for users to create and

A. Holzinger and K.-M. Simonic (Eds.): USAB 2011, LNCS 7058, pp. 471–481, 2011.

maintain symbolic links [2]. However, studies like those of Barreau [3], Teevan et al. [4], Bergman et al. [1], or Alvarado et al. [5] have shown that users prefer navigation over searching. The method and software discussed in this paper therefore focuses on navigation and not search.

Unfortunately, hierarchical folder structures do not scale well [6, 7], suggesting that alternative navigational structures need to be investigated. Since the 1980s, numerous research tools for personal information management (PIM) have been developed, but none of them have made it onto the typical user's desktop of today: some reasons for this are described in Voit et al. [8].

This paper describes a new concept for storing and retrieving local files called TagTree. TagTree takes user-supplied tags and automatically generates and maintains a navigational tree (folder) structure of tags. The TagTree concept is implemented in a prototype called *tagstore*, which serves as a flexible testbed framework.

2   Related Work

WorkspaceMirror [9] introduced unified hierarchies across email folders, web page bookmarks, and personal document folders, allowing the user to benefit by reusing the same mental model to navigate through distinct information spaces.

Most research software products introduce some kind of new file browsing interface to the desktop. Interfaces providing spatial cues for orientation within a users' information space draw on real-world spatial metaphors. However, Lansdale [10] states that: "assertions made about the inherent value of visio-spacial information represent a simplistic view of human cognition and no guarantee of good design". He further remarks that pictures are less well-suited for recall than for differentiation between items.

Besides the definition of arbitrary attributes per item, the Presto system [11] allowed users to place documents in collections and workspaces. Presto also provided dynamic collections based on queries, later introduced in Apple's Mac OS X as "smart folders". In addition to its main interface based on Java Swing, Presto provided NFS-based shared network folders, which mapped collections for legacy applications.

With the File Attribute Browser [12], users can navigate files by selecting properties such as "modified this week", by selecting certain file types, or by specifying document sizes.

The Phlat interface presents a desktop search window containing the user's email, calendar events, local documents, and web history. The user is able to sort query results by columns such as title, date, author, email recipient, and so forth.

Feldspar [13] allows users to define relations to search within emails, files, web history, calendar events, and more. This approach supports the expression of access criteria such as the first email from a certain person met at a particular conference last May.

Other research tools provide an overview of user data using a timeline. Lifestreams [14] presented a visual timeline of every document and email a user ever send, received, or edited. MyLifeBits [15] provides an advanced interface which tries to combine as much personal information as possible. It even includes telephone conversations, radio and television programs, mouse and keyboard events, audio- and video recordings, and periodic screenshots of the desktop. The goal of MyLifeBits is to record the whole life of a user and to visualise all the accumulated data on a single timeline.

PersonalBrain [16] allows the users to link between documents. In contrast to other mind mapping software products, PersonalBrain is not limited to strictly hierarchical structures, but items can be linked together in arbitrary ways.

The Haystack project [17] provided a framework to define semantic relations between objects, more fine-grained than files. The relation structure was kept separately from its user interface. An interface called Ozone provided navigation in the object space and users could define collections like in Presto.

Nepomuk [18] attempted to realise a social semantic desktop using the Resource Description Framework (RDF). Besides technological challenges, users do not seem quite ready for semantic technologies. RDF notation requires a radically new way of thinking and semantic tools like Nepomuk might only become of general interest in the far future.

There are also some lower-level attempts to provide better user experience in information access. The idea of a semantic file system was discussed in Gifford et al. [7]. It introduced an NFS-based file system which allowed interactive search requests to be represented by dynamic folders. The semantic metadata of files was automatically extracted using format-dependent transducers. This work was remarkable in its approach, because there was no need for a new interface: the semantics of the file system and its folder structure were simply extended with a new concept, from which all existing applications could benefit without modification.

A more recent attempt to develop a semantic file system like Gifford et al. [7] is TagFS [19]. Using RDF, TagFS provides a semantic framework which allows tags to be attached to files within a special file system.

3   Tagging

Files in strict hierarchies of folders are insufficient for modern demands (Seltzer and Murphy [20], Fertig et al. [21], Shirky [22], Freeman and Gelernter [23]). The file system is the basic common interface shared by all software products. Although several projects promote semantic relations like Nepomuk [18], users are not yet ready to embrace such a radically new concept. However, in the context of Web 2.0, users have already widely adopted the practice of adding metadata to information in the form of tags. Studies show that tagging is a promising approach to handling multiple contexts related to information [7, 22, 24]. Tagging can be considered as a kind of semantic relation, but with only one fixed predicate "has_tag".

TagTree is a new concept for storing and retrieving files and folders using a tagging mechanism mapped to the file system hierarchy. Certain folders in the local folder hierarchy of the user's computer have alternative semantics conferred upon them, in a manner similar to Gifford et al. [7]. The TagTree

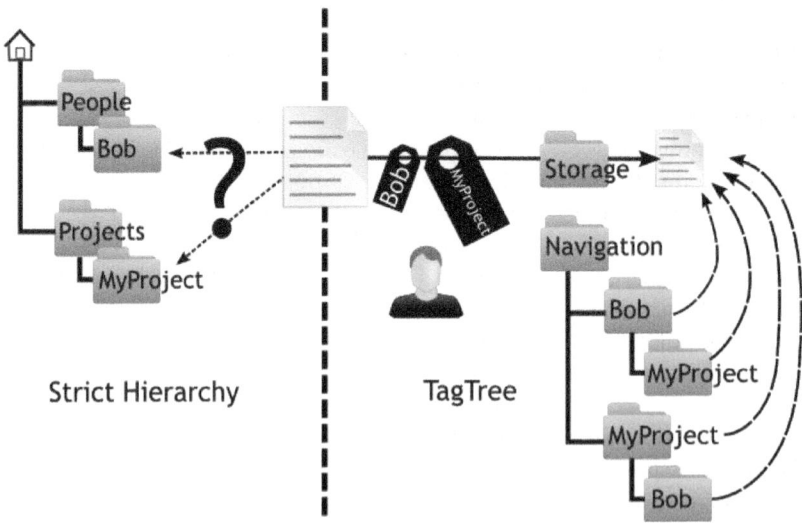

Fig. 1. The TagTree concept when storing a file `Bob's ideas about MyProject.txt`

concept is implemented in a software framework called *tagstore*. Instead of providing a special search interface, TagTree provides an alternative navigational folder structure based on user-supplied tags.

Since it is mapped to a standard folder hierarchy, TagTree is compatible with all standard applications, and the user is not confronted with a special navigational interface.

4 TagTree and tagstore

The concept of TagTree is illustrated in Figure 1. Rather than having to choose a destination folder within the folder hierarchy, the user stores all new items (files or folders) in a single folder, the central tagstore storage folder. When a new item is saved in this folder, a tagging dialog pops up and the user is able to enter one or more tags related to the item (see Figure 2).

After confirmation, tagstore creates a corresponding TagTree folder hierarchy in the tagstore navigation folder. The TagTree folder hierarchy consists of one folder path for each permutation of the tags associated with the item. Within each folder along each path, a symbolic link is created pointing to the original item stored in the central tagstore storage folder.

For example, to store a file `Bob's ideas about MyProject.txt` in a tagstore, a user would first put the file into the central tagstore storage folder. In the tagging dialog, tags such as `Bob` and `MyProject` might be given to the file. Henceforth, the single target file may be found along any one of four possible paths `Bob`, `MyProject`, `Bob/MyProject`, and `MyProject/Bob`, as well as directly in the central tagstore storage folder itself. Figure 3 shows the corresponding, fully expanded TagTree.

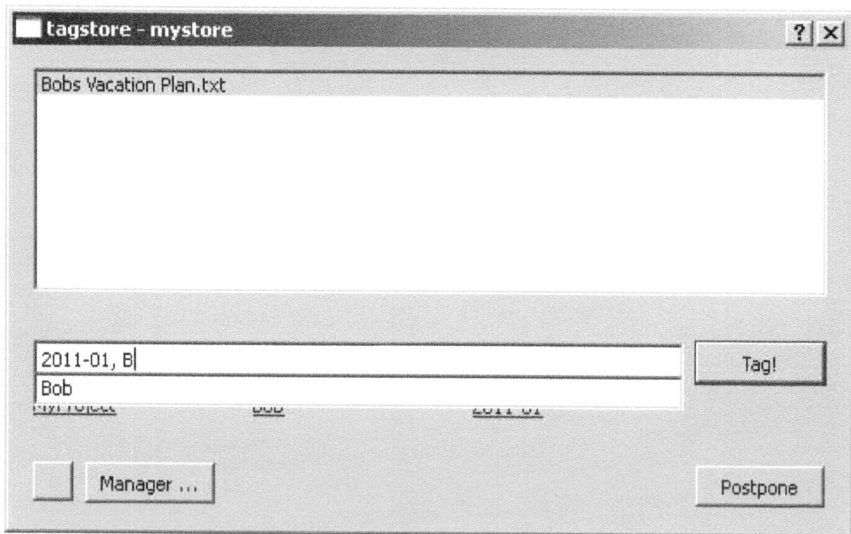

Fig. 2. The tagstore dialog window. The user has started typing a new tag beginning with "B", so tagstore pops open a window showing all previously used tags with that prefix (here "Bob")

When the user wants to access the item, it is not necessary to remember a single strict series of folder names. Navigation can begin using any of the associations connected with the item. The more tags the user can remember, the more specific the implicit query becomes, and the fewer items are presented at that level. The user does not even have to finish navigating the entire path down to a folder leaf: whenever an item in the current list of matching items is recognised, it can be accessed directly.

5   The Benefits of tagstore and Tagging

The concept of storing items in TagTrees provides several improvements compared to classical folder hierarchies. Metadata is added by the user during the storing process, a time when the user has a maximum of contextual information about the item available. Using a tagging mechanism supports the expression of a rich variety of metadata. Typical folder structures and item names do not support a large variety of metadata.

The tagstore implementation supports the user with features such as automatic datestamps. If enabled, datestamps are written as default tags into the tagline. Similarly, the user is able to define expiry dates for items added to a tagstore. After an expiry date is reached, the corresponding item is moved automatically into a special folder called **expired items**. Users tend to keep files for a long time and do not delete them, even when they are only for temporary

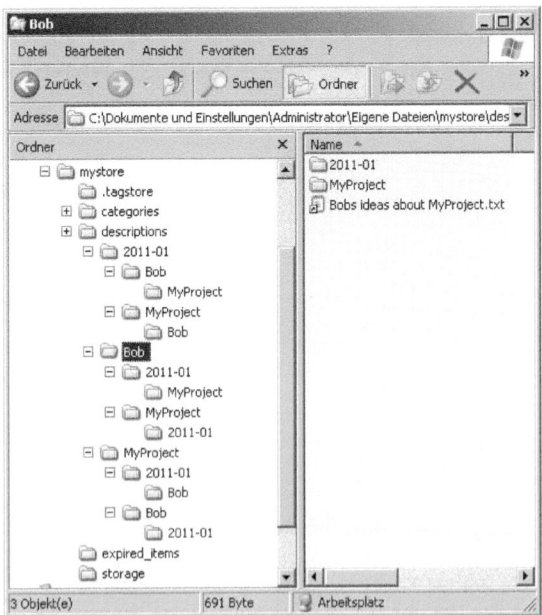

Fig. 3. Windows Explorer with the expanded TagTree of the file `Bobs ideas about MyProject.txt` tagged with the tags `2011-01`, `Bob`, and `MyProject`

use [3]. With this feature, users are able to define explicit temporal ranges of interest for information [25].

Path names and file names mostly reflect a single dimension of contextual information, such as the document's title. Tagging offers the possibility to use multi-dimensional metadata, such as an arbitrary combination of dates, authors, project, events, and so forth.

6   Limitations of tagstore

The current implementation of tagstore has some technological limits. Items with many tags result in a large number of folders and links. Current file systems have a fixed number of possible file or folder entries (inodes) per hard disk partition. Therefore, a reasonable upper bound of items per tagstore is only a few thousand items. For testing purposes, this limit should be no problem.

There is an exponential relation between the number of tags of an item and the number of folders and links that have to be created. This results in a performance problem when tagging an item with many tags. On conventional hardware, a reasonable upper bound of tags per item is six. Currently, if a user enters more than six tags, a warning message appears and disables the Tag button. The button is re-enabled, when the user reduces the number of tags to six or fewer. Several studies have shown that the number of tags users assign to items is generally below six in the vast majority of tagging tasks [26, 27].

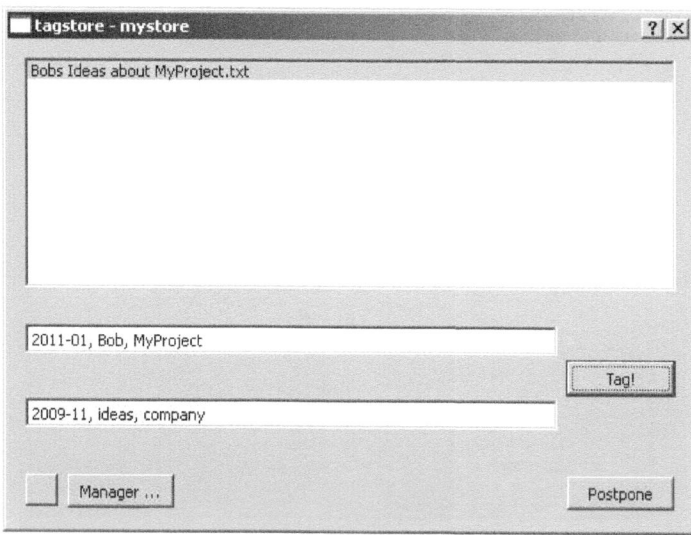

Fig. 4. The tagstore dialog window showing two separate taglines for categorising tags and describing tags

7 Preliminary Results

A formal experiment (counterbalanced 2×2 repeated measures) was conducted in January 2011. A total of 18 participants compared storing and then re-finding files in Windows Explorer using folder hierarchies and with tagstore using tags.

Two task sets were prepared. In the first task set, the participant had to store thirty files of a general nature into a folder hierarchy also constructed by the user. In the second task set, the same set of files had to be added to a tagstore and appropriately tagged. The order of the two task sets was counterbalanced between two groups of 9 users each. The files consisted of ten PDF text documents, ten (computer generated) graphics, and ten photographs.

The dependent variables measured were time to file/tag, time to re-find, number of navigation subtasks to re-find files, depth of folder hierarchy per file, and the number of tags assigned.

The preliminary results appear to show no statistically significant differences for filing or re-finding files. The feedback questionnaire showed a statistically significant ($p < 0.05$) subjective preference of the users for the tagstore method over the folder hierarchy: 14 users (77.8 %) preferred tagstore and only 4 users (22.2 %) preferred folders. This result is remarkable, since the experiment was the first time participants had seen tagstore or the TagTree concept and half of the users had previously never used any form of tagging.

Comments made by the participants suggest that field studies might show even better acceptance and re-finding performance. Several users suggested that

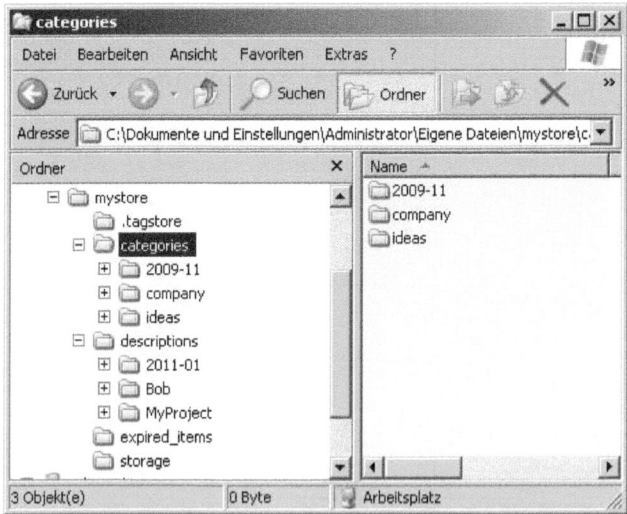

Fig. 5. Windows Explorer showing separate TagTrees for categorising tags and describing tags

using tagstore on their own files (rather than the generic files provided in the study) might provide even more benefit.

8   Future Work

The TagTree concept and its tagstore implementation are not an exhaustive solution for information storage and retrieval. As Lansdale [10] states, tools for information retrieval have to be constantly enhanced and can never be complete.

Further formative usability tests (thinking aloud tests, heuristic evaluations) are planned to improve the usability of tagstore. Further comparative studies (formal experiments) will test the effectiveness of controlled vocabularies, multiple taglines, and tag recommendations. In addition, it is intended to run longer-term field tests with tagstore, over a period of several weeks or months. An instrumented version of tagstore will allow log files to be generated and collected for analysis.

In the current tagging dialog, users are offered suggestions for tags based on the most recently used and most often used tags. In future, a more sophisticated recommender system will be used to generate tag suggestions.

Recent studies of social tagging systems [28] shows that tags might be able to be split up into categorizing tags and describing tags. The current implementation of tagstore also provides the possibility for multiple taglines to test the benefits of separate tag categories (Figures 4 and 5).

The problem with homonyms and synonyms of tags is an important issue for persons using tagging systems. Controlled vocabularies, where users are able to define their own set of allowed tags, can help to alleviate this problem.

9 Concluding Remarks

Information re-finding is a crucial part of our daily work. Studies show that navigation is preferred to search by users. Items located in strict hierarchies of folders are insufficient for modern demands.

TagTree is introduced as a new method to organize items (files or folders) for re-finding by navigation. Tags entered by the user generate navigational folder structures. Within TagTree structures, users are able to re-find items by association. This method is implemented in a research framework called tagstore.

Using tagstore as a research framework, a wide range of research topics can be investigated: tag management needs, tag vocabulary and tag taxonomy issues, the tagging behaviour of users over time, differences between users, and so forth.

It is hoped that the research results emanating from tagstore can lead to improvements in the user experience concerning personal information storage and retrieval. To have any widespread impact, though, these results will need to find their way into user applications, operating systems, and file systems of the future.

References

1. Bergman, O., Beyth-Marom, R., Nachmias, R., Gradovitch, N., Whittaker, S.: Improved search engines and navigation preference in personal information management. Transactions on Information Systems 26(4), 1–24 (2008) ISSN 1046-8188, doi:10.1145/1402256.1402259
2. Gonçalves, D.J., Jorge, J.A.: An Empirical Study of Personal Document Spaces. In: Jorge, J.A., Jardim Nunes, N., Falcão e Cunha, J. (eds.) DSV-IS 2003. LNCS, vol. 2844, pp. 46–60. Springer, Heidelberg (2003), http://virtual.inesc.pt/dsvis03/papers/05.pdf, doi:10.1007/b13960
3. Barreau, D.: The persistence of behavior and form in the organization of personal information. Journal of the American Society for Information Science and Technology 59(2), 307–317 (2008) ISSN 1532-2882, doi:10.1002/asi.20752
4. Teevan, J., Alvarado, C., Ackerman, M.S., Karger, D.R.: The perfect search engine is not enough: a study of orienteering behavior in directed search. In: Proceedings of the SIGCHI Conference on Human Factors in Computing Systems, CHI 2004, pp. 415–422. ACM, New York (2004), http://people.csail.mit.edu/teevan/work/publications/papers/chi04.pdf, doi:10.1145/985692.985745
5. Alvarado, C., Teevan, J., Ackerman, M.S., Karger, D.: Surviving the information explosion: How people find their electronic information. AI Memo AIM-2003-006, MIT AI Laboratory, Department of Computer Science (2003), http://hdl.handle.net/1721.1/6713
6. Dourish, P., Edwards, W.K., LaMarca, A., Salisbury, M.: Presto: An experimental architecture for uid interactive document spaces. Transactions on Information Systems 6(2), 133–161 (1999), http://www.dourish.com/publications/1999/tochi-presto.pdf, ISSN 1073-0516, doi:10.1145/319091.319099

7. Gifford, D.K., Jouvelot, P., Sheldon, M.A., James, W., O'Toole, J.: Semantic file systems. In: Proc. 13th ACM Symposium on Operating Systems Principles (SOSP 1991), pp. 16–25. ACM (October 1991), http://cgs.csail.mit.edu/history/publications/Papers/sfs.ps, doi:10.1145/121132.121138

8. Voit, K., Andrews, K., Slany, W.: Why personal information management (pim) technologies are not widespread. In: ASIS&T 2009 Workshop on Personal Information Management (PIM 2009) (November 2009), http://pimworkshop.org/2009/papers/voit-pim2009.pdf

9. Boardman, R., Sasse, M.A., Spence, B.: Life beyond the mailbox: A crosstool perspective on personal information management. In: Proc. CSCW 2002 Workshop on Redesigning Email for the 21st Century. ACM (November 2002), http://www.iis.ee.ic.ac.uk/~rick/research/pubs/email-cscw2002.pdf

10. Lansdale, M.W.: The psychology of personal information management. Applied Ergonomics 19(1), 55–66 (1988), http://simson.net/ref/1988/Lansdale88.pdf, ISSN 0003-6870, doi:10.1016/ 0003-6870(88)90199-8

11. Dourish, P., Edwards, W.K., LaMarca, A., Salisbury, M.: Using properties for uniform interaction in the presto document system. In: Proc. 12th Annual ACM Symposium on User Interface Software and Technology (UIST 1999), pp. 55–64. ACM (November 1999), http://www2.parc.com/csl/projects/placeless/papers/uist99-presto.pdf, doi:10.1145/320719.322583

12. Marsden, G., Cairns, D.E.: Improving the usability of the hierarchical file system. In: Proc. Annual Research Conference of the South African Institute of Computer Scientists and Information Technologists on Enablement through Technology (SAICSIT 2003), South African Institute for Computer Scientists and Information Technologists (SAICSIT), pp. 122–129 (September 2003), http://pubs.cs.uct.ac.za/archive/00000190/01/saicsit2003-dec.pdf, ISBN 1581137745

13. Chau, D.H., Myers, B., Faulring, A.: What to do when search fails: Finding information by association. In: Proc. 26th SIGCHI Conference on Human Factors in Computing Systems (CHI 2008), pp. 999–1008. ACM (April 2008), http://www.cs.cmu.edu/~dchau/feldspar/feldspar-chi08.pdf doi:10.1145/1357054.1357208

14. Freeman, E., Fertig, S.: Lifestreams: Organizing your electronic life. In: AAAI Fall Symposium 1995. AAAI (November 1995), http://www.aaai.org/Papers/Symposia/Fall/1995/FS-95-03/FS95-03-007.pdf

15. Gemmell, J., Bell, G., Lueder, R.: Mylifebits: A personal database for everything. Communications of the ACM 49(1), 88–95 (2006), http://research.microsoft.com/pubs/64157/tr-2006-23.pdf, ISSN 0001-0782, doi:10.1145/1107458.1107460

16. Hugh, H.: Personal brain (November 2010), http://www.thebrain.com/

17. Huynh, D., Karger, D.R., Quan, D.: Haystack: A platform for creating, organizing and visualizing information using rdf. In: Proc. International Workshop on the Semantic Web (WWW 2002) (May 2002), http://semanticweb2002.aifb.uni-karlsruhe.de/proceedings/Research/huynh.pdf

18. Bernardi, A.: Nepomuk: The social semantic desktop (November 2010), http://nepomuk.semanticdesktop.org/

19. Blochdorn, S., Görlitz, O., Schenk, S., Völkel, M.: Tagfs — tag semantics for hierarchical file systems. In: Proc. 6th International Conference on Knowledge Management (I-KNOW 2006), pp. 304–312 (September 2006),
http://triplei.tugraz.at/blog/wp-content/uploads/2008/11/37tagfs.pdf

20. Seltzer, M., Murphy, N.: Hierarchical file systems are dead. In: Proceedings of the 12th Workshop on Hot Topics in Operating Systems HOTOS 2009, Monte Verita, Switzerland (May 2009)

21. Fertig, S., Freeman, E., Gelernter, D.: Finding and reminding. reconsidered. SIGCHI Bulletin 28(1), 66–69 (1996) ISSN 0736-6906, doi:10.1145/249170.249187

22. Shirky, C.: Ontology is overrated: Categories, links and tags (2005),
http://www.shirky.com/writings/ontologyoverrated.html

23. Freeman, E., Gelernter, D.: Lifestreams: A storage model for personal data. ACM SIGMOD Bulletin 25, 80–86 (1996)

24. Quan, D., Bakshi, K., Huynh, D., Karger, D.R.: User interfaces for supporting multiple categorization. In: Proc. 9th IFIP TC13 International Conference on Human-Computer Interaction (INTERACT 2003), pp. 228–235. IOS Press (September 2003), http://www.idemployee.id.tue.nl/g.w.m.rauterberg/conferences/INTERACT2003/INTERACT2003-p228.pdf, ISBN 1586033638

25. Mayer-Schönberger, V.: Delete: The Virtue of Forgetting in the Digital Age. Princeton University Press (October 2009) ISBN 0691138613

26. Hsieh, J.L., Chen, C.H., Lin, I.W., Sun, C.T.: A web-based tagging tool for organizing personal documents on pcs. In: International Conference of Computer-Human Interaction 2008 (CHI 2008), Florence, Italy (April 2008),
http://works.bepress.com/lucemia/18/

27. Pak, R., Pautz, S., Iden, R.: Information organization and retrieval: A comparison of taxonomical and tagging systems. Cognitive Technology 12(1), 31–44 (2007),
http://business.clemson.edu/Catlab/pubs/pak-pautziden-2007.pdf

28. Strohmaier, M., Koerner, C., Kern, R.: Why do users tag? detecting users' motivation for tagging in social tagging systems. In: Proc. 4th International AAAI Conference onWeblogs and Social Media (ICWSM 2010). Association for the Advancement of Artificial Intelligence (May 2010),
http://www.aaai.org/ocs/index.php/ICWSM/ICWSM10/paper/viewFile/1497/1892

Detecting Cognitive Impairment Using Keystroke and Linguistic Features of Typed Text: Toward an Adaptive Method for Continuous Monitoring of Cognitive Status

Lisa M. Vizer[1] and Andrew Sears[2]

[1] UMBC, Information Systems Department, Baltimore, MD, USA
vizer1@umbc.edu
[2] Rochester Institute of Technology, B. Thomas Golisano College of Computing and Information Sciences, Rochester, NY, USA
andrew.sears@rit.edu

Abstract. Perception, attention, and memory form the foundation of human cognition, and are functions that most people take for granted. However, factors such as environment, mood, stress, education, trauma, aging, or disease can impact cognitive function both positively and negatively. For example, working memory capacity generally declines somewhat with age, but a particular individual's accumulated knowledge and skills usually remain intact and can continue to grow. Current methods of monitoring persons for cognitive decline use only normative data and do not take individual differences into account. Given that early intervention can lessen the impact of cognitive decline, concern that current cognitive assessments do not adequately address individual differences, and growing technology use by older adults, this paper investigates a more effective method for monitoring cognitive function using everyday interactions with IT.

Keywords: Keystroke dynamics, Behavioral biometrics, Stress, Cognitive decline.

1 Introduction

Continued health and independence are key goals for many older adults [41]. Research shows that both older adults and their loved ones desire peace of mind regarding cognitive health in aging [41, 44]. Furthermore, patients and medical professionals need tools to manage cognitive health and to allow patients to be active participants in care [1, 41]. However, mainstream assessments of cognitive function exhibit shortcomings in light of these motivating factors.

The most commonly administered tests for assessing cognitive function typically include measures of functional operation such as verbal fluency, working memory, attention, and planning [1, 36]. These tools have long been established as valid and reliable for discrete testing and for identifying cognitive functioning outside of the

A. Holzinger and K.-M. Simonic (Eds.): USAB 2011, LNCS 7058, pp. 483–500, 2011.
© Springer-Verlag Berlin Heidelberg 2011

normative standards. Nevertheless, there are several drawbacks when it comes to continuous monitoring and detecting change. First, the required equipment, personnel, and time represent significant investments for assessment practitioners. Second, assessment appointments can be inconvenient for the patient. As a result, assessments are administered infrequently and only in reaction to a concern, providing no baseline for comparison. Therefore, scores are only compared to normative data, and the resulting conclusions do not take individual differences into account and cannot be used to ascertain a change in the individual's status. In addition, measurements are sufficiently course-grained that the lack of sensitivity makes it difficult to identify subtle changes between successive assessments. In light of these shortcomings, the customary assessments are ill-suited for early detection of changes in function that are due to disease.

While the assessment tools used by the majority of practitioners have not changed significantly in the last 30 years, the information technology (IT) landscape has changed considerably during that time. According to the Pew Research Center, 83% of Americans own mobile phones and 74% use the Internet [46]. Among working adults 96% use either the Internet or a mobile phone [37]. Younger generations are the leading technology users, but older adults show the highest rates of new Internet adoption [29]. The Pew Internet & American Life Project [29, 46] showed that 38% of older adults use the Internet, and 74% of Internet users over the age of 64 used email. Furthermore, these percentages will soon increase as Baby Boomers [28], who have much more computer experience in the workplace than prior generations, begin to retire.

Given that early intervention can lessen the impact of cognitive decline, concern that current cognitive assessments can be ineffective, and growing technology use by older adults, this research will investigate how attributes of everyday interactions with IT can be leveraged to proactively and continuously monitor cognitive function.

2   Impacts on Cognitive Function

Models of health and functioning [50, 65] demonstrate that cognitive function can be impacted by two categories of issues: health conditions and contextual factors. Health conditions are diseases, disorders, and injuries while contextual factors are external and internal influences.

Cognitive functions, including memory and processing, are utilized extensively during interactions with Information Technology (IT), as illustrated by the Model Human Processor [6]. For that reason, any factor that impacts cognitive function can impact performance on tasks involving technology. This section will discuss how various factors impact cognition, and how those impacts relate to technology use.

2.1   Health Conditions

Health conditions are diseases, disorders, and injuries that may influence a person's functioning. For this research, the focus is on the functional impacts of age-related cognitive changes and cognitive impairment.

Aging. Normal aging is associated with changes in cognitive, motor, social, emotional, and sensory functions [8]. These changes begin to be most noticeable after about age 65 [12, 32, 69]. Although there is a degree of decline that occurs normally with age, individual differences in performance are significant, even more so among the older adult population than among younger adults [51, 52, 64]. Given the high variability in performance both between and within individuals, solutions that adapt to each person and modify the system response to changes in performance are essential.

Specific cognitive impacts include declines in information processing capabilities and speed, working and episodic memory, attention, and visual search [49, 61], with both the degree and rate varying from person to person. However, while working memory capacity and processing speed decrease with age, crystallized intelligence or knowledge base, stays intact or may even increase [12, 49, 69]. Motor movements slow as one ages so execution of manual tasks may take longer, with the possible exception of highly practiced tasks [48]. Vision also declines due to changes in visual functions such as visual acuity, contrast sensitivity, and near vision [42, 43].

While these cognitive, motor, and sensory functions are directly involved in IT interactions, social and emotional functions are involved in communication. Changes in any of these functions can affect IT performance, especially those interactions involving spontaneous thinking, information processing, and interpersonal communication, such as generating email correspondence.

Changes in cognitive function associated with aging are illustrated by an update to the MHP using data from older adults [25]. Each parameter value in the model was estimated using data from studies identified through a literature review. The revised model was then validated with additional data from a study of performance on mobile phone tasks. Results showed different slowing factors for the cognitive (1.7), perceptual (1.8), and motor (2.1) information processing categories. The keystroke-level model's predictions were consistent with the empirical results of the experiment. Depending on the specific information processing demands involved in a task, time estimates are 20% to 100% longer for older adults than for younger adults. Based on this model, a task involving a high number of motor movements will take about twice as long for an older adult to perform, while a task with a large number of eye movements relative to motor movements will take only about twenty percent longer.

These results are consistent with those from standard finger-tapping tests of motor movement speed which show that motor speed declines significantly as individuals age. Keele [32] cites data from a large study of tapping speed with persons ranging from 17 to 81 years of age that showed tapping rates begin to decrease noticeably after about age 55. In a variant of the tapping task with participants from age 20 to 70, Welford et al. [61] studied movement time between targets and found that speed declined after about age 60.

Cognitive Impairment. Cognitive impairment is defined as a deficit in cognitive faculties. Mild Cognitive Impairment (MCI) is impairment greater than that associated with normal aging, but not so severe as to impact routine daily activities, and not as advanced as dementia [57]. Persons with MCI can live independently but may notice some difficulty recalling names or other words. According to the American

College of Physicians [44], the current prevalence of MCI for those over age 70 is 22%, and 12% of that population convert to dementia each year. Given the high rate of conversion from MCI to dementia, more effective techniques for identifying the development of MCI or changes in the cognitive status of individuals with MCI that may be indicative of the onset of dementia are of particular interest.

Jimison et al. [27] draw a connection between cognitive impairment and performance on a computer game task. They found that variability in scores could discriminate between participants with and without MCI. Further exploratory studies [26] also suggest that variability in keying speed during the login sequence might be useful in discrimination between these populations as well, though data and results were not published.

2.2 Contextual Factors

The World Health Organization defines contextual factors as encompassing external environmental factors and internal personal factors. External environmental factors include social structures, physical environs, tasks, and equipment features. Internal personal factors include such things as gender, age, disposition, coping skills, educational and professional background, character, and experience.

External Factors. A variety of features external to a person can impact his or her cognitive function. Examples include the activities in which he or she is engaged, the tools he or she is using, as well as the physical and social environment in which he or she is operating. When these factors compete for cognitive resources [9], cognitive function can change, and may result in deficits in concentration, short-term memory, fine motor control, reasoning, and verbal performance [10, 16, 35]. The following sections discuss the impact of situationally-induced and experimentally-induced cognitive stress.

Situationally-Induced Stress. Perhaps the clearest examples of external factors impacting performance are situationally-induced impairments and disabilities (SIID). SIIDs occur when an individual's capabilities are negatively impacted or rendered inadequate by the environment or task [50]. These types of impairments or disabilities are by nature temporary, intermittent, and highly variable. Two general examples are the impact of loud music on a student's ability to process study material, or the impact of multitasking on performance of any particular single activity. For example, every person has a unique typing pattern that is sufficiently stable to strengthen security systems, but there are inherent pattern fluctuations that have been attributed to situational stress, including the task environment [40]. Another example is the decreased performance experienced when using a hand-held device while walking [34].

Experimentally-Induced Stress. Studies have validated the ability of certain tasks and conditions to induce acute psychological stress. These tasks and conditions are used extensively in psychological and cardiovascular research. Methods fall into five categories [55]: (1) problem-solving tasks, (2) information-processing tasks, (3) psychomotor tasks, (4) affective conditions, and (5) aversive or painful conditions. Methods are selected based on the desired response and other practical and theoretical considerations.

Derakshan and Eysenck [9] review results of several studies and conclude that processing efficiency is impaired regardless of whether the distraction is from a cognitive task or external condition. Since each method induces stress that interferes with cognitive processing, each method should also impact performance.

In a study of a text composition task, Vizer et al. [59] found that cognitive stress affects linguistic and keystroke attributes of typed text. In this study, psychological stress was induced using mental multiplication [2] and 3-back number recall [12] tasks.

Internal Factors. A person's reactions to stress and other environmental and health factors are mediated by individual characteristics. Some features, such as age, educational and professional background, and experience, are easily measured while others, such as disposition, coping skills, and general character, are more abstract. The interaction of each individual's unique characteristics with features of his or her environment and health will in turn affect performance on tasks.

In a review of research on the impact of trait anxiety on task performance, Eysenck et al. [13] find that studies show significant differences in task performance between persons with high trait anxiety versus those with low trait anxiety. Findings suggest that individual differences in trait anxiety affect components of the working memory and attentional control in stressful situations, thus impacting performance.

In addition, Sliwinsky et al. [52] studied individual differences in performance on an n-back memory task relative to subjective assessments of daily stress. The study found that performance was better on low-stress versus high-stress days, and that within-person effects were larger for older adults than for younger adults.

In the Vizer et al. [59] study of typing performance, accuracy of the data analysis improved significantly when individual differences were controlled for through normalization of data per participant. Participant demographics were fairly homogeneous with regard to quantifiable variables such as age, experience, and education level, however, so dissimilarities might be due to trait factors that were not assessed.

3   Assessment of Cognitive Function

Assessment of cognitive function is becoming more important as the population ages and lifespan increases, and monitoring of cognitive function is central to the care of those with cognitive decline [1]. More frequent and convenient monitoring of the status of cognitive function is desirable, but existing solutions rely on methods that are inadequate. One critical barrier is that current tests are usually administered in a physician's office or a rehabilitation facility, causing inconvenience for the patient, utilizing valuable healthcare resources, and making frequent monitoring unrealistic. The following sections describe current methods and research into technologies to address the limitations of existing solutions.

3.1   Assessment of Cognitive Function Related to Health Conditions

Cognitive function is usually assessed by health professionals in a medical setting, but only when a health condition impacts an individual's cognition. Established neuropsychological tests are the most common assessment method. Examples of test applications in Human-Centered Computing (HCC) are given at the end of the discussion.

Neuropsychological Measures. Traditionally, medical and psychological professionals assess cognitive function during office visits or through in-home nursing visits. Several methods are well-accepted and widely used [1, 36], including short interviews and tests such as the Mini-Mental State Examination (MMSE) [14], the Abbreviated Mental Test (AMT) [23], the Mental Status Questionnaire (MSQ) [30], and the Symbol Digit Modalities Test (SDMT) [53], as well as more extensive tests such as the Wechsler scales of intelligence and memory [60], the Halstead-Reitan battery [47], and the Benton tests [4]. Test results are correlated to cognitive facility and can be used to assess cognitive function or diagnose cognitive dysfunction. Depending on the purpose of the evaluation, practitioners choose the instrument according to desired test domain, resource constraints, availability of normative data, reliability, and validity [1].

Health Assessment and Human-Centered Computing. Research indicates that embedded assessment is desired by older adults and their caretakers, and can prompt earlier interventions and treatment, thus improving health outcomes [41]. However, most research has focused on monitoring overt indicators such as mobility and very little has examined monitoring of cognitive function. While detection of gross motor dysfunction is necessary, more studies are needed to assess the subtle signs of cognitive aging and dysfunction.

Jimison et al. [26, 27] found connections between cognitive impairment and performance on computer tasks. Their first study [27] showed increased variability in scores on an instrumented computer game for older adults with MCI, demonstrating that interactions with technology might be used to discriminate cognitive function. Exploratory studies with keystroke sequences during login [26] suggested that variability in keystroke timings might also differentiate individuals with MCI from those without MCI, though no results were published.

3.2   Assessment of Cognitive Function in Context

When contextual factors impact cognition, cognitive function must be assessed in context. Common methods for assessing function in context are neurophysiological measures, performance measures, and self-report instruments [5]. Examples of the successful application of these methods in HCC are given at the end of the section.

Neurophysiological Measures. Humans exhibit similar outwardly visible signs in response to both physical and cognitive stress, but those signs are caused by different physiological changes in the nervous system [10]. During physical stress a sympathetic nervous response is dominant, while an adrenal response is dominant during cognitive stress. Although the hormonal response to the two types of stress differs, the outward manifestations are very similar [10, 56]. Therefore, it is difficult to attribute changes in the readily measured outward signs as coming from one specific type of stress or from a combination of both types of stress. An example is "white coat hypertension" [3] where the cognitive stress associated with simply being in a physician's office can lead to changes in blood pressure. In this situation, without measuring stress hormone levels immediately, the physician cannot be sure whether an individual's elevated blood pressure should be attributed to the stress of the office visit, an underlying medical condition, or both.

Physiological measurements are the most common method for detecting changes in stress level. Increases in stress hormone levels, heart rate, blood pressure [7], pupil dilation, and galvanic skin response [18] can all be used to indicate the presence of stress. Healey and Picard [21] leveraged the physiological response to stress, instrumenting cars to detect driver stress. Analysis of data from a car outfitted with electromyogram, electrocardiogram, galvanic skin response, and respiration sensors achieved a correct recognition rate of 88.6% using an optimal set of features.

Performance Measures. Performance measures are a means of gauging function under stress through overt output on a task. Measures of accuracy, errors, and efficiency capture the level of execution in a stress situation. Common methods for manipulating stress in a task include varying load, varying speed, or introducing any of a number of secondary tasks [17].

Many studies have also investigated the effect of stress on work performance [18, 38]. Increases, decreases, and no differences in productivity and performance have all been observed in the presence of stress. This variation among results may be explained by differences in levels of stress, individual differences, and the inverted U-shaped stress-performance curve [19]. These differences will cause slight variations in the width and shape of the curve. For example, some persons might have a narrower comfort zone or a lower rate of performance decline. However, the general trend is of maximal performance when there is a moderate level of stress with lower levels of performance occurring at hypostress and hyperstress.

Self-report Instruments. Self-report instruments for stress are subjective questionnaires that assess the level of workload, distress, and other indicators. Examples include the NASA-TLX [20], the Pressure Management Inventory [63], the Dundee Stress State Questionnaire [39], and the Job Content Questionnaire [31]. The NASA-TLX, in particular, has been researched extensively and validated repeatedly. It takes very little time to administer, especially the unweighted version, and has proven to be robust under diverse administration circumstances. Each of these questionnaires is sensitive to the experience of stress, but putting them into practice is outside the normal routine and requires a time commitment.

Assessment in Context and Human-Centered Computing. Affective computing considers changes in an individual's affect, or observable manifestations of emotion, to detect stress. Current affective computing research that addresses stress assessment includes automatic optical recognition of facial expressions [11], pressure-sensing mice to detect frustration [45], and automatic speech analysis [66]. Automatic optical facial expression recognition currently has an accuracy rate of 68% when classifying stress versus non-stress conditions [11]. Analysis of pressure applied to a computer mouse produces an accuracy of 88% [45], and speech analysis gives a correct classification rate of 71% when data are collected during tasks that induce mental stress [66].

Physiological measures and affective computing methods are well-studied and usually achieve high accuracy rates, but the approaches employed typically measure overt and predictable reactions to acute events during the course of the event. The assessments can be obtrusive, require supplementary equipment, and are often labor or computationally intensive. Keystroke and linguistic analysis of typed text circumvents these drawbacks because they examine the text produced by everyday interactions with information technology.

Keystroke dynamics is the study of *how* a person types. Typing samples are evaluated based on features including keystroke durations, keystroke latencies, input rates, and key rates. Statistical methods for analyzing spontaneously generated text can discriminate between known users of a system with research in network security confirming fluctuations in keystroke pattern due to stress, environment, and change in function [40]. These results were subsequently validated by a study from Vizer et al. [59] that found that cognitive stress affected keystroke attributes of spontaneously typed text. The models showed that some keystroke dynamics features were discriminators between text samples produced under control conditions and after exposure to cognitive stress with machine learning analysis achieving 75% correct classification of stress versus non-stress samples. Features used in the machine learning analysis included pause metrics, input rates, correction key frequencies, and navigation key frequencies.

Linguistic analyses examine *what* is typed rather than *how* it is typed. Features are extracted from the text and analyzed for different purposes, including deception detection. Deception detection in text-based computer-mediated communication exploits the idea that deception is cognitively stressful [70] to differentiate truthful messages from deceptive messages. Text is analyzed for linguistic and paralinguistic cues that indicate deceptive intent [68] (Table 1), and messages can be classified as truthful or deceitful with a wide range of correct classification rates from 57.4% to 88.5% [15, 67]. The Vizer et al. [59] study showed that cognitive stress impacted linguistic attributes of spontaneously generated text, similar to the impact of stress from engaging in deception. Cues such as negativity, content diversity, and lexical diversity changed after exposure to cognitive stress induced by psychologically stressful tasks.

Table 1. Linguistic cues related to deception detection in computer-mediated communication (adapted from [68])

Linguistic cues and descriptions	As compared to truth tellers, deceivers...
Quantity – the amount of information in text messages	use more words and sentences
Word diversity – the ratio of unique words	have lower lexical and content diversity
Language complexity – average sentence length, average word length, pausality	use less complex language
Expressivity – the frequency of adjectives and adverbs	have greater expressivity
Non-immediacy – expression to disassociate oneself from his/her message content	use fewer self-references and more modal verbs
Informality – typographical error ratio	are more informal
Cognitive complexity – the ratio of cognitive operations	use words that involve higher cognitive complexity
Affect – positive and negative emotions	produce more positive and negative affect
Spontaneous correction – ratio of immediately corrected messages	are less likely to spontaneously correct errors in messages
Uncertainty – verbal uncertainty indicating the lack of sureness	are more uncertain in their wording

3.3   Assessing Change in Cognitive Function

Assessing change in cognitive function is important in the context of caring for those at risk for dementia and other age-associated cognitive decline. Changes are detected by administering tests at intervals of several months to a year and comparing results. However, it can be difficult to detect the subtle changes that may signal the beginning of age- or disease-related cognitive decline because the tests are not sufficiently sensitive, the testing interval is too long, and baseline data are often not available. Another consideration is the learning effects that occur when the same assessment is given multiple times. Research shows that the learning effect can persist even when assessment administration is separated by years, thus confounding results [24]. Assessments employed for detection of cognitive decline must test a range of cognitive domains, have adequate age-adjusted normative data, and be standardized, reliable, valid, and resistant to learning effects [1]. Though many tests are used for repeated measures of cognitive ability, none are expressly developed for detecting change. Rather, they have been developed for static assessment of cognitive function and practitioners rely on score comparisons to demonstrate change.

Keystroke dynamics and deception detection research illustrate the possibility of employing everyday keyboard interactions for unobtrusive monitoring of cognitive function. Keystroke and linguistic analyses can be applied to keyboard interactions to identify important information about the user. Features of timing and language are extracted with changes in these features corresponding to changes in cognitive function due to either contextual or health factors.

4   Proposed Solution

Monitoring of cognitive function is central to the care of individuals diagnosed with or at risk for cognitive decline, regardless of etiology [1]. The population is aging at an unprecedented rate, and the first members of the Baby Boomer generation [28], born from 1946 to 1964 [58], are beginning to reach retirement age, and memory preservation is a chief concern among older adults [41]. Because early detection of cognitive impairment can lead to better outcomes, the need for effective assessment becomes more urgent as the population ages. Studies have shown that care providers, elders, and medical professionals desire embedded assessment so that changes in health can be detected as early as possible to allow for appropriate interventions and effective treatment [41].

The motivating factors mentioned at the beginning of this paper are continued health and independence for older adults, peace of mind regarding cognitive health for older adults and loved ones [41, 44], and cognitive health management and collaboration tools for patients and medical professionals [1, 41]. In light of these motivating factors, the current assessment methods each suffer from one or more shortcomings. Examples include that they depend on impact factor, depend on functional domain, are obtrusive and inconvenient, require specialized equipment and training, are only suited to infrequent administration, are scored against normative data, lack baseline data, and are subject to learning effects. A functional monitoring approach using text-based computer interactions has the potential to address all of these shortcomings as well as empower medical professionals and older adults in the management of cognitive health.

Information technology offers a unique vehicle for assessment since computer and technology use is widespread and growing. The Pew Research Center found that 83% of Americans own mobile phones and 74% use the Internet [46]. Among working adults, 96% use either the Internet, email, or a mobile phone [37]. In addition, interviews with older adults and their loved ones found that they were very enthusiastic about email, usually checking it daily, and were increasingly using computers and the Internet [22]. Recent studies from the Pew Internet & American Life Project [29, 46] show that this trend continues with 38% of older adults using the Internet. Between 2005 and 2009, those aged 70 to 75 years posted the highest rates of new Internet adoption. Furthermore, 74% of Internet users over the age of 64 used email, making it the most pursued Internet activity for that cohort. These percentages will expand as Baby Boomers [28], a generation of about 80 million persons [58], begin to retire. This generation has much more computer experience than prior generations, primarily due to their exposure to information technology in the workplace.

The preceding discussion outlined the need for more sensitive, convenient, and frequent assessments to monitor cognitive status. Cognitive impairment causes changes in cognitive function, including deficits in concentration, short-term memory, fine motor control, reasoning, and verbal performance [10, 16, 35]. Each of these functions is utilized during interactions with IT, as illustrated by the Model Human Processor [6]. Previous research supports this link between changes in cognitive function and changes in IT interactions [59]. Insights from keystroke dynamics and deception detection research illustrate the possibility of leveraging everyday keyboard interactions for unobtrusive monitoring of cognitive function. Over time, changes in salient keystroke and linguistic features could indicate changes in cognitive function due to contextual or health factors.

In an exploratory study of this concept, Vizer et al. [59] confirmed a link between the presence of cognitive stress and changes in features of spontaneously typed text. The research found that cognitive stress affects both linguistic and keystroke attributes of the text and that models can be improved significantly when individual differences are controlled for through normalization of data per participant. In addition, analysis established that certain keystroke dynamics and linguistics features were promising discriminators between text samples produced under control conditions and after exposure to cognitive stress.

4.1   Research Questions

It is expected that cognitive stress and cognitive impairment will induce changes in timing, keystroke, and linguistic patterns. A set of timing, keystroke, and linguistic features will be adopted from keystroke dynamics and deception-detection research [59, 68] for study. The following research questions stem from gaps in the literature on cognitive assessment and human-centered computing solutions.

1. Can typing samples be classified as being produced
    (a) under stress vs. no-stress conditions?
    (b) by young adults vs. older adults?
    (c) by older adults with vs. without cognitive impairment?
2. What keystroke and linguistic features differ between
    (d) stress and no-stress conditions?
    (e) young adults and older adults?
    (f) older adults with and without cognitive impairment?
3. Do cognitive stress and cognitive impairment lead to changes in the same or different features?

4.2   Analysis

Text samples can be analyzed to establish models of keystroke and linguistic features drawn from the literature. The classification models would form the basis for answering the research questions. After each typing sample, participants will complete the NASA-TLX to assess task workload. For comparisons across individuals, keystroke and linguistic features and NASA-TLX scores from the control and experimental samples will be normalized to z-scores using means and standard deviations calculated per feature or score from the baseline samples. Logistic regression can be used to build and test models for discriminating between classes of samples including classification of stress versus no-stress samples, and classification of samples from individuals with and without cognitive impairment (Fig. 1).

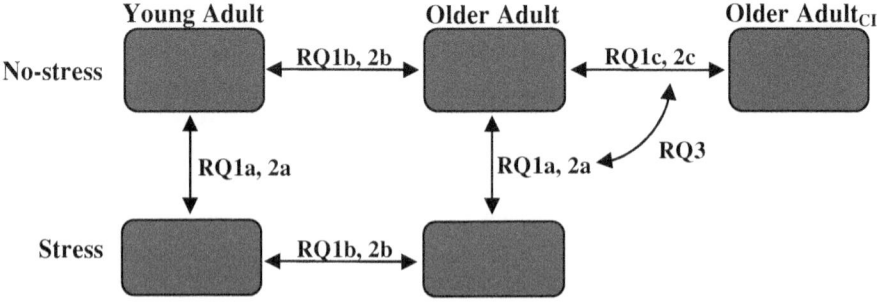

Fig. 1. Data analysis plan for groups

This same process can also be used to build and test models to discriminate between stress and no-stress samples for individual participants (Fig. 2). For comparisons within the data from each individual participating in the extended protocol, features do not need to be normalized since each participant is his or her own control.

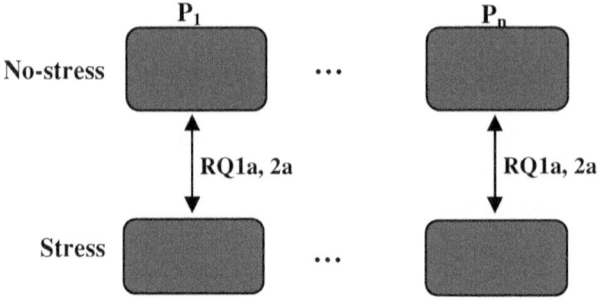

Fig. 2. Data analysis plan for individuals

5   Discussion

This research will result in a better understanding of how changes in cognitive function affect interactions with technology and can lead to a method for improved monitoring of cognitive function. The examination of text samples with a focus on both cognitive stress and cognitive impairment facilitates understanding of the specific keystroke and linguistic features valuable in discriminating cognitive stress and cognitive impairment from normal function. Investigation of changes per person enables further insight into individual differences in responses to cognitive stress and cognitive decline. The proposed solution has the potential to:

1. unobtrusively gather data about function, regardless of the type of impact factor;
2. facilitate the gathering of baseline data;
3. capture data continuously over a length of time;
4. leverage behaviors in which the individual is already engaged;
5. avoid learning effects;
6. use readily available equipment;
7. automatically adjust to the unique characteristics of each individual; and
8. allow for early detection of changes.

In addition to cognitive decline, a degree of physical decline occurs in normal aging [54]. To mitigate against physical decline having an undue effect on the data analysis, scores will be normalized per individual and NASA-TLX scores of physical effort will be analyzed as a covariate. While this approach does not completely remove the effect from physical decline, it reduces the influence on an individual basis. We believe this will result in more robust models since the analysis incorporates variation that is consequent to normal physical decline in aging. Furthermore, there is evidence that decline in motor function is concomitant with and a significant feature of cognitive decline [33]. This suggests that rather than attempting to separate the two types of decline, a comprehensive analysis must consider them together.

Privacy is also an issue to older adults concerned with the intrusiveness and loss of control that can be associated with a monitoring system. However, research suggests that older adults are willing to trade some privacy for systems that ensure safety and foster greater independence [62]. In light of these concerns, it is important to consider data utility, analysis, and control in any monitoring system. We believe that our approach would be acceptable to older adults because it offers high utility, objective computerized data analysis, and could be tailored to each individual's preferences for the control of raw data and generation of alerts. This approach is high utility because it has the potential to detect the early signs of cognitive decline, a vital facet of effective memory care that is also notoriously difficult to accomplish [62]. Second, the objective computerized analysis method examines aggregate features of the text and does not need to retain the text after features are extracted. This reduces the intrusive nature of monitoring. Last, users could choose how and what data is retained as well as to whom alerts are directed. Users might wish to retain text for later use or prefer to retain only the extracted features and end analysis. If the analysis reveals an issue that should be communicated, users might also choose to whom that information is directed, such as to a loved one or a medical professional, and whether that choice is based on the suspected issue. Each of these considerations is critical in empowering healthcare consumers to be active participants in their own care.

6   Conclusion

Given the relationship between cognitive processes needed to use technology and those impacted by cognitive impairment and stress, this research will explore keystroke and linguistic attributes of spontaneously typed text as a possible approach for monitoring cognitive changes. This approach has several advantages over traditional methods of monitoring cognitive function because it is unobtrusive and gathers baseline data for comparison and diagnosis as well as continuous data for day-to-day monitoring. This study will form the basis for longer-term studies of change in cognitive function over time, culminating in an unobtrusive method for cognitive monitoring that leverages everyday computer interactions.

Acknowledgements. This material is based upon work supported under an NSF Graduate Research Fellowship and NSF Grant No. CNS-0619379. Thanks to those who have provided insight and guidance for this work, including Drs. Lina Zhou, Ant Ozok, Sara Czaja, Kate DeMedeiros, Jason Brandt, and Kathleen Price.

References

1. American Psychological Association. Guidelines for the evaluation of dementia and age-related cognitive decline, Washington, DC: American Psychological Association (1998)
2. Ashcraft, M.: Cognitive arithmetic: A review of data and theory. Cognition: International Journal of Cognitive Science 44, 75–106 (1992)
3. Ayman, D., Goldshine, A.D.: Blood pressure determinations by patients with essential hypertension: the difference between clinical and home readings before treatment. American Journal of the Medical Sciences 200, 465–470 (1940)
4. Benton, A., Hampshire, K.d.S., Varney, N., Spreen, O.: Contributions to neuropsychological assessment. Oxford University Press, New York (1983)
5. Bourne, L., Yaroush, R.: Stress and cognition: A cognitive psychological perspective, NASA (2003)
6. Card, S., Moran, T., Newell, A.: The Model Human Processor: An Engineering Model of Human Performance. In: Boff, K., Kaufman, L., Thomas, J. (eds.) Handbook of Perception and Human Performance, pp. 1–35. John Wiley & Sons, New York (1986)
7. Cohen, S., Kessler, R., Gordon, L.U.: Strategies for Measuring Stress in Studies of Psychiatric and Physical Disorders. In: Cohen, S., Kessler, R., Gordon, L.U. (eds.) Measuring Stress: A Guide for Health and Social Scientists, pp. 3–28. Oxford University Press, New York (1995)
8. Craik, F., Salthouse, T.: The handbook of aging and cognition. Lawrence Erlbaum Associates, Mahwah (2000)
9. Derakshan, N., Eysenck, M.: Anxiety, Processing Efficiency, and Cognitive Performance: New Developments from Attentional Control Theory. European Psychologist 14(2), 168–176 (2009)
10. Dimsdale, J.E., Moss, J.: Plasma catecholamines in stress and exercise. Journal of the American Medical Association 243, 340 (1980)

11. Dinges, D.F., Venkataraman, S., McGlinchey, E.L., Metaxas, D.N.: Monitoring of facial stress during space flight: Optical computer recognition combining discriminative and generative methods. Acta Astronautica 60(4-7), 341–350 (2007)
12. Dobbs, A.R., Rule, B.G.: Adult Age Differences in Working Memory. Psychology and Aging 4(4), 500–503 (1989)
13. Eysenck, M., Derakshan, N., Santos, R., Calvo, M.: Anxiety and cognitive performance: Attentional control theory. Emotion 7, 336–353 (2007)
14. Folstein, M., Folstein, S., McHugh, P.: Mini-mental state. A practical method for grading the cognitive state of patients for the clinician. Journal of Psychiatric Research 12(3), 189–198 (1975)
15. Fuller, C., Biros, D., Wilson, R.: Decision support for determining veracity via linguistic-based cues. Decision Support Systems 46, 695–703 (2009)
16. Gauthier, S., Reisberg, B., Zaudig, M., Petersen, R.C., Ritchie, K., Broich, K., Belleville, S., Brodaty, H., Bennett, D., Chertkow, H., Cummings, J.L., de Leon, M., Feldman, H., Ganguli, M., Hampel, H., Scheltens, P., Tierney, M.C., Whitehouse, P., Winblad, B.: Mild cognitive impairment. Lancet 367(9518), 1262–1270 (2006)
17. Gawron, V.: Human performance measures handbook. Lawrence Erlbaum Associates, Mahwah (2000)
18. Goldberger, L., Breznitz, S.: The Handbook of Stress. The Free Press, New York (1993)
19. Hancock, P.A., Warm, J.S.: A Dynamic Model of Stress and Sustained Attention. Human Factors 31(5), 519–537 (1989)
20. Hart, S., Staveland, L.: Development of NASA-TLX (Task Load Index): Results of empirical and theoretical research. In: Hancock, P., Meshkati, N. (eds.) Human Mental Workload, pp. 139–183. Elsevier, Amsterdam (1988)
21. Healey, J., Picard, R.W.: SmartCar: detecting driver stress. In: 15th International Conference on Pattern Recognition, pp. 218–221 (2000)
22. Hirsch, T., Forlizzi, J., Hyder, E., Goetz, J., Kurtz, C., Stroback, J.: The ELDer project: social, emotional, and environmental factors in the design of elder technologies. In: 2000 Conference on Universal Usability, pp. 72–79. ACM Press, New York (2000)
23. Hodkinson, H.: Evaluation of a mental test score for assessment of mental impairment in the elderly. Age and Ageing 1(4), 233–238 (1972)
24. Houx, P., Shepherd, J., Blauw, G.-J., Murphy, M., Ford, I., Bollen, E., Buckley, B., Stott, D., Jukema, W., Hyland, M., Gaw, A., Norrie, J., Kampr, A., Perry, I., MacFarlane, P., Edo Meinders, A., Sweeney, B., Packard, C., Twomey, C., Cobbe, S.M., Westendorp, R.: Testing cognitive function in elderly populations: the PROSPER study. Journal of Neurology, Neurosurgery, and Psychiatry 73, 385–389 (2002)
25. Jastrzembski, T., Charness, N.: The Model Human Processor and the Older Adult: Parameter Estimation and Validation With a Mobile Phone Task. Journal of Experimental Psychology: Applied 13(4), 224–248 (2007)
26. Jimison, H., Jessey, N., McKanna, J., Zitzelberger, T., Kaye, J.: Monitoring Computer Interactions to Detect Early Cognitive Impairment in Elders. In: First Distributed Diagnosis and Home Healthcare Conference, Arlington, VA (2006)
27. Jimison, H., Pavel, M., McKanna, J., Pavel, J.: Unobtrusive Monitoring of Computer Interactions to Detect Cognitive Status in Elders. IEEE Transactions on Information Technology in Biomedicine 8(3), 248–252 (2004)
28. Jones, L.Y.: Great Expectations: America and the Baby Boom Generation. Coward McCann, New York (1980)
29. Jones, S., Fox, S.: Generations Online in 2009. Pew Internet & American Life Project, Pew Research Center, Washington, DC (2009)

30. Kahn, R., Goldfarb, A., Pollack, M., Peck, A.: Brief objective measures for the determination of mental status in the aged. American Journal of Psychiatry 117, 326–328 (1960)
31. Karasek, R., Brisson, C., Kawakami, N., Houtman, I., Bongers, P., Amick, B.: The Job Content Questionnaire (JCQ): An instrument for internationally comparative assessments of psychosocial job characteristics. Journal of Occupational Health Psychology 3, 322–355 (1998)
32. Keele, S.: Motor Control. In: Boff, K., Kaufman, L., Thomas, J. (eds.) Handbook of Perception and Human Performance. John Wiley & Sons, New York (1986)
33. Kluger, A., Gianutsos, J., Golomb, J., Ferris, S., George, A., Franssen, E., Reisberg, B.: Patterns of motor impairment in normal aging, mild cognitive decline, and early Alzheimer's disease. Journals of Gerontology: Series B 52B(1), 28–39 (1997)
34. Lin, M., Goldman, R., Price, K., Sears, A., Jacko, J.: How do people tap when walking? An empirical investigation of nomadic data entry. International Journal of Human-Computer Studies 65(9), 759–769 (2007)
35. Lupien, S.J., Maheu, F., Tu, M., Fiocco, A., Schramek, T.E.: The effects of stress and stress hormones on human cognition: Implications for the field of brain and cognition. Brain and Cognition 65(3), 209–237 (2007)
36. MacKenzie, D., Copp, P., Shaw, R., Goodwin, G.: Brief cognitive screening of the elderly: A comparison of the Mini-Mental State Examination (MMSE), Abbreviated Mental Test (AMT), and Mental Status Questionnaire (MSQ). Psychological Medicine 26, 427–430 (1996)
37. Madden, M., Jones, S.: Networked Workers. Pew Internet & American Life Project, Pew Research Center, Washington, DC (2008)
38. Mandler, G.: Thought, memory, and learning: Effects of emotional stress. In: Goldberger, L., Breznitz, S. (eds.) The Handbook of Stress. The Free Press, New York (1993)
39. Matthews, G., Joyner, L., Gilliland, K., Campbell, S., Falconer, S., Huggins, J.: Validation of a comprehensive stress state questionnaire: Towards a state "Big Three"? In: Mervielde, I., DeFruyt, P., Ostendorf, F. (eds.) Personality Psychology in Europe. Tilburg University Press, Tilburg (1997)
40. Monrose, F., Rubin, A.: Keystroke dynamics as a biometric for authentication. Future Generation Computer Systems 16(4), 351–359 (2000)
41. Morris, M., Intille, S.S., Beaudin, J.S.: Embedded Assessment: Overcoming Barriers to Early Detection with Pervasive Computing. In: Gellersen, H.-W., Want, R., Schmidt, A. (eds.) PERVASIVE 2005. LNCS, vol. 3468, pp. 333–346. Springer, Heidelberg (2005)
42. Owsley, C., Sekular, R., Siemsen, D.: Contrast sensitivity throughout adulthood. Vision Research 23, 689–699 (1983)
43. Pitts, D.: The effects of aging on selected visual functions: Dark adaptation, visual acuity, stereopsis and brightness contrast. In: Sanders, M., McCormick, E. (eds.) Human Factors in Engineering and Design. McGraw Hill, New York (1982)
44. Plassman, B., Langa, K., Fisher, G., Heeringa, S., Weir, D., Ofstedal, M., Burke, J., Hurd, M., Potter, G., Rodgers, W., Steffens, D., McArdle, J., Willis, R., Wallace, R.: Prevalence of Cognitive Impairment without Dementia in the United States. Annals of Internal Medicine 148(6), 427–434 (2008)
45. Qi, Y., Reynolds, C., Picard, R.W.: The Bayes Point Machine for Computer-user Frustration Detection via PressureMouse. In: 2001 Workshop on Perceptive User interfaces. ACM, New York (2001)
46. Rainie: Internet, broadband, and cell phone statistics. Pew Internet & American Life Project, Pew Research Center, Washington, DC (2010)

47. Reitan, R.: Halstead-Reitan Neuropsychological Test Battery. Western Psychological Services, Los Angeles (1993)
48. Salthouse, T.: Effects of Age and Skill in Typing. Journal of Experimental Psychology: General 113(3), 345–371 (1984)
49. Salthouse, T., Babcock, R.: Decomposing adult age differences in working memory. Developmental Psychology 27, 763–776 (1991)
50. Sears, A., Young, M.: Physical Disabilities and Computing Technologies: An Analysis of Impairments. In: Jacko, J., Sears, A. (eds.) The Human-Computer Interaction Handbook, New York, pp. 829–852 (2008)
51. Sliwinski, M., Buschke, H.: Modeling Intraindividual Cognitive Change in Aging Adults: Results from the Einstein Aging Studies. Aging, Neuropsychology, and Cognition 11(2-3), 196–211 (2004)
52. Sliwinski, M., Smyth, J., Hofer, S., Stawski, R.: Intraindividual Coupling of Daily Stress and Cognition. Psychology and Aging 21(3), 545–557 (2006)
53. Smith, A.: The symbol-digit modalities test: a neuropsychological test of learning and other cerebral disorders. In: Helmuth, J. (ed.) Learning Disorders, pp. 83–91. Special Child Publications, Seattle (1968)
54. Smith, C., Cotter, V.: Age-related changes in health. In: Capezuti, E., Zwicker, D., Mezey, M., Fulmer, T. (eds.) Evidence-Based Geriatric Nursing Protocols for Best Practice, pp. 431–458. Springer Publishing Company, New York (2008)
55. Steptoe, A., Vögele, C.: Methodology of Mental Stress Testing in Cardiovascular Research. Circulation 83(suppl. II), II-14–II-24 (1991)
56. Swaab, D.F., Bao, A.M., Lucassen, P.J.: The stress system in the human brain in depression and neurodegeneration. Ageing Research Reviews 4(2), 141–194 (2005)
57. Torpy, J., Lynm, C., Glass, R.: Mild Cognitive Impairment. Journal of the American Medical Association 302(4), 452 (2009)
58. US Census Bureau. Selected Characteristics of Baby Boomers 42 to 60 Years Old in 2006, Washington, DC (2006)
59. Vizer, L.M., Zhou, L., Sears, A.: Automated Stress Detection Using Keystroke and Linguistic Features: An Exploratory Study. International Journal of Human-Computer Studies 67(10), 870–886 (2009)
60. Wechsler, D.: A standardized memory scale for clinical use. Journal of Psychology 19, 87–95 (1945)
61. Welford, A., Norris, A., Shock, N.: Speed and accuracy of movement and their changes with age. In: Koster, W. (ed.) Attention and Performance II. North Holland, Amsterdam (1969)
62. Wild, K., Boise, L., Lundell, J., Foucek, A.: Unobtrusive In-Home Monitoring of Cognitive and Physical Health: Reactions and Perceptions of Older Adults. Journal of Applied Gerontology 27(2), 181–200 (2008)
63. Williams, S., Cooper, C.: Measuring occupational stress: Development of the pressure management indicator. Journal of Occupational Health Psychology 3, 306–321 (1998)
64. Wilson, R., Bienias, J., Evans, D., Bennett, D.: Religious Orders Study: Overview and Change in Cognitive and Motor Speed. Aging, Neuropsychology, and Cognition 11(2-3), 280 (2004)
65. World Health Organization. Towards a Common Language for Functioning, Disability and Health: ICF, Geneva (2002)
66. Yin, B., Ruiz, N., Chen, F., Khawaja, M.A.: Automatic cognitive load detection from speech features. In: OzCHI 2007, Adelaide, Australia, pp. 249–255. ACM, New York (2007)

67. Zhou, L., Burgoon, J.K., Twitchell, D., Qin, T., Nunamaker, J.F.: A comparison of classification methods for predicting deception in computer-mediated communication. Journal of Management Information Systems 20(4), 139–165 (2004)
68. Zhou, L., Zhang, D.: Following Linguistic Footprints: Automatic Deception Detection in Online Communication. Communications of the ACM, 119–122 (2008)
69. Zimprich, D., Martin, M., Kliegel, M., Dellenbach, M., Rast, P., Zeintl, M.: Cognitive Abilities in Old Age: Results from the Zurich Longitudinal Study on Cognitive Aging. Swiss Journal of Psychology 67(3), 177–195 (2008)
70. Zuckerman, M., DePaulo, B., Rosenthal, R.: Verbal and nonverbal communication of deception. In: Berkowitz, L. (ed.) Advances in Experimental Social Psychology, pp. 1–57. Academic Press, New York (1981)

Electronic Rating of Objective Structured Clinical Examinations: Mobile Digital Forms Beat Paper and Pencil Checklists in a Comparative Study

Felix M. Schmitz[1], Philippe G. Zimmermann[1], Kevin Gaunt[2], Markus Stolze[2], and Sissel Guttormsen Schär[1]

[1] Institute of Medical Education, University of Bern, Konsumstr, 13,
3010 Bern, Switzerland
{felix.schmitz,philippe.zimmermann,
sissel.guttormsen}@iml.unibe.ch
[2] Institute for Software, University of Applied Science, Oberseestr, 10,
8640 Rapperswil, Switzerland
{kevin.gaunt,markus.stolze}@hsr.ch

Abstract. During a two-day objective structured clinical examination (OSCE), we compared two types of checklists for student performance ratings: paper & pencil vs. digital checklists on iPads. Several subjective and objective measures from 10 examiners were collected and computed. Data showed that digital checklists were perceived as significantly more usable and less exertive and were also preferred in overall ratings. Assessments completed with digital checklists were found to have no missing items while assessments completed with paper checklists contained more than 8 blank items on average. Finally, checklist type did not influence assessment scores even though when using digital checklists more item-choice changes were produced.

Keywords: electronic assessments, OSCE, iPad, checklists, data quality, effort, perceived usability, preference.

1   Introduction

In 1975 Harden and his colleagues introduced the Objective Structured Clinical Examination (OSCE) at which medical students rotate around a series of stations in the hospital ward (Fig. 1) [1]. At these stations, the candidates are asked to perform a procedure with a standardized patient (e.g. perform an anamnesis) or with an anatomical model (e.g. clinical examination). The student's performance is observed and scored by an examiner using a standardized checklist. Hence, the students' final scores are usually calculated based on the score sheets handed in by every examiner. Since all students are assessed based on identical content by the same examiners using predetermined guidelines, OSCE can be an objective, valid and reliable method of assessment [1-3]. Today OSCE is an established tool in the repertoire of clinical assessment methods in many medical schools around the world [2].

A. Holzinger and K.-M. Simonic (Eds.): USAB 2011, LNCS 7058, pp. 501–512, 2011.
© Springer-Verlag Berlin Heidelberg 2011

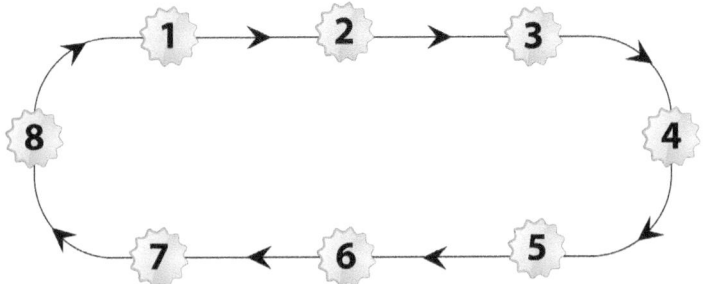

Fig. 1. OSCE consists of a circuit of stations usually manned with an examiner and a standardized patient. Students move from station to station, where they perform medical procedures.

The main drawback of OSCE is "the increased preparation required" ([1], p. 451): case-based tasks and the according checklists must be created (iteratively), standardized patients and examiners must be acquired, selected and carefully trained, students must be randomly assigned into rotation groups, and so on. Furthermore, carrying out the exam is time and resource consuming. The packed schedule requires the examiners' full attention and time, during which they are missing at the clinic. Additionally, the process of extracting the examiners evaluations is very time consuming: up to 60% of the paper checklists must be manually verified in order to ensure the assessments contain no missing data. Then they have to be transformed into digital representations by scanning the paper checklists. This error-prone transformation from paper-based information to digital data is the standard procedure used today. Summing up: OSCE is a time and resource-intensive form of examination (e.g. [2], [4]).

This unsatisfactory process has motivated us to start a project titled *Electronic Registration of Objective Structured Clinical Examination (e-OSCE)* which aims for a more efficient and entirely digital preparation, execution and analysis process of OSCEs (Fig. 2) [5], [6].

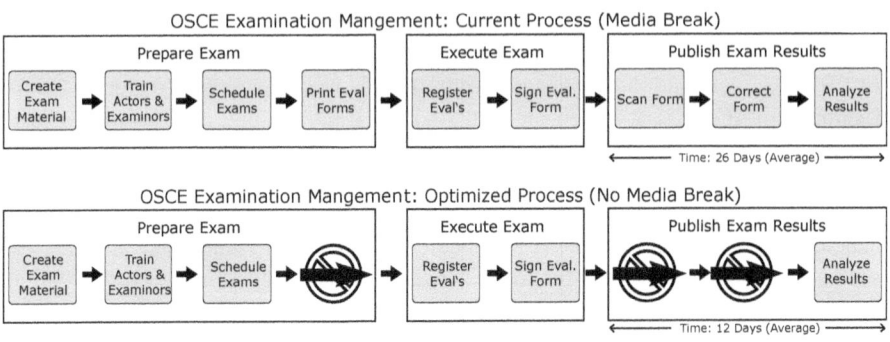

Fig. 2. The project e-OSCE aims for an optimization of the preparation and analysis process and for a facilitation of scoring the candidates' performances by introducing digital checklists running on iPads

Our literature research revealed that a few previous attempts to perform OSCE evaluations digitally exist [7-9]. These projects were promising with regard to effectiveness, efficiency, and user satisfaction. However, none of the investigated systems have been established as tools for real exams so far, as these projects applied devices that are outdated (i.e. PDAs) by today's standards. The current generation of tablet PCs is thin, light and cheap. This convinced us that it was worthwhile to revisit this challenge in our project. The project went through several stages. The first stage included the development of an exam client interface for Apple iPhones. Our usability tests and in-depth interviews soon revealed that the display size was too small for the intended content. The second stage addressed this issue by developing a Windows tablet PC client. First experiences in a field test showed that this hardware form factor was better suited to displaying the medical checklists. However, the power consumption of the available hardware at that time (2010) was insufficient and the test subjects deemed the devices too uncomfortable (due to weight and heat emission) to use for the intended time period. Hence in the third and current stage of the e-OSCE project we switched to Apple iPads as client devices. We developed an exam client named *OSCE-Eval*, a JAVA based server component for delivery and reception of examination data and a web-based exam management component. All of these components have been undergoing various laboratory and field tests [10].

Besides the technical maturity of the system concerning stability, speed and security, several subjective and objective characteristics of the client application are a major focus of the user tests mentioned above. Due to the examiners high cognitive load during the exam and the long examination time, the system has to be usable with minimal effort and has to support the user throughout the examination process. Furthermore, a major focus of the project is to improve the unsatisfactory data quality of the paper-based evaluations. Hence, the digital checklists have to reduce or eliminate input errors by preventing missing, unreadable or ambiguous data input. Since the change from paper checklists to a digital evaluation process is challenging for the OSCE examiners, we are interested in how well they accept the new system in comparison to the paper version.

In the following chapters we present the results of our study investigating subjective and objective characteristics of OSCE-Eval in comparison to paper-based checklists. This study was conducted during a real OSCE.

2   Hypotheses

As previously stated, the usability of OSCE-Eval is crucial for two reasons: to validate that the examiners are able to adequately operate the application and to minimize the induced cognitive load for examiners. Compared to the existing paper and pencil checklists (PCL), OSCE-Eval offers more guidance and support through on-screen messages, time tracking with audio-visual feedback, graphical accentuation of blank items, indication of already processed and prospective forms, etc. (for an overview of the features, see [10]). Moreover, the application is built for touch screen devices (i.e. Apple iPads) that are "the most natural of all input devices" ([11], p. 387; see also [12]). In other words, touch screens are intuitive, but PCLs are self-explanatory instruments, too. We consider the benefits associated with OSCE-Eval to outperform PCL in respect to perceived usability. This leads us to our first hypothesis (H1).

H1: Compared to PCL the perceived usability of OSCE-Eval is more satisfying

The examiners' tasks result in a high mental effort during an OSCE day: they consistently observe and evaluate students' performances and therefore need to be attentive for longer time spans. Consequently, it is important to assist them as much as possible in order to keep them focused. The evaluation of a student's performance during an OSCE is similar to a repetitive non-sequential selection task. This is because candidates usually do not adhere to diagnosing in the same order as the checklist would indicate. OSCE-PCLs used at the medical faculty of the University of Bern are typically between two to four pages long. Thus finding the right item is a search task that regularly involves turning pages (PCL) or scrolling (OSCE-Eval). In this context, scrolling seems to be more convenient, because one doesn't have to search through a stack of several pages. Moreover, OSCE-Eval uses popovers (also known as callouts; see Fig. 3) to represent the available choices for each checklist item (e.g. *yes*, *partial* and *no*). When performing non-sequential selection tasks, popovers have been found to deliver better performance and evoke more user-confidence compared to using inline radio buttons in electronic forms [13]. Obviously popovers can't be used in PCLs, leaving a checkmark design as the only alternative. Therefore scrolling and the use of popovers are unique to OSCE-Eval and could result in lower mental effort. On the other hand, computer anxiety could be evoked when using OSCE-Eval. Computer anxiety increases stress during the usage of digital devices, e.g. [14-15]. However, following [16] we expect iPad devices to be inviting (playful) tools for the examiners and thus decrease the likeliness of computer anxiety to occur. For this reason we postulate that the examiners will experience less mental effort by using OSCE-Eval.

H2: The experienced mental effort is lower when using OSCE-Eval than when using PCL

In regard to data quality, missing data (i.e. blank items) are unlikely when using OSCE-Eval. This is because the system enables the use of input validation and visual feedback for unprocessed checklist items. Of course, with PCL this level of support is not possible. This leads us to our third hypothesis (H3).

H3: Using OSCE-Eval results in less missing data than by using PCL

The evaluation process must not be influenced by checklist type (objectivity). Despite both checklist types consisting of the identical set of items, we expect the checklist type to have an impact on scoring results. The reason for this is that the systems obviously feel different and therefore could influence the examiners' scoring behavior (see H4).

H4: Evaluation results differ between checklist types.

Finally, we are interested in which checklist type (OSCE-Eval vs. PCL) will be preferred by the end-user (i.e. the examiners). We postulate that examiners either prefer OSCE-Eval or PCL (see H5).

H5: Preference of the two checklist types is different.

3   Method

3.1   Sample and Design

Participants were 10 physicians (2 women) from the medical faculty of the University of Bern acting as examiners in a two-day OSCE (5 participants per examination day). The examiners' age ranged between 34 and 50 years. The mean age was 40.20 years ($SD = 5.87$). All examiners were fluent in German.

To test our hypotheses, we conducted a within-subject study with the factor "checklist type" comprised of two levels: (1) OSCE-Eval (running on iPad) and (2) paper and pencil checklist (PCL). In order to avoid a sequence effect, we counterbalanced the checklist type order (see Procedure). Overall, the examiners executed a total of 240 evaluations.

3.2   Material

The checklists used in this study consisted of 36 items that had been used in previous OSCEs. Both checklist types featured the same items in the same order according to the same evaluation dimensions: *anamnesis* (15 items), *exploration* (10 items), *diagnosis* (5 items), *communication* (5 items), and *overall impression* (1 item). The checklist items were typeset in Helvetica 9 pt. for PCL (printed at 300 dpi) and Helvetica 13 pt. for OSCE-Eval (using a 132 ppi screen). The PCL was a total of three pages long and the choices available were presented by the use of multiple checkbox lists (Fig. 3). Depending on the iPad's orientation, OSCE-Eval displayed either 789 characters (portrait) or 607 characters (landscape) on screen. The available choices per item were presented using popovers (Fig. 3). All examiners operated OSCE-Eval on identical first generation Apple iPad (2010) devices.

To familiarize the examiners with the usage of OSCE-Eval (see Procedure) we prepared a 12 minutes introductory video. The video is available online at [10] (in German). Since we needed training material on how to cope with the checklists, we also filmed two 5 minutes videos showing either a "bad" or a "good" performance of a student (played by an actor).

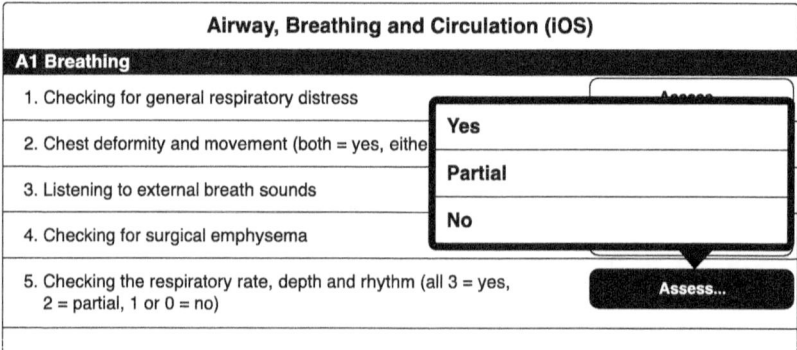

Fig. 3. Schematic comparison of checklist types: PCL uses a checkbox design (top) and OSCE-Eval uses a popover design (bottom). The items were identical for OSCE-Eval and PCL.

3.3   Measurements

Subjective Usability. To test which checklist type was perceived to be more usable (see H1), the examiners were presented with an adapted version of the Post-Study System Usability Questionnaire (PSSUQ) [17]. The original PSSUQ is a 19-item instrument for assessing user satisfaction with system usability. The reliability of its overall scale has been found to be excellent (*Cronbach's Alpha* = .97) [17].

We selected a subset of 16 PSSUQ items suitable for both OSCE-Eval and PCL and translated them into German. All items were 7-point Likert scales ranging from *1 = strongly disagree* to *7 = strongly agree*. An example for one of the items is *Overall, I am satisfied with how easy it is to use OSCE-Eval [PCL]*.

Experienced Mental Effort. To test how intensely the examiners experienced the effort of their task (observing and evaluating candidates' performances) (see H2), we used the German version of the Rating Scale Mental Effort (RSME) [18]. The German RSME is an analogous 220 mm long one-item graphic scale anchored at its end points with the values *0* and *220*. Between the end points 7 written terms were displayed additionally in order to enrich the scale semantically. The terms ranged from *barely exertive* for *20* and *extremely exertive* for *205*. Examiners were asked to do the following: *Please specify how exertive your task (observing and evaluating) was by marking a point on the continuum with a cross.* We evaluated the examiners input by measuring the cross' offset distance in millimeters from 0 by using a ruler. According to [19] "The Rating Scale Mental Effort proved to be a reliable and valid instrument measuring psychological costs" (p. 139).

Missing Data. To test which checklist type contained less missing data (see H3), we manually counted unanswered evaluation items for PCL and entered the results into SPSS. For OSCE-Eval, before transposing data to SPSS, we queried the application's database for unanswered questions. To do that, the test software recorded every one of the examiners' choices and stored them locally inside a database.

Scoring Results. To test if the checklist type influenced scoring results (see H4), we analyzed the scores of 5 of the checklist items used in the forms. All of these items were global scales of the evaluation dimensions *anamnesis, exploration, diagnosis, communication,* and *overall impression.* All 5 items were 5-point rating scales ranging from *1 = very bad* to *5 = very good*.

In order to compare data from both checklist types, we scanned the PCLs. From the resulting Microsoft Excel file we then computed the mean scores for all 5 global ratings per examiner and entered them into SPSS. OSCE-Eval stored all of the examiners' choices in XML files for each candidate. To extract the mean ratings from OSCE-Eval, it was necessary to parse the XML forms and sort them by examiner. A script was developed for this purpose.

Preference Ratings. After using both OSCE-Eval and PCL, examiners were asked with which checklist type they would prefer to work in the future (see H5). The choices for this question were either *OSCE-Eval* or *paper and pencil checklist.*

Subjects. During the examiners' training session, that took place two days before the exam (see Procedure), we handed out a questionnaire. It contained questions regarding their gender, age and handedness as well as their experience with iPads, iPhones, and touch screens in general. We also wanted to know if they had prior experience as OSCE examiners (all 7-point rating scales from *1 = not experienced at all* to *7 = very experienced*). Finally, we were interested in how comprehensible and effective the instruction video demonstrating the usage of OSCE-Eval was: (1) *The training video is comprehensible* and (2) *I think I am able to use OSCE-Eval without problems because of the training video.* Both items were 7-point Likert scales from *1 = strongly disagree* to *7 = strongly agree*.

3.4   Procedure

OSCE Training. Two days before the examination was conducted, all 10 examiners were introduced to their tasks by communicating the aims, procedures and rules of OSCE. Then the examiners were given a sample paper and pencil checklist consisting of 5 items from the evaluation dimension *communication*. The investigator made sure that every examiner understood the scope of each item. Then examiners watched the video of a student performing badly at an examination station and had to evaluate that student's performance by rating the 5 items on their checklist. This was followed by a public discussion moderated by the investigator. The discussion finished when the examiners reached a consensual evaluation result. A similar private evaluation and validating discussion followed after the second video was shown. This time it showed the student performing well.

After this introduction the examiners watched the 12 minutes OSCE-Eval training video. We then handed out the questionnaire to collect data regarding the examiners demographics, ICT and OSCE experience, and their perception of the training video. After all examiners had completed their questionnaires, we answered open questions about the usage OSCE-Eval. Once the examiners felt reasonably comfortable two hands-on trainings took place in two different rooms. Half of the sample ($n = 5$) operated OSCE-Eval while observing a re-enacted scene played by two actors, one in the student's and the other in the patient's role. The scene was based on a cased-based example matching the items of the form. The other half of the sample used PCL while observing a comparable re-enacted scene. After finishing the evaluation using either OSCE-Eval or PCL the two groups changed checklist type and completed the same tasks with a comparable scene.

Finally, the examiners were informed about the dates of the their OSCE and the type of checklist they will be using first during the examination.

OSCE Examination. The examination spanned two days, with the procedure on either day being identical: 30 minutes prior to the start of the examination 5 examiners were seated at their stations. They were introduced to the standardized patient acting out a patient case. Then we handed out either an iPad running OSCE-Eval or the PCL. Each examiner started evaluating the performance of 12 candidates by using either checklist type. Subsequent to the evaluation of 12 students examiners completed the questionnaires on usability satisfaction and mental effort. After lunch we exchanged the checklist type so the accordant examiners evaluated another 12 students by using the opposed system (see Table 1). Then they filled out the questionnaires on usability satisfaction and mental effort for the second time. Additionally, the examiners had to state whether they would prefer OSCE-Eval or PCL as an instrument in further evaluations.

Each evaluation lasted for 15 minutes including a 2-minute break to allow for the students changing stations and for examiners to complete the evaluation. The schedule was structured into different rotations, each consisting of 4 evaluations. After each

Table 1. Schedule for examiners either starting with the OSCE-Eval application or the PCL

Day of run	Examiner (ID)	Checklist type used for first 12 evaluations	Checklist type used for last 12 evaluations
1	1	OSCE-Eval	PCL
1	2	PCL	OSCE-Eval
1	3	OSCE-Eval	PCL
1	4	PCL	OSCE-Eval
1	5	OSCE-Eval	PCL
2	6	PCL	OSCE-Eval
2	7	OSCE-Eval	PCL
2	8	PCL	OSCE-Eval
2	9	OSCE-Eval	PCL
2	10	PCL	OSCE-Eval

rotation the examiners were granted a 15-minute break. After the first 3 rotations, the examiners had a 30-minute lunch break. After lunch the checklist type was interchanged and the exam continued for another 3 rotations. In total, an examination day spanned approximately 8 hours, including the time for answering the questionnaires.

4   Results

All examiners were either right-handed or ambidextrous. Before participating in the study, examiners had little experience using iPads. In fact they were more experienced using iPhones and other touch screen-based devices (see Table 2). Furthermore, most participants were novices in regard to acting as examiners within an OSCE (Table 2). The OSCE-Eval instruction video was perceived as comprehensible and effective (Table 2).

Table 2. Overview of the examiners' ICT experience, OSCE experience and OSCE-Eval training video evaluation

Variable	N	Min	Max	M	SD	Mode	Mdn
iPad usage experience [i]	10	1	7	3.00	2.36	1	2
iPhone usage experience [i]	10	1	7	5.20	2.39	7	6
Touch-screen usage experience [i]	10	4	7	5.80	1.14	5; 7	5.5
OSCE-examiner experience [i]	10	1	7	2.50	2.17	1	1
Comprehensibility of training video [ii]	10	4	7	6.30	.95	7	6.5
Ability to use OSCE-Eval due to video [ii]	10	3	7	5.40	1.43	7	5.5

[i] Scale from *1 = not experienced at all* to *7 = totally experienced*.
[ii] Scale from *1 = strongly disagree* to *7 = strongly agree*.

To test our first 4 hypotheses, we computed Wilcoxon tests for paired samples (the non-parametric equivalent of the paired samples t-test).

The satisfaction with system usability (overall scale) was higher for OSCE-Eval (M = 6.36, SD = .54) than for PCL (M = 5.60, SD = .88). This difference is statistically significant (z = -1.94, $p_{(1-tailed)}$ = .027). Therefore, we accept our first hypothesis (H1). The experienced mental effort was lower using OSCE-Eval (M = 71.30, SD = 32.96) than using PCL (M = 89.20, SD = 38.85). This difference is significant (z = -1.84, $p_{(1-tailed)}$ = .033) and the reason why we also accept our second hypothesis (H2). As expected, when using OSCE-Eval, examiners did not miss to fill in any data (i.e. blank items). In contrast, examiners left open between 1 and 27 blank items (M = 8.40, SD = 7.58) by using PCL. Wilcoxon test statistics showed that this distinction is highly significant (z = -2.81, $p_{(1-tailed)}$ = .0025). We consequently accept our third hypothesis (H3). Data further showed that evaluation results did not significantly differ between checklist types for any of the 5 evaluation dimensions (Table 3). Thus, we reject our fourth hypothesis (H4).

Table 3. Comparison of scoring results

Score dimension	N	$M_1 (SD_1)$ [i]	$M_2 (SD_2)$ [ii]	SS+	SS-	Z	$P_{(2-tailed)}$
Anamnesis	10	3.52 (.23)	3.45 (.53)	31	24	-.357	.721
Exploration	10	3.41 (.33)	3.30 (.35)	39	16	-1.173	.241
Diagnosis	10	3.87 (.40)	4.02 (.45)	13	42	-1.480	.139
Communication	10	3.95 (.31)	3.96 (.37)	24	21	-.178	.859
Overall impression	10	3.67 (.27)	3.61 (.48)	24	21	-.178	.859

[i] Parameters M_1 and SD_1 based on scores transmitted by operating OSCE-Eval.
[ii] Parameters M_2 and SD_2 based on scores transmitted by operating PCL.

In order to test which checklist type was preferred by the examiners (see H5) we conducted a Chi-square test. Our data shows that 8 examiners (out of 10) preferred OSCE-Eval as an evaluation instrument. 1 examiner abstained from voting and 1 preferred using PCL. Consequently, the number of observations per cell significantly differs from the expected number per cell ($Chi^2(1, N = 9)$ = 5.44, p = .02). For this reason we accept our fifth and final hypothesis.

5   Discussion

In this study, we investigated whether commonly used paper and pencil checklists (PCL) or item-identical digital checklists running on Apple iPads (OSCE-Eval) are the more suitable instrument when applied within the medical assessment framework Objective Structured Clinical Examination (OSCE).

Our comparative study provides the following five results regarding our initial hypotheses. First, the experienced usability differed between checklist types. In particular, examiners perceived the usability of OSCE-Eval as to be significantly more satisfying compared to PCL. Second, the usage of OSCE-Eval decreased the examiners' perceived mental effort significantly in comparison with the usage of PCL. Third, examiners did not leave any blank items when using OSCE-Eval. In contrast, when using PCL examiners sometimes failed to provide an input for every checklist item. This difference is strongly significant. Fourth, checklist types did not have an impact on scoring results (H4 rejected) why we assume OSCE-Eval to be a non-distracting evaluation instrument. Fifth, a statistically significant difference in the examiners' preference benefitting OSCE-Eval was found.

Examiners justified their clear preference by underlining the simplicity of the touch screen, the ability to observe performances from multiple views by walking around the station while using the iPad for scoring, and the provided support and feedback associated with OSCE-Eval (e.g. highlighting blank items). Examiners also mentioned that when using OSCE-Eval, it is easier to correct previously processed checklist items simply by tapping the accordant item again and then selecting another choice. When using PCL, already processed items must be crossed out before ticking off another choice, so corrections are more tedious. In this respect, we also extracted data from log files as well as from the paper forms and found that there was a significantly higher occurrence of evaluation changes when examiners used OSCE-Eval ($M = 35.80$, $SD = 17.68$) as when they worked with PCL ($M = 9.50$, $SD = 5.52$) ($z = -2.703$, $p_{(2\text{-}tailed)} = .007$). Apparently examiners were more conservative selecting choices when using PCL. We assume the higher effort in modifying an answer and the limited number of changes (before the form becomes unreadable) are possibly attributable to this.

The limitation of the present study is its small sample size ($N = 10$). As already pointed out, OSCE is a costly form of examination for medical faculties. That is why we were not able to invite more physicians joining as examiners. However, we see these preliminary results as promising, which is why we intend to replicate the present study in a bigger exam with more subjects.

In conclusion, the digital checklist type OSCE-Eval running on iPad outperformed the commonly used paper and pencil checklist in respect to all subjective dimensions surveyed in this study, i.e. subjective usability, experienced effort and preference. Further, when examiners used OSCE-Eval, the data quality was much better than when using the paper version of the form (i.e. no blank items). Finally, OSCE-Eval did not influence examiners' scoring behavior. Thus we regard this type of checklist as a non-distracting evaluation instrument. Based on the results of this study we are looking forward to apply OSCE-Eval to productive OSCEs in the near future and are exited to expand our findings.

Acknowledgments. The E-OSCE project is funded by SWITCH through the AAA (E-Infrastructure for E-Science) research program as well as by the University Bern and the University of Applied Science Rapperswil (HSR).

References

1. Harden, R.M., Stevenson, M., Downie, W.W., Wilson, G.M.: Assessment of clinical competence using objective structured examination. Br. Med. J (Clin. Res. Ed.) 1, 447–451 (1975)
2. Barman, A.: Critiques on the objective structured clinical examination. Ann. Acad. Med. 34, 478–482 (2005)
3. Harden, R.M., Gleeson, F.A.: Assessment of clinical competence using an objective structured clinical examination (OSCE). Med. Educ. 13, 41–54 (1979)
4. Gupta, P., Dewan, P., Singh, T.: Objective Structured Clinical Examination (OSCE) Revisited. Indian Pediatr. 47, 911–920 (2010)
5. Serving Swiss Universities (SWITCH), http://www.switch.ch/aaa/projects/detail/FHO.2
6. Serving Swiss Universities (SWITCH), http://www.switch.ch/aaa/projects/detail/UNIBE.4
7. Schmidts, M.B., http://m3e.meduniwien.ac.at/resources/e_osce.pdf
8. Treadwell, I.: The usability of personal digital assistants (PDAs) for assessment of practival performance. Med. Educ. 9, 855–861 (2006)
9. Hatfield, C.L., Bragg, H.H.: Utilizing Electronic Objective Structured Clinical Exam (eOSCE) Stations for College-Wide Assessment Purposes. In: 109th Annual Meeting of the American Association of Colleges of Pharmacy, Chicago, Illinois, p. 81 (2008)
10. E-OSCE official Website, http://www.e-osce.ch
11. Holzinger, A.: Finger Instead of Mouse: Touch Screens as a Means of Enhancing Universal Access. In: Carbonell, N., Stephanidis, C. (eds.) UI4ALL 2002. LNCS, vol. 2615, pp. 387–397. Springer, Heidelberg (2003)
12. Holzinger, A., Hoeller, M., Schedlbauer, M., Urlesberger, B.: An Investigation of Finger versus Stylus Input in Medical Scenarios. In: ITI 30th International Conference on Information Technology Interfaces, pp. 433–438. IEEE Press, New York (2008)
13. Gaunt, K., Schmitz, F.M., Stolze, M.: Choose Popovers over Buttons for iPad Questionnaires. In: Campos, P., Graham, N., Jorge, J., Nunes, N., Palanque, P., Winckler, M. (eds.) INTERACT 2011, Part II. LNCS, vol. 6947, pp. 533–540. Springer, Heidelberg (2011)
14. Hudiburg, R.A.: Psychology of Computer Use.7. Measuring Technostress - Computer-Related Stress. Psychol. Rep. 64, 767–772 (1989)
15. Anderson, A.A.: Predictors of computer anxiety and performance in information systems. Computers in Human Behavior 12, 61–77 (1996)
16. Webster, J., Martocchio, J.J.: Microcomputer Playfulness - Development of a Measure with Workplace Implications. Mis. Quart. 16, 201–226 (1992)
17. Lewis, J.R.: Ibm Computer Usability Satisfaction Questionnaires - Psychometric Evaluation and Instructions for Use. Int. J. Hum.-Comput. Int. 7, 57–78 (1995)
18. Eilers, K., Nachreiner, F., Hänecke, K.: Entwicklung und Überprüfung einer Skala zur Erfassung subjektiv erlebter Anstrengung (The development and testing of a scale to validation for recording subjectively experienced effort). Zeitschrift für Arbeitswissenschaft 40, 215–224 (1986)
19. Zijlstra, F.R.H.: Efficiency in Work Behaviour; A Design Approach for Modern Tools. Delft University Press, Delft (1993)

What Determines Public Perceptions of Implantable Medical Technology: Insights into Cognitive and Affective Factors

Anne Kathrin Schaar and Martina Ziefle

Communication Science, RWTH Aachen University,
Theaterplatz 14, 52062 Aachen, Germany
{schaar,ziefle}@humtec.rwth-aachen.de

Abstract. Medical Technology is one of the rising branches of technology development within the last decades. Especially device miniaturization is enormously progressing what makes implantable technology to a promising approach for the future. Especially in times of the demographic change implantable medical technology could play its part in the delivery of healthcare services, supporting an independent and mobile aging. From a technical point of view, implants are far-developed and will enter the market in the next years. From a human factors' point of view, there is a considerable lack of acceptance-related knowledge and understanding of perceived benefits and barriers across a diverse population. Using a qualitative approach, this study gains insights into public perceptions of implantable medical technology, the level of information revealing misconceptions and basic fears. It thus explores cognitive and affective factors that form the acceptance of implantable medical technology. Results allow the identification of information and technical communication deficits in order to derive a sensitive information and communication policy.

Keywords: Public perception, Acceptance, Implants, Medical Technology.

1   Introduction

Medical Technology is one of the rising technology branches within the last decades. Miniaturization of technology enables new implants, like for example medical stents, that can be positioned deeper and more precisely into sensitive body areas, as into the brain, ears, eyes, or just into small blood vessels, with a broad application field. The stents may take over different functions within medical treatment and care, as e.g. drug delivery [1], monitoring reasons [2] [3] or medical information storage [4]. Beyond medical stents, there are other implantable medical devices, as e.g. pacemaker, cochlear implant or deep brain stimulation, which are used in the medical sector since a few years and are thus fairly known in the public.

The progress in medical invasive technology opens up a large space between different poles, ranging from new possibilities to keep ill patients independently living (new technological innovation), keeping people alive which would have died

A. Holzinger and K.-M. Simonic (Eds.): USAB 2011, LNCS 7058, pp. 513–531, 2011.
© Springer-Verlag Berlin Heidelberg 2011

otherwise (medical necessity) up to overstepping personal, physical and private limits. So far, innovations in this sector are predominately driven by technical, medical and legal aspects as well as the necessity of medical treatment and care. On the contrary, the human factor and the prevailing extent of acceptance or aloofness towards new medical technology fall short. The same applies for the underdeveloped public awareness that any technical innovation is exigently needed, especially in this sensitive field that breaks – be it necessary or not – into persons' intimate spaces.

The discussion about the importance of users' attitude towards and acceptance of new medical products is slowly influencing mainstream acceptance studies in different contexts [5] [6]. So far we learned that - opposite to Information and Communication Technologies [ICT] - which are mostly perceived as useful - the acceptance of medical technology is much more complex and strongly affected by health status, age, gender roles, culture, personal living conditions or care situation [7] [8] [5]. Especially in situations of health threats, acceptance patterns might change and common acceptance habits are losing their validity. From a psychological point of view it is decisive that acceptance follows users' knowledge about technology, what they think technology offers them or in which way a new technology may hinder or restrain them. Thus, cognitions and mental models of technology as well as assumptions about consequences of technology and accompanied risks form acceptance patterns.

This study aims to uncover cognitions, public opinions and mental models of invasive medical technology. Using qualitative methods, we wanted to find out what "average" users expect from implantable technologies. Learning the impact of different technology types, that are known to a different extent in the public, perceptions, perceived benefits and fears of four implantable medical devices were gathered and possible influence of individual factors on attitudes were analyzed.

1.1   Implantable Medical Technologies

Medical technologies in general, and implantable devices in particular show a great variety regarding application fields and device types, ranging from chips in the context of electronic patient records to be placed directly under the skin, up to devices implantable into hearts or brains. Due to device miniaturization, most of the surgeries are accomplished minimal-invasive. Figure 1 illustrates the selection of implants that are under study in this research.

Pacemaker: The first pacemaker was implanted in 1958 [9]. Its transvenous implementation was first introduced in 1968. Since pacemakers are established for more than 50 years now, pacemakers are widely known. Pacemakers consist of two main parts: A subcutaneous implantable device (Fig. 1.1: http://www.pflegewiki. de/wiki/Herzschrittmacher), equipped with an aggregate with two electrodes (dual chamber pace maker) or one electrode (one chamber device). The electrodes are touching the wall coated with Purkinje Fibers, providing the impulse over the heart muscle to evoke a total contraction of the heart chamber. The size of the aggregate is about four to five centimeters, consists of a lithium battery and control electronics, which are housed in a titanium case [9]. Modern pacemakers allow an individual adaption of the hearts' special performance requirements. The battery's endurance is about eight years.

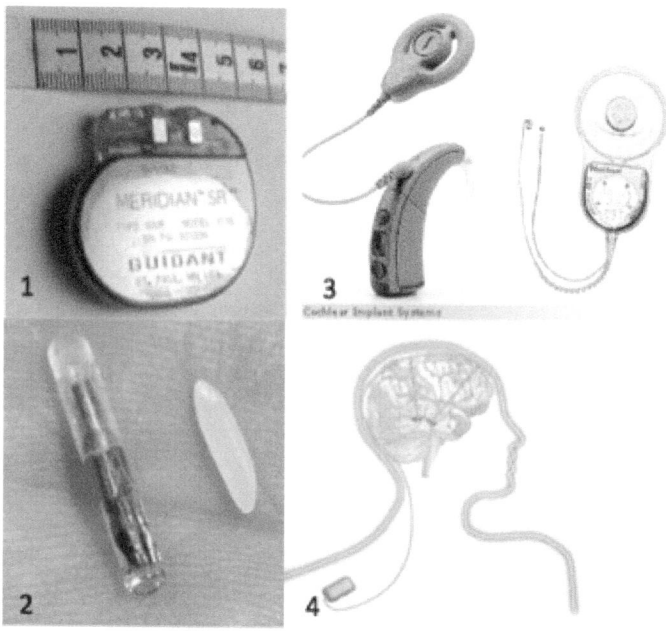

Fig. 1. Implants (1.1pace maker, 1.2 medical chip, 1.3 cochlear implant, 1.4 Deep-Brain-Stimulation

Cochlear Implant: The cochlear implant represents a device for recovery of the hearing of profoundly deaf or severely hard hearing persons. In 1984, first preclinical tests were run, the first successful surgery was accomplished in 1986. The implant is located into the cochlear, which is a part of the inner ear that is the receptor field for the hearing perception. The cochlear areal is coated with about 16000 hearing cells that are not regenerative once destroyed. The implantable part has two subparts: a number of electrodes that are insert and fixed in the cochlear and a coil that is implanted under the scalp behind the ear [9] , plus a processor for data management. The external part of the implant has a microphone, a speech processor, a battery and a coil that is fixed at the place of the implanted coil via magnetism (Fig 1.3 implant: www.htz-potsdam.de/ci.htm). The microphone records audible signals translated into electronically signals and transported via internal and external coils. Impulses are sent via the implanted electrodes to the remaining nerve stumps of sensory cells. From there, signals are transported to the brainstem, re-modeled and sent to the audio and speech centre via auditory pathway.

Medical Chips: Medical chips or stents are implanted for several reasons: data storage [4], monitoring [3] [2], drug-delivery and tracking [10]. In the United States, the invasive chip technology was for the first time licensed in 2004 (Food & Drug Administration), after filing the application in 2002. The invasive chip for measuring vital parameters (e.g. blood pressure, blood sugar) was first presented by the German Fraunhofer Institute for Microelectronic Circuits and Systems in 2008. These medical chips have nearly the size of a rice grain (Fig. 1.2 (http://post.cloudfront. goodinc.com/MastheadImage/17037/org_chip) and can be implanted at many places in the human body. In cases of RFID-Chips that are used for tracking or data storage the chips can be implanted directly under the patients' skin without difficult or complex surgeries. For the measurement of blood pressure or bladder volume, chips are implanted into the corresponding body-areas.

Deep-Brain-Stimulation: Deep-Brain-Stimulation [DBS] is a quite risky surgical operation within the brain, in which a so-called "brain pacemaker" is implanted. The pacemaker is a hair-fine electrode that sends electronically impulses to specific brain parts. The DBS is especially used for the treatment of Parkinson patients, where the electrode is placed in the Substantia Nigra (midbrain). Stimulating this brain area reduces an excessive distribution of dopamine, which is responsible for the typical Parkinson tremor and paralysis. The brain pacemaker consists of the electrode and another internal and external part [9]. The internal part includes a controller as well as a battery (endurance 3-5 years [9]. The controller is implanted under the collarbone and connected to the electrode [10] (Fig. 1.4: http://neuro2.med.uni-magdeburg. de/neurologie/document/bilder/tiefen). The external part of the implant is the general controller for the brain pacemaker and able to switch the device on and off. The external controller modulates frequency and current. Initially the DBS was tested for the treatment of pain and spastic paralysis. Later, it was used for the treatment of Parkinson disease. The first DBS surgery for Parkinson therapy happened in 2001 [9], although the underlying technology is already known since the 1960ies. Furthermore, DBS is also used for the treatment of depressions and obsessive-compulsive disorders [10].

1.2   Perception and Acceptance of Medical Technologies

There is a lot of evidence that the perception of technical devices as well as their cognitive representation has a huge influence on device interaction and the openness of users to accept it and integrate objects into their daily routines. In the context of ICT it could be shown [11] that persons with an appropriate mental model of how a device works and how a technical menu might be structured show a considerably better effectiveness and efficiency when interacting with the device. In addition, a proper mental model of the device also positively influences technology acceptance [11]. However, the publicity of a technology is another factor that is decisively impacting the acceptance [12]. Relatively unknown medical technology evokes perceptions of risks that are detached from real risks but though are influencing the acceptance of medical technology. Recently [12], users' attitudes and the acceptance of a medical stent implanted directly under the skin (monitoring of vital parameters) had been examined. It was found that a lot of misconceptions, felt risks and fears were prevailing that dramatically influenced acceptance patterns, especially in female users and users with only little technical knowledge. The findings are especially noteworthy as they show that the novelty of such medical technologies and the small factual knowledge of participants how a specific medical technology could affect normal living at home is considerably decreasing acceptance. Though, the reluctance of people is not literally a refusal to use these systems, but more probably a global insecurity of how these systems work and an uncertainty whether these systems bring more negative effects than benefits, what is definitely a lack of appropriate in information policy. Furthermore, recent studies show that health consciousness [8] and a positive general attitude toward the own body as well as appropriate coping strategies [13] do considerably impact acceptance patterns.

Furthermore, the acceptance of medical technology is correlated with user diversity [5] [14] [15] [16]. Among individual factors, age, gender and technical expertise are crucial variables modulating acceptance. A closer look reveals technical expertise (in both, perceived as well as factual levels) is the most critical one as it correlates to age (with increasing age technical expertise decreases) and gender (women usually report lower levels of technical expertise and show a lower self competence when handling technology) [16]. On the basis of the outcomes and the specificity of the medical technology acceptance, existing acceptance models like the Technology Acceptance Model (TAM) [17] [18] and its refinement (Unified Theory of Acceptance and Use of Technology, UTAUT) [19] should be further elaborated and, if appropriate, extended.

1.3   Questions Addressed and Logic of Empirical Procedure

The aim of this study was thus to analyze cognitive conceptions and prevailing information levels with respect to implantable medical technology. There is a huge knowledge gap about the public discourse, and possibly ambivalent attitudes to implantable medical technologies. This is of specific impact as the public opinion also considerably impacts the cognitive mind setting of future users. In order to collect comprehensive opinions and to reflect them across a broader sample of women and men of different ages, we chose the questionnaire-method. Though, as the acceptance for future medical technology is a sensitive issue, we were also interested to gather qualitative insights to understand individuals' attitudes and barriers.

2   Method

In this section, the questionnaire instrument is outlined. A first remark addresses the recruitment rationale of participants and population characteristics.

2.1   Recruitment Rationale of Participants

The recruitment rationale was to survey basically healthy people in order to explore opinions about future electronic solutions in healthcare. The study was executed in different classes at a German vocational college. Vocational colleges combine a wide range of educational qualifications. Therefore participants with different educational backgrounds (social and technical professions) can be reached and collect unbiased opinions in a natural environment. The survey took place during class and implied a short introduction into the topic of implantable devices that had to be evaluated in the questionnaire. At the end of the test sessions, a closing discussion in the plenum was initiated.

2.2   The Questionnaire

The questionnaire was divided into three main parts: (1) *Demographic variables*: the first section included questions about demographic data as well as information about the health status, experience with diseases (self and family members). (2) *Public knowledge and attitudes toward implants*: The second part dealt with incorporated medical technology. Participants were instructed to list known implants. They were encouraged, to list as many as they would know (allowing us to estimate the degree of public knowledge and, also, to analyze which of the devices would be dropped most frequently, and, also, which of the devices would be mentioned first).   Also, participant's general attitudes toward implants were quantitatively assessed, using four items (6-point scale, 1 = full agreement, 6 = full rejection, Table 1).

Table 1. Items regarding general attitudes towards implantable technology

Please rate the following statements (1 = full agreement 6 = full rejection)
For me, persons with an implant can be regarded as healthy
For me, implants may compensate illness, but are never able to heal
For me, implants are very valuable and should be developed and investigated in the future
For me, implants do exceed ethical boundaries and highly prone arbitrariness

(3) *Cognitive Models and Perceptions*: In the third section, cognitive models and perceptions were collected. First, participants were asked to envision that they would need and have such an implant, to note their first associations related to the devices as well as their envisioned function. Then, participants estimated the size of the devices, and its assumed location. The assessment of the perceived location and size referred to the hypothesis that the sensitivity of the body location (as e.g. brain, heart [12]) in combination with the size would considerably impact participants' perception (4) At the end, participants were requested to rank the different implants according to a) the perceived dangerousness of the operation, b) the perceived usefulness (in case of being ill) as well as c) the most important concern or fear in the context of implants in general and d) the most important benefit. After data collection, the experimenter answered upcoming questions and filled potential knowledge gaps (e.g. the real size and position of the devices under study).

2.3   Participants

A total of N=72 respondents participated in this survey, between 16 and 27 years of age (M=19; SD=2). The gender distribution was quite asymmetrical, with 78.9% women (N=56) and 21.1% men (N=16). Regarding health states, it can be noted that the sample reported to be quite healthy. The health status had to be answered on a 6-point scale (from 1: very good to 6: very poor). 25% (N=18) reported to be in a "very good" health status, 44.4% (N=32) evaluated their health status as "good". Further, 20.8% (N=15) described their own health status as "rather good" and 9.7% (N=7) reported to be in a "quite poor" health status. None reported to be in a poor or very poor health status. We also assessed the awareness of the importance of a good health (also to be answered on a 6-point Likert scale (1= very strong, 6= very low). Only 12.8% (N=2) reported to have a "very strong" level of awareness. 33.8% (N=24) reported to have a "strong", and further 32.4% (N=24) "rather strong" health awareness. 26.8% (N=19) reported to have a "quite low" and 2.8% (N=2) a "low" health awareness. None of the respondents described his/her health awareness as "very low".

3   Results

Due to the exploratory approach, the focus was set on a detailed description of the outcomes, learning about the prevailing opinions, misconceptions, fears and benefits. Also, correlations (Spearman rank analyses, significance level 5%) were run, reflecting potential relations between user characteristics, device types and attitudes. We present participants' perceptions of implantable medical technology in general as well as conceptions about size and assumed body localizations. Also we report the perceived concerns and benefits that are related to implantable medical technology.

3.1   Common Attitude and Knowledge about Implants in General

First, the information level and the publicity of the implants are described. Participants were asked to write down implants they would know (several mentions were allowed). In Figure 2 outcomes are depicted. We received 182 mentions: Most of the participants wrote down 2-3 different implants (or, what they regarded an implant would be), however, there were also three participants out of 72, which did not know any implant (no mentions). Figure 2 shows that breast implants were most common (N=41, 26 times mentioned first, 10 times second, and 5 times third), followed by dental implants with 29 mentions (7 times mentioned first, 12 times second and 10 times third) and the pacemaker on the third place (total: N=18, with 8 times mentioned first, 5 times second and 5 times third). In the centerfield there are knee, hip, skin and hair implants (with 13 to 10 mentions).

Overall, we see a quite diverse information level. Mentions covered medical devices (e.g., "heart valve", "pacemaker"), but also devices for beautification (e.g., "breast implant", "cosmetic surgery"). Noticeably, often no factual devices were mentioned, but just body regions (e.g., "hip", "breast", "face" "shoulder") or even materials (e.g., "silicon", "metal plate") connected to implants. Misconceptions were also prevalent: "Botox", is of course no implant, but a culturally related beautification measure.

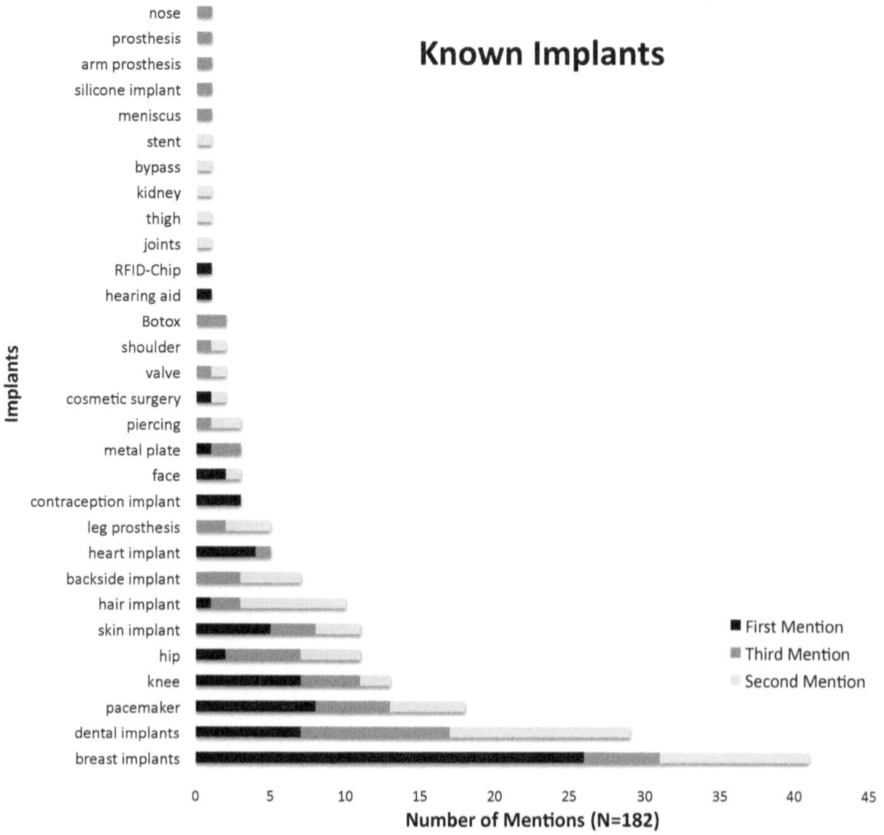

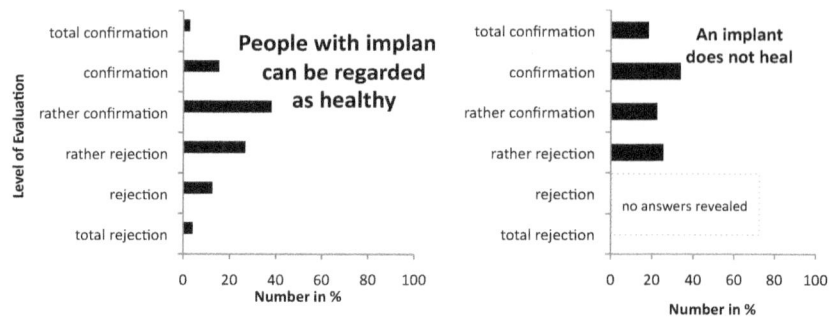

Fig. 2. Known implants, classified according to mentioning order

Furthermore, general attitudes towards implants have been assessed. Figure 3a and 3b and 4a and 4b show the descriptive outcomes regarding participants' level of confirmation. 56.3% of the sample confirmed to varying degrees that implants are able to make person healthy again, though 43.7% reject this claim (Fig. 3a).

Fig. 3a. People with implants can be regarded as healthy   **Fig. 3b.** Implants do not heal

Most respondents (91.7%) confirmed that further research in the field of implantable technologies should be done (Fig. 4a). Regarding the question if implants are touching ethical boundaries, 70.4% did not agree, 29.6% of respondents though believed this to be the case.

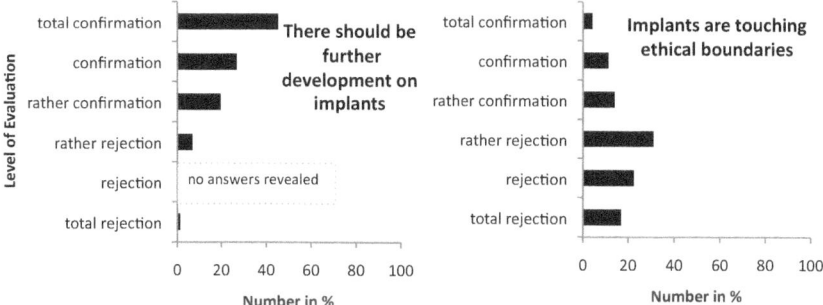

Fig. 4a. General attitude towards implants: There should be further developments on implants

Fig. 4b. General attitude towards implants: Implants are touching ethical boundaries

Stopover: Concluding so far it was found that three devices show a prominent publicity: The breast implant as a beautification measure, dental implants, representing both, medical devices and beautification measure, as well as the pacemaker, which belongs to the most established medical device. Furthermore, the majority of respondent does not expect any ethical harm and votes for further development in this section. Attitudes whether implants may restore perceived frailness into a healthy overall constitution are inconclusive.

3.2   Cognitive Model of the Pacemaker

In this section, we report on cognitive models of pacemakers. Respondents were requested to name the assumed function, the device's body position as well as its size (Fig. 5a).

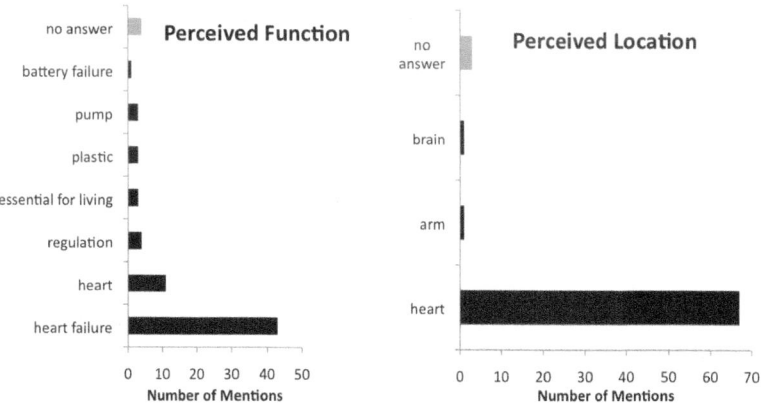

Fig. 5a. Perceived function of pacemaker

Fig. 5b. Perceived location

The majority showed to be well informed, classifying the pacemaker as a device to support the heart (N=43). 11 participants knew at least the organ. The location for the pacemaker was correctly identified by most of the participants. Regarding the perceived size, a high insecurity about real size of a pacemaker can be determined, with answers ranging from 0.3 to 30 cm (Fig. 6).

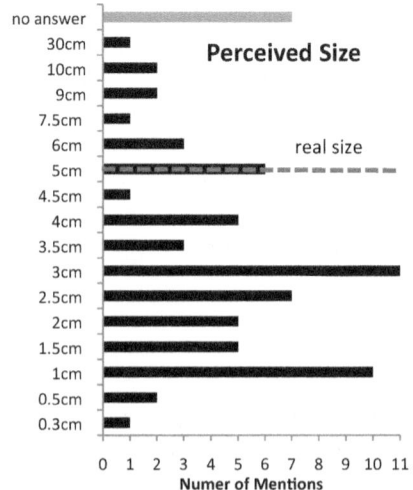

Fig. 6. Perceived function of a pacemaker

3.3 Cognitive Model of the Medical Chip

Now, cognitive models with respect to medical chips are focused. Asked for the assumed function, many participants assume diabetes as the key application, while the majority though seems not know the chip's function at all (no answers, Fig. 7a). The location is mostly ascribed to inner organs, what more or less match reality. It is noticeable that most respondents have no clue about the chip's location (Fig. 7b).

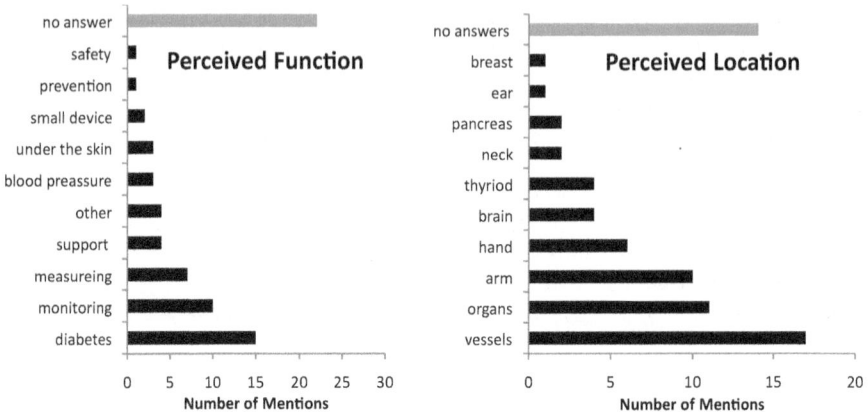

Fig. 7a. Perceived function of a medical chip   **Fig. 7b.** Percevied location

With respect to the assumed size (Fig. 8), the dominant part of the sample is not able to indicate the size of the medical chip (N=20). 18 out of 57 participants that had given an answer to this question though assume 1 cm as the probable size of the medical chip (what is correct). It is though astounding how large the variety about the chip's size is (range between 1mm and 15 cm!).

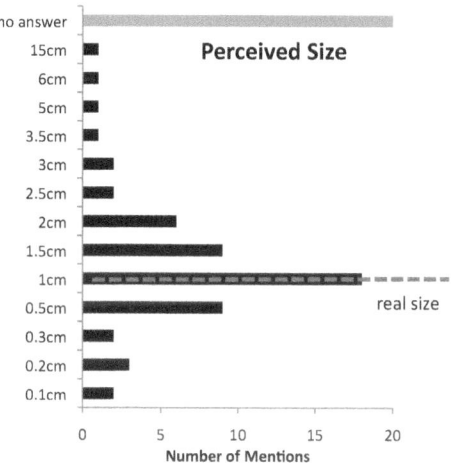

Fig. 8. Perceived size of a medical chip

3.4   Cognitive Model of the Cochlear

Asking for the function of the cochlear, the majority of participants knows the correct function respective the target organ (N=41, Fig. 9a). Also the location – the ear – is mostly correctly indicated (N=53, Fig. 9b). Some users (N=16) assume the brain to be the target location for the cochlear.

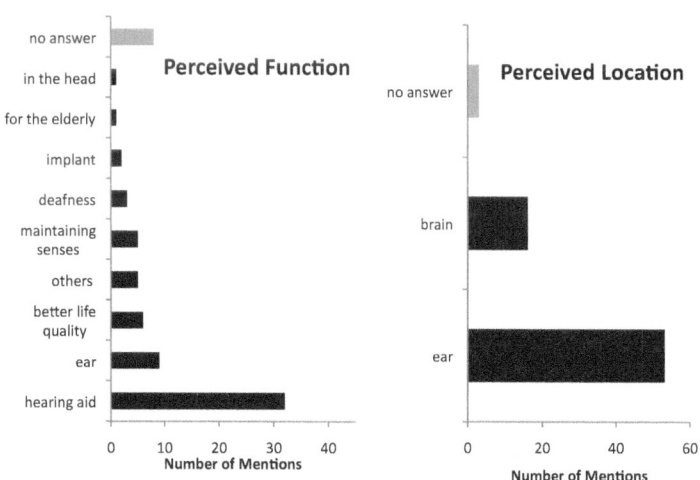

Fig. 9a. Perceived function of the cochlear   **Fig. 9b.** Perceived location

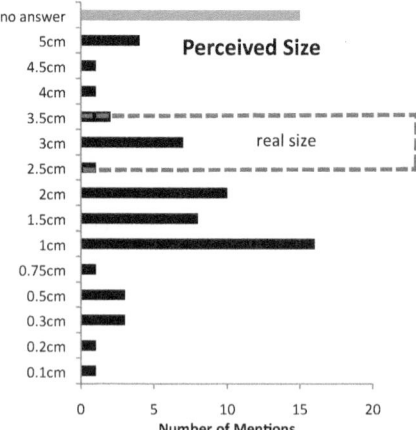

Fig. 10. Perceived size of the cochlear implant

How large are cochlear devices in the cognitive model of participants? Though respondents showed to be well informed about function and location of the cochlear, their assumptions of the appropriate size varies considerably, ranging from 1mm to 5 cm, while the real size is about 2.5-3.5 cm (Fig. 10). Nearly 20% of respondents did not have a clue about how large a cochlear would be.

3.5   Cognitive Model of Deep-Brain-Stimulation

DBS are - due to the riskiness and costliness of surgeries very rarely. The low familiarity with DBS was reflected by the vagueness of mentions (Fig. 11a).

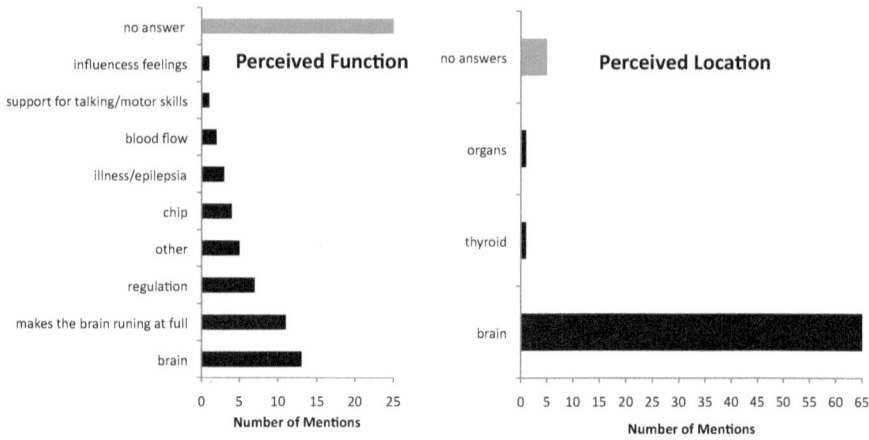

Fig. 11a. Perceived function of the DBS   **Fig. 11b.** Perceived location DBS

Most participants do not know the specific function (no answer), though it can be taken from answers that participants know somehow that DBS has something to do with regulation support of the brain, but also "chip", "illness/epilepsies" and "influences feelings" were associations in the context of DBS. However, most of respondents (N=65) do correctly identify the brain as appropriate location/organ.

The perceived size of an implant for DBS again shows a considerably variation, ranging from very small (smaller than 1 cm) up to 6cm, with 1cm as the most frequent answer (N=18), yielding a solid underestimation of the real size (5 cm).

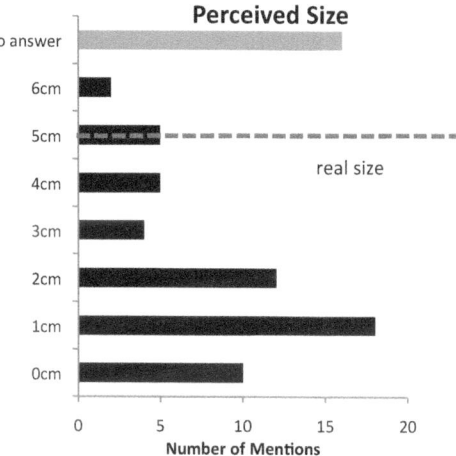

Fig. 12. Perceived Size of the DBS

3.6   Perceived Risk, Benefits and Concerns

At the end, participants were requested to rank the evaluated devices according to the perceived riskiness or danger for them (Fig. 13).

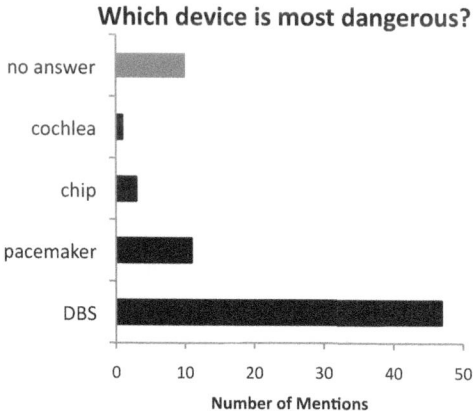

Fig. 13. Most dangerous device (first mentions) ranking

As Figure 13 illustrates there is no doubt: The DBS is evaluated as the most risky device (N=47). Though considerably lesser mentions (N=11), the pacemaker is ranked on second position, followed by the medical chip (N=3). Apparently, the cochlear is not connected to risk and danger (with one 1 mention). In addition, we asked participants to note the biggest concern on the one hand but also the biggest benefit of medical implants in general (Fig. 14a and b). Regarding the biggest concern (N=72), the biggest perceived barrier relates to the risk of the surgery (N=18), followed by concerns about technical problems and negative side effects. When looking at perceived benefits by having medical implants, the most often mentioned benefit is the higher life quality (N=21). But also the normalization of living ("normal life") by help of an implant in spite of chronic illness is an advantage, which is important to participants as well as the possibility of "repair of dysfunctions" in combination with a general "support" by medical technology.

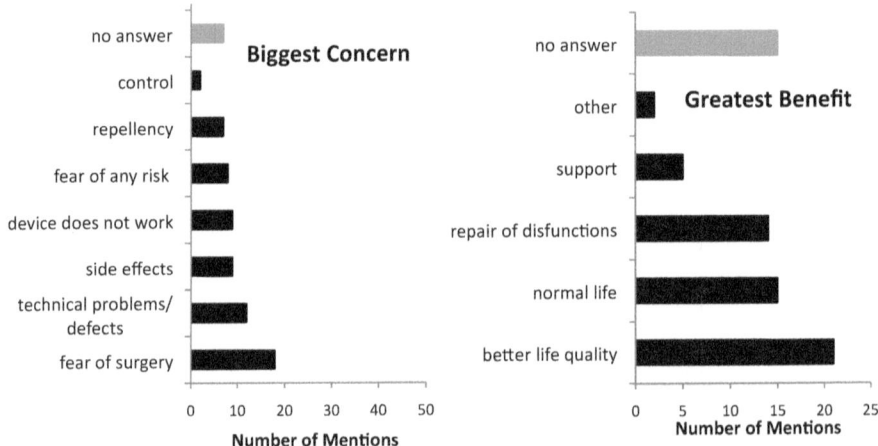

Fig. 14a. Biggest concern in the context of implants   **Fig. 14b.** Greatest benefit

Finally, we looked for inter-correlations between user characteristics (gender, health status, health awareness, self-reported technical expertise) and ratings regarding the perceived dangerousness of the four devices, as well as concerns and benefits seen in implants. It is an astounding finding that the given answers did not correlate with user diversity, showing that the outcomes reported here can be regarded as kind of universals. Only the self-reported technical expertise of participants seem to impact the perceived risk brought by implants (r=.026; p<.05). With increasing technical expertise, the lower are the perceived risks connected to medical implants.

3.7   Qualitative Findings

So far, we concentrated on a descriptive quantitative analysis on ratings. Though, participants also had the chance to comment spontaneously on possible thoughts at different places within the questionnaire. In the following, some of the comments of participants are quoted in order to illustrate the underlying cognitions or affective statements.

In these free comment fields both pro-using statements were given as well as contra using statements. Arguments, which were given by participants in the category "pro's", reveal first and foremost that implants compensate illness and help patients to live "healthy". This is illustrated by the following original comments.

> "Even though implants are foreign particles inside the body, they then belong to own body and help to live an independent life" (female, 17 years).

> "Medical implants are "good", they can safe life, can help people and allow to live independently even after traumatic accidents (male, 26 years).

However, there were also pensive statements, which do reflect substantial normative and ethical questions. They show that implants are perceived only as desirable and - from an ethical point of view justifiable – whenever they address medical issues, justified by handicaps, accidents or illness. Conversely, whenever they are used for beautification reasons, things change. The following comment illustrates this:

> "Implants in the context of health = good; implants in the context of "looks and beauty = bad" (female, 29 years).

One male respondent also argues that further developments in implants - even though necessary- would represent the wrong focus of efforts. Instead he argues to research on the pathogenesis and the aetiology of diseases in order to minimize the necessity to use implants.

However, some participants reported that they would use implants only under certain circumstances, and that wearing an implant would be their last alternative when would see no other opportunities.

Possibly, such an attitude might be due to the relative youth and the solid health state of participants here, however, the underlying norms which shine up seem have other routes, which are often used in the public media in the context of privacy and the feeling of control by others. This is illustrated by the following comment of a male participant:

> "Misuse in general can neither be excluded nor is misuse controllable. For example, radio tags could be connected to the implant, without informing the patients. Similarly, governments also do betray citizens quite frequently"(male, 23 years).

Even though such a comment is of course quite arbitrary and reflects a high degree of simple-mindedness and a low level of sophistication, it is though precarious in which mental mindset a technology development as a medical implant is evaluated.

Stopover. Looking at the perceptions of different implants we saw on the one hand that there is a clear view of established implants, like the pacemaker. Also, the perception of a medical chip, as e.g. a medical stent, was obviously related to existing mental models. This can be taken from a quite homogenous answering pattern that is in touch with reality (regarding function, size and location of the chip). When it comes to more unknown implants, as the cochlear that only affects a specific patient group, but an implant with a well conceivable function (hearing discovery), we also see quite sufficient mental models, at least with respect to its core functionality (hearing aid). The fact that the cochlear is also a neuronal implant, with complex functions and influencing of neuronal processes, participants are not aware of. The DBS revealed to be the most unknown device. For sure the naming of the device provokes specific cognitions and leads to threat and the feeling of riskiness, even though the factual function of the DBS is broadly unknown.

4   Discussion

The present paper was concerned with young persons' perception of implantable medical technology. We addressed a young and healthy sample of students of vocational trainings in order to reveal prevailing knowledge and attitudes toward medical technology. Four medical implant technologies were selected (pacemaker, medical chip, cochlear and deep brain stimulation) which vary not only with respect to the familiarity and implementation frequency (with the pacemaker as the most often used and therefore convenient technology on the one end and the deep brain stimulation as the most rarely used technology at the other end). Participants' knowledge about the devices' function, their assumptions about the device location and the assumed size of the device were assessed. The latter was related to the hypothesis that the sensitiveness of the body location in combination with and presumptions of the physical size should impact the risk perception.

Outcomes revealed that young persons knowledge of implants show a broad range. On the one hand, pacemaker and cochlear implant are quite familiar and known with respect to their core functionality and its disease-specifics. In contrast, the chip and the deep brain stimulation are not known and the assumptions about their function revealed to be quite vague. When it comes to the evaluation, it was found that risk perceptions relate to a lesser extent to device familiarity and implementation frequency of devices, but more strongly to what participants' know from cosmetic surgery and the perceived body location and the felt invasiveness. This can be taken from the fact that the pacemaker – targeting the heart as a highly sensitive organ, but broadly known is ranked on the second place in the dangerousness-rating, directly behind the deep brain stimulation, that addresses the brain as another highly sensitive organ, but in addition suffers from its unfamiliarity in public perceptions. Clearly it could be revealed that the less the knowledge about the device the bigger are unspecified concerns. Generally hopes in the context of implants are related to a general improvement of the living conditions and the wish for healing. Concerns are in the first place related to surgery risks and only in a second step to technical defects of the implants.

The fact that the perceptions were not impacted by user diversity, show the universal character of outcomes. Thus, when comprising the duties for a transparent information and communication strategy we do not have to consider specific using roles, user groups or personal abilities, but are able to derive the information needs for the whole group of young and healthy people. The main message in the context of acceptance of medical implant technology is that a missing awareness seems to support the rejection or distance of/to the medical technology. With a enlightened population and an active communication about new technologies it could be avoided that unspecified fears and negative attitudes and perceptions coming from nothing concrete but mental models are hindering the benefit of implantable medical technology in the future.

This is especially precarious as the public discussion about cosmetic surgery, the societal pressure to look young and healthy on the one hand and the smouldering stigma when being old, frail and ill on the other hand form the underlying cognitive models of people. When facing the demographic change and the factual increase in the portion of old and increasingly older people, which are naturally ill, old and frail, this is completely irrational. Beyond the absurdity of this attitude given the natural life course, we should be aware that people often react to a global insecurity of societal change with general fears and ascribe their affect-laden attitudes to single technologies even though they do not need to be necessarily connected [20-24]. In this context, the sometimes hysterical and lurid press coverage of privacy protection and innovative technologies within the public media plays a prominent role. Even though it is naturally a high value that body and private limits are treated with caution and respect, any undifferentiated public discussion fails to form a responsible, fair and objective information and communication of medical implants, which considers benefits and risks and the sensitive trade-off between both at the same time [25].

Future studies have to investigate whether these perceptions are limited to the young and healthy group examined here and to what extent they change when older persons are under study. One could expect that ageing and illness change these attitudes, as older persons might be more aware of the general need of medical technology and of the fact that they themselves could need technologies like this in the near future. Also, the cultural dependency of the public perception in combination with societal values should not be underestimated [8]. Finally, future research has to find out in which ways public perception differs when not the medical necessity case (using implants for medical reasons and compensation of handicaps) is of interest, but for enhancement or even beautification reasons.

Acknowledgements. The authors would like to thank directors, teachers as well as the students of the Käthe-Kollwitz-Schule Berufskolleg der StädteRegion Aachen. They all showed a high openness to research issues and willingness to participate. In addition, many thanks go also to K. Peirera for her research assistance. This research was supported by the excellence initiative of the German federal and state governments.

References

1. Trenk, D., Neumann, F.-J.: Drug-eluting coronary stents: as safe as bare-metal stents, but optimized antiplatelet therapy further improve clinical outcome. Eur. J. Clin. Pharmacol. 64, 227–232 (2007)
2. Schnakenberg, U., Krüger, C., Pfeffer, J.-G., Mokwa, W., vom Bögel, G., Günther, R., Schmitz-Rode, T.: Intravascular pressure monitoring system. Sensors and Actuators A: Physical. 110, 61–67 (2004)
3. Schmitz-Rode, T.: Vascular capsule for telemetric monitoring of blood pressure. RöFo. Fortschritte auf dem Gebiete der Röntgenstrahlen und der Nuklearmedizin. 175, 282–286 (2003)
4. Smith, A.D.: Evolution and acceptability of medical applications of RFID implants among early users of technology. Health Mark Q 24, 121–155 (2007)
5. Wilkowska, W., Gaul, S., Ziefle, M.: A Small but Significant Difference – The Role of Gender on Acceptance of Medical Assistive Technologies. In: Leitner, G., Hitz, M., Holzinger, A. (eds.) USAB 2010. LNCS, vol. 6389, pp. 82–100. Springer, Heidelberg (2010)
6. Scheermesser, M., Kosow, H., Rashid, A., Holtmann, C.: User acceptance of pervasive computing in healthcare: Main findings of two case studies. In: Second International Conference on Pervasive Computing Technologies for Healthcare, PervasiveHealth 2008, pp. 205–213 (2008)
7. Arning, K., Gaul, S., Ziefle, M.: "Same Same but Different" How Service Contexts of Mobile Technologies Shape Usage Motives and Barriers. In: Leitner, G., Hitz, M., Holzinger, A. (eds.) USAB 2010. LNCS, vol. 6389, pp. 34–54. Springer, Heidelberg (2010)
8. Alagöz, F., Ziefle, M., Wilkowska, W.: Openness to accept medical technology – a cultural view. Full paper submitted to the 7th Conference of the Austrian Computer Society: Human-Computer Interaction: Information Quality in eHealth. Springer, Berlin
9. Fiedeler, U.: Stand der Technik neuronaler Implantate. Forschungszentrum Karlsruhe, Karlsruhe (2008)
10. European Group on Ethics in Science and New Technologies to the European Commission (ed.) The ethical aspects of ICT implants in the human body. In: Proceedings of the Roundtable Debate. Office for Official Publications of the European Communities, Luxembourg (2005)
11. Arning, K., Ziefle, M.: Effects of age, cognitive, and personal factors on PDA menu navigation performance. Behaviour Information Technology 28, 251–268 (2009)
12. Ziefle, M., Schaar, A.K.: Gender differences in acceptance and attitudes towards an invasive medical stent. eJournal Health Informatics 6(2), e13, 1–18 (2011)
13. Wilkowska, W., Ziefle, M.: User diversity as a challenge for the integration of medical technology into future home environments. In: Ziefle, M., Röcker, C. (eds.) Human-Centred Design of eHealth Technologies, Concepts, Methods and Applications, pp. 95–126. IGI Global, Hersehy
14. Ziefle, M., Röcker, C.: Acceptance of Pervasive Healthcare Systems: A comparison of different implementation concepts. In: 4th ICST Conference on Pervasive Computing Technologies for Healthcare (2010)
15. Ziefle, M., Wilkowska, W.: Technology acceptability for medical assistance. In: 4th ICST Conference on Pervasive Computing Technologies for Healthcare (CD Rom) (2010)

16. Ziefle, M., Schaar, A.K.: Technical Expertise and Its Influence on the Acceptance of Future Medical Technologies: What Is Influencing What to Which Extent? In: Leitner, G., Hitz, M., Holzinger, A. (eds.) USAB 2010. LNCS, vol. 6389, pp. 513–529. Springer, Heidelberg (2010)

17. Davis, F.D.: Perceived Usefulness, Perceived Ease of Use, and User Acceptance of Information Technology. MIS Quarterly 13, 319–340 (1989)

18. Davis, F.: User acceptance of information technology: system characteristics, user perceptions and behavioral impacts. International Journal of Man-Machine Studies 38, 475–487 (1993)

19. Venkatesh, V., Morris, M.G., Davis, G.B., Davis, F.D.: User Acceptance of Information Technology: Toward a Unified View. MIS Quarterly 27, 425–478 (2003)

20. Siegrist, M.: The Influence of Trust and Perceptions of Risks and Benefits on the Acceptance of Gene Technology. Risk Analysis 20(2), 195–204 (2000)

21. Peters, E., Slovic, P.: The Role of Affect and Worldviews as Orienting Dispositions in the Perception and Acceptance of Nuclear Power. Journal of Applied Social Psychology 26(16), 1427–1453 (1996)

22. Covello, V.T.: The perception of technological risks: A literature review. Technological Forecasting and Social Change 23(4), 285–297 (1983)

23. Otway, H.J., Pahner, P.D.: Risk assessment. Futures 8(2), 122–134 (1976)

24. Slovic, P., Fischhoff, B., Lichtenstein, S.: Why Study Risk Perception? Risk Analysis 2(2), 83–93 (1982)

25. Ziefle, M., Röcker, C., Holzinger, A.: Medical Technology in Smart Homes: Exploring the User's Perspective on Privacy, Intimacy and Trust. In: The 3rd IEEE International Workshop on Security Aspects of Process and Services Engineering (SAPSE 2011), 35th Annual IEEE Computer Software and Applications Conference, Munich, Germany, July 18-22 (2011)

Assessing Medical Treatment Compliance Based on Formal Process Modeling*

Reinhold Dunkl, Karl Anton Fröschl,
Wilfried Grossmann, and Stefanie Rinderle-Ma

University of Vienna, Austria
Faculty of Computer Science
{firstname.[midname.]lastname}@univie.ac.at

Abstract. The formalization and analysis of medical guidelines play an essential role in clinical practice nowadays. Due to their inexorably generic nature such guidelines leave room for different interpretation and implementation. Hence, it is desirable to understand this variability and its implications for patient treatment in practice. In this paper we propose an approach for comparing guideline-based treatment processes with empirical treatment processes. The methodology combines ideas from workflow modeling, process simulation, process mining, and statistical methods of evidence-based medicine. The applicability of the approach is illustrated based on the Cutaneous Melanoma use case.

Keywords: Healthcare Processes, Process Modeling, Process Mining.

1 Introduction

Clinical practice is based upon medical knowledge, relating healing interventions causally to diseases, as well as upon clinical treatment routines integrating medical/pharmaceutical theory with best practices of patient care [5]. Medical guidelines, or standard operation procedures, codify the implementation of such clinical routines, in order to raise the specificity of patient care, to reduce the burden of medical decision making by defining applicable diagnostic criteria and intervention patterns, and to accumulate past experience in patient care as the state-of-the-art. In spite of their *prescriptive* intent, however, medical guidelines by necessity leave much room to adapt to specific circumstances and interpretations. Thus, while clinical evidence mirrors the conduct of patient care as defined through guidelines, empirical records of treatment rather reflect, in a *descriptive* way, the practical consequences of guideline implementation.

In what follows, the question is raised if there is anything to be learned from systematically contrasting medical evidence with guidelines and, as a prerequisite, which methodological frame, or toolbox, is required to support such a kind of comparison. To this end, it is hypothesized that, because of their inexorably

---

* The work presented in this paper was conducted in the context of the EBMC^2 project that is co-funded by the University of Vienna and the Medical University of Vienna.

A. Holzinger and K.-M. Simonic (Eds.): USAB 2011, LNCS 7058, pp. 533–546, 2011.

generic nature, guidelines give rise to different ways and conditions of (compliant) implementation, the variability of which is becoming apparent only through the statistical analysis of formal reconstructions of clinical treatment processes. For one thing, it is to be expected that guideline implementation, on the level of the individual patient receiving a guideline-controlled treatment, undergoes manifold refinements accounting for the immanent variability of patients' health conditions, anamnestic peculiarities, adverse drug effects, and so forth.

In order to account for this empirical variability of patient treatment processes, a representation language providing sufficient level of descriptive detail, including diagnostics, interventions, medications, etc., in conjunction with a means to express the dynamics of treatment processes is essential. This requirement is met best by some formal process modeling language equipped with a temporal calculus [22,3]. Depending on the respective domain of investigation, once the specific vocabulary of the medical domain is identified, individual clinical treatment processes can be restated formally as sentences of the process language, thus constituting the sample of process instances amenable to statistical scrutiny. On top of this symbolic reconstruction of empirical treatment processes, statistical analysis – more specifically, process mining methodology – is used to separate structural from (in principle) random components of process descriptions. At this stage, critical *structural* variations (if any) in guideline implementation are detected. Provided that medical guidelines themselves are restated in terms of formal process models (that is, as treatment process schemata), the formal difference between these "reference processes" and evidence-based process schemata becomes tractable. Furthermore, a suitable logic of comparison established between symbolically represented process schemata admits formal interpretation of differences in terms of a measure of (process) compliance. As yet, however, within the Evidence Based Medicine Compliance Cluster (EBMC^2) project, an *analytical model* is developed first, adapting and extending already existing simulation-based process mining proposals (for instance, such as [1]) with apt process distance measures and an exploratory mechanism for candidate substantiations of empirical process alterations; this conceptual approach is argued and presented subsequently.

Section 2 gives an overview of the proposed methodological framework and its reasoning, and links the proposal to related work in the field. In particular, the role and structure of formal modeling of medical treatment processes is introduced. Next, Section 3 turns to a practical illustration example, the case of Cutaneous Melanoma treatment, presenting a pertinent guideline in order to sketch approaches towards formal guideline representations. Based on Sections 2 and 3, Section 4 presents the main functional building blocks of the proposed framework used to simulate synthetic treatment processes on top of (i) formalized guideline-based process models, and (ii) patient samples. Furthermore, suitable process log data structures are considered, and data-analytical techniques of process aggregation and comparison, respectively, based on log data are discussed. The concluding section of the paper briefly discusses expected benefits of the framework, indicates how the conceptual approach is linked to pertinent data, and points out still open issues in need of further research within the EBMC^2 project.

2   Methodologies of Modeling Clinical Routine

2.1   From Medical Evidence to Medical Guidelines

Medical evidence draws on empirical results about different treatments. PICO (cf. e.g., [21]: 113) is a standard scheme for obtaining such evidence from analyzing alternative therapies, prognosis of recovery/survival, diagnosis of health status, prevalence studies, etc. Using appropriate study designs, the PICO scheme produces, ideally, significant statistical evidence in terms of likelihoods, p-values, area under the ROC, sensitivity and specificity, or various risk measures. Methodological rigor of study design decides about the strength of evidence attainable (cf. [20,26]), but yields rather isolated evidence:

- study focus is a single, well-defined question in order to obtain an accurate as possible answer;
- results are of a *statistical* nature, providing, at best, a numerical quantification of degrees of evidence over well-defined populations;
- integral treatment processes are dealt with in piecemeal fashion under standard conditions and, in particular, treatment *interactions* are barely addressed.

As a response, and remedy, medical *guidelines* seek to integrate the bits and pieces of medical evidence studies into coherent treatment processes in order to provide assistance to health professionals towards effective, high quality medical practice according to the best medical knowledge available from both, clinical research and expert consensus [10]. Formally, guidelines are composed of *key actions*, typically recommended conditionally depending on patients' socio-demographic and medical attributes (e.g., prior diagnoses), and usually indicating a degree of recommendation depending on the particularities of treatment instances and the medical setting. In general, key actions also carry some outcome measure impacting on future actions, perhaps supplemented with a quality measure.

Medical guidelines may be represented in varying degrees of formalization, from plain narrative to highly structured [25]. Workflows provide a rather natural means of expression, highlighting the "algorithmic" flavor of treatment processes and permitting a stepwise refinement of abstraction levels [23] including the annotation of branching and looping conditions. Fig. 1 sketches a top-level treatment flow pattern with building blocks to receive case-dependent iterative refinement (cf., e.g., Fig. 3 and 4 below).

Formal process modeling, however, has to account for a variety of flow conditions (such as unexpected treatment termination), the incidental interleave of concurrent treatment processes (e.g., in intensive care), as well as other contingencies, entailing discrepancies between ideal guideline implementation and

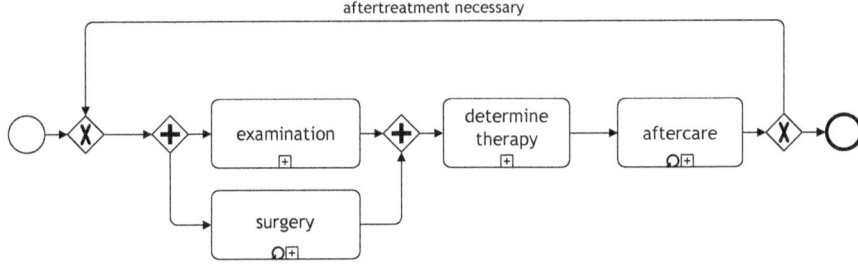

Fig. 1. A High-level Treatment Process Flow Representation

actual clinical care practice. This is reflected in multifarious activities in guide-line formalization [19]. In contrast to that, much less attention has been devoted to a systematic comparison of guideline-based treatment processes with actual clinical treatment processes.

2.2 Analyzing Treatment Processes

The general strategy of comparing medical guidelines to clinical treatment prac-tice is depicted in Fig. 2. First, a guideline is converted into a guideline-based process model composed of key actions. An actual treatment process depends on patient attributes X as well as institutional parameters θ reflecting the per-sonal decisions and institutional environment of the acting health professional (cf. Subsection 2.1). With respect to the personal attributes we have to take into account that only a subset of these attributes is used as decision parameters for treatment according to the guidelines. Hence we split this patient attributes in diagnostic attributes X_d and personal attributes X_p, i.e. $X = (X_d, X_p)$. Indi-vidual attributes of a patient are denoted by (x_p, x_d). Treatment of a patient with diagnostic attributes x_p within a given institutional setting θ according to a guideline would result in so called *synthetic* log data denoted by $l_g(x_d, \theta)$. If we know the distribution $P(X_d)$ of the diagnostic attributes in a population of interest, we can simulate the distribution of possible synthetic treatment logs for this population for any given institutional setting θ. Accordingly, the random function of these synthetic logs is denoted by $l_g(X_d, \theta)$. In order to obtain the distribution $P(X_d)$, we use epidemiological data about the health status of the entire population, e.g., from prevalence studies.

Application of the guidelines in the treatment process of a patient depends usually not only on diagnostic attributes x_d but also on some of the personal attributes x_p. Hence, we denote in contrast to simulated process log data, clin-ical log data for a patient with attributes $x = (x_d, x_p)$ by $l_e(x_d, x_p, \theta)$, and the random function describing the empirical treatments for a patient collective by $l_e(X_d, X_p, \theta)$. Now, provided that both clinical and simulated synthetic log data are represented in a unified format (cf. Subsection 4.2), the problem of treat-ment compliance assessment can be (re-)stated as one of analyzing the deviance

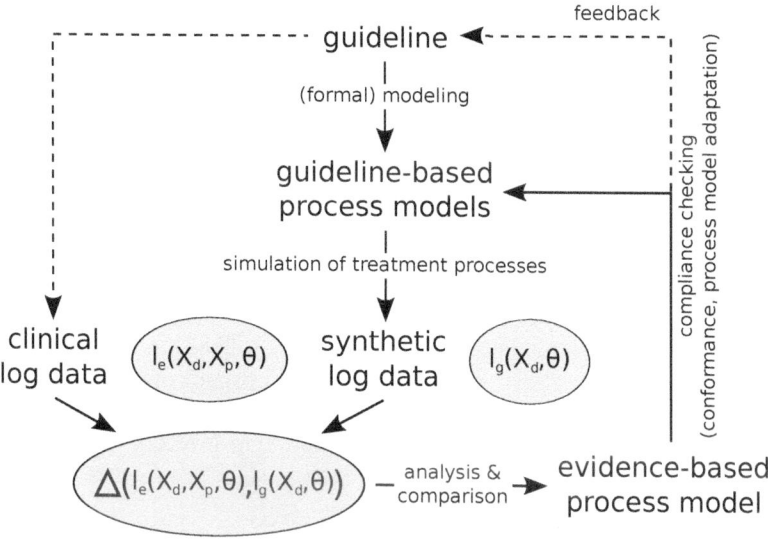

Fig. 2. Overall Methodology

$\Delta(l_e(X_d, X_p, \theta), l_g(X_d, \theta))$. More specifically, depending on available knowledge about $P(X_d)$ and the choice of the health system parameter, θ, typical research inquiries are as follows:

Distribution of clinical log data. Given X_d for a well-defined population, the degree of deviation of $l_e(X_d, X_p, \theta)$ from $l_g(X_d, \theta)$ can be analyzed, and whether such deviations can be explained in terms of X_p. Deviations of interest could be, e.g., partial compliance to the guidelines (such as patients modifying the intake of medication, delaying follow up, or exiting from after-care altogether). Formally, analysis – using traditional statistical techniques adapted to process data – results in distributions of clinical log data relative to specific patient sub-collectives defined by synthetic data.

Estimation and comparison of institutional parameters, θ, if unknown, from clinical log data. Prior to such an estimation, of course, each instance of clinical log data has to be assigned to one class of synthetic log data, using traditional machine learning methods in combination with process mining ([1,18]).

Outcome analysis, seeking to figure out in how far realizations of different classes of synthetic log data, defined by the conditional process logic, influence the outcome of the treatment, and the sensitivity of the deviations from the clinical log data with respect to the outcome. Note that, contrary to traditional medical evidence (cf. Subsection 2.1), rather complex temporal treatment patterns (rather than well-defined treatments) have to be be evaluated using techniques of process mining, adding considerable analytical value compared to more conventional statistical approaches.

So far, we have formulated these research questions from a formal analytical point of view. Yet from practical point of view, evaluation of *medical conse-quences* of these analyses is of utmost importance. In particular, the method may be used for evaluating which differences between synthetic treatment processes are of relevance from medical point of view. Eventually, as result of the analysis, *evidence-based process models* ensue, feeding back to the compliance evaluation of underlying medical guidelines.

Another issue of interest concerns the application of the approach for improving the quality of information about treatment processes. The simulated synthetic log data $l_g(X_d, \theta)$ based on a guideline give a rather complete picture of possible results. Comparison with the empirical treatment data $l_e(X_d, X_p, \theta)$ can identify incomplete medical treatment data as well as differences in the granularity of different data sources. In that way, the approach opens the opportunity to identify "blind spots" in documentation systems. Sometimes methods for data imputation and transformations for aligning different levels of detail can help to improve data quality for existing data about treatment processes.

2.3   Related Work

The EBMC^2 project in general and the methodology presented in this paper in particular are related to the areas of evidence-based medicine, medical guidelines, medical and healthcare processes, as well as process mining. Related work in the transition from evidence-based medicine to medical guidelines has been discussed in Section 2.1; medical and healthcare processes emerge as research topics in different domains. The Evimed project [12], for example, addresses literature research as to how guidelines relate to medical evidence. Apparently, these activities are rather orthogonal to the focus of the EBMC^2 project.

Process mining refers to a bundle of techniques to discover and analyze different facets of business processes. Some of these techniques have been applied to different application scenarios, particularly in the healthcare domain [17] where in case studies, mostly, hospital processes were discovered (mined) from process logs. Process discovery could be useful in the context of the EBMC^2 project, too; however, the main focus will be on *process synthesis* based on guidelines and delta analysis of synthetic and clinical processes. In general, simulation is an effective method to gain insights into real-world processes [1]. In the EBMC^2 project, we investigate the applicability of simulation and delta analysis in the healthcare domain. Specifically, we aim at analyzing the causes for deviations between guideline-based processes and clinical processes.

3   Cutaneous Melanoma as a Case in Point

For the sake of illustration, a sample medical guideline concerning the diagnosis and treatment (but not prevention) of Cutaneous Melanoma [9] is used. Clearly, the narrative nature of the guideline addresses the physician in summarizing, based on studies and data available at the time of preparation, best practices of diagnostic approaches as well as a variety of established therapies including advanced stages of the disease. It is important to keep in mind that it "... may be necessary or even desirable to deviate from these guidelines in the interest of specific patients or under special circumstances." ([9]: 271), emphasizing the generic character of the guideline as a set of – sometimes rather soft – constraints on advisable treatment decisions, and progressions, respectively. In spite of this generality, the overall structure of the guideline can be captured formally in the three-phase process skeleton exhibited in Fig. 1, of which Fig. 3 excerpts the aftercare phase expressed in a widespread standard of business process modeling, BPMN (Business Process Modeling Notation), chosen from amongst a set of equivalent alternatives such as GLIF, Asbru, EON, PROforma, GUIDE, or PRODIGY, all demonstrably "... close to traditional workflow languages" [16], as a direct comparison between BPMN and PROforma confirms that business process modeling languages can cope quite well with requirements of the health care domain [7].

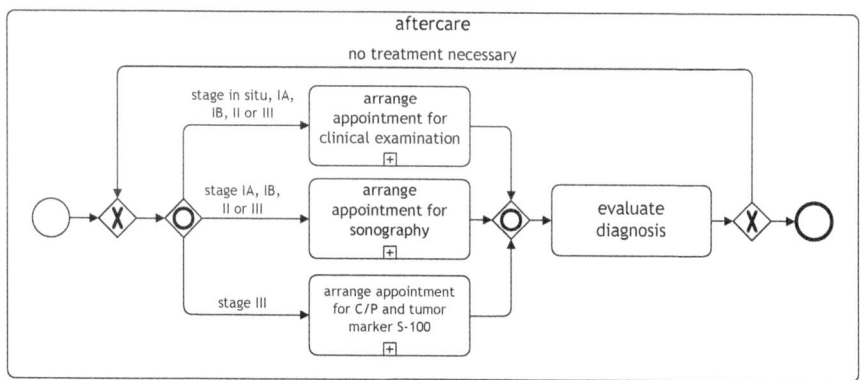

Fig. 3. BPMN Model: Melanoma Aftercare Phase

The example highlights both, the conditional branching and looping of progressions within a guideline as well as the nesting of subprocesses, admitting a successive refinement of process models while retaining their fundamental, non-recursive block structure. Fig. 4 illustrates refinement by nesting for the case of repeated *sonography* appointments in patient aftercare, stating the suggested choice of appointment intervals dependent on melanoma stage and the time lapse since last tumor diagnosis; again, however, it must be stressed that the guideline admits "considerable variation in follow-up approaches" ([9]: 279) because of an apparent lack of empirical data legitimating any particular recommendation, and that the depicted subprocess is but a debatable variant.

Regardless of the preferred modeling stance, particularly the branching decisions of treatment progressions may refer to patient characteristics and conditions beyond those stated explicitly in the guideline, like the staging of melanoma,

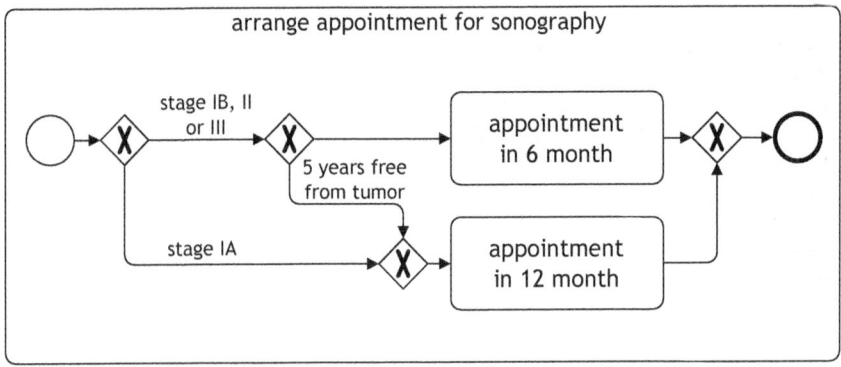

Fig. 4. BPMN Model: Sonography Aftercare Subprocess

tumor thickness, etc. ([9]: 273f). Accordingly, with respect to both, diagnostics and therapeutic actions, the representation language used to model patient treatment processes has to encompass a broader range of expressive elements, including typical clinical parameters (such as lab readings), patient characteristics (such as demographic variables, anamnesis, survival time, etc.), and medical interventions, in order to account appropriately for the cited "interest of specific patients or ... special circumstances." Moreover, if treatment process schemata are to be induced from medical patient records by means of process, or decision, mining methods, salient distinctions between actual treatment progressions, and branchings therein, may escape recognition simply because of an undue scarcity of formal expression.

4   Guideline-Based Simulation and Analysis of Medical Treatment Processes

The overall methodology for modeling, simulating, and analyzing medical guidelines and clinical treatment processes is shown in Fig. 2. Deriving formal process models based on medical guidelines is illustrated by the Cutaneous Melanoma guideline in Section 3. In this section we focus on the generation of synthetic treatment processes based on the guideline process models and sketch how possible analysis and comparison of these data with clinical treatment processes can be conducted. Fig. 5 depicts the different levels: a) medical guidelines setting out a "frame" for possible treatment processes, b) synthetic treatment processes that reflect possible process executions based on the medical guidelines and can be created using simulation techniques, and c) the clinical processes, i.e., the processes implicitly executed or explicitly supported by a process-aware information system (PAIS) within the hospital or clinic. Comparing a) and c) leads to insights in how far the clinical treatment processes follow their corresponding guidelines and – in case they do not – find out about the reasons why. This corresponds to the questions set out by the area of business process compliance (BPC) [15]. Here focus is on developing (semi-)automatic techniques to check compliance of real-world processes with guidelines, regulations, and compliance rules.

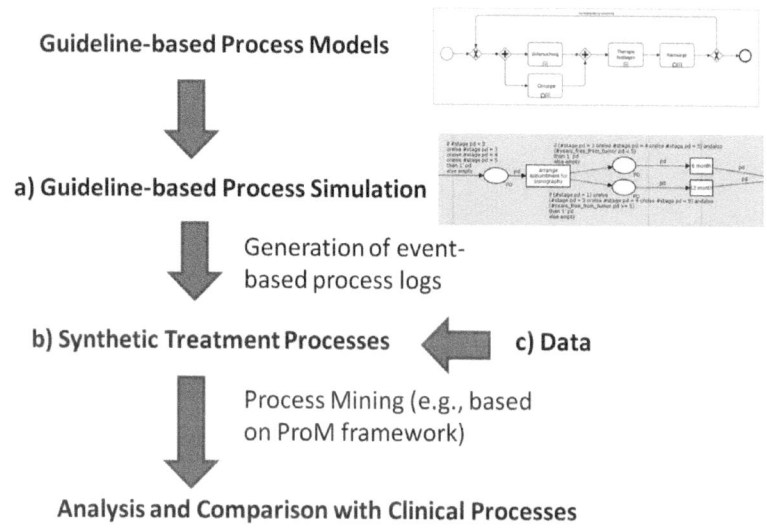

Fig. 5. Basic Modules of Simulation

Based on the guideline process models b) synthetic treatment processes can be generated using simulation tools such as CPN-Tools [13]. Generally, such simulation tools can take different parameters into account for which, e.g., certain probability distributions can be defined [2]. Hence, first of all, we can generate the possible interpretation of the guideline by generating possible process executions based on the guideline process models. As illustrated in Fig. 6B, the relevant process data elements are *stage* and *years_free_of_tumor*, since all decisions within the guideline depend on them. However, other clinical data might be available such as *age* or *gender*. Feeding these additional data into the simulation reveals possible influences on decision points within the treatment processes. Finally, comparing synthetic and clinical treatment processes b) and c) might yield additional insights if, e.g., synthesized processes considering additional data elements correspond, but also deviate from the real-world processes.

4.1   Generating Synthetic Evidence

As discussed before, for synthesizing treatment processes based on guideline process models, a suitable process simulation tool should offer facilities to define conditions to control the process flow depending on patient treatment data.

Additionally, it is required that the tool is able to transport these patient treatment data through the process. Reviewing possible alternative tools for process
simulation [13] and the aim for using the synthesized process data for process
mining we decided to use CPN-Tools for our illustration. We use the approach
described by [2] to create computable log files out of the CPN-Tools simulation.

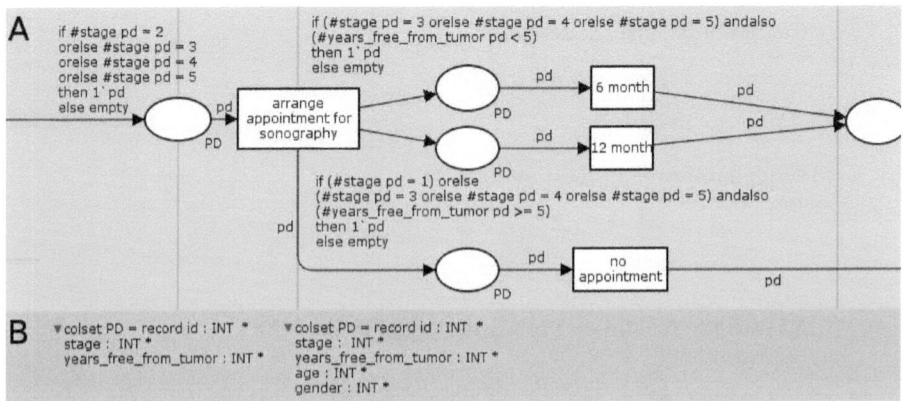

Fig. 6. Colored Petri net model in CPN-Tool: Sonography Appointment Subprocess

Figure 6A shows the subprocess (cf. Fig. 4) now modeled as a colored Petri
net within CPN-Tools. We first use a record-typed color set (cf. Fig. 6B) as
a token that holds patient data which include the two parameters *stage* and
years_free_of_tumor that are used for the decisions within the Melanoma guideline. A simulation on this Petri net followed by analyzing with process mining
tools will result in a guideline compliant process model.

As motivated in Section 3, typically a patient data record includes more information than considered within the guideline. To simulate this fact we add
additional data elements such as *age* and *gender* to our simulation by extending
the patient data record (cf. Fig. 6B). As a result we can determine if the process
mined model will differ from the guideline, moreover we can identify where and
why the simulated – and in case of real-world data the real – treatment processes
deviate from the guideline. Note that another possible way to simulate processes
that deviate from the guideline is an alteration of the colored Petri net by manipulating the model itself (e.g., by adding a 9 month activity for arranging an
appointment). Finally, the simulation model can be extended by "predictable"
exceptions that are not included within the guideline, but are valuable to analyze, e.g., patient behavior. In Melanoma aftercare, one possibility is that no
arrangement for the next check-up is made since the patients may not show up
(see the additional exit transition "no appointment" in Fig. 6).

4.2   Representing Process Evidence

The comparison and statistical analysis of both, clinical and synthetic treatment process data, necessitates a simple yet versatile data structure using some unified, flexible format capable to represent all process-contingent patient data. Essentially, a *medical biographic store* (MBS, for short) is arranged as a logical data frame recording process log data originating from both, clinical care documentation (empirical log data from clinical treatment processes, such as electronic patient records) and simulation runs using guideline-based process models. More specifically, with respect to the notation introduced above, a clinical treatment process produces, for some patient taken care of, a trace $y(x_d, x_p)$ of log data, whereas "applying" some guideline-based process model g to this patient yields a trace of synthetic log data $g(x_d, \theta)$.

The MBS relates to electronic health record approaches (cf. ISO/CEN EN 13606; [4,6,8,11,14]), yet without committing itself to any particular syntactic standard of health data representation. Rather, the data structure of the MBS annotates each elementary entry, or *protocol particle*, with a spatio-temporal and subject-matter reference to account for a variety of modes of subsequent data selection and aggregation operations, yielding a quadruple structure

$$\langle pid, \langle temp, loc, type \rangle, feat, value \rangle$$

where *pid* signifies an (MBS-)internal patient identifier, *temp* the temporal and *loc* the location references, respectively, of the *value* field, while *type* annotates the origin, or context (such as diagnosis, medication, intervention, ...) of the recorded *value*, and *feat* represents the clinical, or medical, feature (of the patient *pid*) the *value* is the recorded value of. Ontologically, protocol particles record *partial* discontinuities of patient (health) states, assuming that absence of such evidence implies the steadiness of state. As an example from the application domain, a protocol particle

$$\langle \#2006.184.277, \langle 2007\text{-}09\text{-}17, AKH\ Wien\text{-}Derma, dgn \rangle, melanoma\text{-}stage, IIC \rangle$$

would record the clinical documentation entry for (real) patient *#2006.184.277* diagnosing a stage *IIC* melanoma on *Sept. 17, 2007*, at the *Dermatological Clinic* of the General Hospital Vienna. Technically, each particle component may in turn bear a rich (that is, nested) formal substructure as mandated by particular data-analytical investigations, notably process and decision mining to discover actual patient treatment process schemata, and entailed by the semantics of *feat* entries.

For purposes of statistical analysis, it is mandatory that case-by-variate structures can be derived easily from the MBS by (i) converting MBS extractions into "flat file" views by simply selecting subsets of *feat* fields recorded in protocol particles, and (ii) facilitating the formal addition of further variables by defining various temporal etc. predicates on the annotation fields of a patient's protocol particles (e.g., in order to investigate the temporal dynamics of an event sequence, etc.).

4.3   The Analysis Dimension: Compliance

After simulating a medical guideline the basic hypothesis about $l_g(X_d, \theta)$ assumes that clinical log data (that is, actual treatment processes) do not depend on personal attributes such as *age* and *gender* (cf. Fig. 6). One technique to analyze this hypothesis on decision points and possible exit states within the synthetic treatment processes is provided by decision mining [24]. Decision mining is implemented within process mining frameworks, such as ProM [16]. Using the reporting tools of ProM, we can produce the following report table summarizing the outcomes of the treatment processes (i.e., 'dead', 'healed', 'no show', 'keep appointment') grouped by, e.g., age and gender classes (cf. Tab. 1). Under the basic hypothesis, there should be no significant differences in the exit state distributions, of course. Otherwise, one has to think about a reformulation of the guideline considered in terms of personal attributes X_p, or through improving the implementation strategy of the treatment process.

Table 1. Example Report Structure

	dead	healed	no show	keep appointment
age < 20	x %	...	...	...
20 ≤ age ≤ 30	y %	...	...	...
...	...	...	...	...
gender = f	z %	...	...	...

5   Conclusions and Outlook

The virtues of the proposed approach towards assessing the guideline-compliance of clinical treatment processes can be summarized as follows: (i) formalizing the representation of clinical treatment processes amounts to a rigorous process view on medical evidence; (ii) formalizing clinical treatment processes as well as medical guidelines allows to restate the concept of process compliance in a more precise fashion than before; and (iii) evidence-based data-driven compliance assessment highlights the actual scope of guideline implementations, whether compliant or not. Obviously, formal compliance assessment drives the understanding of clinical practice, and, in doing so, feeds back to the maintenance and evolution of guidelines in the light of empirical evidence.

As it stands, though, the outlined methodology is but a research program, entailing a range of research issues including, to name just the most important ones, the development of a modeling framework for patient treatment processes accounting for a wide variety of conditions and exceptions typically not even mentioned in the narratives of medical guidelines, effective approaches towards wrapping and integrating available patient record data from various – and often scattered – clinical documentation and electronic health record infrastructures, strategies for deciding about the scope of medical evidence to be included in the analyses at all, the tuning of the simulation apparatus generating synthetic evidence from formal process models for selected patient population collectives, and both, statistical process mining and decision mining techniques, applied to available data bodies.

Obviously, theoretical advancement of the topic will have to be paralleled by extensive practical experimenting with a range of medical guidelines in the light of different bodies of medical and epidemiological evidence. For the time being, within the EBMC^2 project, three valuable data sources are investigated thoroughly, namely (i) a detailed data collection of clinical Cutaneous Melanoma stage 4 protocols, (ii) a vast body of administrative data of the Austrian Main Association of Social Insurers comprising a comprehensive picture of medical patient treatments, and (iii) Melanoma-relevant excerpts of the Austrian cancer register. Currently, much effort is devoted to the formal process-focused integration of these (as well as further) sources of patient-related Melanoma data as an indispensable, yet non-trivial prerequisite to process mining and, at a more general level, to the validation of the proposed EBMC^2 analytical methodology of comparing medical treatment practice with medical guidelines.

Acknowledgements. We thank all our collaborators in the EMBC^2 project: Michael Binder, Wolfgang Dorda, Georg Duftschmid, Walter Gall, Milan Hronsky, Christoph Rinner, and Stefanie Weber.

References

1. van der Aalst, W.M.P.: Process Mining – Discovery, Conformance and Enhancement of Business Processes. Springer, New York (2011)
2. Alves De Medeiros, A.K., Günther, C.W.: Process mining: Using CPN tools to create test logs for mining algorithms. In: Proceedings of the Sixth Workshop and Tutorial on Practical Use of Coloured Petri Nets and the CPN Tools, pp. 177–190 (2005)
3. Benthem, J.V.: The Logic of Time. Reidel, Dordrecht (1983)
4. Blobel, B.: Advanced EHR architectures – promises or reality? Methods Inf. Med. 45(1), 95–101 (2006)
5. Cochrane, A.: Effectiveness and Efficiency – Random Reflections on Health Services. Royal Society of Medicine Press, London (1972)
6. Eichelberg, M., Aden, T., Riesmeier, J.: A survey and analysis of electronic healthcare record standards. ACM Computing Surveys 37(4), 277–315 (2005)
7. Fox, J., Black, E., Chronakis, I., Dunlop, R., Petkar, V., South, M., Thomson, R.: From guidelines to careflows: Modelling and supporting complex clinical processes. In: Computer-Based Medical Guidelines and Protocols: A Primer and Current Trends, pp. 44–61. IOS Press, Netherlands (2008)
8. Gall, W., Grossmann, W., Duftschmid, G., Wrba, T., Dorda, W.: Analyses of EHRs for research, quality management and health politics. In: Proc. MIE 2008, XXIst International Congress of the European Federation for Medical Informatics. Studies in Health Technology and Informatics, vol. 136, pp. 425–430 (2008)
9. Garbe, C., Peris, K., Hauschild, A., Saiag, P., Middleton, M., Spatz, A., Grob, J., Malvehy, J., Newton-Bishop, J., Stratigos, A., Pehamberger, H., Eggermont, A.: Diagnosis and treatment of melanoma: European consensus-based interdisciplinary guideline. European Journal of Cancer 46(2), 270–283 (2010)

10. Guyatt, G., Oxman, A., Schüneman, H., Tugwell, P., Knottnerus, A.: Grade guidelines: A new series of articles in the journal of clinical epidemiology. Journal of Clinical Epidemiology 64, 380–382 (2011)
11. Häyrinen, K., Saranto, K., Nykänen, P.: Definition, structure, content, use and impacts of electronic health records: A review of the research literature. Int. J. Medical Informatics 77, 291–304 (2008)
12. Hunter, A., Williams, M.: Using clinical preferences in argumentation about evidence from clinical trials. In: Proc. 1st ACM Int'l. Health Informatics Symposium (2010)
13. Jansen-Vullers, M., Netjes, M.: Business process simulation – a tool survey. In: Workshop and Tutorial on Practical Use of Coloured Petri Nets and the CPN Tools, Aarhus, Denmark (2006)
14. Koch, O.: Process-based and context-sensitive information supply in medical care. In: Proc. 2nd Int. Workshop on Context-Based Information Retrieval. Computer Science Research Report 114, pp. 93–104. Roskilde University, Denmark (2007)
15. Ly, T., Rinderle-Ma, S., Göser, K., Dadam, P.: On enabling integrated process compliance with semantic constraints in process management systems – requirements, challenges, solutions. Information Systems Frontiers, 1–25 (2009)
16. Mans, R.: Workflow Support for the Healthcare Domain. Proefschriftmaken.nl, Netherlands (2011)
17. Mans, R.S., Schonenberg, M.H., Song, M., Aalst, W.M.P., Bakker, P.J.M.: Application of process mining in healthcare – a case study in a dutch hospital, vol. 25, pp. 425–438 (2009)
18. Marsland, S.: Machine Learning – An Algorithmic Perspective. Chapman & Hall/CRC, Boca Raton (2009)
19. OpenClinical, http://www.openclinical.org/gmmintro.html (accessed July 28, 2011)
20. Oxford Centre for Evidence-Based Medicine, http://www.cebm.net/index.aspx?o=5653 (accessed July 28, 2011)
21. Perleth, M., Busse, R., Gerhardus, A., Gibis, B., Luhmann, D.: Health Technology Assessment: Konzepte, Methoden, Praxis für Wissenschaft und Entscheidungsfindung. Berliner Schriftenreihe Gesundheitswissenschaften, Medizinisch Wissenschaftliche Verlagsgesellschaft (2008)
22. Rescher, J., Urquhart, A.: Temporal Logic. Springer, New York (1971)
23. Rosenfeld, R., Shiffman, R.N.: Clinical practice guideline development manual: A quality driven approach for translating evidence into action. Otolaryngol. Head. Neck Surg. 140(6 suppl. 1), 1–43 (2009)
24. Rozinat, A., van der Aalst, W.M.P.: Decision Mining in ProM. In: Dustdar, S., Fiadeiro, J.L., Sheth, A.P. (eds.) BPM 2006. LNCS, vol. 4102, pp. 420–425. Springer, Heidelberg (2006)
25. Shiffman, R.N., Karras, B., Agrawal, A., Chen, R., Marenco, L., Nath, S.: Gem: a proposal for a more comprehensive guideline document model using xml. Journal of the American Medical Informatics Assoc. 7, 488–498 (2000)
26. The Cochrane Collaboration, http://www.cochrane.org/ (accessed July 28, 2011)

An Enhanced Approach to Supporting Controlled Access to EPRs with Three Levels of Identity Privacy Preservations

Rima Addas and Ning Zhang

School of Computer Science,
University of Manchester,
Manchester, UK

Abstract. The emergence of e-health has put an enormous amount of sensitive data in the hands of service providers or other third parties, where privacy risks might exist when accessing sensitive data stored in electronic patient records (EPRs). EPRs support efficient access to patient data by healthcare providers and third party users, which will consequently improve patient care. However, uncontrolled access to distributed EPRs can introduce serious concerns related to patient privacy. This indicates that there is a need for a stronger fine-grained access control mechanism to be used in e-health applications. This paper, therefore, presents a novel method to support access to distributed EPRs with three levels of patient identity privacy preservation. The method offers a number of significant features: (1) it makes use of credentials to support the three-levels of accesses; (2) it simplifies key management distribution; (3) it allows better performance; (4) it supports separation of duties among trusted third parties (ensuring accountability); (5) it improves scalability. The method makes use of cryptographic primitives. In comparison with related work, the method supports three levels of access requirements while preserving data owner's privacy on a single platform.

Keywords: e-Health, Distributed EPRs, Identity Privacy (Anonymity), Linkability, Credentials, Performance, Security.

1 Introduction

e-Health is the use of the Internet or other electronic media to deliver health related information and services. Patient data can be collected, stored and managed at a single site or distributed sites. The important implications of e-health are becoming more and more apparent to patients, health service providers (HSPs) and third party users. e-Health facilitates the provision of medical support remotely at any time and enables access to, and exchange of, patient health data on demand [1]. For example, patients can access their recent test results outside of office hours. They can also update their demographic information remotely using their home computers.

A. Holzinger and K.-M. Simonic (Eds.): USAB 2011, LNCS 7058, pp. 547–561, 2011.
© Springer-Verlag Berlin Heidelberg 2011

In addition, e-health can also bring benefits to HSPs. For example, e-Health enables HSPs to gain rapid access to patient information that can aid in the diagnosis of any medical condition or the development of suitable treatment plans. It can make patient medical history, test results and practice guidelines obtainable from an operation room. Easy and instant access to EPRs, and efficient sharing of medical information, regardless of their locations, can prevent paper mix-ups, and allow physicians to make more accurate decisions [2]. Furthermore, e-health can improve clinical research by allowing the integration of databases for developed analysis, allowing linked simulations and enabling remote control of medical research implements. Thus, clinical researchers could more quickly work out a cure for a disease, which will in turn lead to a better patient health care. All these benefits will lead to better quality and management of health data as well as care delivery and health system management thus saving patients' lives [3].

While e-health can provide these benefits, it also introduces a number of challenging issues. One of these issues is how to preserve patients' privacy while allowing authorized access to their data. In real life situations, there are various scenarios, where different user groups have legitimate reasons for accessing patient EPRs. Based on the principle of least privilege, each user group should only be granted with an access right that is just sufficient for them to perform an assigned task. To facilitate this minimum access right management, we have identified three distinctive user groups [4], each with a defined level of access. The first group users are given rights to access anonymised data. In other words, they are not allowed to link multiple EPR objects of the same patient, nor link a record to the patient's real identity. The second group users, for legitimate reasons, are allowed to access multiple objects of the same patient, but are not allowed to link the objects to their owner's (i.e. the patients') identity. In other words, users in this group are allowed to link the multiple objects of the single patient but without being able to identify the patient. Finally, the third group users are allowed to access patients' records as well as identify the owners of the records.

To achieve these 3-level privacy-preserving accesses, patients' records need to be de-identified and indexed with proper pseudonyms. De-identification means that patient identifiable information is removed from the records [5]. There are three de-identification methods, anonymization, depersonalization and pseudonymization. Anonymization is the process of hiding (or removing) a patient's identification data and only make other information (i.e. de-identified information) available for access [6]. Depersonalization is a process similar to anonymization. But, it comprises the removal of as much identification information as necessary to protect patient identification data [7]. However, in practice, there are times when, for legitimate reasons, multiple de-identified records of the same patient may need to be linked (e.g. when we need to study the history of a patient's medical condition). In such cases, methods should be in place to allow de-identified records to be linked together and to the owner's identity in a controlled manner. The two methods mentioned above do not support this linkability requirement. To facilitate this, pseudonyms can be used to index a patient's de-identified record. Pseudonymization is the process of adding an identifier (a pseudonym) into a patient's de-identified record. The association between a real identity and the associated pseudonym or between two or more associated pseudonyms can be done in a controlled manner, e.g. by using a cryptographic key [8].

Most pseudonym generation methods used in supporting privacy preserving EPR access [9], [10], [11], focus on preserving patient anonymity. They use irreversible pseudonyms to index de-identified records. This type of pseudonyms only supports anonymous data access. Though the pseudonym generation methods in [12], [13], have considered the linkability requirement, they do not support a secondary use of patient information. That is they do not allow linking of multiple pseudonyms of the single patient without revealing the patient's identity. A notable method that has addressed this limitation is LIPA [14]. Yet, LIPA supports this linkable privacy preserving data access, but assuming that patient records managed by different HSPs are stored in a single repository. The solution does not support distributed data access. To the authors' best knowledge, the works that are most related to our work are Deng's method [15] and the PIPE method [16]. Both methods aim to securely integrate primary and secondary usage of distributed medical data without compromising the patient's identity privacy. This paper describes an alternative method with the aim of reducing access delays. In other words, the method described in this paper is more efficient than Deng's and PIPE methods.

The method is an improved version of the method proposed in [4]. It supports distributed EPR access with three levels of patient identity privacy protections:

- *L1: Linkable access:* At this level, multiple data objects of the same patient can be linked, and this set of objects can be linked to the patient's identity. L1 should be limited to L1 users (i.e. users with linkable access privilege).
- *L2: Linkable anonymous access:* At this level, multiple data objects of the same patient can be linked, but this set of objects cannot be linked to the patient's identity. L2 should be limited to L2 users (i.e. users with linkable anonymous access privilege).
- *L3: Anonymous access:* At this level, multiple data objects of the same patient cannot be linked, nor the patient's identity is exposed. L3 should be limited to L3 users (i.e. users with anonymous access privilege).

The access privileges may be granted to users, depending on their respective roles or job functions, and/or can be granted based upon patients' (i.e. data owners') consents.

This paper describes a novel three-level identity privacy preservation (3LI2P) method. To distinguish this method from an earlier method that we have designed, we call this method 3LI2P version 2 (3LI2Pv2). The 3LI2Pv2 method makes use of multiple layers of pseudonym generations to protect the patient's identity privacy. In this method, cryptographic primitives are used to generate patient pseudonyms. Although cryptographic primitives are complex, they provide rigid services for privacy and security implementations, which cannot be provided by any other scheme.

The rest of the paper is organized as follows. Section 2 outlines the design preliminaries. Section 3 gives an overview of the 3LI2Pv2 method before describing the method in detail in Section 4. Section 5 analyses our method and finally, Section 6 concludes the paper and outlines the future work.

2 Design Preliminaries

The design preliminaries include the assumptions, notation and requirements used in the design of the 3LI2Pv2 method.

2.1 Assumptions

The design of the 3LI2Pv2 method was based on the following assumptions.
(A1). Patients' records have already been de-identified.
(A2). Entities with higher privileged credentials do not pass their credentials to entities with lower ones.
(A3). Each entity, z, generates its own public/private key pair (PU_z and PR_z), and PU_z will be certified by a trusted third party (TTP) and PR_z is known only to entity z.
(A4). Communication channels between entities are resilient. That is, messages sent will eventually be received by their intended recipients.
(A5). Communication channels are authentication, confidentiality and integrity protected. This can be achieved by using the Secure Socket Layer (SSL) protocol.
(A6). A central trusted third party (C-TTP) is trusted by all the participants (e.g. HSPs).

2.2 Notation

The notation used throughout the rest of this paper is summarized as follows.

- C-TTP: The method makes use of a unique central trusted third party (C-TTP).
- H-TTP_j: A local TTP associated to HSP j, $j \in (1, m)$.
- PID_i: Patient i's unique identity (e.g. NHS number).
- $O_{i,r}$: Patient i's object/record r, $r \in (1, n)$.
- $PS_{1,i}$: Patient i's L1 pseudonym.
- $PS_{2,i,j}$: Patient i's L2 pseudonym generated for HSP j.
- $PS_{3,i,c}^{L1}$: Patient i's L3-Type-I pseudonym, generated by C-TTP for L1 access.
- $PS_{3,i,c}^{L2}$: Patient i's L3-Type-II pseudonym, generated by C-TTP for L2-inter-HSP access.
- $PS_{3,i,j}^{L2}$: Patient i's L3-Type-III pseudonym, generated by H-TTP_j for L2-intra-HSP access.

- SK_c: A symmetric key only known by C-TTP.
- $PU_P=(e_P, n_P)$, $PR_P=(d_P, n_P)$: Party P's public and private RSA keys, $P \in \{z, \text{C-TTP}, \text{H-}TTP_j\}$, where z is a user.
- $PU_{j,c}=(e_{j,c}, n_{j,c})$, $PR_{j,c}=(d_{j,c}, n_{j,c})$: HSP j's public/private keys generated by C-TTP.
- $H(m)$: A collision-resistant one-way hash function (e.g. SHA-256).
- $E(SK_P, m)$ and $D(SK_P, m)$: Encryption and decryption of a data item m using symmetric key, SK_P, of a party P and a symmetric cipher, e.g. AES [17].
- $E(PU_P, m)$: The cipher-text of data item, m, encrypted with a public key PU_P of a party, P, using RSA cryptosystem [18].
- $x||y$: Concatenation of data items, x and y.

2.3   Design Requirements

The requirements are specified for the design of the 3LI2Pv2 described in Section 3.

(R1) Linkability: With an L1 credential, an authorized L1 user should be able to re-identify a patient from the patient's pseudonyms. In our approach, this linkability is achieved by applying cryptographic operations to a patient's multiple level pseudonyms.

(R2) Anonymous Linkability: With an L2 credential, authorized L1 and L2 users should be able to link multiple de-identified objects of the same patient without identifying the patient. In our approach, this requirement is met by using L1 and L2 pseudonyms.

(R3) Anonymous Access: With an identity credential, authorized L1, L2 and L3 users can access a patient's de-identified objects without being able to link them nor to learn the patient's identity. In our approach, this is achieved by using L3 pseudonyms.

(R4) Minimizing Access Delay: Access delay is defined as the time elapsed from submitting an access request to the time the access request is responded. This metric measures the method's access performance. This delay should be kept as low as possible.

(R5) Optimising 3LI2Pv2 Performance: The performance is measured by:

- *Computational cost:* is measured in terms of the number of cryptographic operations necessary for generating the three-level pseudonyms per patient.
- *Communication cost:* is measured in terms of the number and the size of transactions/messages exchanged between protocol entities for the issuance of the three-level pseudonyms per patient.
- *Storage cost:* is measured in terms of the number of pseudonyms and keys required per patient per HSP.

(R6) Ensuring Accountability: The involvement of TTPs (C-TTP/H-TTP_j) in facilitating privacy preserving access to EPRs should be accountable. In our approach, this is achieved by using the principle of the septation of duties among

TTPs. That is each TTP maintains its own secret keys, and does not share the keys with another TTP.

(R7) Scalability: The approach should be scalable. In other words, the addition of a patient or a patient's record should not introduce excessive overheads into the solution.

3   An 3LI2Pv2 Method Overview

The idea of our 3LI2Pv2 method is to allow access to a patient's EPR objects with multiple levels of identity privacy preservation. To facilitate this idea, three levels of pseudonym generations are introduced, which made the method offers important features:

-**(F1) Support 3-level of Controlled Access.** This is achieved by: (1) for L1 access, only one entity can recover the patient's real identity. (2) for L2 access, two features are supported: (2.1) L2-Inter-HSP linking (i.e linking objects of the same patient in a single HSP), and (2.2) L2-Intra-HSP linking (i.e linking objects of the same patient in multiple HSPs). Finally, (3) for L3 access, we make use of the minimum disclosure principle.

-**(F2) Support 3LI2Pv2 Credentials.** This is achieved by granting users with different access credentials based on their appropriate roles.

-**(F3) Optimize Performance.** This is achieved by minimizing the storage, computational and communication costs.

-**(F4) Ensure Accountability.** This is achieved by supporting the separation of duties among entities (TTPs and users). In other words, secret keys and patient pseudonyms (except for L2 pseudonyms) are not distributed or shared between entities.

-**(F5) Improve Scalability.** This is achieved by minimizing the number of keys necessary for generating the patient's multiple layers of pseudonyms.

-**(F6) Prohibit Unauthorized Linkage by HSPs.** This is achieved by prohibiting HSPs from sharing each others' patients' pseudonyms.

-**(F7) Simplify Key Management.** This is achieved by reducing the number of keys (necessary for generating patients' pseudonyms) that needs to be managed.

-**(F8) Pseudonyms Indistinguishably.** This is achieved by having each level of a pseudonym uniquely generated by a respective TTP with a respective key.

In the 3LI2Pv2 method, we design a hierarchy of three-level pseudonyms. That is higher-level pseudonyms are built on lower-level ones. To clarify this hierarchy, we have shown the structure of the pseudonyms in Figure 1. The hierarchy is described in detail in Section 4. The design considerations for this 3-level pseudonyms hierarchy are:

- The purpose of the L1 pseudonym is to hide a patient's real identity. It is also used as a common identifier to index a particular patient's data objects stored in multiple sites.

- The L2 pseudonym is built on L1 pseudonym. The purpose of the L2 pseudonym is to hide L1 pseudonym from unauthorized entities (i.e. restrict L2-inter-HSP access), and to facilitate L2-intra-HSP access, as the multiple objects of the same patient in a HSP is indexed with a unique L2 pseudonym.

- The L3 pseudonyms are built on lower-level pseudonyms (L1 and L2). The purpose of them is to protect lower-level pseudonyms from unauthorized entities, and to support different access credentials. Because different access levels require different credentials, we have designed three types of L3 pseudonyms: **(a) L3 Type-I Pseudonym Generation:** This pseudonym is built on L1 pseudonym (because L1 pseudonym has a direct link to the patient's real identity). It is generated to provide L1 access credential, and is given to L1 users as a part of their credentials. **(b) L3 Type-II Pseudonym Generation:** This pseudonym is also built on L1 pseudonym. We choose to build this pseudonym on top of L1 and not on top of L2 pseudonym because we want to minimize the decryption operations performed (i.e. minimize the computational cost). It is generated to provide L2-inter-HSP access credential, and is given to L1/L2 users as a part of their credentials.

(c) L3 Type-III Pseudonym Generation: This pseudonym is built on L2 pseudonym (as L2 pseudonym can directly support L2-intra-HSP access). It is generated to provide L2-intra-HSP access credential, and is given to L1/L2 users as a part of their credentials.

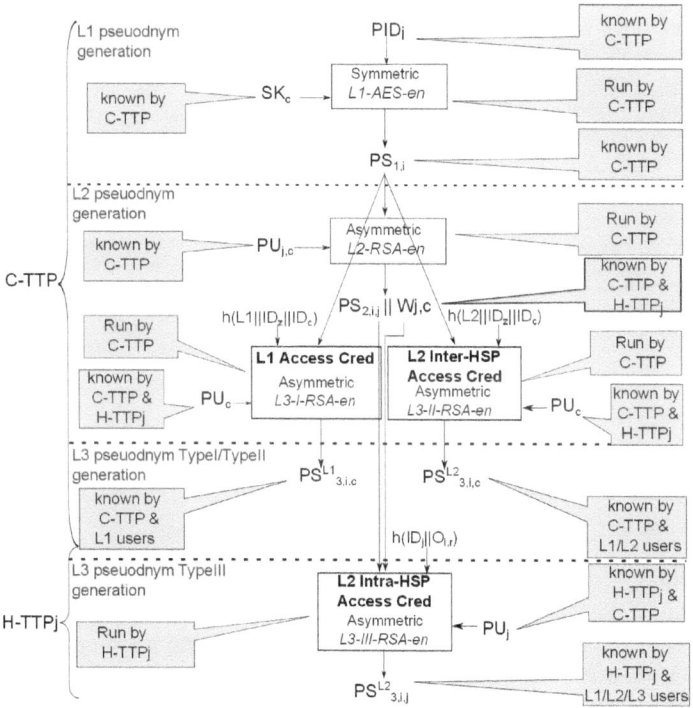

Fig. 1. Hierarchy of The Three-level Pseudonyms

4   The 3LI2Pv2 Method in Detail

The 3LI2Pv2 method mainly consists of three methods of pseudonym generation and reversal. A Level-1 Pseudonym Generation and Reversal (L1-PGR) method, a Level-2 Pseudonym Generation and Reversal (L2-PG) method and a level-3 Pseudonym Generation and Reversal (L3-PGR) method. Each method consists of a key generation method, a pseudonym generation algorithm and a pseudonym reversal algorithm. The pseudonym generation methods are depicted in Figure 2.

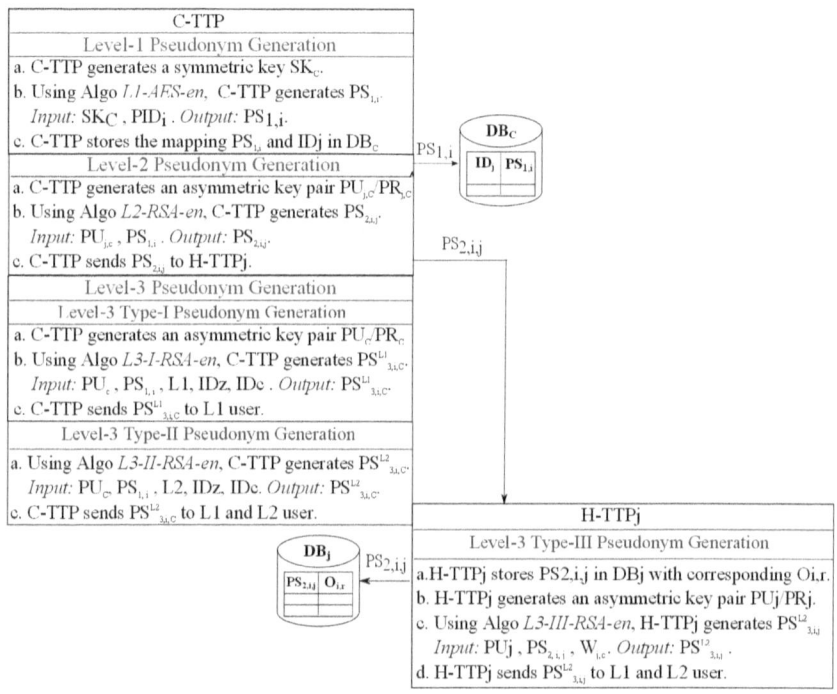

Fig. 2. Generation of The Three Levels Pseudonyms

4.1   Level-1 Pseudonym Generation and Reversal (L1-PGR) Method

This method is executed by C-TTP. It generates and reverses a unique L1 pseudonym, $PS_{1,i}$, for each patient i. A symmetric cryptosystem is used to generate the L1 pseudonyms. The reasons behind using a symmetric cryptosystem rather than a hash function is that the method needs to support (R1), i.e. to allow the recovery of a patient's original identity from his/her pseudonym. Although hash functions are more efficient than symmetric cryptosystems, they are one-way, and do not support this linkability requirement. The reason for choosing a symmetric cryptosystem instead of an asymmetric cryptosystem is because the former is more efficient. L1 pseudonyms, for all patients, are generated by C-TTP regardless of their being managed by one HSP or multiple HSPs. So it is necessary to make sure that the pseudonym generation and reversal operations are performed in the most efficient manner. The chosen symmetric cipher is Advanced Encryption Standard (AES). The following describes how L1 pseudonyms are generated and reversed.

- **Level-1 Pseudonym Key generation (L1-PKG) Method:** The key used to generate the patients' L1 pseudonyms is a single symmetric key, SK_c. The reason behind using a single symmetric key here is because we want to reduce the computational burden on C-TTP. So only a single SK_c is necessary in the generation of the patients' L1 pseudonyms, regardless how many EPR objects they have, and where these objects are managed. C-TTP will generate this key and the knowledge of SK_c is limited to C-TTP.

- **Level-1 Pseudonym Generation (L1-PG) Algorithm:** This algorithm generates an L1 pseudonym to protect the patient's identity. It is executed by C-TTP. This pseudonym generation is depicted in Algorithm L1-AES-en in Figure 1 and in Equation 1. C-TTP then stores the mapping of $PS_{1,i}$ and the HSP's identity in its database (DB_c).

$$PS_{1,i} = E(SK_c, PID_i) \tag{1}$$

- **Level-1 Pseudonym Reversal (L1-PR) Algorithm:** This algorithm reverses the patient's $PS_{1,i}$ to retrieve the patient's real identity. It is executed by C-TTP when an L1 access is requested by an L1 user. So only C-TTP can retrieve the patient's real identity. Equation 2 depicts this reversal operation.

$$PID_i = D(SK_c, PS_{1,i}) \tag{2}$$

4.2   Level-2 Pseudonym Generation and Reversal (L2-PGR) Method

This method is executed by C-TTP. It generates and reverses patients' L2 pseudonyms. The L2 pseudonyms are generated using an asymmetric cryptosystem, because: (1) although asymmetric ciphers are more computation costly than symmetric ones, asymmetric ciphers are necessary here, as C-TTP needs to generate a unique key pair for each HSP to achieve *(F6)*. However, C-TTP need not store the HSPs' corresponding private keys, as it relies on a technique that can manage this issue in an effective manner (described below). As a result, we simplify key management, achieving *(F7)*. (2) The asymmetric keys are generated for HSPs and not for patients. As the number of participating HSPs is usually less than the number of patients, the number of keys would be reasonable to manage thus asymmetric cryptosystem would be reasonable here. The following describes L2 pseudonym generation and reversal.

- **Level-2 Pseudonym Key Generation (L2-PKG) Method:** This method generates an RSA key pair ($PU_{j,c}/PR_{j,c}$) for each H-TTP_j. This key pair is generated by C-TTP for H-TTP_j. H-TTP_j does not have the knowledge of the key pair. The key used to generate the patient's L2 pseudonym is the public key ($PU_{j,c}$), as described below.

- **Level-2 Pseudonym Generation (L2-PG) Algorithm:** This algorithm generates patients' L2 pseudonyms to protect the L1 pseudonyms. It is executed by C-TTP, as shown in Algorithm L2-RSA-en in Figure 1, Figure 2 and in Equation 3.

$$PS_{2,i,j} = E(PU_{j,c}, PS_{1,i}) \tag{3}$$

To achieve $F7$, C-TTP relies on a technique (the W technique) to manage the recovery of the HSP's private key ($PR_{j,c}$) needed to unwrap L2 pseudonym. The idea of this technique is to computationally link the HSP's public key ($PU_{j,c}$) with C-TTP's private key (PR_c). Where $W_{j,c} = (h(PR_c||PU_{j,c})^{-1}d_{j,c}) \bmod n_{j,c}$. So after generating $PS_{2,i,j}$, to facilitate the recovery of the HSP's private key, C-TTP will concatenate $W_{j,c}$ with the resulted pseudonym. C-TTP then will send it ($PS_{2,i,j}||W_{j,c}$) to the respective HSP. C-TTP can later recover the private key ($PR_{j,c} = (d_{j,c}, n_{j,c})$) by computing $d_{j,c} = (h(PR_c||PU_{j,c})W_{j,c}) \bmod n_{j,c}$. Each H-$TTP_j$ then, stores the $PS_{2,i,j}||W_{j,c}$ in its H_{DB} along with the corresponding patient's EPR object.

- **Level-2 Pseudonym Reversal (L2-PR) Algorithm:** This algorithm reverses an L2 pseudonym to retrieve the corresponding L1 pseudonym. It is executed by C-TTP when an L2-inter-HSP access is requested by L1 or L2 user. The algorithm is performed using the RSA private key ($PR_{j,c}$) controlled by C-TTP. First, C-TTP will recover the key, as described above, and then uses this key to unwrap $PS_{2,i,j}$, as shown in Equation 4.

$$PS_{1,i} = D(PR_{j,c}, PS_{2,i,j}) \tag{4}$$

4.3 Level-3 Pseudonym Generation and Reversal (L3-PGR) Method

In this method, three types of L3 pseudonyms ($PS_{3,i,c}^{L1}$, $PS_{3,i,c}^{L2}$, $PS_{3,i,j}^{L2}$) are generated. They are generated by different TTPs for different access levels (as described in Section 3). These L3 pseudonyms are generated using asymmetric cryptosystem. The reason behind this decision is because these L3 pseudonyms are distributed to users (as they are handed out to them as part of their access credentials), and the corresponding private keys of these L3 pseudonyms need to be strictly secured. In other words, the private keys should be only known by respective TTPs, and not shared among any other entities, to ensure septation of duties $(F4)$, thus using asymmetric cryptosystem would be essential here. The following shows the generation and reversal of the three types of L3 pseudonyms.

- **L3 Type-I Pseudonym Generation and Reversal Method:** This method is executed by C-TTP. It generates and reverses a patient's L3-Type-I pseudonym ($PS_{3,i,c}^{L1}$). This pseudonym is generated for L1 access credential (as described in Section 3). The following shows how this pseudonym is generated and reversed.

A - **L3 Type-I Key Generation Method.** This method generates an asymmetric key pair (PU_c/PR_c) to generate/reverse $PS_{3,i,c}^{L1}$. This key pair is generated by C-TTP. Only C-TTP knows the corresponding private key. The key used to generate $PS_{3,i,c}^{L1}$ is PU_c.

B - **L3 Type-I Pseudonym Generation Algorithm.** This algorithm is executed by C-TTP when C-TTP needs to generate an L1 access credential for L1 user. The algorithm generates $PS_{3,i,c}^{L1}$. As shown in Equation 5, it encrypts the L1 pseudonym concatenated with the hash of L1, the user's identity (ID_z) and the C-TTP's identity (ID_C) using C-TTP's public key. The purpose of the concatenation is to differentiate between Type-I and Type-II L3 pseudonyms.

$$PS_{3,i,c}^{L1} = E(PU_c, PS_{1,i}||h(L1||ID_z||ID_C)) \tag{5}$$

C - **L3 Type-I Pseudonym Reversal Algorithm.** This algorithm is run by C-TTP when C-TTP needs to verify the L1 user' L1 access credential before allowing the access. The algorithm performs the reversal operation (using the C-TTP's private key), i.e, unwraps $PS_{3,i,c}^{L1}$ to get the patient's $PS_{1,i}$, as shown in Equation 6.

$$PS_{1,i}||h(L1||ID_z||ID_C) = D(PR_c, PS_{3,i,c}^{L1}) \tag{6}$$

- **L3 Type-II Pseudonym Generation and Reversal Method:** This method is also executed by C-TTP. It generates and reverses an L3 Type-II pseudonym $(PS_{3,i,c}^{L2})$. This pseudonym is generated for L2-intra-HSP access credential (as described in Section 3). The following shows how this pseudonym is generated and reversed.

A - **L3 Type-II Key Generation Method.** This method is similar to the L3 Type-I Key Generation Method. The key used to generate $PS_{3,i,c}^{L2}$ is PU_c.

B - **L3 Type-II Pseudonym Generation Algorithm.** This algorithm is executed by C-TTP when C-TTP needs to generate an L2-inter-HSP access credential for L1 or L2 user. The algorithm generates $PS_{3,i,c}^{L2}$, as shown in Algorithm L3-TypeI-RSA-en in Figure 1, Figure 2 and in Equation 7.

$$PS_{3,i,c}^{L2} = E(PU_c, PS_{1,i}||h(L2||ID_z||ID_c)) \tag{7}$$

C - **L3 Type-II Pseudonym Reversal Algorithm.** This algorithm is run by C-TTP when C-TTP needs to verify the L1/L2 users' L2-inter-HSP access credentials. The algorithm retrieves the patient's L1 pseudonym, as shown in Equation 8.

$$PS_{1,i}||h(L2||ID_z||ID_c) = D(PR_c, PS_{3,i,j}^{L2}) \tag{8}$$

- **L3 Type-III Pseudonym Generation and Reversal Method:** This method is performed by H-TTP_j. It generates and reverses an L3 Type-III pseudonym $(PS_{3,i,j}^{L2})$. This pseudonym is generated for L2-Intra-HSP access credential (as described in Section 3). The following shows how this pseudonym is generated and reversed.

A - **L3 Type-III Key Generation Method.** This method generates a key pair (PU_j/PR_j) for $PS_{3,i,j}^{L2}$ generation and reversal. The key pair is generated by H-TTP_j. Only H-TTP_j knows the corresponding private key. The key used to generate this pseudonym is H-TTP_j's RSA public key (PU_j).

B - **L3 Type-III Pseudonym Generation Algorithm.** This algorithm is executed by H-TTP_j when H-TTP_j needs to generate the L2-intra access credentials for L1/L2 users. The algorithm generates $PS_{3,i,j}^{L2}$, as shown in Equation 9.

$$PS_{3,i,j}^{L2} = E(PU_j, PS_{2,i,j}||W_{j,c}||h(ID_j, O_{i,r}))$$ (9)

C - **L3 Type-III Pseudonym Reversal Algorithm.** This algorithm is only executed by H-TTP_j when H-TTP_j needs to verify the L1/L2 users' L2-intra access credentials before allowing the access. The algorithm unwraps $PS_{3,i,j}^{L2}$ to get the patient's L2 pseudonym, as shown in Equation 10.

$$PS_{2,i,j}||W_{j,c}||h(ID_j, O_{i,r}) = D(PR_j, PS_{3,i,j}^{L2})$$ (10)

5   The Method Analysis

The method analysis includes requirements and performance analysis.

5.1   Requirements Analysis

This section analyses the 3LI2Pv2 method against the requirements set in Section 2.3.

- Generating reversible $PS_{1,is}$ using a symmetric cryptosystem, the patient's identity can be traced using the right key. The knowledge of this key is limited to C-TTP. Thus linkability (R1) is achieved in a controlled manner.
- Having $PS_{1,i}$ to be the common identifier of a patient's multiple EPR objects managed by multiple HSPs allows linking objects of a single patient without identifying the patient. Thereby supporting anonymous linkability (R2).
- Since patients' EPR objects are stored in a de-identified manner, and no linkability can be achieved without providing valid credentials, anonymous access (R3) is fulfilled.
- Our method proposed three-level pseudonym generations, which normally, add overheads to the solution. However, our method maintained a good performance supporting (R4/R5). This is due to reducing access delays by minimizing computational, communication and storage costs. A detailed performance analysis is described in Section 5.2.
- Only C-TTP holds SK_c (knows the mappings between $PS_{1,i}$ and PID_i). Only C-TTP holds $PR_{j,c}$ (knows the mapping between $PS_{1,i}$ and $PS_{2,i,j}$). Thus, any malicious release of patient identity/pseudonyms can be prevented. This ensures separation of duties (R6).
- In our method, all patients are allocated a single SK_c to reveal their identity. Also, all patients are only allocated a single $PR_{j,c}$ to unwrap the $PS_{2,i,j}$ in a specific HSP. When a new patient's data set is added, no additional keys will be required. This is because the same HSP's $PU_{j,c}$ is used to generate the patient's

L2 pseudonym. Even when a new patient is added to the HSP's database, no additional key (SK_c) is required, for generating L1 pseudonym, and no additional key $(PU_{j,c})$ is required for generating L2 pseudonym. So if the increase in the performance cost is linear then scalability (R7) can be met.

- To increase the security level of the solution, legitimate users are granted with different levels of access, by granting them with different credential types. In addition, the users are not given any secret keys to perform the access operations. The secret keys are only known by respective TTPs. Finally, the most sensitive secret key (SK_c), which reveals a patient i's identity, PID_i, is only known to C-TTP and no other entity can obtain this key. From this, it is evident that our method provides a high level of security.

5.2   Performance Analysis and Comparison with Related Work

This section presents a theoretical performance analysis of our solution. Performance is measured in terms of: (1) computational cost, (2) storage cost, and finally, (3) communication cost. Communication cost will be described in the prototype model.

-**Computational Cost:** Computation cost is measured here by calculating the number of cryptographic operations used for the generation of the three levels pseudonyms. A comparison between our solution and other two methods (Deng's and PIPE methods) is performed in terms of computational cost. We show this in table 1 when a patient has his/her data managed by a single HSP and multiple (m) HSPs.

Table 1. Computational Cost Comparison with Related Work

Methods	Crypto Operations	Enc/Dec Ops 1 patient in 1 HSP	Enc/Dec Ops 1 patient in m HSPs	Levels
Deng's Method	HMAC Symmetric	i obj Enc 2(i obj) Enc/1(i obj)Dec	m(i obj) Enc 2m(i obj) Enc/m(i obj)Dec	L1, L3
PIPE Method	Hash Function Symmetric Asymmetric	1 Enc 1+1(no of key shares) Enc/Dec 2+1(no of key shares) Enc/Dec	m Enc 1+m(no of key shares) Enc/Dec 2+m(no of key shares) Enc/Dec	L1, L3
Our Method	Hash Function Symmetric Asymmetric	3 Enc 1 Enc/Dec 4 Enc/Dec	2+m Enc 1 Enc/Dec 4m Enc/Dec	L1, L2, L3

From the table, it can be seen that our method supported three levels of access while the other methods supported only two levels. Taking this into consideration, our method performed better than the others. The extra exponentiation operations (from the asymmetric cryptosystems) in our solution are due to: (1) granting legitimate users with distinct access credentials (which is not considered in the other methods); (2) simplifying key management distribution; and (3) supporting separation of duties.

-**Storage Cost:** Storage cost is measured in terms of the number of pseudonyms/ keys needed for each patient in a single HSP/s. Table 2 shows a storage cost

Table 2. Storage Cost Comparison with Related Work

Methods	No. of HSP	No. of Pseudonyms	No. of Keys	Levels
Deng's Method	1 patient/1 HSP	2(i obj)	2	L1, L3
	1 patient/mHSPs	2m (i obj)	2m	
PIPE Method	1 patient/1 HSP	1+i obj	3	
	1 patient/mHSPs	m+i obj	3m	L1, L3
Our Approach	1 patient/1 HSP	5	4	
	1 patient/mHSPs	3+2m	3+2m	L1, L2, L3

comparison between our solution and the other methods (Deng's and PIPE). From the table, it can be seen that our solution introduced fewer storage costs than in the other methods. This is because the number of pseudonyms generated in our solution is fewer than in the others. Besides, considering that our solution facilitated three access levels, the number of keys generated, especially when a patient has his/her objects managed by (m) HSPs, is reasonable.

6 Conclusion

This paper has presented an enhanced method for supporting access to distributed EPRs with three levels of identity privacy preservation. The novelty of our method is reflected by the three levels of pseudonym generations, which have made our solution offers a number of interesting features, including: (1) the method is designed to allow legitimate users to perform different levels of access to a patient's distributed EPRs, without compromising his identity privacy. This was achieved by the multiple layers of patient pseudonym generations, and by granting users with proper credentials that is suitable for their roles; (2) it allows better performance by minimizing storage, computational and communication costs; (3) it protects patient identification data from malicious entities by controlling the disclosure of patient pseudonyms and secret keys, and not sharing them between entities. This was achieved by providing separation of duties among local/global TTPs, thereby supporting accountability; (4) it handles the growth of patients and patients' data while maintaining a reasonable performance. This was achieved by the reducing the number of keys needed to generate the patients' pseudonyms, thereby supporting scalability.

For future work, we include the design of the three access protocols making use of the three levels of patient pseudonyms.

References

1. Katzenbeisser, S., Petkovic, M.: Privacy-preserving recommendation systems for consumer healthcare services. In: Proceedings of the 2008 Third International Conference on Availability, Reliability and Security, pp. 889–895. IEEE Computer Society, Washington, DC, USA (2008)

2. Yang, Y., Han, X., Bao, F., Deng, R.H.: A smart-card-enabled privacy pre-serving eprescription system. IEEE Transactions on Information Technology in Biomedicine 8(1), 47–58 (2004)

3. Bloom, B.S.: Crossing the quality chasm: A new health system for the 21st century. JAMA 287(5), a-646–a-647 (2002)

4. Addas, R., Zhang, N.: Support access to distributed EPRs with multiple levels of identity privacy preservation. In: Proceedings of the 2011 Sixth International Conference on Availability, Reliability, and Security, Vienna, Austria, pp. 9–16. IEEE Computer Society (2011)

5. Pfitzmann, A., Hansen, M.: Anonymity, unlinkability, undetectability, unobserv-ability, pseudonymity, and identity management - a consolidated proposal for ter-minology. Technical report (February 2008)

6. Clayton, R.: Anonymity and traceability in cyberspace. Technical report, Univer-sity of Cambridge, Computer Laboratory, Darwin College (2005)

7. Rogers, J., Puleston, C., Rector, A.: The clef chronicle: Patient histories derived from electronic health records. In: ICDEW 2006: Proceedings of the 22nd Inter-national Conference on Data Engineering Workshops, p. 109+. IEEE Computer Society, Washington, DC, USA (2006)

8. Alhaqbani, B., Fidge, C.: Privacy-preserving electronic health record linkage using pseudonym identifiers, pp. 108–117 (July 2008)

9. Pommerening, K., Reng, M.: Secondary use of the ehr via pseudonymisation. Stud-ies in Health Technology and Informatics 103, 441–446 (2004)

10. Slamanig, D., Stingl, C.: Privacy aspects of ehealth. In: ARES 2008: Proceedings of the 2008 Third International Conference on Availability, Reliability and Security, pp. 1226–1233. IEEE Computer Society, Washington, DC, USA (2008)

11. Iacono, L.: Tmulti-centric universal pseudonymisation for secondary use of the ehr. In: Proc. of HealthGrid, pp. 239–247 (2007)

12. Schartner, P., Schaffer, M.: Unique User-Generated Digital Pseudonyms. In: Gorodetsky, V., Kotenko, I., Skormin, V. (eds.) MMM-ACNS 2005. LNCS, vol. 3685, pp. 194–205. Springer, Heidelberg (2005)

13. Elger, B.S., Iavindrasana, J., Lo Iacono, L., Müller, H., Roduit, N., Summers, P., Wright, J.: Strategies for health data exchange for secondary, cross-institutional clinical research. Computer Methods and Programs in Biomedicine 99(3), 230–251 (2010)

14. Zhang, N., Rector, A., Buchan, I., Shi, Q., Kalra, D., Rogers, J., Goble, C., Walker, S., Ingram, D., Singleton, P.: A linkable identity privacy algorithm for healthgrid. In: From Grid to Healthgrid: Proceedings of Healthgrid 2005, pp. 234–245 (2005)

15. Deng, M., DeCock, D., Preneel, B.: Towards a cross-context identity management framework in e-health. Online Information Review 33(3), 422–442 (2009)

16. Riedl, B., Grascher, V., Fenz, S., Neubauer, T.: Pseudonymization for improving the privacy in e-health applications. In: Hawaii International Conference on System Sciences, p. 255+ (2008)

17. Blömer, J., Seifert, J.-P.: Fault Based Cryptanalysis of the Advanced Encryption Standard (AES). In: Wright, R.N. (ed.) FC 2003. LNCS, vol. 2742, pp. 162–181. Springer, Heidelberg (2003)

18. Rivest, R.L., Shamir, A., Adleman, L.: A method for obtaining digital signatures and publickey cryptosystems. Commun. ACM 21, 120–126 (1978)

SemScribe: Automatic Generation
of Medical Reports

Lukas C. Faulstich[1], Kristin Irsig[1], Malik Atalla[1], Sebastian Varges[2],
Heike Bieler[2], and Manfred Stede[2]

[1] ID GmbH & Co. KGaA, Berlin, Germany
[2] Applied Computational Linguistics Lab, University of Potsdam, Germany

Abstract. Images and videos resulting from diagnostic imaging procedures such as echocardiography need to be analyzed and interpreted by
physicians in order to diagnose diseases of the patient. This process can
be split into two steps: in a first step, various morphological features depicted in the images have to be interpreted and described. Then, a diagnostic conclusion has to be drawn from these observations. The first step
can be facilitated by offering a structured entry form and some means to
generate textual descriptions from the data entered in this form. While it
is straight-forward to implement some basic text generation functionality
using hard-wired text templates, the generation of fluent, well-readable
text from structured data is much harder. In this collaboration we have
combined advanced methods from computational linguistics and medical
knowledge resources to solve this problem. We have built a prototype for
the domain of echocardiography and evaluated it in a clinical setting.

1 Introduction

We present an implemented system that automates the mapping from individual
medical observations to a medical report in natural language, and thus eliminates the need for a distinct text production step on the side of the physician.
The doctor enters observations into a structured entry form, and the corresponding text is produced instantaneously. Our approach, however, does not rely on
precoded segments of "canned text"; instead, we employ *natural language generation* technology for a fully automatic mapping between non-linguistic input
and linguistic output. This idea is inspired by the SUREGEN system [3,4], but
adds an emphasis on re-usable generation components as well as a grounding
in a (pre-existing) domain ontology, which facilitates the transfer of the system
to other medical domains as well as to other target languages (at present, we
generate German text only).

The paper is structured as follows. Section 2 provides more details about our
task, and Section 3 describes the overall architecture of the system. Next, Section
4 focuses on the language generation module and outlines the sequence of steps
necessary for mapping non-linguistic observation data to text. Finally, Section
5 discusses related work, and Section 6 presents our conclusions and some tasks
for future work.

A. Holzinger and K.-M. Simonic (Eds.): USAB 2011, LNCS 7058, pp. 563–573, 2011.

2   Task Description

Our project addresses a subtask of the larger endeavor of intelligent assistance for the production of doctor's letters. Depending on the particular clinical domain, the texts to be produced are more or less stereotypical, thus suggesting different methods for creating them. Our project focuses on cardiology, and the first step was to obtain a corpus of authentic doctor's letters, in order to study the linguistic phenomena and then to devise appropriate production strategies.

In the various cardiological diagnoses, one general finding is a very high density of information, which leads to a relatively telegraphic style of concatenated noun phrases, rather than full-fledged sentences. Consider the example in Figure 1, taken from an echocardiography diagnosis. By 'informational density', we refer to the fact that individual units of information (measurements, observations) are typically fused into complex noun phrases, which, as we argue in this paper, has consequences for deciding on the best strategy of production.

The most trivial setting for our task would be a mapping from each individual observation (roughly speaking, from each physician's mouse click) to a German sentence or phrase, with the "text" resulting from a simple concatenation of those phrases. However, this is unlikely to work since

- the physician will favour a particular ordering of information in the text, which need not correspond to the order of *entering* the information (i.e., taking measurements, making observations);
- as indicated above, information that conceptually belongs together, needs to be *aggregated* into more complex information units, so that a coherent, readable text results.

A solution based on text blocks can easily accommodate the first problem (by pre-storing the final order of phrases) but has problems with the second one. While it is in principle possible to manage a large set of text blocks that accounts not only for individual observations but for particular *combinations* of observations/measurements and expresses such information bundles in corresponding text bundles, this approach becomes inflexible and extremely difficult to port to other domains, where the problems are similar yet require a complete new set of text blocks.

Our solution therefore opts to employ *natural language generation* technology (see, e.g., [12]), which in a sequence of three steps systematically maps non-linguistic information to linguistic output, i.e., text:

1. Document planning: Serializing the information units into an appropriate order.
2. Sentence planning: "Chunking" the information into bundles that will later be expressed as individual sentences; deciding on words to use for conveying the information; deciding on how to bundle information units into appropriate linguistic phrases; deciding specifically on the words for referring to concepts/entities in the domain (so-called *referring expressions*: in/definite noun phrases, proper names, pronouns).

(1) a. Beide Ventrikel und der rechte Vorhof sind normal dimensioniert.
     b. (Both ventricles and the right atrium are of normal size.)

(2) a. Sämtliche LV-Wände sind leichtgradig verdickt.
     b. (All LV-walls are mildly thickened.)

(3) a. Der linke Vorhof ist mit 53 mm mittelgradig dilatiert bei unauffälliger globaler
        und regionaler linksventrikulärer Pumpfunktion.
     b. (The left atrium is moderately dilated at a size of 53mm and exhibits an un-
        remarkable global and regional ventricular pumping function.)

Fig. 1. Example sentences from the corpus of medical reports

3. Realization: the morphosyntactically-correct expression of the sentence plan
   as a sentence (even if telegraphic) in the target language (here: German);
   this involves fixing word order, insertion of function words, producing proper
   inflection.

The overall setting for our project therefore comprises a user interface allowing
the physician to enter information, mapping this information to a standardized
representation, and then starting the text generation component. A central aspect is the possibility of flexible adaptation of the generation decisions to the
physician's needs and preferences. Therefore, the scenario also involves a toolbox
for defining and editing both the document plans (i.e., defining the ordering of
information in the text) and the devices for mapping non-linguistic information
to linguistic expressions (of different types); these devices we call *frames*. The
second central aspect is the overall portability: Obviously, developing the text
generation component is initially more costly than a simple text block system.
It is thus of utmost importance to ensure the portability and adaptability of the
various sub-components to other clinical domains, so that overall a cost-effective
solution results.

   In the next section, we first explain the overall system architecture in detail,
and thereafter turn specifically to the natural language generation component.

3   SemScribe System Overview and Architecture

The architecture of the SemScribe system is depicted in figure 2. Semscribe
assumes an IT environment where general patient data and diagnostic images
are available from a hospital information system (HIS) or a picture archiving
and communication system (PACS).

   SemScribe is comprised of

- a GUI for structured data entry,
- the Natural Language Generation (NLG) component proper,
- medical and linguistic knowledge stored in the ID MACS terminology server,
- authoring tools for creating and editing linguistic knowledge, and

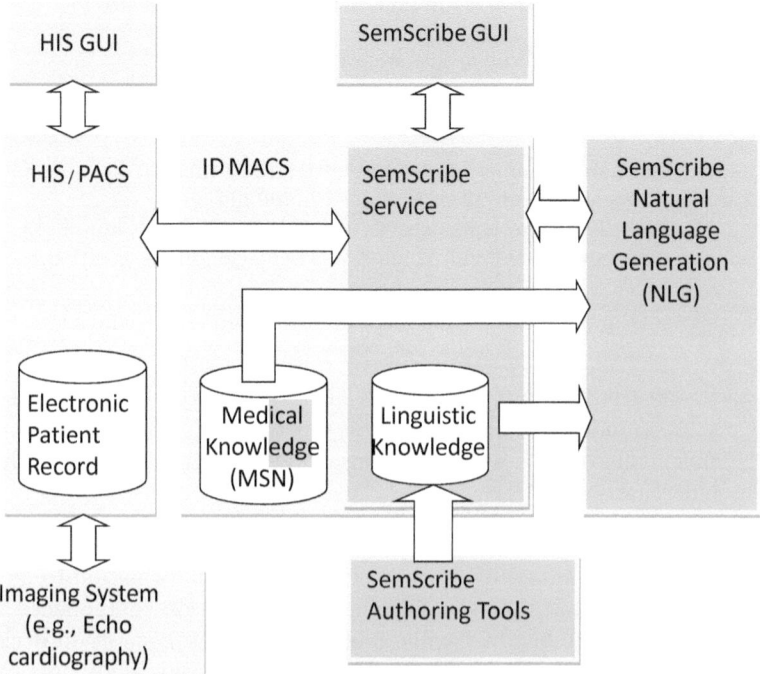

Fig. 2. The architecture of the SemScribe system. Components of the SemScribe project proper are shown in green.

- a communication module within the ID MACS® terminology server that makes data and knowledge available to the NLG component and delivers generated text to the GUI.

SemScribe uses the ID MACS® – medical semantic network – by ID as a general source of medical knowledge, which has been extended with special cardiological knowledge to cover the application domain of SemScribe.

3.1 User Interface and Data Format

A screenshot of the graphical interface for data entry that will be verbalized as *'Both ventricles and the right atrium are of normal size.'* is shown in figure 3.

The output of structured data entry – and hence, the input to the language generator – can generally be described as a list of triples *(object,attribute,value)* where the object typically is an organ, the attribute a property (e.g. length) and the value the actual measurement or interpretation, for example *(leftVentricle, size, normal)*. We refer to these triples as observations.

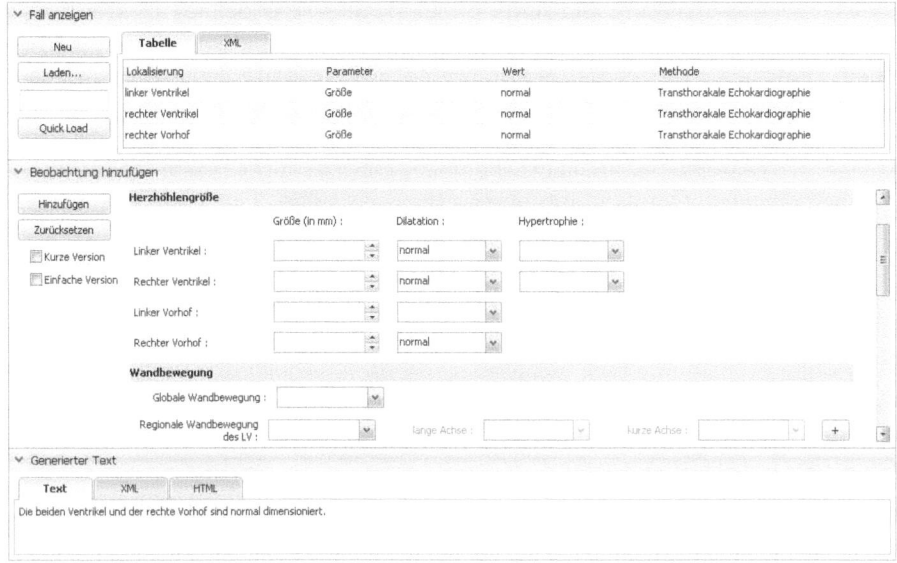

Fig. 3. Screenshot of the graphical interface for data entry (output text in German)

4   Natural Language Generation

In the SemScribe approach, natural language generation is sentence-wise incremental, driven by the input of the user interface. For architectural simplicity, we currently explore the use of a 'slim' processing pipeline [11] in which partial solutions are passed from one processing module to the next. The processing pipeline is structured as follows:

1. Data entry: user enters input via a web form (section 3.1 above),
2. Document planning (section 4.1),
3. Sentence planning including aggregation, frame instantiation and sentence construction, amongst others (section 4.2),
4. Referring expression generation including logical inferencing over the ontology (section 4.3),
5. Morphological realization (section 4.4).

This processing pipeline will be described in the next sections.

4.1   Document Planning

The document planner defines the overall structure of the document. This concerns paragraphs, headlines and content order. The planner can be configured individually according to the needs of the application and the preferences of the hospital or physician.

The general structure and order of the document is defined in a document template. This organizes hierarchical paragraphs, headlines and the order of the final content. To this end, abstract *content elements* are defined as containers for observations, which may be arranged within the same sentence.

The document planner does not have to be adjusted to process other languages. To generate texts in another domain, the user supplies new configurations of the document template and observation mappings. The result of document planning is the document template filled with the input observations.

4.2   Sentence Planning

The sentence planning task includes aggregation, lexicalization of observations, and referring expressions planning. Sentence planning is performed by recursively composing partially specified syntactic trees, similar in spirit to the SPUD [14] and PROTECTOR [8] systems.

The sentence planner works on all observations within a content element, resulting in one or more sentences for each content element. The linguistic knowledge used for sentence planning is organized in frames and concept entries, which control the lexicalization of the input. Each frame describes a specific aspect of the domain language and contains a set of templates, each one representing a syntactic tree as a possible sentence plan for the aspect considered in the frame. Templates may recursively invoke other frames, thus constructing the final sentence plan for an observation from multiple substructures.

In this section, we describe the overall sentence planning process for a content element from observations to sentence plan.

Concepts. The input observation contains codes for *attribute*, *object* and *value* (see section 3.1). The codes point to concepts in the ontology. A dictionary represents a set of variants for each concept of the domain. Each variant represents a syntactic tree which will be adjoined to the sentence plan. The advantage of using a tree structure rather than a plain string is that different inflectional forms can be realized for the same entry.

Aggregation. Multiple observations are aggregated by identical attributes and values or by object, i.e. different observations were made about the same organ(s).

Frame Instantiation. The next step is to construct a sentence plan for each aggregated observation. This is done by selecting and filling *templates*. Templates are syntactic structures with variables (*slots*) to be filled. They are organized in frames; each frame describes an aspect of the domain.

The initial frame for processing an observation is determined by the observation attribute. Thus, an observation with attribute 'size' will use the 'size'-frame. The frame contains several templates, each one producing a clause for describing the size of an object. Template selection is generally controlled by the object and value of the input observation. A template requires input slots and restricts them to specific values, such as a specific code or a syntactic category for realization. Next, the slots are filled with the concept dictionary entry for the corresponding input code. Input concepts of organs are marked as referring expressions and a convenient realization variant will be selected later (see Section 4.3). The result of frame instantiation is a syntactic tree usually representing a clause.

The frame instantiation mechanism works language independently. It can combine any syntactic tree of the frame and concept lexicons without making any assumptions about the grammar. Adapting it to other languages entails preparing the appropriate linguistic resources.

Variants Ranking. The selection of the best template or realization variant is based on a ranking of the variant's features. The linguistic resources are annotated with predefined feature-value-pairs. Currently, we use the boolean features *'short'* and *'simple'*. The GUI provides to the user a selection of a short version with abbreviations and compact sentences (often without a verb) and a simple version for the patient instead of the version with medical terms for the physician. The variants are ranked by weight and the best variant is used for realization. Figure 4 shows different versions for the same input.

1. Die beiden Ventrikel und das rechte Atrium sind normal dimensioniert.
   (Both ventricles and the right atrium are of normal size.)
2. Die beiden Herzkammern und der rechte Vorhof sind normal dimensioniert.
   (Both heart chambers and the right atrium are of normal size.)
3. LV, RV und LA normal dimensioniert.
   (LV, RV and LA of normal size.)

Fig. 4. Example for different text versions for the same input

Sentence Construction. Frame instantiation supplies a list of syntactic clause trees. For each clause, the system can generate a simple sentence. In some cases, two or more clauses can be combined.

At this stage in the pipeline we obtained most of the final sentence plan with only the referring expressions still remaining variables. Figure 5 shows the sentence plan at this stage for the example input.

4.3   Referring Expression Generation

The task of generating referring expressions (GRE) can be characterized by the following question: given a domain model – in this case the medical ontology – and a set of referents, how can we uniquely identify the referent(s) using natural language? This task has often been combined with the requirement to be minimal, i.e. to use only a minimal number of properties, and with considerations of computational complexity. Early work often centered around the 'incremental algorithm' [2] which incrementally 'intersects' attributes until the referent is

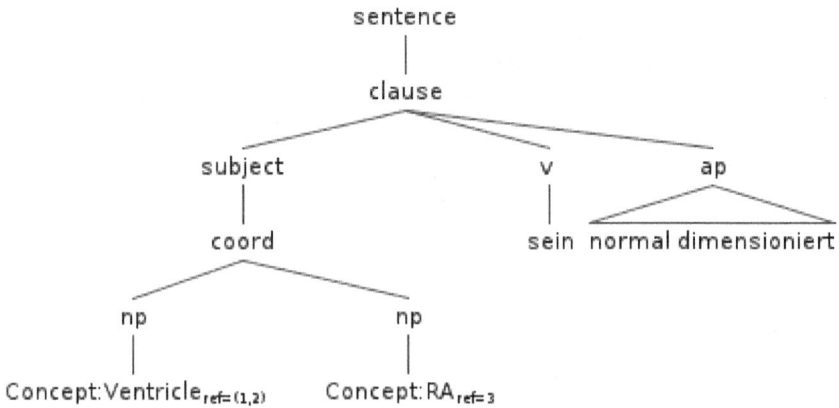

Fig. 5. Sentence plan before referring expression generation

uniquely identifiable. Due to the importance of GRE to the field of language generation in general, several alternative approaches to GRE have been developed, e.g. the graph algorithm of [5] or the 'overgeneration and ranking' approach of [15].

In SemScribe, where domain knowledge is available in the form of a medical ontology that includes ISA relationships between concepts, we often need to model reference to several objects by the name of a dominating concept. The resulting, possibly generalized concept can be used in combination with attributes identified with a standard GRE approach such as the incremental algorithm.

Ontological Inference. In example 1, the use of *'both ventricles'* presupposes that the objects in question are of type 'ventricle' and that there can only be two of them. The required knowledge is part of the ISA relation of a medical ontology of about 80000 concepts/nodes. Nodes/concepts in the ontology are concept classes (TBox), not instances of a particular patient's organ (ABox). The input to NLG, on the other hand, is interpreted as being at the instance level (note the case ID). Ontological inference takes place before the frame/template is selected because it influences the selection.

In the ontological inference stage, we generally search for a concept/node in the ontology that dominates as many input concepts as possible without dominating any other nodes not mentioned in the input. The ISA graph of the ontology is queried by an algorithm that performs a mixed-order traversal for each input concept in turn by walking 'bottom-up' from the input concepts to higher-level concepts and then 'top down' to the sisters of that input concept.

Referring Expression Specification. After syntactic template selection, i.e. with the syntactic constraints known, the referring expression structure can be specified further and inserted into the sentence plan. For generalized concepts, an appropriate quantifier needs to be selected based on the size of the extensions:

'*both [ventricles]*', '*all four [heart chambers]*'. Furthermore, the inner structure of the referring expression is used to determine the need of a conjunction.

4.4 Morphological Realization

The last generation step is the construction of the actual language output for the sentence plan. This is done by the realization module XBarGen [13]. This module constructs from a sentence plan a binary syntactic tree and moves each constituent into its language specific location. The location and the morphological features of the sentence plan (derived from templates and concept entries) determine the final inflection of the words. The tree will be realized by generating a flat string from the tree and replacing each leaf with its correct inflectional form. To this end a full form dictionary established from Morphisto[1] with 16.500 base forms of German general language is used, as well as standard inflection rules for words missing in the dictionary. The realizer is specialized to German language. Although it is domain independent, the dictionary has to be extended with domain specific terms.

5   Related Work

All of the reporting modules we have seen in clinical systems so far rely on text templates or canned text. These mechanisms have the disadvantage of low expressivity and high redundancy. They require either considerable configuration effort or manual editing of the generated text to ensure a fluent and correct result. Still, template-bases approaches have the advantage that their configuration requires only a minimum of training. On the other hand, we are confident that the authoring tools we have developed for internal use in the project will evolve into configuration tools that can be used easily by medical staff without expert linguist knowledge.

In the computational linguistics community, natural language generation has been employed in the past in the health care sector. Cawsey *et al.* [1] describe a system for generating tailored text that explains treatments, diseases etc. to patients. Reiter *et al.* [10] generate customized letters that encourage people to stop smoking. Both these approaches have a different focus (patients/end users). Regarding the architecture of language generation systems, like [1,10] we chose a slim pipeline over more complex approaches such as 'overgeneration and ranking' [6,16] or machine learned committed choice models [9,7].

6   Conclusions and Future Work

Natural language generation can be a powerful means to communicate complex structured data in a concise and effective way. The actual effectiveness of this

---

[1] http://www1.ids-mannheim.de/lexik/TextGrid/morphisto/

method depends on the quality of the text generation algorithms and the linguistic and domain-specific knowledge used. In this work, we described the application of methods from computational linguistics, in particular natural language generation, to the domain of echocardiology findings. Currently, the SemScribe prototype is evaluated in the cardiology department of our clinical partner. We intend to incorporate the text generation technology developed in SemScribe in future clinical documentation products by ID. An important challenge is to develop user-friendly configuration tools that allow users to customize medical text generation solutions without linguistic expertise while retaining the advantages of our computational linguistics approach.

Acknowledgments. The SemScribe project presented here has been funded by the German Ministry of of Economics and Technology[2]. We wish to express our thanks to Dirk Hüske-Kraus for supporting the project with valuable advice and providing examples of cardiologic discharge letters. We also thank our clinical partners from Klinikum Ernst von Bergmann, Potsdam, for fruitful discussions, example data, deployment and evaluation of the prototype: Yvon Franke, Klaus Bonaventura, Frank Suckrow, Markus Weber.

References

1. Cawsey, A., Jones, R., Pearson, J.: The Evaluation of a Personalised Health Information System for Patients with Cancer. User Modeling and User-Adapted Interaction 10(1), 47–72 (2000)
2. Dale, R., Reiter, E.: Computational Interpretations of the Gricean Maxims in the Generation of Referring Expressions. Cognitive Science 19, 233–263 (1995)
3. Hüske-Kraus, D.: Suregen-2: A shell system for the generation of clinical documents. In: 10th Conference of the European Chapter of the Association for Computational Linguistics (EACL 2003), Budapest, Ungarn (2003)
4. Hüske-Kraus, D.: Text Generation in Clinical Medicine. Methods of Information in Medicine (Methods Inf. Med.) 42(1), 51–60 (2003)
5. Krahmer, E., Verleg, A., van Erk, S.: Graph-based Generation of Referring Expressions. Computational Linguistics 29(1), 53–72 (2003)
6. Langkilde, I., Knight, K.: Generation that Exploits Corpus-based Statistical Knowledge. In: Proceedings of COLING/ACL 1998, Montreal, Canada, pp. 704–710 (1998)
7. Mairesse, F., Walker, M.: Controlling User Perceptions of Linguistic Style: Trainable Generation of Personality Traits. Computational Linguistics 37(3) (2011)
8. Nicolov, N., Mellish, C.: PROTECTOR: Efficient Generation with Lexicalized Grammars. In: Recent Advances in Natural Language Processing (RANLP), vol. II, pp. 221–243. John Benjamins, Amsterdam (1999)
9. Paiva, D.S., Evans, R.: Empirically-based Control of Natural Language Generation. In: Proceedings of the 43rd Annual Meeting of the ACL, pp. 58–65 (2005)

[2] Gefördert durch: Bundesministerium für Wirtschaft and Technologie aufgrund eines Beschlusses des Deutschen Bundestags. Förderkennzeichen KF2604501RR0 und KF2262302RR0.

10. Reiter, E., Robertson, R., Lennox, S., Osman, L.: Using a Randomised Controlled Clinical Trial to Evaluate an NLG System. In: Proceedings of the Annual Meeting of the Association for Computational Linguistics (ACL) (2001)
11. Reiter, E.: Has a Consensus NL Generation Architecture Appeared, and is it Psycholinguistically Plausible? In: Proceedings of the Seventh International Workshop on Natural Language Generation (INLG 1994), Kennebunkport, Maine, USA, pp. 163–170 (1994)
12. Reiter, E., Dale, R.: Building Applied Natural Language Generation Systems. Cambridge University Press, Cambridge (2000)
13. Sawitzky, D.R.: Generierung deutscher Sätze nach dem X-Bar-Schema: Entwurf und Implementierung, BA thesis, University of Potsdam (2011)
14. Stone, M., Doran, C.: Sentence Planning as Description Using Tree-Adjoining Grammar. In: Proceedings of ACL 1997, pp. 198–205 (1997)
15. Varges, S., van Deemter, K.: Generating referring expressions containing quantifiers. In: Proceedings of the 6th International Workshop on Computational Semantics (IWCS-6), Tilburg (2005)
16. Varges, S., Mellish, C.: Instance-based Natural Language Generation. Journal of Natural Language Engineering 16(3), 309–346 (2010)

Accessibility Evaluation for Open Source Word Processors

Christophe Strobbe, Bert Frees, and Jan Engelen

Katholieke Universiteit Leuven, Kasteelpark Arenberg 10,
B-3001 Heverlee-Leuven, Belgium
{christophe.strobbe,bert.frees,jan.engelen}@esat.kuleuven.be

Abstract. In parallel with the products of Microsoft's Office suite, two open source word processors are gaining popularity. OpenOffice.org Writer and its more recent alternative (or "fork") LibreOffice Writer both implement as their default storage format the OpenDocument Text format (ODT, a subset of ODF) and support various output formats including the Portable Document Format (PDF) and XHTML. Through the extensions "odt2daisy" and "odt2braille", developed within the European ÆGIS project, both Writers can also export ODT documents to DAISY (audio books, talking books) and to printable Braille, taking into account its language and country dependent formatting rules. This contribution focuses on the accessibility evaluation software that was developed in the same European ÆGIS project, intended to support authors in creating accessible ODT documents that can be converted error-free into DAISY and/or Braille.

Keywords: Accessibility, accessibility evaluation, office documents, OpenOffice.org, LibreOffice, Evaluation and Report Language (EARL).

1 Introduction

Digital accessibility, i.e. a usable access to ICT based information, covers many areas. The E-ACCESSIBILITY POLICY TOOLKIT FOR PERSONS WITH DISABILITIES developed by the International Telecommunication Union (ITU) and the GLOBAL INITIATIVE FOR INCLUSIVE ICTS (G3ICT), created to support the implementation of the UN CONVENTION ON THE RIGHTS OF PERSONS WITH DISABILITIES [17] cover the following technology areas: wireless phones, radios, television, remote consoles, land line phones, Web sites, personal computers, software, electronic kiosks, broadband services and access to published works [6]. Access to office formats used for word processing, spreadsheets and presentations is a superset of and a precondition for "access to published works".

In practice there are considerably fewer guidelines and tools related to the accessibility of office formats than for web content. However, office formats are often used as a source for web content, for example by exporting word processing files as HTML or PDF. Office formats also need to be accessible in order to constitute a suitable source for formats aimed at persons with disabilities, notably audio books (typically DAISY books [7]) and Braille.

A. Holzinger and K.-M. Simonic (Eds.): USAB 2011, LNCS 7058, pp. 575–583, 2011.
© Springer-Verlag Berlin Heidelberg 2011

It is also anticipated that the future DAISY standard will be closely linked with ePUB, the most popular e-book standard [18]. ODF can then also be used as a basis for e-book publishing.

Authors therefore would greatly benefit from guidance for accessible authoring that is integrated into an office suite. The accessibility checker for OpenOffice.org and LibreOffice Writer developed in the framework of the ÆGIS project [3] provides this kind of guidance.

The remainder of this paper describes the background for this tool, how it is implemented and what functionality it offers. It also explains why a taskpanel was chosen as user interface, describes how authors can use this taskpanel to repair errors and warnings, gives examples of the automatic and semi-automatic repairs supported by the checker and describes very briefly which errors and warnings are implemented. For a more technical approach we refer to [16].

2   Accessibility of Office Formats

2.1   Existing Accessibility Evaluation Tools

Since the publication of the Web Content Accessibility Guidelines (WCAG) 1.0 in 1999 [4], many tools for the evaluation of web content have been developed. The website of the World Wide Web Consortium (W3C) contains a database of Web accessibility evaluation tools that currently lists a few dozen tools [14]. These tools range from simple colour contrast checkers to "web accessibility managers" for website administrators. Compared to this database, the list of accessibility evaluation tools for office formats is very short.

A few tools for the evaluation of PDF documents are available (Adobe Acrobat Pro, NetCentric's CommonLook Section 508 for Adobe Acrobat, the freeware PDF Accessibility Checker [PAC] by the Swiss organisation Zugang für Alle/Access for All and the web-based PDF accessibility checker by the eGovMon project in Norway), but these tools cover PDF as a final-form output format that cannot be easily edited.

As stated above, tools that evaluate accessibility of word processing files are very scarce:

- aDesigner is a tool that was originally developed by IBM Tokyo [11] and later donated to the Eclipse Foundation [5]. This tool is a disability simulator for web content that also helps users check the accessibility of OpenDocument Format (ODF) and Flash content.
- The accessibility checker introduced in Microsoft Word 2010, PowerPoint 2010 and Excel 2010, which provides errors, warning and tips [13], is the first evaluation tool that is built directly into an office suite.

aDesigner is therefore the only tool that evaluates the accessibility of ODF content. Other checkers that were developed in the past have since been abandoned. The OPEN DOCUMENT FORMAT ACCESSIBILITY EVALUATION TOOL developed by a team of students at the University of Illinois at Urbana-Champaign under the supervision of Dr. Jon Gunderson came online in 2006 [8] but has not been available for several years. The SourceForge project hosting site contains at least 9 ODF accessibility checkers that were started in 2006 as part of the "IBM Accessibility Phase 2 Contest" in Japan. These projects have names such as "ODT Accessibility Checker", "ODT Checker", "Simple ODT Validator" and "ODF Accessibility Validator" but all have been abandoned.

2.2 LibreOffice/OpenOffice.org as a Source for Accessible Formats

OpenOffice.org is probably the most widely used open source office suite. Both OpenOffice.org and its recent fork LibreOffice can be used to create accessible content. Guidance is available in various locations, including the ODF ACCESSIBILITY GUIDELINES by the Accessibility subcommittee of the OASIS Open Document Format for Office Applications (OpenDocument) TC [12], the AUTHORING TECHNIQUES FOR ACCESSIBLE OFFICE DOCUMENTS by the Accessible Digital Office Document (ADOD) Project [2] and OPENOFFICE.ORG AND ACCESSIBILITY by Web Accessibility in Mind (WebAIM) [15].

Thanks to the recent availability of the open source extensions odt2daisy [10] and odt2braille [9], both developed in the framework of the ÆGIS project, OpenOffice.org and LibreOffice Writer can export OpenDocument Text (ODT) to DAISY books and to Braille, respectively. However, in order to create valid and usable DAISY books or Braille documents, the ODT source documents need to fulfil a number of criteria, for example,

- images and other objects need a text alternative, which can be rendered for visually impaired readers as synthetic speech or Braille,
- headings need to be styled with Heading styles instead of big bold text or other visual characteristics that suggest headings,
- the default language of the document and any language changes inside the document need to be identified in order to select the correct speech synthesis engine or Braille translation table during the conversion process,
- images need to be in JPEG or PNG (Portable Network Graphics) format when exporting to DAISY. This is a constraint of the DAISY standard.

Some accessibility criteria are easy to fulfil, while others are easily overlooked, for example, because they have no visual effect (e.g. adding text alternatives to objects, accidentally creating empty headings). Some criteria are only relevant when exporting to specific other formats, for example, the restriction on image formats in DAISY.

It is clear that integrating support for accessible authoring into OpenOffice.org/LibreOffice Writer would make it easier for authors to meet the accessibility criteria.

3 The ODT Accessibility Checker

3.1 General Approach

In the previous chapter the need for an accessibility checker was clearly demonstrated. Within the framework of the European Ægis project, such a checker was developed by the authors at K.U.Leuven.

3.2 User Interface

The goal of the accessibility checker is to make users aware of accessibility issues in their content. Ideally, this should be as straightforward as checking the spelling, a feature that is built into several office suites, but ***accessibility is more complex than spelling***. There are several ways in which authors could be alerted to accessibility issues. Several methods were explored in the initial stages of the project.

The *first* option consisted in adding a new layout mode, similar to the Print Layout and Web Layout that can be found in Writer's View menu. This new "Accessibility View" would make authors aware of how assistive technologies (AT) "perceive" the document. For example, where an image has no text alternative, there would be nothing (or just an empty frame). Where headings are faked by means of big bold text instead of the appropriate Heading styles, the content of these headings would be rendered as normal text. Where tables are "faked" by paragraphs of tab-separated columns, the text of the "columns" could simply run together. However, such an Accessibility View would be incomplete without guidance on how to repair the issues. There was also a technical barrier: the accessibility checker is developed as an extension, and extensions for OpenOffice.org or LibreOffice cannot create new layout modes.

The *second* option consisted in adding errors and warnings to the source document by means of highlighting and/or some type of comments or notes. When using highlighting, removing the highlighting should be as simple as clicking a button. Unfortunately, adding such highlighting can only be done by modifying the document; the accessibility checker would then need to remove any remaining highlighting when the user closes the document without repairing all the issues (and in this process distinguish between its own highlighting and highlighting added by the user!). The same is true for underlining: the type of underlining that is used by the spelling checker cannot be created by an extension, and the type of underlining that can be created by an extension would become part of the document (unlike the wavy underlining that most word processors use for spelling errors). Using OpenOffice.org's built-in comment system to provide information on accessibility issues was judged too technical and insufficiently user-friendly.

The different options were extensively discussed within the group of ÆGIS software specialists and the project finally settled on the use of a ***taskpanel*** to display a list of errors and warnings and all the other required information. The taskpanel is a component that has been available in Writer only since OpenOffice.org and LibreOffice 3.3 (late 2010).

The taskpanel of the accessibility checker consists of three parts (cf. figure 2).

Fig. 1. Part of a text document in which a table layout is suggested by using visual clues (spaces and tabs)

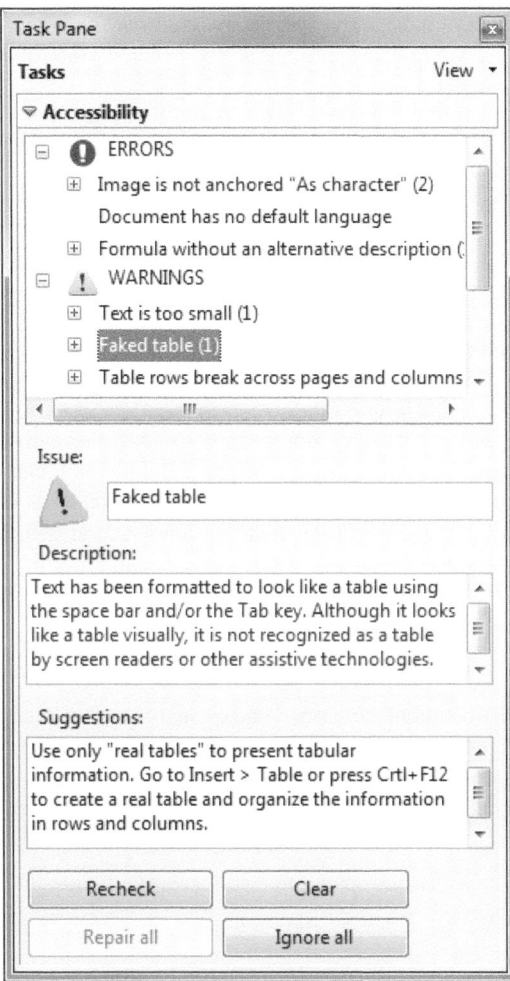

Fig. 2. Taskpane of the Accessibility checker, displaying the problems with the texts shown in fig. 1

The top part displays a list of errors and warnings for issues detected in the document. When the author selects an error or warning, the relevant section of the document is highlighted (in a way similar to the highlighting used by the Accept or Reject changes dialog). The middle part displays three types of information for the error or warning currently highlighted in the top part: the name of the issue, a description (which usually explains why something is an accessibility issue) and suggestions for repair. The bottom part contains four buttons: a 'Recheck' button to trigger the accessibility evaluation, a 'Clear' button to clear the list of errors and warnings, a 'Repair' button to repair issues that can be fixed automatically or semi-automatically, and an 'Ignore' button that can be used to delete a false positive. The

Repair button only becomes active when an issue can be repaired automatically or semi-automatically. Examples of automatic repair include the following:

- When the checker finds an empty heading (i.e. an empty paragraph with a Heading style), activating Repair replaces the Heading style with the Default style.
- When a table allows rows to break across pages and columns, activating Repair unchecks the option "Allow row to break across pages and columns" that authors would otherwise need to find in the Table Format dialog.

Examples of semi-automatic repair include the following:

- When the document has no default language, activating Repair opens the language settings dialog, where authors can set the default language for documents.
- When an image or other object has no text alternative, activating Repair opens the Description dialog, where authors can enter the object's title (which would match HTML's alt attribute) and description.
- When the document's title field is empty, activating Repair opens the document properties dialog, where authors can enter this metadata item. The document title is required by odt2daisy when converting the document to an audio book.

Many repairs cannot be performed automatically or semi-automatically, for example,

- When the document contains images in formats not supported by DAISY, the author needs to convert the images to JPEG or PNG outside Writer and re-insert the new image.
- When a table contains merged cells, the author must decide whether to split to individual cells again or to simplify the table in a different way.

In each of these instances, the repair suggestions explain what the author can do to fix the issue.

3.3 Implemented Issues and Warnings: Some Examples

Web developers and web accessibility advocates can refer to the W3C's Web Content Accessibility Guidelines (WCAG) as the generally accepted reference for web accessibility. Authors of office formats are not so fortunate. They can refer to Accessibility Guidelines Version 1.0 prepared by the ODF Accessibility subcommittee or the Authoring Techniques for Accessible Office Documents by the ADOD project (see above), but these documents don't have a structure based on testable and easily reference-able success criteria that is attractive to evaluation tool developers. The table below gives a few examples of a mapping between WCAG 2.0 success criteria, the Authoring Techniques for Accessible Office Documents from the ADOD project and the ODF checks that are currently implemented in our tool. The evaluation tool can perform checks that are applicable only to Braille or to DAISY; these checks can be enabled or disabled in Writer's options dialog. Some checks do not map to any WCAG 2.0 criterion, for example the check for image formats that are not supported by DAISY. Note that the accessibility checker currently only evaluates

OpenDocument Text (the word processing format); there is no support for presentations or spreadsheets yet.

Table 1. Mapping between WCAG 2.0, ADOD and ODF accessibility checks (a few examples)

WCAG 2.0	ODF Check(s)	Comments
1.1.1 Non-text Content	Error: formula has no text alternative. Warnings: image has no text alternative; object has no text alternative; special characters or symbols are rendered by means of a special font instead of Unicode.	ADOD Technique 3 Some images may be for decoration only and therefore do not require a text alternative.
1.3.1 Info and Relation-ships	Warnings: table contains merged cells; table cell contains another table; table has no repeatable heading row(s); table rows break across pages or columns; table is very long; long table has caption below table instead of above; caption is not linked to any image or table; text formatting (e.g. big bold text) suggests that a paragraph should have a Heading style.	ADOD Technique 6 (using named styles instead of direct formatting) ADOD Technique 7.1, 7.2, 7.3, 7.4
1.4.8 Visual Presentation (AAA)	Warnings: text is justified; font size is smaller than 9 points; long span of text in all caps, underlined or italic.	ADOD Technique 9.1 WCAG does not require a minimum font size or prohibit text that is in all caps, underlined or italic.
2.4.5 Multiple Ways (AA)	Warning: Braille edition has no table of contents.	ADOD Technique 7.5, 7.6
2.4.6 Headings and Labels (AA)	Errors: empty Heading style; incorrectly ordered headings; heading inside a frame (DAISY check). Warnings: document contains no Heading styles; document has more than 6 levels of headings (which is not acceptable for a DAISY document).	ADOD Technique 5 Some documents may not require headings, e.g. letters.
3.1.1 Language of Page	Error: document has no default language	ADOD Technique 2

Remark: this table is an excerpt of the full, extensively annotated table that will appear in [16].

For various reasons, some WCAG 2.0 success criteria are not listed in our full list. Furthermore some warnings are issued that do not correspond to any success criterion in WCAG 2.0. A few examples:

- The document contains images in a format not supported by DAISY.
- Material will be omitted in the Braille edition because odt2braille is unable to process it.
- The document contains 8 dot Braille but the embosser does not support it.

4   Evaluation and Report Language (EARL)

OpenOffice.org and LibreOffice both support the use of RDF (Resource Description Framework) for storing metadata inside ODF files. The accessibility checker uses this feature and stores information on errors and warnings as RDF inside the ODT document. The format used for this purpose is the Evaluation and Report Language (EARL)[1], an RDF format for describing test results that is being developed by the World Wide Web Consortium (W3C).

5   Outlook

The current version of the ODF accessibility checker evaluates many criteria for accessible documents. In addition to repair suggestions, it also supports automatic and semi-automatic repair functions whenever feasible. If the accessibility checker becomes an integral part of OpenOffice.org and LibreOffice, it could be situated in the Tools menu, below language-related items such as "Spelling and Grammar".

In autumn 2011 the Accessibility checker will be tested thoroughly with the Ægis user panel and results will be available for discussion at USAB 2011.

The accessibility checker will, depending on further discussions within the Ægis project, most likely be released under an open source license, possibly the Lesser General Public License (LGPL) 3, which is also the license for odt2daisy and odt2braille.

Acknowledgements. This work was partially funded by the EC FP7 project ÆGIS - Open Accessibility Everywhere: Groundwork, Infrastructure, Standards, Grant Agreement No. 224348. Additional funding was provided by the DocArch group at Katholieke Universiteit Leuven.

References

1. Abou-Zahra, S. (ed.) Evaluation and Report Language (EARL) 1.0 Schema - W3C Working Draft, May 10 (2011),
   http://www.w3.org/TR/2011/WD-EARL10-Schema-20110510/

2. Accessible Digital Office Document (ADOD) Project. Accessibility of Office Documents and Office Applications, `http://adod.idrc.ocad.ca/`
3. ÆGIS - Open Accessibility Everywhere: Groundwork, Infrastructure, Standards, `http://www.aegis-project.eu/`
4. Chisholm, W., Vanderheiden, G., Jacobs, I. (eds.) Web Content Accessibility Guidelines 1.0 - W3C Recommendation, May 5 (1999), `http://www.w3.org/TR/WCAG10/`
5. Eclipse Foundation. ACTF aDesigner (no date), `http://www.eclipse.org/actf/downloads/tools/aDesigner/index.php`
6. International Telecommunication Union (ITU) and the Global Initiative for Inclusive ICTs (G3ict). Technology areas (no date), `http://www.e-accessibilitytoolkit.org/toolkit/technology_areas`
7. National Information Standards Organization (NISO). ANSI/NISO Z39.86-2005. Revision of ANSI/NISO Z39.86-2002. Specifications for the Digital Talking Book, `http://www.daisy.org/z3986/2005/Z3986-2005.html`
8. Korn, P.: Accessibility test tool for OpenDocument files. Peter Korn's Weblog, December 8 (2006), `http://blogs.oracle.com/korn/entry/automated_testing_of_opendocument_files`
9. odt2braille, `http://odt2braille.sf.net/`
10. odt2daisy, `http://odt2daisy.sf.net/`
11. International Business Machines Corporation (IBM). IBM aDesigner (no date), `http://www-03.ibm.com/able/accessibility_services/adesigner.html`
12. Microsoft Corporation. Accessibility Checker (no date), `http://office2010.microsoft.com/en-us/starter-help/accessibility-checker-HA010369192.aspx`
13. OpenDocument - Accessibility SC, `http://www.oasis-open.org/committees/tc_home.php?wg_abbrev=office-accessibility`
14. World Wide Web Consortium (W3C). Web Accessibility Evaluation Tools: Overview, `http://www.w3.org/WAI/ER/tools/` (last updated March 17, 2006)
15. Web Accessibility in Mind (WebAIM). OpenOffice.org and Accessibility (no date), `http://webaim.org/techniques/ooo/`
16. Strobbe, C., Frees, B., Engelen, J.: An Accessibility Checker for OpenOffice.org and LibreOffice Writer. Paper accepted for the second Ægis Conference, Brussels, December 1-2 (2011)
17. United Nations CONVENTION on the RIGHTS of PERSONS with DISABILITIES (December 2006), `http://www.un.org/disabilities/convention/conventionfull.shtml`
18. EPUB standard for electronic books, `http://en.wikipedia.org/wiki/EPUB`

A Touch Sensitive User Interface Approach on Smartphones for Visually Impaired and Blind Persons

Elmar Krajnc, Mathias Knoll, Johannes Feiner, and Mario Traar

FH JOANNEUM, Internet Technology
Werk-VI-Straße 46, 8605 Kapfenberg, Austria
{elmar.krajnc,mathias.knoll,johannes.feiner,
mario.traar.itm08}@fh-joanneum.at
http://www.fh-joanneum.at/itm

Abstract. This paper presents a user interface concept for touch screens which enables visually impaired or blind people to control applications. More and more people tend to switch to advanced smart phones with touch screen technology. So do blind people in order to have a powerful computer in their hands to support them. Unfortunately, a touch interface is not as easy to control as classical hardware buttons with a fixed location and haptic feedback. With advanced frameworks it should be possible to modify applications in a way to support the usage of touch screens for the visually impaired. The suggested new solution for Android mobile phones is to provide specialised "talking touch" views, such as a "talking touch list", which allow fast input with audio feedback. An early prototype version showed an already promising positive response on first usability studies with the target group.

Keywords: Touch, Accessibility, Mobile Computing, Visually Impaired, Android, iPhone, GUI.

1   Introduction

Nowadays the most common personal information devices are mobile phones. Today about 20% of the phone owners use smart phones and the number is rising [2]. Modern smart phones provide much CPU power and users have thousands of applications at their fingertips. Fingers are also important for the user interface. Normal mobile phones with a small display and a keypad are getting rare. Smart phones with only a few keys or buttons and a large touch screen are now state of the art technology. Mobile operation systems which support mostly touch screens represent about 50% of the market and it is predicted that in 2015 about 80% of all smart phones will run a touch screen supported OS [6]. For blind people the transition to up-to-date handhelds means to switch from classical phones with hardware buttons to new phones with touch technology. This shift is a huge step further from configurable "soft keys", where users do not know the meaning of a key in advance. Soft keys require to read the text (the title of the

A. Holzinger and K.-M. Simonic (Eds.): USAB 2011, LNCS 7058, pp. 585–594, 2011.

button) which describes the current action. Therefore blind people have to guess from the current context what a button is for. That kind of navigation through applications is more difficult, but with touch screens phone users have no idea at all, whether there are any buttons to click on, or where the buttons are located on the current user interface.

Android phones using the Google frameworks and Apple iPhones have some assisting technology built in (see Section 2). For others, as for example Microsoft Win Phone 7, not even screen readers are available at the moment.

1.1   Hypothesis and Expected Results

The idea to provide visually impaired and blind people with new ways to interact with the applications on their phones. This requires the improvement of the software which controls the input and output for each navigation step within an application. Selecting options and entering information should be as easy and as accurate as possible. A framework should provide developers with the required functionality. Adapting existing applications for blind people should not be too difficult. Implementing only a few modifications, by using the framework described in Section 3.2, should be enough.

The following chapters describe the context of our studies including the usage and the development constraints (Section 3.1). The current state of the art of research and also the existing support on different smart phone platforms is explored in Section 2. The overall design, the concept and the prototype development are laid out in Section 3.2. Finally, the consequences of using the new "talking touch" framework can be found in Section 3 (which describes the feedback of the usability tests also), and the outlook of ongoing development is in the last Section 5.

2   Related Work

Different aspects of usability for visually impaired people have been research topics for a long time. Audio based navigation support is discussed by Sánchez et al. [13]. Several smartphone based assistive technologies are compared in [11]. See Krajnc et al. [9] for a developer's view on mobile software development for blind people, especially the user centred interaction design for the target group. General usability standards have been set by Nielsen [12] back in 1993 and most of them still apply to interfaces on mobile phones. Special design guidelines for mobile computers are also given by Holzinger and Errath [4].

Web accessibility[1] (e.g. set text size, contrast, flash built for screen readers, image alternatives) is important, but not enough to handle modern touch screen

---

[1] Accessibility standards for people with disabilities can for instance be found e.g. in U.S. Section 508 where Standard 1194.26 focuses especially on desktop and portable computers (keyboards and other mechanically operated controls, touch screens, biometric identification, and ports and connectors) http://www.uspto.gov/web/offices/cio/s508/08desktops.htm.

mobile phones. The American Foundation for the Blind (AFB) still does not list any touch screen phone on their "cell phones and related software" web pages[2].

For people with impaired vision the modern smart phones provide different accessibility technologies such as screen readers and physical feedback. The *iPhone*, for example, provides a screen reader called "Voice Over"[3] which can also be controlled by gestures. If Voice Over is switched on the clicking differs from normal mode, i.e. when touching a button a corresponding description can be heard and on double-tap the button gets activated. Often, additional feedback such as a sound is generated when moving from one button to another. Gestures like swiping help to move back and forth between items or screens. Text input of long text is done by moving one finger over the soft keys and by confirming with a tap of another finger.

Simple other features like switching to "white on black" or zoom functionality are available. On powerful devices even (limited) voice control is available. The iPhone provides only music and phone book support.

The biggest problem is still to provide enough orientation and context on the screen. Fitting out smart phones with internationalisation features – providing automated spoken text in different languages – is even more difficult and expensive. Getting used to and learning the ins and outs of screen readers is not too big a problem for disabled people. Initial training pays off for blind people very soon. So hardware buttons with tactile feedback can indeed be replaced by advanced touch screen functionality. Support by means of vibration, spoken text and sounds is possible. On request bluetooth hardware can be attached. On the Apple pages a list of more than 30 supported braille devices[4] can be found.

Several assistive technologies are available for the *Android* phones, but they are neither built into the system nor are they activated by default. Users choose from different libraries for supporting their applications. On the Android, unlike on the iPhone, the developers are requested to put much effort into adapting each and every application they implement to the special needs of the visually impaired. End users must even check if any text-to-speech library is installed.

An advanced library is the "eyes free"[5] software which replaces the normal graphical interface with an eyes-free shell. The main idea is to provide radial stroke-based gestures to trigger a certain functionality. For example, the "Talking Dialer" lets users enter numbers via those gestures. On the one hand, vibrating

---

[2] The American Foundation for the Blind lists cell phones and related software at http://www.afb.org/ProdBrowseCatResults.asp?CatID=74.

[3] Voice Over: http://www.apple.com/accessibility/iphone/vision.html

[4] iPhone supported braille devices: http://www.apple.com/accessibility/iphone/braille-display.html.

[5] Find eyes-free for android at http://code.google.com/p/eyes-free or download TalkBack/Kickback/Soundback from https://market.android.com/details?id=com.google.android.marvin.talkback.

feedback assures proper selection and mistakes can be corrected (unintended input undone) by shaking the phone. Developers can look up good practices[6] for coding against the accessibility layer. This software layer provides APIs to text-to-speech, haptic feedback and trackball or directional controller (d-pad) navigation.

Windows Mobile 6.5 phones can use some accessibility features with screen readers such as Talks[7] or Mobile Speak[8]. Win Phone 7 does not offer accessibility features (except for TTY support and speech recognition). Hopefully more features will be provided in the upcoming versions[9].

Several aspects of routing (visually) impaired people are addressed by Bradley and Dunlop [3]. They focus on the human-computer-interaction (HCI) point of view, especially on the mental and physical demands for people with special needs.

Mobile or smart phones are cost-effective assistive technologies for blind people [11], therefore suitable software is requested. For visually impaired and blind people a lot of research has been done in various areas like e-learning or medicine. Only few special surveys in the field of touch screens for blind people have been performed. See for example Bigham and Cavender [1] for audio captchas which allow blind people to use this way of secure login. Holzinger et al [5] describe aspects of improving mobile applications for elderly and Sánchez et al. [13] for an approach of navigation through audio-based virtual environments for blind people. Findings about developments employing user centred design (UCD) for visually impaired people can be found in Krajnc et al. [9].

Approaches for alternative input methods include special ways to enter letters. Even special writing concepts have been invented as such as EdgeWrite [14] which introduces a mobile device friendly unistroke font. Blind Sight [10] offers auditory feedback to this users and allows them to interact with the mobile phone without looking at the screen.

Some of these related projects offer the opportunity to interact with keys and buttons. To provide an accessible user interface on touch screens we need new forms of interaction. In Slide Rule [8] the touch screen is operated with multi touch gestures. With the help of a touch screen and vibration V-Braille [7] represents Braille characters on a standard mobile phone.

---

[6] It is good practice on Android to make input elements focusable and provide every input widget with a content description. See at http://developer.android.com/guide/practices/design/accessibility.html.

[7] Nuance Talks http://www.afb.org/prodProfile.asp?ProdID=752&SourceID=74

[8] http://www.optelec.nl/hulpmiddelen-voor-blinden_slechtzienden-en-dyslectici/producten/toegankelijke-mobiele-telefoon/spraaksoftware/mobile-speak.html

[9] For accessibility on Win Phone 7 see http://www.microsoft.com/windowsphone/en-us/howto/wp7/basics/ease-of-access-on-my-phone.aspx. Mango Update is scheduled for fall 2011 http://www.microsoft.com/windowsphone/en-us/cmpn/mango-overview.aspx.

3   Conception and Implementation Results

3.1   Conception

For this paper we assume the following context: the target group comprises blind or visually impaired people who use an application for way finding (indoor and outdoor navigation). For the development of this application open source software development was used to make the results available to the community. The Android[10] framework is the first choice for developers who seek a maximum of flexibility. The development kits allow software to be run on the broadest range of hardware. In future work software for the iOS platform might be coded also, but the "experimental possibilities" on iPhones and iPads much more limited.

Once the design of the GUI was finished, its implementation started. The milestones were on the one hand providing an easy to use framework of menu and list interfaces and on the other hand the completion of one menu feature as a proof of concept. Figure 1 shows a diagram of the task at hand. A demo of the talking touch list view is shown in Figure 3.

3.2   Implemented Prototype with "Talking Touch List View" and "Talking Touch Menu View"

Views are the visible part of an activity in an Android application. They can either be defined in XML files or in source code. Due to the fact that the "Talking Touch View" is created to be used by blind and visually impaired people, distinct classes had to be designed. They provide the functionality needed. The main task for the view is inherent in the "text-to-speech" functionality, which is initialised in one abstract class called "AbstractWays4AllView". Derived from it are the classes "AbstractTalkingTouchView" and "AbstractTalkingTouchListView". The first is responsible for the menu interface and the second for the list interface. Whenever an activity is in need of one of these views, it will implement a view derived from the abstract classes (see Figure 2).

The touchable menus are highly dynamic. A menu implementation contains four areas where the user may be directed to another activity by double tapping them. Aside from menus, lists constitute a major and vital ingredient for graphical user interfaces. In order to create a list component, especially for blind people, certain conditions had to be met.

Firstly, the default list representation in Android comes along with a neat scrolling feature. Visually impaired users depend on element's with fixed positions. So this kind of scroll list is not usable for them, because they cannot remember an element's location. For this reason it was decided to build a new type of list which is presented as a set of pages.

The advantage of the list implementation is its independency from resolutions of different devices. The touchable areas are highly dynamic, too. All the features of the menu representation (e.g. text-to-speech capabilities) are also part of the

---

[10] Find the documentation — especially about accessibility — in the SDK online http://developer.android.com/sdk.

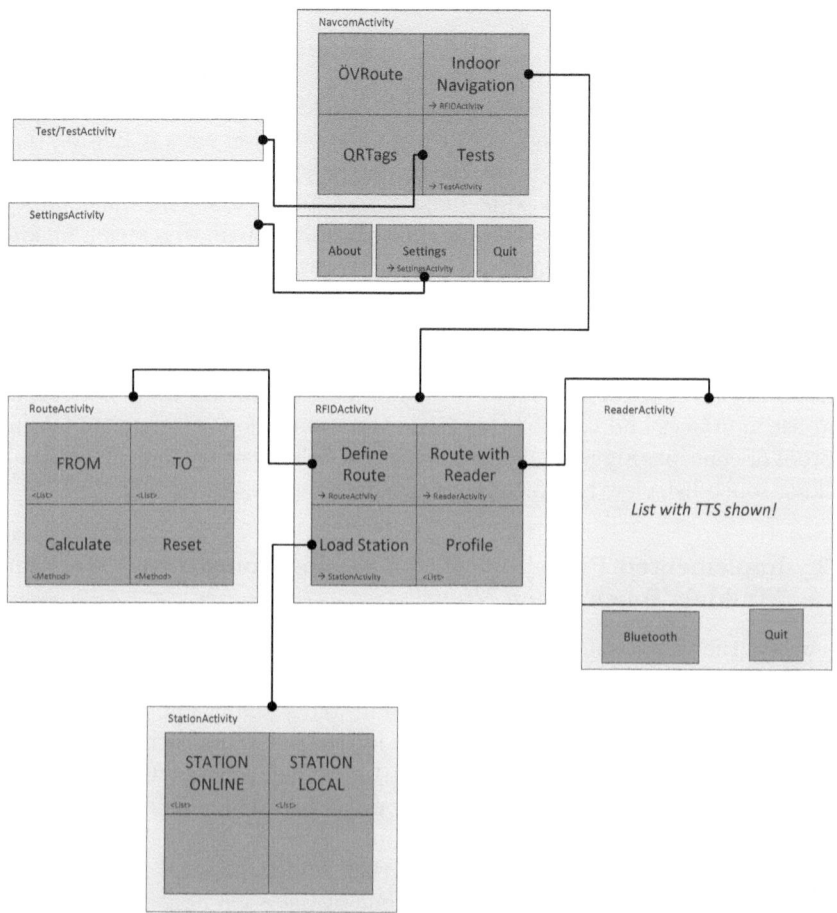

Fig. 1. The diagram showing the GUI sections

list view. A vital functionality is to provide the information where the list starts, ends, to which page someone may proceed and how many pages are left.

When starting the application the first time, a surface with several logos appears. As this is an application for visually impaired people, no further graphics are needed. For development and documentation reasons, it is however, possible to switch to a visual representation of the touchable areas of the application.

3.3   Implementation of Talking Dialer Gesture Input

Inputs from the user have so far not been covered by the concept of the Talking Touch View. There are some approaches that facilitate the textual input by blind people. For instance the Talking Dialer of the Eyes-Free project offers a special

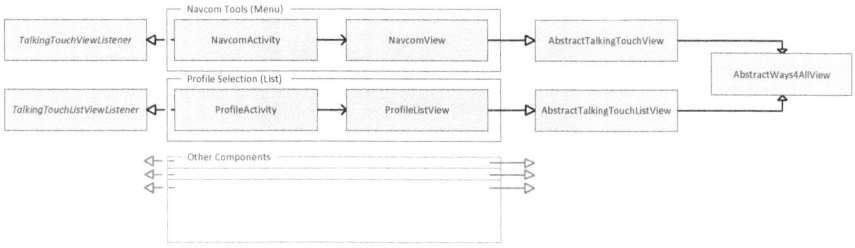

Fig. 2. Classes building one GUI element

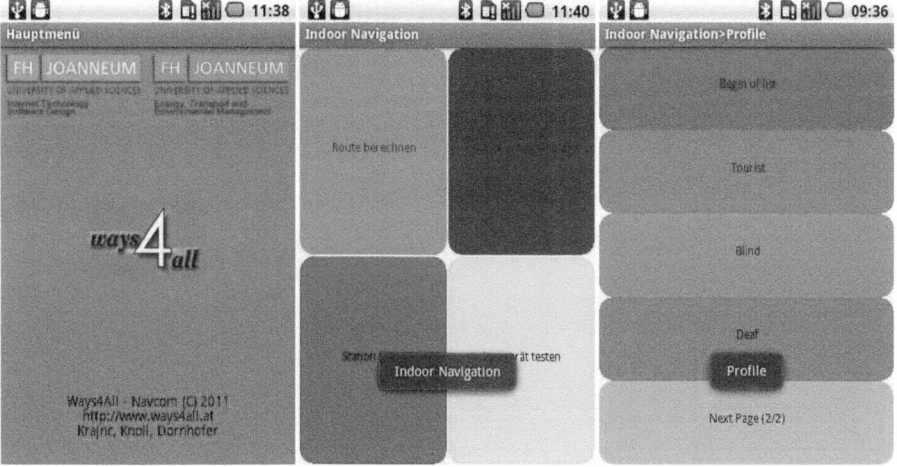

Fig. 3. The 3 screenshots of the actual application are showing the main screen, the menu areas of the "Indoor Navigation" menu and the list of profiles

input scheme or user input by means of the android gestures. In this application we made the text input method exchangeable. For example, one might choose to input via the Talking Dialer Gesture Input (see Figure 4). If the user prefer one special kind of textual input, she can change it in any way.

4 Evaluation of the User Interface

To evaluate our user interface we conducted a usability study. We recruited seven users to perform a usability test [12]. There were two blind participants, two participants with a visual disorder and three with no visual restraints. Five out of the seven persons were male and had experiences with smart phones. Two were female and had no experience with smart phones (detail see table 1).

To test the user interface we prepared a Thinking Aloud (TA) test [12]. After a short introduction to the touch screen device the participants got assignments.

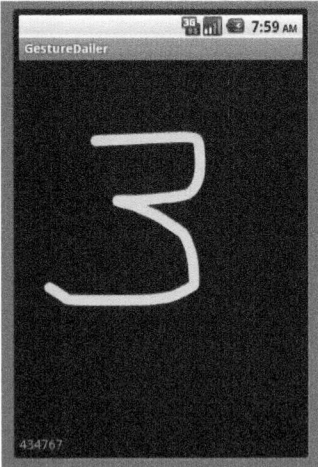

Fig. 4. The screenshots of the textual input with gestures

Table 1. Test participants

	Age	Gender	Visual Faculty	Experience with Usability Testing	Experience with Smart Phones
Testperson 1	31	m	blind	yes	yes
Testperson 2	29	f	Blind	no	no
Testperson 3	26	m	normal	no	yes
Testperson 4	30	f	visual disorder	no	no
Testperson 5	23	m	normal	no	yes
Testperson 6	22	m	normal	yes	yes
Testperson 7	35	m	visual disorder	no	yes

They had to perform six different tasks on the talking touch user interface and four tasks on the gesture interface. They were, for instance, asked to "change the profile to *Blind*" or to "enter the telephone number *543289*". Four testers could successfully finish all tasks of the test. The Talking Touch Interface had a success rate of 88% and the gesture application had a success rate of 89% (find the details in Table2).

According to the feedback given by the participants after the usability test, the navigation and the position of the items were rather simple and easy to access. The selection with a double click is very intuitive and was recognised without any explanation. Some minor problems occurred when the users switched from the four-items menus to the list menu. Also the speed of the voice output was sometimes too fast, but the speech rate could be changed in the general settings. The feedback given after selecting a menu item was sometimes not precise enough.

Table 2. Testresults

	TP1	TP2	TP3	TP4	TP5	TP6	TP7
Ways4All Task 1	ok	ok	ok	ok	ok	ok	ok
Ways4All Task 2	ok	ok	ok	ok	ok	ok	ok
Ways4All Task 3	ok	-	ok	ok	-	ok	ok
Ways4All Task 4	ok	-	ok	ok	-	ok	ok
Ways4All Task 5	ok	ok	ok	ok	ok	ok	ok
Ways4All Task 6	ok	ok	ok	ok	-	ok	ok
Gesture Dailer Task 1	ok	ok	ok	ok	ok	ok	ok
Gesture Dailer Task 2	ok	ok	ok	ok	-	-	ok
Gesture Dailer Task 3	ok	ok	ok	-	ok	ok	ok
Gesture Dailer Task 4	ok	ok	ok	ok	ok	ok	ok

The feedback of the gesture input was good. It was very intuitive and most participants had no problems (One problem was reported, which depends on various writing styles of numbers and letters). All the reported problems did not stem from the basic concept. Therefore, any necessary adaptations can be implemented in future versions of the software without much effort.

5   Future and Outlook

Further research with additional output and input facilities is necessary and already planned as the next steps. For example, the force feedback (vibration) and audible output (fait or loud sound in low or high frequency) will be used as feedback to users. With different shake gestures users can provide input (acknowledge or reject the current selection). The visually impaired - as a marginal group in our society - are awaiting the results which can really improve their mobility and independency in their daily lives.

References

1. Bigham, J.P., Cavender, A.C.: Evaluating existing audio CAPTCHAs and an interface optimized for non-visual use. In: Proc. 27th International Conference on Human Factors in Computing Systems (CHI 2009), pp. 1829–1838. ACM (2009)
2. BITKOM: Jeder fünfte handynutzer besitzt ein smartphone (telekommunikation und neue medien e.v. bundesverband informationswirtschaft. presseinformation) (October 2010), http://www.bitkom.org/de/themen/54894_65506.aspx
3. Bradley, N.A., Dunlop, M.D.: An experimental investigation into wayfinding directions for visually impaired people. Personal Ubiquitous Computing 9(6), 395–403 (2005)
4. Holzinger, A., Errath, M.: Mobile computer web-application design in medicine: some research based guidelines. Univers. Access Inf. Soc. 6, 31–41 (2007), http://dl.acm.org/citation.cfm?id=1283708.1283718

5. Holzinger, A., Searle, G., Nischelwitzer, A.: On some aspects of improving mobile applications for the elderly. In: Proc. 4th International Conference on Universal Access in Human Computer Interaction (UAHCI 2007), pp. 923–932. Springer, Heidelberg (2007)

6. IDC: Idc forecasts worldwide smartphone market to grow by nearly 50 (March 2011), http://www.idc.com/getdoc.jsp?containerId=prUS22762811

7. Jayant, C., Acuario, C., Johnson, W., Hollier, J., Ladner, R.: V-braille: Haptic braille perception using a touch-screen and vibration on mobile phones. In: Proc. 12th International ACM SIGACCESS Conference on Computers and Accessibility (ACCETS 2010), pp. 295–296. ACM (2010), http://doi.acm.org/10.1145/1878803.1878878

8. Kane, S.K., Bigham, J.P., Wobbrock, J.O.: Slide rule: Making mobile touch screens accessible to blind people using multi-touch interaction techniques. In: Proc. 10th International ACM SIGACCESS Conference on Computers and Accessibility (AS-SETS 2008). pp. 73–80. ACM (2008)

9. Krajnc, E., Feiner, J., Schmidt, S.: User Centred Design Interaction Design for Mobile Application Focused on Visually Impaired and Blind People. In: Leitner, G., Hitz, M., Holzinger, A. (eds.) USAB 2010. LNCS, vol. 6389, pp. 195–202. Springer, Heidelberg (2010), http://www.springerlink.com/content/c3813w7857315241/

10. Li, K.A., Baudisch, P., Hinckley, K.: Blindsight: Eyes-free access to mobile phones. In: Proc. 26th Annual SIGCHI Conference on Human Factors in Computing Systems (CHI 2008), pp. 1389–1398. ACM (April 2008)

11. Narasimhan, P., Gandhi, R., Rossi, D.: Smartphone-based assistive technologies for the blind. In: Proc. 2009 International Conference on Compilers, Architecture, and Synthesis for Embedded Systems (CASES 2009), pp. 223–232. ACM (2009)

12. Nielsen, J.: Usability Engineering. Morgan Kaufmann (1993)

13. Sánchez, J., Sáenz, M., Pascual-Leone, A., Merabet, L.: Navigation for the blind through audio-based virtual environments. In: Proc. 28th International Conference Extended Abstracts on Human Factors in Computing Systems (HIEA 2010), pp. 3409–3414. ACM (2010)

14. Wobbrock, J.O.: EdgeWrite: A Versatile Design for Text Entry and Control. Ph.D. thesis, Human-Computer Interaction Institute School of Computer Science Carnegie Mellon University (July 2006), http://reports-archive.adm.cs.cmu.edu/anon/hcii/CMU-HCII-06-104.pdf

Added Value of In-Situ Methods in Usability Evaluation of a Self-service Ticketing Machine with a View on Elderly Users: A Case Study

Elke E. Mattheiss[1], Johann Schrammel[1], and Manfred Tscheligi[1,2]

[1] CURE – Center for Usability Research and Engineering, Vienna, Austria
{mattheiss,schrammel}@cure.at
[2] ICT&S, University of Salzburg, Austria
manfred.tscheligi@sbg.ac.at

Abstract. Self-service systems are very common in the public space and usability plays a crucial role for user acceptance. We describe the evaluation of a self-service ticketing machine installed in trams in the city of Graz. Two in-situ methods (behavior observation, contextual interview) and an online survey were used. We discuss advantages of the different methods experienced in the present study according to effort and output. Unsurprisingly online survey was advantageous in terms of time effort. Concerning output, behavior observation identified the most issues with specific interface objects of all methods. Furthermore we were able to identify usage information about the user group of elderlies. Online survey provided a higher number of general issues with the machine and recommendations for change than the two in-situ methods. Further results are discussed and limitations of the study are described in the paper.

Keywords: Usability evaluation, in-situ, behavior observation, contextual interview, online survey, self-service ticketing, case study, elderly users.

1 Introduction

Self-service systems are considered to be modern and efficient and are widely used in public transport. As they need to be operated by a broad range of users with heterogeneous technical abilities, the usability of these systems is essential.

There are various approaches how usability evaluation of computer systems can be performed. The Human-Computer Interaction (HCI) community has brought forth a large diversity of evaluation methods, whose suitability depends on the concrete situation of the evaluation including the computer system to evaluate, the context of use, and the kind of results striven for. Various classifications to categorize these methods according to key aspects can be found in previous literature, like user involvement (required, not required), context of evaluation (generic, application specific), type of results (qualitative, quantitative) [1], objective versus subjective measures, targeted usability aspect (effectiveness, efficiency, satisfaction) [2], study setting (laboratory, field), and target groups (e.g. elderly users [3]). In the present work we used two in-situ methods (behavior observation, contextual interview) and

A. Holzinger and K.-M. Simonic (Eds.): USAB 2011, LNCS 7058, pp. 595–606, 2011.

an online survey. The *behavior observation* consisted of twelve hours observing the buying process at the ticketing machine in the tram. For the *contextual interview* users were asked in the tram about issues with and attitudes towards the ticketing machine right after they used it. The *online survey* was retrievable for a week and the link was distributed by e-mail among acquaintances with prior experience with the ticketing machine. Therefore in-situ methods and online survey differed in the participants' context while they took part in the evaluation: *in the context of system use* (in the tram, nearby the ticketing machine, right after a buying process) and *outside the context of system use* (not in the tram, not right after a buying process). Another difference between the methods relate to the kind of information they are able to provide. Only behavior observation can provide *performance data* (number of specific kinds of errors in a given time period, duration of the buying process) but on the other side only contextual interview and online survey can assess the *users' attitudes and opinions.*

The focus of the present paper is on the advantages of each of the three used methods in terms of effort and output in the evaluation of a self-service ticketing machine. The evaluation was undertaken to find usability issues associated with the ticketing machine. However the focus of this case study is to report and reflect on the used methods in the particular context of a self-service ticketing machine and with a view on elderly users of the system. We describe the time effort for the evaluators and the participants in the different evaluation methods. Furthermore we consider the amount of different kinds of information (interface design issues, general issues with the machine, metric data, user ratings, and user recommendations) which the different methods are able to provide in our specific evaluation.

2   Self-service in Public Spaces

Self-service machines are becoming wide-spread in the public space. Using self-service machines is frequently more time and cost efficient than service by employees. Self-service technology has already transformed entire industries, and nowadays users are confronted with them at airport and travel kiosks, vending machines, food-ordering kiosks, self-checkouts, health care kiosks, and retail kiosks [4]. As self-service systems are intended to be handled without assistance, the usability of the systems plays an important role. [5] provides a review of design guidelines for public information kiosk systems dealing with recommendations for location, physical access, language selection, privacy, help, and input to the system.

Another crucial issue for the design of self-service systems is that they should be accessible for all kinds of users including those having physical or cognitive disabilities. Research efforts target this challenge by intelligent designs which are able to adapt their user interfaces to user characteristics like user heights, seeing ability, and motor abilities influencing the target hitting accuracy (e.g. [6]). Considering elderly people in the design of self-service system is crucial not only because they typically face a variety of impairments but also because age was found to have a negative influence on the preference for service technology over contact to personnel [7].

Researchers investigated the users' interaction with self-service systems in the public space. In [8] and [9] an extensive study about a ticketless travelling system in an airport train is presented. Using behavioral observations they found that users of the system did not actively request assistance and got quickly annoyed when they had problems to operate the machine [8]. That emphasizes the importance of designing easy to understand and operate systems. Usability is also one important factor contributing to the users' acceptance towards a system. According to the prominent Technology Acceptance Model [10] the perceived usefulness and the perceived ease of use are of primary relevance for the attitude towards using a system, which again is a factor for the actual system use. However, research work in the field of self-service ticketing systems (e.g. e-ticketing [11] and mobile ticketing [12]) claim that in addition to ease of use and usefulness also other factors like subjective norm, technology trust [11], social influence, cost, prior experience, risk, and use context [12] are important for the use intention. [13] found that the users' attitude towards self-service in railway ticketing and travel information was more positive when there was offered an interaction with an employee as a fall-back option.

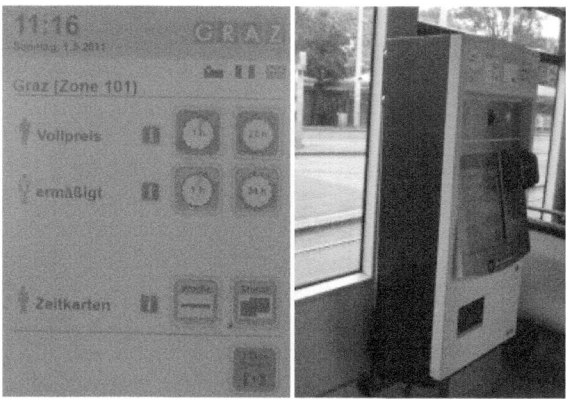

Fig. 1. User interface (left) and positioning (right) of the self-service ticketing machine

In our case the ticket machines were installed in the trams, usually at the second entrance, oriented towards the left side of the tram (see Fig. 1). In this position the users' interaction with the ticketing machine is visible to bystanders. This is relevant for the user interaction because users may be embarrassed when struggling with the machine. As an alternative to using the machine, tickets are available in pre-sale. At the ticketing machine the users have the possibility to buy full fair and reduced tickets for one hour, 24 hours, 3 days (tourist ticket), a week, and a month (see Fig. 1 left). It is possible to pay with coins, credit card, or debit card. Since paying with card requires entering a PIN, trust and risk factors may be important for the user acceptance, because other passengers could potentially see the PIN. To enhance accessibility for a broader range of users the buying procedure is explained at the top of the machine, different languages can be selected, and the contrast settings can be changed. The specifics of the ticketing machine influenced the selection of appropriate evaluation methods, which are described in the next section.

3 Research Method

For the evaluation of a self-service ticketing machine located in the trams not only the interface design, but also a lot of contextual aspects may contribute to the perceived usability of the system. Context is described in [14] as "...the sum of relevant factors that characterize the situation of a user and an application, where relevancy implies that these factors have significant impact on the user's experience when interacting with that application in that situation". In the present evaluation relevant context factors are for example sunlight towards the display, number of people in the tram, and movement of the tram. According to [15] a frequent reason for system failure is the fact that designers do not pay enough attention to the context of system use. Therfore we decided against conducting a traditional usability study in a laboratory setting, because the above stated context factors would be hard to simulate.

In-situ methods have the advantage to consider such context factors as they are conducted directly in the context of system use, and therefore overcome the problem of neglecting it. An example for an in-situ approach is *ethnography* which is roughly characterized by field work in a natural setting, providing a more complete context of activity [16], and typically consisting of a prolonged activity with a discursive and lengthy output [15] like rich descriptions of interactions. An obvious issue with this kind of traditional ethnography is the amount of time it requires. Therefore a "quick and dirty" ethnographic approach, with days of observation sparsely spread over a period of twelve months to evaluate a ticketless travelling system, was used in [8]. By these means it was possible to have a short and focused study. The authors gained with it a general understanding of the situation as well as a reality-check of the system in terms of an evaluation [9]. The authors present excerpts of their observations illustrating several problems and incidents as well as design implications.

Another cost efficient ethnographic approach named *rapid ethnography* is proposed by [17]. We considered some key aspects of this approach to develop our research method. The considered key aspects are to define specific questions (prior to the evaluation) that should be answered (to facilitate motivated looking and avoid a wide-angle lens approach), to choose a reasonable time sample (to ensure a representative and large sample of observations), and to use interactive research approaches like interviews (to understand the user behavior more rapidly in the field). We used the two methods *behavior observation* and *contextual interviews* as an approach of rapid ethnography. This combination of methods allowed us to gather behavioral data from the observations like performance data (e.g. task completion time, number of errors) as well as subjective attitudes and opinions of the users.

A *survey* is a completely different evaluation approach than ethnographic methods. A self-administered mail survey distributed to a random sample of 1000 users was used in [12]. Even less effort is needed when the survey is applied via an online survey tool and the link is distributed to acquaintances, asking them to forward the link to other potentially interested people. This approach was used by us for time and cost reasons. An obvious disadvantage of the survey approach is that it is only possible to gather subjective data about the users' attitudes without being able to capture time measurements and other performance data.

The Present Study. In the following paragraphs the participants and the procedure of the conducted evaluation methods are described in detail. Behavior observation and contextual interview were conducted in-situ at the same time. The online survey was distributed a week after the in-situ evaluation was completed.

Setting of Behavior Observation and Contextual Interview. The behavior observations and the contextual interviews were conducted in the same time period by two evaluators in the trams near the ticketing machine. The study took place in June on a weekday and a weekend day at three different times of the day (about 8.00-10.00, 12.00-14.00, 16.00-18.00) to include a preferably broad range of different users regarding demographic characteristics (e.g. age) and travelling aim (e.g. way to work, travel during leisure time). Evaluators travelled for about two hours with a tramline from one final stop to the other.

Behavior Observation. The focus of the behavior observation was on issues with the user interface design and associated errors, but also other incidents were noted on a prepared protocol. Those incidents include duration of the buying process, type and amount of bought tickets, number of people waiting for buying a ticket, social interactions between users of the ticketing machine, sex of the users, and other user characteristics (e.g. children who are estimated by the observers to be aged under 14 years, elderlies estimated to be aged above 65 years, and physical limitations, foreign language as mother tongue) as effectively as possible. The evaluator observed the buying process of the users from behind. Participants of the behavior observation were all people who used the ticketing machine during the approximately twelve hour observation period. Altogether the buying processes of 122 (50 male, 72 female) users were observed, eight of them were classified according to their appearance as an elderly person older than 65 years. Table 1 lists characteristics of all the participants.

Contextual Interview. For the contextual interview the evaluator asked a user who just finished the buying process to answer some interview questions. Participants were chosen by chance and with a targeted rate of four interviews per hour. Alltogether 45 (25 male, 20 female) users with a mean age of 32 (standard deviation (SD) = 13.96) years were interviewed. One of them was aged above 65 years. The interview took about two-to-three minutes and included nine questions covering problems with the buying process, rating of the usability of the machine, rating of the design, frequency of using the ticketing machine, preference for buying the ticket from the tram driver instead of the machine, proposed changes, and accessibility for users with physical impairments. The answers of the interviewee were recorded with a dictation machine or noted down, if the user was not agreeable with the recording.

Table 1. Characteristics of the participants of the different methods

	Behavior Observation	**Contextual Interview**	**Online Survey**
Number	122	45	26
Sex	50 male, 72 female	25 male, 20 female	10 male, 16 female
Mean Age	-	32.00 years (SD*=13.96) min=12, max=73	33.81 years (SD=13.00) min=17, max=70
Elderlies (65+)	8	1	1

*SD = Standard Deviation

Online Survey. The online survey was created with the open source survey application LimeSurvey [18]. The link to the survey was distributed in terms of a cost and time efficient approach to acquaintances of the authors' private and professional environment that were assumed to have prior experience with the ticketing machine in Graz. Moreover recipients of the link were asked to forward it to potentially interested people of their environment. By these means we aimed to spread the survey out to a more comprehensive sample. The survey took about ten minutes to be completed and covered in addition to the questions of the contextual interview also some questions related to demographic information and usage of the public transport system in general. The survey was online retrievable for one week and in this time period 26 participants completed it. This relatively small number of participants seems to be due to the instance that we announced the link by e-mail and in postings at social networking sites for only one time. Most participants completed the survey right after they received the link. Therefore if a larger sample is targeted the survey should be announced multiple times. In our case 26 participants (10 male, 16 female) with a mean age of 33.81 (SD = 13.00) years sufficed. One participant aged above 65 took part in the survey.

4   Costs and Benefits of the Used Methods

In this part we present and discuss the used methods behavior observation, contextual interview, and online survey in terms of time effort (for evaluators and participants of the study) and output (number of identified usability issues, performance data, ratings, user recommendations). Furthermore we take a closer look on the data related to the elderly users. Because of the prevalence of qualitative data, the results remain mainly on a descriptive level.

4.1   Time Effort

When applying methods to evaluate a technology, there is always the question about which method suits best to obtain the highest output with the lowest effort. Reflecting on the methods used within the present evaluating study we collected the time effort we experienced in our specific evaluation. The extent of the applied methods are twelve hours behavior observation, 45 contextual interviews lasting two-to-three minutes (in our case accomplished in a twelve hour time period – but in principle also in less time possible), and 26 completed online surveys lasting about 10 minutes. Table 2 provides an overview about the time efforts for the three applied methods separated for the evaluation activities (preparation, execution for evaluator and participants, data entry, and data analysis). We classified the time effort into "none", "small", "medium", and "large". This classification is for comparing the time effort of the three methods in the different evaluation activities but not to compare the time effort between evaluation activities.

It is not surprising that overall the online survey has an advantage compared to the in-situ methods in terms of time effort for the evaluator. There is no time effort for the evaluator for execution and data entry, because this is accomplished automatically by the LimeSurvey application. The clear structure of the online form also facilitates the data analysis compared to the contextual interview, which is more opened and therefore often results in more chaotic data. Only the preparation time is higher than for the in-situ methods, because the online survey has – besides being planned content wise - also set up technically with the LimeSurvey application. For the participants filling out the online survey requires the greatest time effort.

We experienced the greatest time effort for the evaluator in the execution of the *behavior observation*. Of course the duration of observation was chosen to be twelve hours, but in the given context a significantly shorter observation period would have not been sufficient to gain an overview of the situation and observe enough buying processes to collect a reasonable number of usability issues.

Table 2. Overview of the time effort (classified into none, small, medium, and large) for the different methods experienced in the evaluation used

Evaluation Activity	Behavior Observation	Contextual Interview	Online Survey
Preparation	Small	Small	Medium
Execution			
Evaluator	Large	Medium	None
Participant	None	Small	Medium
Data entry	Medium	Large	None
Data analysis	Medium	Large	Medium

4.2 Output

The most crucial aspect of evaluation methods is the output they produce in terms of how many problems and recommendations for change are they able to identify. Since methods differ naturally in the kind of information they can provide (e.g. behavior observation cannot provide user ratings of usability) we reflect on the methods separately for different information types. For the analysis we collected all information gathered by the three evaluation methods in one list. Then we checked for each entry of the list from which methods they were identified. Finally we classified the information on the list according to their content into the five types: interface design issues, general issues with the ticketing machine, metric data, user ratings, and user recommendations.

Interface Design Issues. To find issues related to the interface design was the main focus of the evaluation and all three methods were potentially able to identify them. We only considered concrete issues with specific aspects of the design and neglected more general statements about the interface (e.g. "it's too complicated") for this analysis.

In sum 14 interface design issues were identified by all three methods together. The percentage of issues observed in the tram and the number of problems reported when the users were asked (in the tram or via online survey) are shown in Fig. 2 (three bars on the on the left side). The behavior observation found eight issues (57.14 %), the contextual interviews seven (50.00 %), and the online survey only three (21.43 %). Having a look on the issues which were not identified by behavior observation, it becomes clear that the six remaining issues would be hard to identify by behavior observation, because they cannot be *observed from the outside* without knowing what the users' think. For example a user who has "problems reading the text in the given font size" looks for an observer from behind just like a user who has troubles with the interface, and would be noted as "being confused" but without having any concrete information about the problem. On the other hand behavior observation identified six issues which were not identified by the other two methods, which relate to *specific interaction steps or objects*. For example although we observed some users having problems with a button for adjusting the number of tickets to buy, none of the users reported a related issue when they were asked in the interview and online survey.

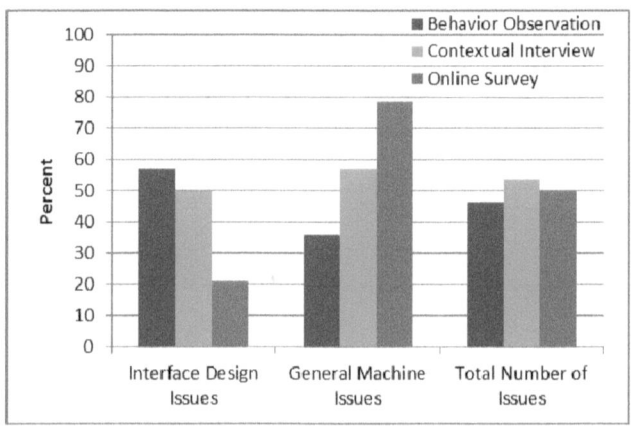

Fig. 2. Percentages of the identified interface design issues, general issues with the machine, and total number of issues (sum of interface design and general machine issues) for the different methods

General Issues with the Machine. This category consists of all usability issues which were not related to the interface of the machine, but to the machine itself (e.g. size, positioning, functioning etc.).

In sum 14 general issues with the machine were identified by all methods together, five (35.71 %) by the behavior observation, eight (57.14 %) by the contextual interviews, and eleven (78.57 %) by the online survey (see Fig. 2 three bars in the middle). The small number identified with behavior observation can be explained by the facts that some issues *did not occur during the observation period* (e.g. "machine did not work", "problem to get to the machine when it's crowded") and that some issues were *not observable from the outside* (e.g. "entering the PIN to pay with card feels unsecure when it's crowded"). Only one of the issues identified by behavior observation was not identified by the two other methods. It relates to a very specific functioning issue of the machine which occurred during the observation ("after canceling the payment a 30 seconds delay occurs until the home screen is displayed again") and which probably only few users experienced.

Other Data. The remaining information categories metric data, user ratings, and user recommendations are measurable with only a part of the three methods.

In the category *metric data* all information is collected which is able to answer questions about how often specific incidents happen or how long they take. Behavior observation is most suitable for this kind of information, because it provides a realistic and objective estimation about for example how often specific problems occur in a given time period, how often users ask for help, how many elderly people use the machine, how long the waiting queues are, and how long the buying process takes with cash or card payment (measured by the evaluator with a stopwatch).

User ratings can only be identified with the subjective methods (contextual interview and online survey). We asked our participants of the contextual interview as well as the online survey to rate the usability and the design of the user interface on a scale from one (best rating) to five (worst rating). To analyze potential differences in the ratings of the interview and the online survey data we used an unpaired two-sample t-test. Looking at the usability ratings of our participants we found a significant difference ($t_{69} = -3.12$, $\alpha < 0.05$) between the ratings in the contextual interview (mean = 1.78, SD = 0.64) and the online survey (mean = 2.35, SD = 0.89). The participants of the online survey rated the usability of the interface significantly worse than the participants of the contextual interview. No such difference was found for the rating of the design ($t_{69} = -1.31$, $\alpha > 0.05$).

Like user ratings also *user recommendations* usually cannot be identified by behavior observation. In sum 34 user recommendations could be collected in the data of the contextual interviews and the online survey. The greater amount of concrete recommendations was provided by the participants of the online survey, who stated 24 (70.59 %). The participants of the contextual interviews provided 16 (47.06 %) recommendations. Interestingly only six issues were identified by both methods, which means that most of the issues were identified by just one of the methods. Having a closer look at the content of the recommendations reveals that 15 (44.11 %) recommendations are related to interface design (e.g. "place the buttons more apart from each other") and 19 (55.88 %) to general characteristics of the machine (e.g. "install the machines at the stations, not in the trams"). As described above we saw for the identified issues that online survey found considerably more general machine issues than the other two methods but less interface design issues. For the recommendations no such difference can be found, since 41.67 percent of the online survey participants' recommendations (and 37.50 percent of the contextual interview participants') are related to interface design.

4.3 A View on Elderly Users and Accessibility

In this section we take a closer look on the elderly users and accessibility aspects evaluated. Due to the limited number of elderly participants we will not reflect on the differences between methods, but highlight findings approachable only by specific methods.

As stated above only it is only assessable by behavior observation how often specific incidents happen. A first result in regard to elderly users is the surprisingly small number of elderlies using the ticketing machine - only 8 of 122 observed users (9.76 %) were classified as elderlies. Another interesting finding of behavior observation is that six of the eight as elderly users had problems with the buying process (75 %), but only 23 of the 114 other users (20.18 %). Furthermore three of the four users (75 %) asking other passengers for help were elderly users. These results point out the difficulties elderly users have with self-service technology very clearly. Another finding of the behavior observation relates to the accessibility features of the machine (changing of language and contrast). In the whole observation period none of the users changed the contrast to the mode which is easier to read for visually impaired. Furthermore only one user changed the language settings, although there were several users observed who had problems with the German language (which became obvious when they were asked for an interview).

5   Conclusions

In the present paper we presented and reflected on three different methods (behavior observation, contextual interview, online survey) used in the evaluation of a self-service ticketing machine in the public transport system of Graz, Austria. The main focus of the evaluation was to identify usability issues with the ticketing machine. Altogether 28 issues (interface design issues and general issues with the machine) were identified, and each method could identify about 50 percent of the issues (see also Fig. 2 three bars on the right side). A closer look on the different types of information reveals some interesting results, which are described in the following paragraphs.

The *in-situ methods* behavior observation and contextual interview identified a higher number of concrete interface design issues than the online survey. Especially *behavior observation* provides valuable information about when and where problems occur in the interface interaction process. When asking users' directly to describe the problems they have with an interface, they are often not more concrete than "it is too complicated" – probably because they are unconscious about the origin of the problem. Another advantage of behavior observation is that it can provide information and metrics about how often problems really occur in a given period of time. This cannot be provided by subjective data and can help not to overestimate the severity of an issue raised by user statements. Furthermore it can tell us something about the behavior of specific user groups like how many elderly users are using the machine and face problems. However, a big disadvantage of behavior observation, which is also reflected in our data, is that it can only capture what is actually observable "from the outside" and happens during the observation period. For a clearer understanding of the users' reasons and difficulties as well as to include also incidents apart the observation period, objective behavior observation should be supplemented with a subjective method.

With *subjective methods* - in contrast to behavior observation - also user ratings and user recommendations are recognizable. Comparing the usability ratings of the participants of *contextual interview* and *online survey* shows a significant difference. One possible explanation for that difference is that participants tend to be more critical in an anonymous online survey than in a one-on-one interview.

The *online survey* found less interface design issues but more general issues with the machine than the behavior observation and the contextual interview. This may indicate that general issues with the ticketing machine are very prominent in the participants' memories, but that interface design issues require some kind of proximity to the subject of interest. However when it comes to recommendations, the online-survey participants target the interface design almost equally often like general characteristics of the machine. Furthermore the participants of the online survey provided the highest number of recommendations for change. The absence of time pressure and the possibility to think carefully about the recommendations may be a factor for that instance.

6   Limitations and Outlook

With the present paper we aim to reflect on our experiences with different common methods (behavior observation, contextual interview, online survey) in the field of self-service evaluation. However, the presented results have some limitations. The most important limitation relates to the *two incomparable samples* of the in-situ method and the online survey due to the different recruiting approach of participants. For the in-situ methods all kinds of users of the ticketing machine were asked by chance to be part of an interview, but the online survey was distributed by e-mail and social network sites only to a selective sample of computer and internet users. Therefore besides the different sample size, we have to assume also differences in user characteristics like technophilia. Technophile people may provide more concrete feedback concerning usability issues due to their advanced experience with technology. Furthermore we cannot assume the same degree of heterogeneity in the online-survey-sample than in the in-situ-sample. Another limitation concerns the *data analysis*. We only considered the number of issues and recommendations identified by the different methods, but not the quality. Involving the usefulness of user statements somehow would be an interesting area of further research. Another area for future investigation could include *different user groups* systematically in the study design. It would be interesting to investigate if the results of the methods differ between elderly and other users. A last limitation concerns the interpretation of the presented results in terms of a case study, which means that they *apply to the present evaluation conducted in the specific context of self-service ticketing*. It is conceivable that the comparison between the methods will lead to other results if the context or concrete procedure changes. Nevertheless it provides valuable information for evaluators and a basis for further investigations in regard to added value of in-situ methods.

Acknowledgments. The research presented is conducted within the Austrian project "AIR – Advanced Interface Research" funded by the Austrian Research Promotion Agency (FFG), the ZIT Center for Innovation and Technology and the province of Salzburg under contract number 825345. We would like to thank Holding Graz Linien for access and assistance in doing the fieldwork.

References

1. Bowman, D., Gabbard, J.L., Hix, D.: A Survey of Usability Evaluation in Virtual Environments: Classification and Comparison of Methods. Presence: Teleoperators and Virtual Environments 11(4), 435–455 (2002)
2. Hornbæk, K.: Current Practice in Measuring Usability: Challenges to Usability Studies and Research. International Journal of Human-Computer Studies 64(2), 79–102 (2006)
3. Holzinger, A., Searle, G., Kleinberger, T., Seffah, A., Javahery, H.: Investigating Usability Metrics for the Design and Development of Applications for the Elderly. In: Miesenberger, K., Klaus, J., Zagler, W.L., Karshmer, A.I. (eds.) ICCHP 2008. LNCS, vol. 5105, pp. 98–105. Springer, Heidelberg (2008)
4. Castro, D., Atkinson, R., Ezell, S.: Embracing the self-service economy. The Information Technology & Innovation Foundation (2010)
5. Maguire, M.C.: A Review of User-Interface Design Guidelines for Public Information Kiosk Systems. Int. J. Hum.–Comput. Stud. 50, 263–286 (1999)
6. Hagen, S., Sandnes, F.E.: Toward Accessible Self-Service Kiosks through Intelligent User Interfaces. Pers. Ubiquit. Comput. 14, 715–721 (2010)
7. Simon, F., Usunier, J.-C.: Cognitive, Demographic, and Situational Determinants of Service Customer Preference for Personnel-in-Contact over Self-Service Technology. International Journal of Research in Marketing 24(2), 163–173 (2007)
8. Kristoffersen, S., Bratteberg, I.: Design Ideas for IT in Public Spaces. Pers. Ubiquit. Comput. 14, 271–286 (2010)
9. Bratteberg, I., Kristoffersen, S.: Irreversibility and Forceback in Public Interfaces. In: Proceedings of NordiCHI 2008, pp. 63–72 (2008)
10. Davis, F., Bagozzi, R., Warshaw, P.: User Acceptance of Computer Technology: A Comparison of Two Theoretical Models. Management Science 35(8), 982–1003 (1989)
11. Lee, C.B.P., Wan, G.: Including Subjective Norm and Technology Trust in the Technology Acceptance Model: A Case of E-Ticketing in China. The DATA BASE for Advances in Information Systems 41(4), 40–51 (2010)
12. Mallat, N., Rossi, M., Tuunainen, V.K., Öörni, A.: An Empirical Investigation of Mobile Ticketing Service Adoption in Public Transport. Pers. Ubiquit. Comput. 12, 57–65 (2008)
13. Reinders, M.J., Dabholkar, P.A., Frambach, R.T.: Consequences of Forcing Consumers to Use Technology-Based Self-Service. Journal of Service Research 11, 107–123 (2008)
14. Jensen, K.L.: RECON - Capturing Mobile and Ubiquitous Interaction in Real Contexts. In: Proceedings of MobileHCI 2009 (2009)
15. Hughes, J., King, V., Rodden, T., Andersen, H.: Moving out from the control room: ethnography in system design. In: Proceedings of the Conference on Computer Supported Cooperative Work, pp. 429–439 (1994)
16. Blomberg, J., Giacomi, J., Mosher, A., Swenton-Wall, P.: Ethnographic Field Methods and Their Relation to Design. In: Dchuler, C., Namioka, A. (eds.) Participatory Design: Principles and Practices, pp. 123–156. Erlbaum, Hillsdale (1993)
17. Millen, D.R.: Rapid Ethnography: Time Deepening Strategies for HCI Field Research. In: Proceedings on Designing Interactive Systems: Processes, Practices, Methods, and Techniques, pp. 280–286 (2000)
18. LimeSurvey open source survey application, http://www.limesurvey.org/

When Your Living Space Knows What You Do: Acceptance of Medical Home Monitoring by Different Technologies

Martina Ziefle, Simon Himmel, and Wiktoria Wilkowska

Communication Science, RWTH Aachen University, 52062 Aachen, Germany
{Ziefle,Himmel,Wilkowska}@humtec.rwth-aachen.de

Abstract. Technology acceptance of conventional Information and Communication technologies (ICT) devices is extensively researched within the last twenty years. However, comparably small knowledge is prevalent with respect to ubiquitous ICT in the living environment. Furthermore, there is nearly no data about user acceptance's dependency of integrated technologies on varying domestic spaces and how acceptance varies regarding user diversity. This study explores the acceptance of home-integrated ICT (hands-free equipment, camera, positioning system). In different domestic spaces (living room, bedroom, bathroom) acceptance for integrated technology was assessed, using qualitative as well as quantitative methods. Results show that users' acceptance differs considerably depending on the room type (acceptance is the highest in the living and the lowest in the bathroom). Moreover, the most disliked technology for home monitoring are camera-based systems, followed by the positioning system and the microphone. Also, there was a significant interacting effect of room type and technology: While none of these technologies is accepted for the bathroom, the living room is less sensitive to their presence with the microphone as the most accepted technology. User diversity does not play a major role hinting at generic acceptance patterns regarding ICT integrated in home environments.

Keywords: Domestic Spaces, Technology Acceptance, Room cartography, Ambient Assisted Living, Ubiquitous Computing, User Diversity.

1 Introduction

Due to a strong attention of research, policy and media, it is meanwhile broadly known that in many countries of the world population characteristics change dramatically, with considerable consequences for social, organizational and political processes and procedures. The consequences of the demographic change are especially visible in the health care sector: Increased life expectancy, improved medical healthcare in combination with a higher living standard as well as reduced fertility rates lead to a growing number of frail older persons, who will need medical treatments and long term care provided by health care systems [1]. It is a central question how these challenges can be mastered sufficiently [2, 3, 4].

A. Holzinger and K.-M. Simonic (Eds.): USAB 2011, LNCS 7058, pp. 607–624, 2011.

Today about 15% of the European population reports difficulties in performing daily activities without professional help due to some form of physical, mental or cognitive disability [5]. Also, the prevalence of chronic diseases is expected to further increase in an aging society (diabetes, cardio vascular diseases and dementia as the age-related diseases with the highest incidence rates world wide). As such, the number of patients suffering from e.g. diabetes is expected to increase by 40 % in the next decennia, and those suffering from cardiovascular diseases by even 50% [6]. Thus, increasingly more seniors are expected to require personal care in the coming years. Due to the shortcomings in the medical supply chain and the care sector, third-party's assistance seems to be unavoidable in many cases [7].

The maturity of information and communication technologies, their ubiquity and easy access in combination with electronic health technology may compensate these shortcomings and will thus play an important role in the near future [8, 9]. In contrast to the advanced technical development and the innovation in technologies to be implantable in the home, still, the knowledge about the human factor is considerably underdeveloped. Aspects of humans' technology acceptance, the detailed study and the willingness to accept technology within living spaces as well as the individual usage motives and barriers are mostly disregarded, or even underestimated so far.

As any successful rollout of such sensitive technologies requires first and foremost users' acceptance and their openness, research should focus not only on the technical part, but it should also consider the way these technologies meet users' needs and wants with respect to privacy, dignity, and their requirements for as useful perceived smart home technologies [7, 10, 11, 12, 13].

1.1   Information and Communication Technologies in the Home Environment

Within the last five to ten years a variety of new healthcare concepts for supporting and assisting users in technology-enhanced environments emerged ([14, 7] for an overview of state-of-the-art applications). These Ambient-Assisted-Living (AAL) applications are characterized by a combined use of ICT and health monitoring devices [15, 16]. They enable autonomous and unobtrusive collection of clinical data and support the continuous transmission of physiological information between patients and remote healthcare providers.

By providing a wide variety of services, including assistance to carry out daily activities, health and activity monitoring, getting access to social, medical and emergency systems, and by this facilitating social contacts, smart healthcare applications are expected to bring medical, social and economical benefits to different stakeholders [17, 18, 19]. Applications and systems mainly focus on four different goals: (1) the detection of emergency situations, (2) long-term treatment of chronic diseases and rehabilitation, (3) early detection of and a timely care for illness, and (4) maintaining health and well-being.

Especially, the first goal, the detection and prevention of emergency is of primary interest, as smart technologies monitor the activities at home and focus on falls and congestive heart failures as their main application areas.

More than 30% of seniors 65 years and about 50% of the people over 80 years fall at least once a year [20]. In 20% to 30% of the cases, people suffer serious injuries with sustaining effects on mobility and independence [21]. As many of these falls happen when people are alone at home, mobile emergency systems and devices had been developed enabling users to call for help in an emergency situation. Such mobile devices worn either at the hip or around the wrist are problematic, though. Empirical evidence shows that patients often do not carry those devices or are simply not able to operate them when medical problems occur. As a consequence, people lie on the floor for hours, sometimes even days, unnoticed. Not unusually, these accidents have lethal consequences.

In order to overcome the shortcomings of mobile emergency transmitters, other systems had been developed. Technological approaches range from wearable sensors, like accelerometers and pressure sensors [22, 23], contact free methods using acoustic (microphone) [24] or visual (video camera) [9, 25, 26] sensors. There are even solutions available, which measure the contact forces that are applied to the ground by the users feet [27, 28]. Each approach offers advantages but also drawbacks in certain scenarios. Wearable sensors are mobile and can be used in various locations, however they are not invisible and require a high amount of care and maintenance of the users. Acoustic and visual sensors provide very reliable information but require visible obtrusive technology that may bring up privacy and intimacy concerns.

1.2   Technologies at Home

Even though no one would really deny the usefulness and the necessity of home care technologies for emergency situations, AAL technologies in the own home are though connected with plenty of emotions: acceptance barriers and restraints on the one hand, as well as the wish to be independent and able to live at home for a longer time in spite of illness on the other hand. Thus, the consideration of users' acceptance and the understanding of the nature of barriers and needs and wants is of major importance.

Yet there is increased research awareness that acceptance for medical technology differs in some aspect from the traditional technology acceptance concept [29]. In contrast to traditional ICT, medical assistance devices address mostly older, frail and diseased people, who have very specific and wide-ranged needs [2, 30, 31, 32, 33]. For instance, there is another need regarding the communication with the system for a mobility-impaired person in comparison to a user with hearing deficiencies but otherwise unlimited mobility. The same problem applies to the cognitive skills and their decline over the life span, the technical self-confidence and the willingness to use such modern technology. Hence, there is a great necessity for a comprehensive and sensible identification of factors that influence acceptance of smart home technologies [34, 35].

In addition, some cautionary notes regard to the smart home approach itself. The omnipresence of information may be perceived as a violation of personal intimacy limits, raising concerns about privacy, and loss of control [36, 10]. So far, we have only limited knowledge about the fragile limits between the different poles: on the one hand the wish to live independently at home feeling safe and secure, and on the other hand the feeling of loss of control and the disliking of intrusion in private spheres [36, 37]. For most people there is no other place, which is more intimate and confiding than "the own four walls". The investigation of functional requirements but also emotional barriers in the domestic home environment is for all persons, but especially for frail seniors of utterly importance [8, 19, 38, 37, 39].

Yet, accommodation is extremely important in human's life for reasons of perceived safety, and it belongs to the basic human needs to feel protected, stable and secure. Moreover, health is the greatest wealth and therefore a very sensitive and delicate topic – there is no higher good than this and everyone tries to protect it as long as somehow possible. Thus, the involvement of end users, their perspectives, whishes and needs, into every step of the development process plays a great role for a successful rollout.

2   Research Approach

As there is only little knowledge about users' acceptance of ubiquitous technologies integrated in their homes the aim of this study was to gain insights in the acceptance of smart home technologies. A two-step procedure was applied, using exploratory (qualitative) methods (focus groups) in a first step, followed by a questionnaire study for verification. The question whether there are any factors influencing the acceptance of these new technologies and if so, which these are should be discussed primarily by older users who would be the first users when shipping the products.

Regarding to the improved technology acceptance model (TAM) by Venkatesh and Davis [29] technology acceptance is influenced by two main factors: perceived usefulness and perceived ease of use, which again are influenced by external social and cognitive factors. The contribution of the latter factors though is controversially discussed by acceptance researchers [38] with respect to the number of factors and their relative contribution to acceptance outcomes.

In this paper we laid focus on analyzing the factors:

- Age
- Gender
- Health status
- Attitudes towards technology
- Frequency of technology usage

In the following we will report if and how these factors are influencing the acceptance of upcoming integrated technologies for home-monitoring technologies.

3   Methodology

The empirical approach entailed a two-step procedure. In a first step, five focus groups were run in order to learn users' perceived concerns with regard to smart home technologies and the individual needs and wants. On the basis of individual argumentations, we identified the crucial factors, which were then taken as a basis for the development of the questionnaire instrument. In a second step, the quantitative survey was applied, in order to validate the findings within a broader sample.

3.1   (Semi-) Qualitative Data Collection – Pre-study Focus Groups

The focus groups (FG) were conducted in order to identify the acceptance of different ICT by (potential) users. Qualitative data from 42 mainly older adults were used in the focus groups. The participants were recruited using the authors' social network. The focus laid on elderly people (FG 1-4, Table 2), however in order to check in how far the discussions and arguments raised are age specific, we also had a focus control group with younger adults (FG 5). Snapshots of the focus groups are given in Figure 1.

Table 1. Characteristics of participants in the different focus groups

# focus groups	composition	total	male	female	age range	Ø age	SD
FG 1	old, mixed	10	6	4	60 - 73	68	3,3
FG 2	old, male	8	6	2	55 - 72	63	5,4
FG 3	old, female	8	0	8	50 - 66	58	5,1
FG 4	old, mixed	10	5	5	56 - 67	60	4,3
FG 5	young, mixed	6	3	3	24 - 28	27	1,5

The educational level of participants was above average: 79% of participants had a university degree. Depending on the individual argumentation lines and the different discussion needs, the duration of the focus groups varied from 1:00 to 1:45h. All focus groups were guided and encouraged by the same moderator.

Three focus groups (FG 1-3) followed a free and open discussion forum, identifying generic attitudes. We collected discussions about

1) Technical devices and technologies participants possess and use at home,
2) Attitudes about a different sensibility of rooms, but also an evaluation which rooms seem to be appropriate for medical home monitoring
3) Privacy, security and trust issues touched by the respective monitoring technology

The purpose of the free approach was to give participants a feeling for the ubiquity of technical devices they are surrounded by at home and how much information of their personal life they gain – or could gain, assumed they were equipped with data collecting memory-chips or transmission technology.

The other two focus groups (FG 4 and 5) followed a scenario-based approach. They started with two short futuristic example-movies showing integrated ubiquitous technologies, one positive ("Ambient Assisted Living" (beginning), Fraunhofer IESE, 2009, (00:00:00-00:04:30h) and one negative example ("The Island" (Scene), Michael Bay, 2005, (00:02:30-00:04:10h).

In all focus groups participants were requested to fill out a "technology-room-acceptance-matrix" (Table 2), which showed the acceptance of technologies in different rooms at home under specific conditions, e.g. "when ill". Each participant had to fill out the technique-room-matrix and to note conditional acceptance criteria, if applicable. Results were discussed afterwards. The whole group had – beyond the individual matrices – to find a consensus about one common group matrix. This was done to learn which arguments were commonly agreed on.

Table 2. "Technology-room-acceptance-matrix" (* example entries)

		Rooms		
		Livingroom	bathroom	Bedroom
Integrated	**microphone**	YES*	when ill*	when ill*
home	**camera**	NO*	NO*	when ill*
technologies	**positioning**	YES*	YES*	when ill*

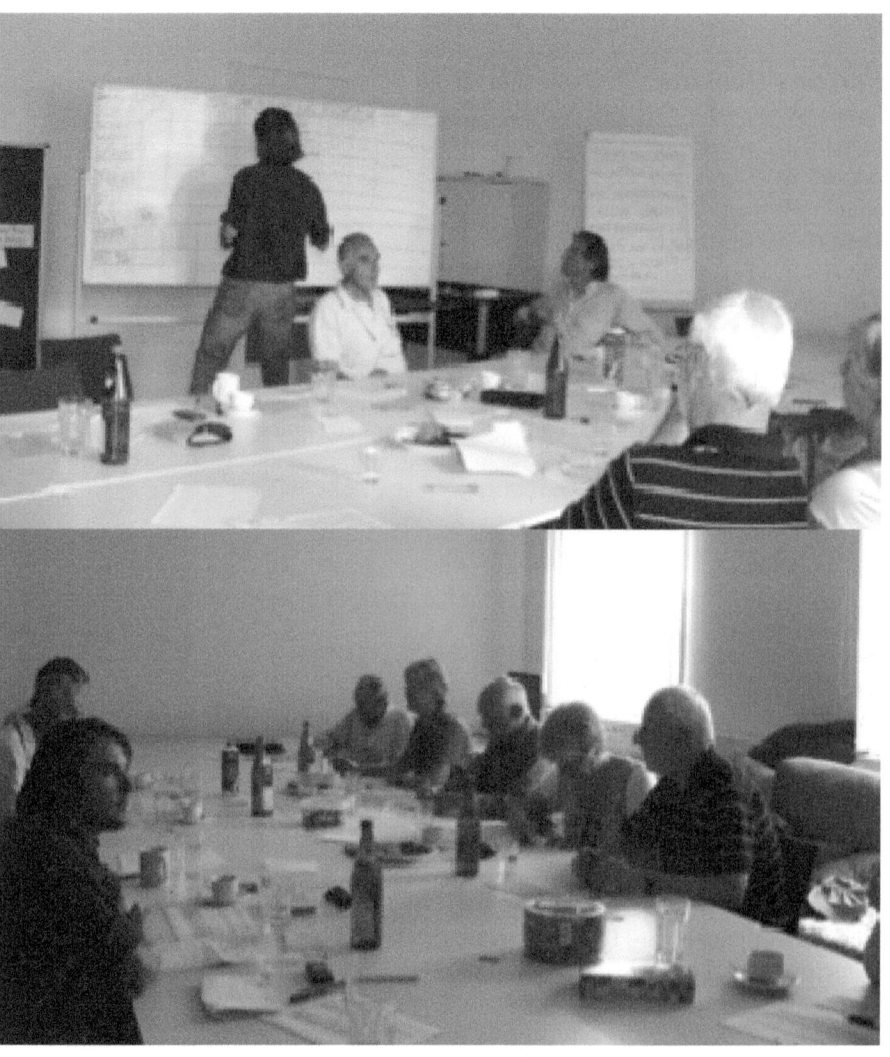

Fig. 1. Snapshot of focus group sessions

3.2   Quantitative Data Collection – Questionnaire

In a next step a questionnaire instrument was designed to validate and supplement the results of the pre-study. 100 adults between 28 – 93 years of age participated. The questionnaire's structure followed five-W-Questions: "*Who*" accepts "*when*" "*what*" (home-integrated technologies), "*where*" under "which conditions"?

"*Who*": The "Who"-part of the questionnaire was arranged in five sections.
- The first part included demographic data with respect to participants' age, gender, educational level and profession.
- The second section applied to person's health status (e.g. present chronicle diseases, dependency on medical devices).
- The third section should figure out person's general attitude towards technique. Five questions addressed interest, stress, trust, fun and distrust on a four-point Likert scale from 1 = "no agreement" to 4 = "full agreement".
- The fourth section focused on the participants' experience with technology in general (usage frequency of popular information and communication devices (PC, mobile phone, video/digital camera, GPS).
- The fifth section should gain information about person's social context (e.g. number of persons at home, dependency on long-term care).

"*When*": The "When"-item determined, if acceptance of integrated technologies is affected by health-status. Therefore all following questions were asked for two scenarios:
- being healthy compared to
- being ill.

Due to space limitations, we report on the results for the ill setting only.

"*When*": The "What"-query determined the kind of integrated information-communication and medical technologies. The three technologies were
- microphone
- camera
- positioning-system.

"*Where*": In this section, three rooms had to be evaluated regarding their sensitivity to technology monitoring
- living room
- bedroom
- bathroom

The questions for the participants' acceptance of technologies in rooms were formulated in personal statements one had to confirm on a four-point scale from "no" = 0 to "yes" = 3.

"*Which conditions*": The conditional acceptance situations, "which" had to be fulfilled to generally accept integrated technologies, were determined in the last section of the questionnaire (privacy concerns, financial burden etc.).

3.3 Participants of the Questionnaire Study

100 younger, adult and elderly persons volunteered to take part in the questionnaire study. Participants were collected mainly by the authors' social network and by announcements in local newspapers. Most questionnaires were distributed in paper-form (partly in senior homes), some online. Three age groups were formed (Table 3).

Table 3. Age group classification of participants in the questionnaire study

	N participants			Age range	M age	SD
	total	Female	Male			
young/middleaged persons	12	8	4	25-38	29	3,5
adult persons	50	29	21	43-64	58	4,4
elderly/retired persons	38	20	18	66-93	75	8

The mean age of the sample was M = 61 years (SD=15,4.) Three age groups were formed: (1) The younger/middle aged persons (aged 20 to 40), (2) adult persons (41 to 65 years of age) and (3) elderly/retired adults (older than 65 years, Figure 3). The latter group referred to the fact that with 65 years the retirement phase starts [39].

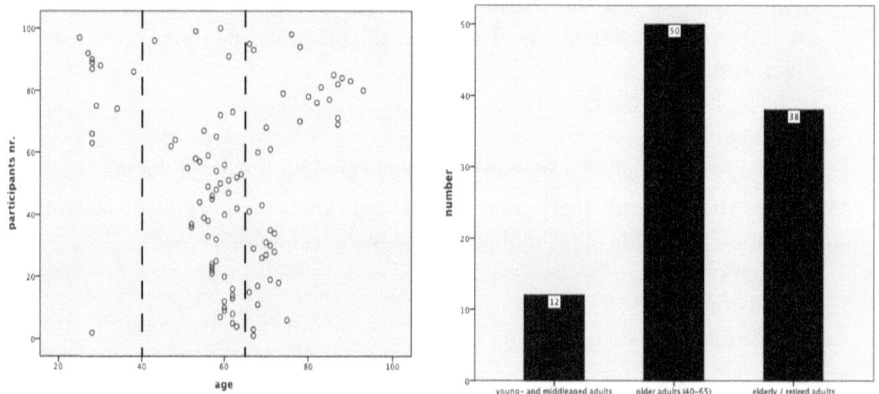

Fig. 2. Distribution of participants' age   **Fig. 3.** Age group classification

As can be seen From Figure 3, the majority of participants belonged to the "adult group", as they are assumed to be the potential users of upcoming new integrated, ubiquitous supporting technologies. Gender (57% female participants) is considered in the analyses due to some substantial differences regarding technology usage [42, 36]. The classification of health status into healthy and ill participants was determined by four questions: (1) Do you have of any chronic diseases? (2) Do you need regularly health check-ups? (3) Are you dependent on any medical devices? (4) Are you dependent on medical care? (5) All people answering positively to at least one of these questions were classified as "ill", in our study 51%.

4   Results

Qualitative data from the focus group study were reported descriptively. Then, quantitative results were analyzed by (M)ANOVA–procedures, referring to effects of room type (contrasting living-, bed-, bathroom), of technology type (contrasting microphone, camera, positioning) as well as interaction effects. For all analyses we also focused on effects of user diversity. The level of significance was set at 5%. Outcomes on the less restrictive significance level of 10% were referred to as marginally significant.

4.1   Qualitative Data: Key Findings from the Focus Groups

The qualitative results of the focus groups were analyzed descriptively. Overall, participants showed a vivid interest in the topic and participated with enthusiasm and high openness. In order to illustrate the individual attitudes, some of the comments of participants are detailed. Answers are categorized by technologies regarding the acceptance in different domestic spaces.

Microphone: The integration of hands-free equipment was mostly accepted in the living room, but was highly controversially discussed for the bed- and bathroom.

> *"From my perspective it is important to have microphones everywhere as you are moving around in your house" (male, FG2)*

> *"And if I'm ill it could be really helpful when somebody could hear me and knows: This guy is still breathing" (male, FG2)*

> *"But I don't want a microphone there and somebody hears me up or down there. That is kind of eavesdropping. Imagine that I have guests and somebody listens to us" (female, FG1)*

Camera: In none of the focus groups, the integration of a camera was accepted for bed- and bathroom, both are perceived as highly intimate. The negative aspects of being watched were frequently compared to future visions of Orwell's "1984, Big Brother is watching you".

> *"Being monitored by camera feels like surveillance" (female, FG2)*

> *"I regard eye contact with camera as highly inappropriate, even when I'm ill" (male, FG2)*

> *"I do not want anybody watching me" (male, FG2)*

> *"I really don't like it. You never know, if there is somebody watching you or not" (male, FG2)*

> *"Recently, I was in the hospital and monitored all the time. I couldn't get over it the whole week. I always felt unpleasant" (male, FG2) (...)*

> *"Well, when was in ICU I felt very guarded and I knew all stand behind me" (male, FG2)*

> *"When I think of communicating with friends and family using the Internet, then they may see me in the living-, or dining room, but they are not able to see me in the bath- or bedroom" (female, FG1)*

Positioning system: The positioning was only conditionally accepted in case of falls. When somebody has fallen and keeps lying on the floor, this system was highly accepted in case of being ill or at fall risk.

> *"When I slip and fall, I would say "yes" to position finding in the bathroom" (female, FG1)*
>
> *"When you are ill and in need of help, then I would accept the positioning in any place" (female, FG3)*

Beyond the different acceptance patterns depending on technology types it was also obvious that personality of participants and general attitudes towards life played a large role within the evaluations of smart home technologies. Overall, two different attitudes were identified: the "Skeptics" and the "Resigned".

The *skeptics* rather declined everything- independently of health state or needs:

> *"Well, I don't want anything at all" (male, FG2)*
>
> *"For me, one negative aspect is the too high reliance on technologies and the lack of respecting persons' personality. (...) That is most important for me when being old and communicating with humans instead of technologies. The real person (contact) is important for me" (female, FG4)*

The *resigned* on the other hand rather accepted all technologies, in case of illness and dependence of care. They seek for the possibility to stay independently at home:

> *"If you tell me that being monitored at home is a real alternative to a retirement home, I would accept it. Then, you don't have to live with the old dodderers" (female, FG2)*
>
> *"If it is necessary and I really need it, when I'm ill, then I would accept any technology anywhere at home" (female, FG3)*

4.2   Quantitative Results of the Questionnaire Survey

Effects of domestic spaces

A first analysis regards the main effect of the type of domestic space, thus addressing the question whether the three rooms under study - living room, bedroom or bathroom - show a different sensitivity towards monitoring through home medical monitoring. It should be noted that for all scenarios the participants had to evaluate they should imagine to be chronically ill. The ANOVA for multivariate measurements revealed a significant omnibus effect of domestic space ($F(2,94) = 30.2$; $p < 0.05$). The descriptive outcomes are visualized in Figure 4 (left side).

Apparently, the living room is the one for which participants would accept home monitoring (M = 2.2 out of 3 points max), followed by the bedroom (though considerably lower with M = 1.8) and last ranked is the bathroom (M = 1.6) which reveals to be most sensitive towards medical monitoring.

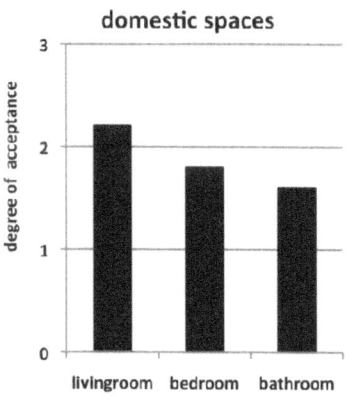
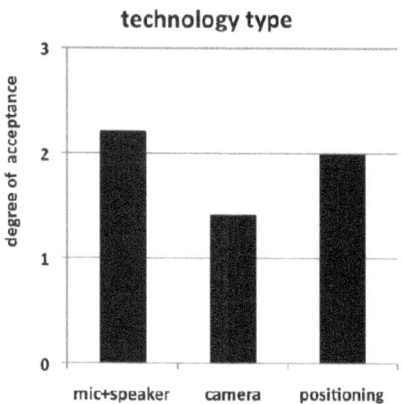

Fig. 4. Left: Main effect of domestic spaces (Means); Right: Main effect of technology types (means). High values represent high levels of acceptance.

Effects of technology type

A second analysis addressed the question whether some of the technologies provoke more concerns than others. In Figure 4 (right), outcomes are illustrated. As can be seen there, there was a significant main effect of technology type ($F(2,94) = 29.4.2$; $p < 0.05$). From all technologies, the microphone (plus speaker) is the most accepted technology (M=2.2/3 points max), followed by the positioning system (M=1.9). The camera is- unequivocally and in a relatively clear distance - ranked last (M = 1.4).

Interacting effects of domestic spaces and technology type

The ANOVA for repeated measurements revealed a significant interaction of domestic space x technology type (Figure 5). The interaction says that the extent of acceptance for a technology also depends on the respective room characteristics. While for the auditory monitoring (microphone and speaker) there is a clear ranking (living room most and bathroom least accepted), the users show an equally low acceptance for camera and positioning system in bathroom and bedroom.

Effects of user diversity

As users might differ in a number of characteristics that should be considered within the cartography of rooms and technology types, we analyzed effects of age groups (contrasting the young, the adult and the older users), gender (contrasting males and females), health states (contrasting the chronically ill vs. the healthy participants) as well as technical experience (contrasting people with a high experience when using conventional information and communication technologies and persons who show a low familiarity with device handling).

In order to come to the point: user diversity did not reveal to be a major factor impacting the acceptance decision which technology type should be used for home monitoring when being ill and which rooms of the house are especially sensitive (no main effects of user diversity). Obviously, there were unequivocal attitudes and answers, showing that "home", "intimacy" and "privacy" are generic categories, which do not vary in a predominant way as a function of different user characteristics. Though, some single interacting effects were found, which were described in the following sections.

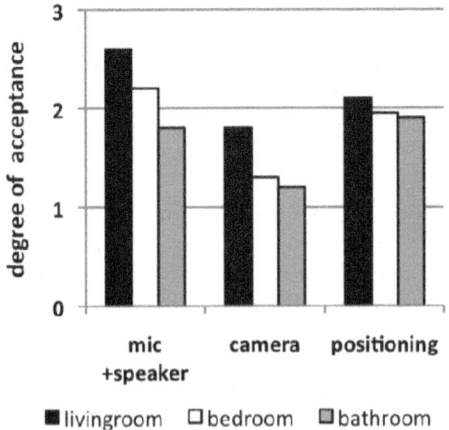

■ livingroom   ☐ bedroom   ▣ bathroom

Fig. 5. Left side: Interacting effect of acceptance of the three different technologies across domestic spaces (Means); Right: Main effect of technology types (means). High values represent high levels of acceptance.

Interacting effect: Age affects the evaluation of technology types in domestic spaces

Statistical testing revealed a marginally significant three-way interaction effect ($F(2,93) = 3.05$; $p < 0.1$) between age, and the evaluation of the technology type in different domestic spaces (Figure 6). As can be seen there, the adult group shows the lowest acceptance from all age groups especially regarding the camera monitoring in bathroom and bedroom.

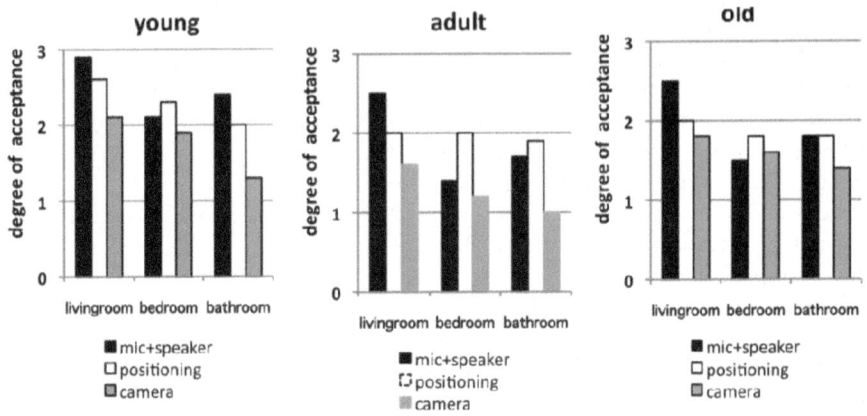

Fig. 6. Marginally significant three-way interaction of age, technology type in different domestic spaces (Means). High values represent high levels of acceptance.

Interacting effect: Gender affects technology acceptance in domestic spaces

Analyses showed a marginally significant three-way interaction $(F(1,93) = 2.045; p < 0.1)$ between gender and technology type in different domestic spaces. Descriptive outcomes are illustrated in Figure 7. From there it can be seen that women tend to accept the microphone monitoring in the living room as well as in the bathroom more strongly than do men.

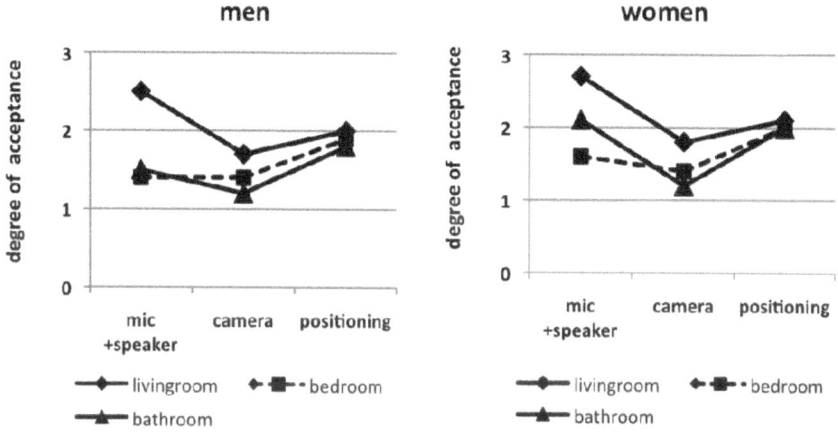

Fig. 7. Marginally significant three-way interaction effect between gender, technology and room type (Means). High values represent high levels of acceptance.

Interacting effect: Health states and the evaluation of technology types

In addition (Figure 8, left side) a significant interacting effect of individuals' health status and the evaluation of the usefulness of the respective technologies were found $(F(1,93) = 4.21; p < 0.05)$.

While the microphone is equally accepted $(M = 2.1)$ 'for ill and healthy persons', the use of the camera and the positioning system would be more strongly accepted for the healthy in contrast to the chronically ill persons, contradicting the expectation that ill persons would more easily accept technology at home. Conversely, for the chronically ill the type of technology is decisive for acceptance.

Interacting effect: Technical expertise and the evaluation of technology types

Participants had been categorized into a group, which reported to be highly familiar with the handling of conventional information and communication technologies and a group, which reports to be quite unfamiliar. As found, the extent of technical expertise shows a marginally significant interacting effect with the evaluation of the technology types under study $(F(2,93) = 2.9; p < 0.1)$. The interaction is depicted in Figure 8 (right side). As can be seen there, both expertise groups are not differing within their low acceptance for the camera as a monitoring technology at home. However, there are distinct differences in the acceptance of the positioning system,

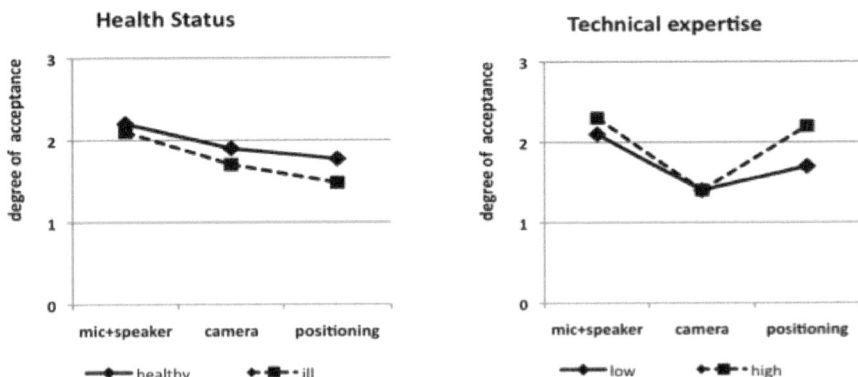

Fig. 8. left side: Interacting effect of health status of participants and the acceptance of technology type (Means); Right side: Interacting effect of technical expertise and technology type (Means). High values represent high levels of acceptance.

which is more strongly accepted by the high technical expertise group compared to the group with low technical expertise.

5   Discussion

In this research, we focused on the technology acceptance for home monitoring technologies. As the "home" is a highly private space, with a specific meaning respecting emotional and social living, we examined if and if so to which extent persons would accept monitoring technologies there, when they would be ill. In order to understand both, universal patterns as well as diversity-prone acceptance answers, we examined 100 users of a wide age range (25-93 years of age). Especially age had been found to severely impact the sensitivity of technology implementation within domestic spaces [38]. But also gender was of interest within acceptance of home monitoring technologies [36, 42]: About one half of the participants were males, the other females. Furthermore, it was a plausible assumption that chronically ill people might have different acceptance patterns than healthy persons, as diseased people know very well the necessity of medical care and also quick care in case of emergency. From this it could be derived that chronically ill persons would more strongly accept home technologies in comparison to healthy people. On the other hand, any disease experienced person handles illness in a much more versed way and knows very well what's going on, possibly much better than any home technology.

Using a scenario based approach all participants had to envisage that they would be ill and need medical care. They were asked to rate the acceptance for three technology types (contrasting technology using the auditory system only, a visual and auditory system (camera in combination with auditory information) and a positioning system, which monitors movements in the room. In order to understand different sensibilities of the rooms itself, three rooms had to be compared respecting the acceptability of home monitoring: The living room, as the most public and representative one, and bed and bathroom, which do have a highly intimate characteristic.

Even though falls are known to happen in all rooms of the house, the most likely places to fall are the bedroom and the bathroom [42]. As many of these falls happen, when people are alone at home, mobile emergency systems should call for immediate help, compensating for long-term consequences of the fall. Unfortunately, bathroom and bedroom are exactly the rooms for which the users would not accept technologies.

Apparently, the feeling of nondisclosure and confidentiality, the emotional and personal activities in these rooms do not tolerate any medical monitoring and need concealment and privacy, independently of the scenario (ill or not), and, independently of health state of participants. The same applies to other user characteristics. Neither gender, nor age was found to seriously impact the acceptance patterns, showing one more the universality of the acceptance outcomes here.

From the technologies under study, the microphone (using only the auditory channel) was the most accepted (especially in combination with the living room). The camera was mostly declined. Here two important motives came into fore. One is that the feeling of being watched provokes feelings of discomfort (rather than feeling of security and safety, what is astonishing especially for the chronically ill persons). The other is that technology still- is regarded as "cold" and "impersonal", and this is highly disliked by participants. If there would be a human being, which would watch that nothing happens, even though this person needs not to be very close to the monitored person, people would prefer this over any technology. Obviously, technology is –at least in this cultural space- not regarded as "helpful", as a "personal safeguard", as "friend", even though this factually is the case. In this context, many more studies have to be carried out, in which the role of technologies at home is carefully studied, and the characteristics technology must have in order to be accepted.

6   Limitations and Future Research Duties

Even though the study provided interesting insights into acceptance of home technologies, this research represents only a first step into a lot bigger room cartography with much more possibly integrated technologies as we singled out just three technologies in three domestic spaces. This regards both, more rooms, and more technologies. Beyond the possibility to integrate more technologies within different rooms one could add portable devices as well as integrating sensors and techniques into furniture, carpets, etc. Possibly, the feeling of mobile technology as monitoring systems would be more easily accepted and not evaluated as "big eye is watching you" as mobility always implies flexibility and While we regarded all use of technologies and acceptance from the viewpoint of one user, the everyday life with partner and family at home means, more than one person could use the technologies at the same time. Therefore it will be really interesting to research acceptance for multi-user purposes.

Also, the investigation of the impact of different using roles on acceptance for medical assistive home technologies is a serious research duty. So far participants had to evaluate that they themselves would have been monitored for the case of emergency rescue. As found, the emergency situation was not taken as equally serious as the fear of violation of own privacy as the most valuable goods. This attitude could change whenever participants would be requested to evaluate the same technologies in the same home environment, but not for themselves, but for the check of the well-being of a close family member or relative, which could live not in the same town or geographical region, but abroad. In this context, we should also focus on more culturally diverse contexts. This demand not only touches different conceptualizations of "home" and "privacy" as well as of the ability to tolerate closeness and sharing of won lives with others. This demands also touches the unawareness of a society, which shows a quite sophisticated customization on a high richness of the care system, an elaborated medical standard, as well as a high density of medical institutions as well as care systems is very high. Acceptance of supporting technologies could be completely different in countries with lower possibilities and economic standards. Also, in sparsely populated or uninhabited areas, as e.g. in the North of Europe, in which people live in remote areas with a long distance to others, acceptance for home monitoring technologies could be evaluated quite differentially.

Acknowledgments. The Authors would like to thank all focus group and questionnaire participants for kindly sharing their opinions on a sensible topic. We also thank Luise and Josef Himmel for their efforts on recruiting and motivating the participants using their social networks. Thanks also to four anonymous reviewers for their critical and constructive comments on an earlier version of this manuscript.

This research was funded by the Excellence Initiative of the German federal and state governments.

References

1. Leonhardt, S.: Personal Healthcare Devices. In: Mekherjee, S., et al. (eds.) Malware, Hardware Technology Drivers of AI, pp. 349–370. Springer, Dordrecht (2006)
2. Arning, K., Ziefle, M.: Different Perspectives on Technology Acceptance: The Role of Technology Type and Age. In: Holzinger, A., Miesenberger, K. (eds.) USAB 2009. LNCS, vol. 5889, pp. 20–41. Springer, Heidelberg (2009)
3. Rogers, Y.: The Changing Face of Human-Computer Interaction in the Age of Ubiquitous Computing. In: Holzinger, A., Miesenberger, K. (eds.) USAB 2009. LNCS, vol. 5889, pp. 1–19. Springer, Heidelberg (2009)
4. Stronge, A.J., Rogers, W.A., Fisk, A.D.: Human factors considerations in implementing telemedicine systems to accommodate older adults. Telemedicine & Telecare 13, 1–3 (2007)
5. Reding, V.: Foreword. In: Roe, P.R.W. (ed.) Towards an Inclusive Future Impact and Wider Potential of Information and Communication Technologies. COST, Brussels, Belgium, pp. i–ii (2007)

6. Heinze, R.G.: Tele-Monitoring@Home. Optionen und Realitäten eines, dritten" Gesundheitsstandortes. In: Proceedings of the Second German Congress on Ambient Assisted Living. VDE Verlag GmbH, Berlin (2009)
7. Schmitt, J.M.: Innovative medical technologies help ensure improved patient care and cost-effectiveness. International Journal of Medical Marketing 2(2), 17–178 (2002)
8. Curry, R., Trejo-Tinoco, M., Wardle, D.: The use of information and communication technology to support independent living for older and disabled people. Department of Health, London (2003)
9. Junestrand, S., Tollmar, K.: Video Mediated Communication for Domestic Environments: Architectural and Technological Design. In: Streitz, N.A., et al. (eds.) CoBuild 1999. LNCS, vol. 1670, pp. 177–190. Springer, Heidelberg (1999)
10. Lalou, S.: Identity, Social Status, Privacy and Face-keeping in the Digital Society. Journal of Social Science Information 47(3), 299–330 (2008)
11. Necheles, T.: Standards of Medical Care: How Does an Innovative Medical Procedure Become Accepted. Medicine & Health Care 10(1), 15–18 (1982)
12. Ziefle, M., Wilkowska, W.: Technology acceptability for medical assistance. Full paper at the 4th ICST Conference on Pervasive Computing Technologies for Healthcare 2010, pp. 1–9 (2010), doi 10.4108/ICST.PERVASIVEHEALTH2010.8859.
13. Zimmer, Z., Chappell, N.: Receptivity to New Technology among Older Adults. Disability and Rehabilitation 21(5/6), 2–230 (1999)
14. Jaehn, J., Nagel, K.: e-Health. Springer, Heidelberg (2003)
15. Aarts, E., Harwig, R., Schuurmans, M.: Ambient Intelligence. In: Denning, P. (Hrsg.) The Invisible Future. The Seamless Integration of Technology into Everyday Life. McGraw-Hill Professional, Lansing (2001)
16. Holzinger, A., Schaupp, K., Eder-Halbedl, W.: An Investigation on Acceptance of Ubiquitous Devices for the Elderly in a Geriatric Hospital Environment: Using the Example of Person Tracking. In: Miesenberger, K., Klaus, J., Zagler, W.L., Karshmer, A.I. (eds.) ICCHP 2008. LNCS, vol. 5105, pp. 22–29. Springer, Heidelberg (2008)
17. Eloy, S., Plácido, I., Duarte, J.P.: Housing and information society: integration of ICT in the existing housing stock. In: Braganca, et al. (eds.) SB 2007, Suistainable Construction, Materials, Practices, Portugal. IOS Press (2007)
18. Eloy, S., Plácido, I., Duarte, J.: Integration of Information, Communication and Automation technologies in Housing Rehabilitation. XXXVII IAHS. In: World Congress on Housing, Santander, Spain, October 26-29 (2010)
19. Lee, M.: Embedded Assessment of Wellness with Smart Home Sensors. In: UbiComp 2010, Copenhagen, Denmark, September 26-29 (2010)
20. Nikolaus, T.: Gait, Balance and Falls - Reasons and Consequences. Deutsche Medizinische Wochenschrift 130(15), 958–960 (2005)
21. de Ruyter, B., Pelgrim, E.: Ambient Assisted-Living Research in CareLab. ACM Interactions 14(4), 3–33 (2007)
22. Lüder, M., Salomon, R., Bieber, G.: StairMaster: A New Online Fall Detection Device. In: 2ndCongress for Ambient Assisted Living, Berlin (2009)
23. Mann, S.: Smart Clothing: The Wearable Computer and WearCam. Personal Technologies 1(1) (1997)
24. Haines, W.D., Vernon, J.R., Dannenberg, R.B., Driessen, P.F.: Placement of Sound Sources in the Stereo Field Using Measured Room Impulse Responses. In: Kronland-Martinet, R., Ystad, S., Jensen, K. (eds.) CMMR 2007. LNCS, vol. 4969, pp. 276–287. Springer, Heidelberg (2008)

25. Khan, S.M., Shah, M.: A Multiview Approach to Tracking People in Crowded Scenes using a Planar Homography Constraint. In: Leonardis, A., Bischof, H., Pinz, A. (eds.) ECCV 2006, Part IV. LNCS, vol. 3954, pp. 133–146. Springer, Heidelberg (2006)
26. Kourogi, M., Kurata, T.: Personal Positioning based on Walking Locomotion analysis with Self-Contained Sensors and a wearable camera. In: Proceedings of the 2nd IEEE/ACM International Symposium on Mixed and Augmented Reality (2003)
27. Klack, L., et al.: Future Care Floor: A Sensitive Floor for Movement Monitoring and Fall Detection in Home Environments. In: Lin, J.C., Nikita, K.S. (eds.) Wireless Mobile Communication and Healthcare (pp, pp. 211–218. Springer, Heidelberg (2011)
28. Leusmann, P., Möllering, C., Klack, L., Kasugai, K., Ziefle, M., Rumpe, B.: Your Floor Knows Where You Are: Sensing and Acquisition of Movement Data. In: Proceedings of the Workshop on Managing Health Information in Mobile Applications (HIMoA 2011), IEEE 12th International Conference on Mobile Data Management (2011)
29. Venkatesh, V., Bala, H.: Technology Acceptance Model 3 and a Research Agenda on Interventions. Decision Sciences 39, 273–315 (2008)
30. Arning, K., Gaul, S., Ziefle, M.: "Same Same but Different" How Service Contexts of Mobile Technologies Shape Usage Motives and Barriers. In: Leitner, G., Hitz, M., Holzinger, A. (eds.) USAB 2010. LNCS, vol. 6389, pp. 34–54. Springer, Heidelberg (2010)
31. Gaul, S., Ziefle, M.: Smart Home Technologies: Insights into Generation-Specific Acceptance Motives. In: Holzinger, A., Miesenberger, K. (eds.) USAB 2009. LNCS, vol. 5889, pp. 312–332. Springer, Heidelberg (2009)
32. Wilkowska, W., Gaul, S., Ziefle, M.: A Small but Significant Difference – The Role of Gender on Acceptance of Medical Assistive Technologies. In: Leitner, G., Hitz, M., Holzinger, A. (eds.) USAB 2010. LNCS, vol. 6389, pp. 82–100. Springer, Heidelberg (2010)
33. Wilkowska, W., Ziefle, M.: User diversity as a challenge for the integration of medical technology into future home environments. In: Ziefle, M., Röcker, C. (eds.) Human-Centred Design of eHealth Technologies. Concepts, Methods and Applications, pp. 95–126. IGI Global, Hershey (2011)
34. Bell, G., Dourish, P.: Back to the shed. Personal and Ubiquitous Computing 11(5), 373–381 (2006)
35. Stewart, J.: The social consumption of ICTs: insights from research on the appropriation and consumption of new ICTs in the domestic environment. RCSS, University of Edinburgh, Edinburgh (2002)
36. Leonardi, C., Mennecozzi, C., et al.: Knocking on elders' door: investigating the functional and emotional geography of their domestic space. In: Proceedings of OZCHI 2009, pp. 1703–1712. ACM (2009)
37. Crabtree, A., Rodden, T., Hemmings, T., Benford, S.: Finding a Place for Ubicomp in the Home. In: Dey, A.K., Schmidt, A., McCarthy, J.F. (eds.) UbiComp 2003. LNCS, vol. 2864, pp. 208–226. Springer, Heidelberg (2003)
38. Dethloff, C.: Akzeptanz und Nicht-Akzeptanz von technischen Produktinnovationen (Acceptance and not-Acceptance of technical product innovations). Pabst Science Publishers (Beiträge zur Wirtschaftspsychologie; 6), Lengerich (2004)
39. Wilhem, H.-J.: Das Alter - ein neuer Lebensabschnitt entsteht. Pr-Internet, HPS-Medienverlag (November 2000)
40. Marquis-Faulkes, F., McKenna, S.J., Newell, A.F., Gregor, P.: Gathering the requirements for a fall monitor using drama and video with older people. Technology and Disability 17, 227–236 (2005)

Identification of School-Aged Children with High Probability of Risk Behavior on the Basis of Easily Measurable Variables

Peter Koncz and Jan Paralic

Technical University of Kosice/Faculty of Electrical Engineering and Informatics/
Dept. of Cybernetics and Artificial Intelligence, Letna 9/B, 042 00 Kosice, Slovakia
peter.koncz@tuke.sk, jan.paralic@tuke.sk

Abstract. The use of the methods of Knowledge Discovery in Databases (KDD) in the domain of public health is still topical. One of the major reasons for its increasing use is the need for an efficient processing of the increasing volumes of data. The aim of our contribution is to analyze the possibilities of the usage of these methods to identify the groups of school-aged children with a high probability of risky behavior. The obtained results are useful for the formation of models applicable for more efficient identification of target groups of prevention programs. In this work we use Slovak national dataset from the international study Health Behaviour in School-Aged Children. The used machine learning methods were Support Vector Machine, Naïve Bayes Classifier and the J48 machine learning algorithm. The results suggest promising possibilities for the use of the machine learning methods to develop classification models useful for public health.

Keywords: Knowledge discovery in databases, machine learning, public health, risky behavior.

1   Introduction

Within the efforts focused on the primary and secondary prevention of risky behavior, the identification of children with a high probability of risky behavior is one of the biggest challenges. It is important because it can provide targeted and thus more effective impact on the current and future behavior of these children. But it is a demanding task, which is also reflected in relatively large target groups of many existing prevention programs. The aim of this paper is therefore to analyze the possibilities of the utilization of machine learning methods to identify school-aged children with a high probability of risky behavior on the basis of easily measurable variables. Easily measurable variables are in the context of this paper defined as variables for which there is little probability of bias due to the provision of socially desirable responses and variables that are easily accessible to the class teachers or educational consultants. The sample used for experiments comes from the international study Health Behaviour in School-Aged Children (HBSC) 2009/2010. The presented results should be used to develop models in order to identify individuals, schools and classes

A. Holzinger and K.-M. Simonic (Eds.): USAB 2011, LNCS 7058, pp. 625–634, 2011.
© Springer-Verlag Berlin Heidelberg 2011

with a high probability of risky behavior in the prevention programs. The rest of the work is structured as follows. The second part describes the existing works focused on the use of KDD in the context of health care with respect to their use in the identification of risky groups. The third section describes our process of models formation and their experimental verification. Finally, the fourth section is devoted to the conclusions and outlines further research.

2   Related Works

Our work can be embedded into the broader context of works devoted to the application of data mining methods to the medical and healthcare data. The increasing attention devoted to the application of data mining techniques to this type of data is significantly influenced by the data availability. During the years, healthcare providers accumulated a huge amount of data related to the patients [1, 2]. Data repositories usually created in association of scientists with academic health centers, governments and also international organizations are another important source of the health related data. An extensive list of such resources, that are publicly available, can be found at Useful Web Resources [3]. The accumulation of medical datasets causes the need for effective methods in order to deal with them. Classical methods based on the hypothesis testing have some weaknesses in this regard. The methods of data mining within the process of KDD represent an alternative approach which can be utilized in the discovery of usable patterns in large datasets with complex relations among variables.

However, the applications of KDD in this domain are limited both in terms of the used methods as well as in terms of the deployment. In terms of the used methods, the logistic regression and induction of decision trees represents the traditional methods of predictive models building in the clinical research [4]. In terms of the deployment, our theoretical analysis findings correspond with findings of Orlygsdottir [5], according to which most of the existing studies using KDD in health care have focused on the prediction of clinical outcomes. KDD has become more and more used also in the field of genomics and proteomics [6]. However, there are only few works focusing on the application of KDD in the research field of the heath related behavior [5, 7]. The disproportionality in the use of the classification and regression trees in the clinical research and in the public health research is reported also in Lemon et al. [8]. Poynton and McDaniel [7] utilized the artificial neural networks trained by the backpropagation of error learning algorithm in their work to classify respondents from "National Health Interview Survey" as a current or former smokers. Orlygsdottir[5] deals with the possibilities of the use of decision trees and logistic regression to predict health promotion behavior of preadolescents. The artificial neural networks were used as a birthing mode predictor by MacDowell et al. [9] and in the similar context there were used different data mining techniques, including logistic regression, neural networks and classification and regression trees by Goodwin et al. [10] in order to identify the accurate predictors of preterm births. The work of Flouris and Duffy [6] is devoted to the use of data mining techniques within the context of epidemiology. Sibbritt and Gibberd [2] proposed in their work a method for data mining in large medical datasets. They propose the method for the generation of decision trees from summary tables, which reduce the amount of processed data. The proposed method was evaluated on the medical record abstracts dataset with over 1.7 million records and twelve variables. The aim was the identification of possible risk factors for an adverse events caused by the health care management. We can also use claims data from the insurance companies that has been shown to be useful for a medical research, however, these databases are designed primarily for the financial reasons [11]. Bertsimas et al. [11] discuss in their work the evaluation of two algorithms for the prediction of health-care costs. The first one is based on the clustering method and the second one is based on the classification tree method. Both methods are showed accurate predictions of health-care costs. Yu et al. [12] used the support vector machine algorithm for the classification of people to those either with undiagnosed diabetes or pre-diabetes and to those without either of these. Their results showed equivalent discriminative performance as the multivariate logistic regression that is a common epidemiological method used for this purpose [12]. They also developed a web-based tool for the classification of diabetes and pre-diabetes. We did not find any other work concerned with the prediction of risky behavior of children.

3   Experiment

This work should help to answer the basic questions related to the capabilities of the classification models to identify the risky groups of school-aged children. These questions are related to the choice of variables and machine learning methods, as well as to the accuracy of the resulted prediction models. The condition of the practical applicability of developed models is the simple measurability of their input variables.

3.1   Sample

Within the frame of this work we use the Slovak national dataset of the Health Behaviour in School-aged Children (HBSC) 2009/2010 study. HBSC is a cross-national research study which aim is to increase the understanding of young health and well-being, health behaviors and their social context [13]. Slovak republic participated in HBSC 2009/2010 together with another 42 countries. The national sample was drawn from the list of schools by taking the size of schools into account. From the approached 108 schools the number of actively participating decreased to 106. The classes within a school were selected by a simple random sampling from a list of classes within schools. One class was selected from all grades that should have been included in the sample. The number of participating classes was 519. The number of students who filled out the questionnaires was 8491. The data collection was realized on each level, i.e. the school, class and individual level. The questionnaires about the school and person level were prepared in agreement with the international guidelines which can be found on the official HBSC site [13].The exact form of the questions related to the variables at the individual and school level can be also found on the official HBSC site [13]. The questionnaires on the level of classes were filled out by the administrators. The variables used in the scope of this work are described in the following subsection. The dataset containing data from individual level were sent for the cleaning process into the international HBSC data center.

3.2   Method

After the reception of cleansed data, we selected the input and output variables, which should have been used during the formation of models. The complete set of variables was formed by three subsets of variables representing the three levels of the measurement: 194 variables at individual level (individual variables), 10 at the level of classes (class variables) and 146 at the school level (school variables). In the selection of the input variables, in accordance with our objectives, we focused on the easily measurable variables enabling the identification of individuals with the various forms of risky behavior. Firstly, we identified variables for which there is a low probability of bias due to the providing of socially desirable responses. For the estimation of this probability, each variable was evaluated by the group of experts. The group of experts was formed by 11 respondents, consisting of researchers from the fields of public health, psychology and concretely health psychology. All respondents were familiar with the problems of bias caused by the provision of socially desirable responses. They were asked to evaluate the different individual level variables with respect to the question "The probability of distortion of variable value due to the provision of socially desirable answers is". Respondents answered on the four-point scale with a forced choice and response options: "very high", "rather high", "rather low" and "very low". Then the variables were ranked according to the average estimated values of the likelihood of distortion. The input variables at the individual level were chosen from the lowest rated variables, i.e. variables with the lowest estimated probability of distortion due to the provision of socially desirable answers.

From the complete set of the individual variables were chosen following variables[1] from the set of variables with lowest rating. Variable M1 (gender), AGE, AGECAT (age category), M5 (breakfast weekdays), M6 (breakfast weekends), M13 (weight), M14 (height), M56 (times injured), M60 – M69 (variables related to number of people living at the main home), M70 (have second home), M88 (talk to best friend), M89 (talk to friend of the same sex), M90 (talk to friend of the opposite sex), M93 (after school with friends), M94 (evenings with friends), M95 (e- & media communication with friends), M96 (headache), M97 (stomach-ache), M98 (back ache), M99 (feeling low), M102 (difficulties with sleeping), PH1 (last week: fit and well), PH3 (last week: felt sad), and group of variables related to motivating factors for physical activity, namely PA1 (to have fun), PA2 (to be good at sport), PA3 (to win), PA4 (to make new friends), PA6(to see my friends), PA9 (enjoy feeling of using body). In addition to these variables we added the variable M106 (academic achievement),

---

[1] Next to the names of variables there are the official variable labels or short descriptions. For exact form of the related questions see official HBSC site http://www.hbsc.org/index.html.

which is directly related to the students current learning outcomes. Each above mentioned variable corresponds to the questionnaire question.

From the complete set of class related variables, we selected variables M2SK (grade), C1 defined as the number of students who are registered in the class, C2 defined as the number of students diagnosed with the learning disorders and C3 defined as the number of students diagnosed with the behavior disorders. The values of these variables were identified, based on the interview with the classroom teachers and recorded by the administrators. This variable set was complemented by two additional variables derived from the questionnaires filled out by students. Variable G1 (average age for class) defined as the average age of respondents from the same class and variable G3 (average academic achievement for class), defined as the average of variable M106 (academic achievement) for the classes.

Subsequently, some other variables were derived and added to the reduced group of individual variables. Variable G4 (individual minus class age), defined as the difference between the respondent age and the value of G1 for respondent class, variable G5 (individual minus grade age) defined as the difference between the respondent age and the average age of respondents within the same grade, variable G6 (individual minus class academic achievement) defined as the difference between the respondent value of the variable M106 (academic achievement) and the value of G3 for respondent class.

Finally, the reduced set of school related variables was formed. This group of variables was formed by variables SLC2 (school location), SLC3 (number of boys at school), SLC4 (number of girls at school), SLC5 (percentage ethnic minority), SLC6 (percentage other 1st language) and own variable REGION defined as the official region where the school is located.

The final reduced set of input variables was formed by 40 individual variables, 6 class variables and 6 school related variables.

As the output variables were selected seven variables from the set of variables with the highest rating, i.e. variables with the highest estimated probability of distortion due to the provision of socially desirable answers. This group of variables was formed by variables M39 (smoked cigarettes last 30 days), M40 (drunk alcohol last 30 days), M41 (been drunk last 30 days), M44 (cannabis last 30 days), M46 (age of first sexual intercourse), M58 (bullied past 2 months) and M59 (bullied others past 2 months). In accordance with the expectations, these variables come from the set of variables related to the risky behavior. The output variables were also discretized, so that the class zero indicated the answer "never" and the class one indicated all other answers, except variable M46, where class one indicated the sexual intercourse before the fifteenth year.

For the formation of models we used three frequently used machine learning algorithms, namely Support Vector Machines, Naïve Bayes Classifier and the machine learning algorithm J48. Support vector machine (SVM) was invented by Vapnik [14]. It is a complex mathematical apparatus, whose detailed description can be found in several monographs, such as in the work of Abe [15]. Essentially, SVM can be characterized as a method for finding the optimal separating hyperplane. This hyperplane separates examples belonging to the different classes in the feature space. If the examples in the original feature space are linearly nonseparable, the feature space can be transformed into the higher dimensional feature space in which these classes are separable. For the purposes of experiments, freely available implementation of SVM libsvm [16] was used. We used SVM type of C-Support Vector Classification with RBF kernel type, epsilon equal to 0.001 and C equal to 0. Naïve Bayes Classifier (NBC) is another popular machine learning method. It is a probabilistic classifier based on the application of Bayesian theorem. NBC uses the naïve and usually not fulfilled assumption that the features used for the classification contribute independently to the final probability of classes. Its more detailed description can be found for example in the work of Paralic et al. [17]. We used it by Laplace correction. The third used machine learning algorithm was the J48 algorithm, which is a freely available implementation of C4.5 algorithm. C4.5 is an algorithm for the formation of decision trees, firstly published in the work of Quinlan [18]. This algorithm uses the value of the normalized information gain. During the training phase the minimum number of cases in the leaf nodes was optimized within the range 10 to 210, while the best results were taken into account. The confidence threshold for pruning was set to 0.25.

During the formation of classification models we used four different sets of input variables in combination with each of the above mentioned methods of the machine learning. The first set was made up of only individual variables, the second was made up by the addition of class level variables to the first set, the third set was formed from the second by addition of school level variables and the fourth set was formed by selection of variables from all three types of variables. The fourth set of variables was formed by variables which are considered to be the most easily measurable, namely AGE, AGECAT (age category), M1 (gender), M106 (academic achievement), and all class and school variables. We removed all records containing missing values from each of used samples.

Table 1. Numbers of records used for different combinations of input and output variables

Output variable	I.	II.	III.	IV.
M39 (smoked cigarettes last 30 days)	1454	1454	1330	1960
M40 (drunk alcohol last 30 days)	2804	2804	2560	3602
M41 (been drunk last 30 days)	934	934	860	1252
M44 (cannabis last 30 days)	138	138	134	176
M46 (age of first sexual intercourse)	162	162	158	216
M58 (bullied past 2 months)	1638	1638	1502	2458
M59 (bullied others past 2 months)	2586	2586	2378	3492

Notes: I. Only individual level variables, II. Individual and class level variables, III. All types of variables, IV. The most easily measurable variables.

From the resulted samples, we formed subsamples containing all records from respondents with the presence of risky behavior what was indicated by the output variables and the equal number of the randomly selected records from the remaining records. The numbers of records used for the different combinations of input and output variables are presented in Table 1. The lower number of records used in variables M44 and 46 is caused by the absence of related questions in questionnaires for younger children.

3.3   Results

The models capability to differentiate between respondents with and without risky behavior, indicated by the output variables, was compared on the basis of average accuracies after 10-fold cross-validation. The average accuracies for each combination of the input and output variables for each machine learning method are shown in Tables 2 to 4. Each table corresponds to one machine learning algorithm and each value represents the achieved average accuracy for different sets of input variables (I. to IV.) and output variable. The description of input and output variables can be found in former part.

Table 2. Average accuracy after 10-fold cross-validation for Support Vector Machine algorithm for different combinations of input and output variables

Output variable	I.	II.	III.	IV.
M39 (smoked cigarettes last 30 days)	73.52	75.31	63.83	60.87
M40 (drunk alcohol last 30 days)	59.41	59.98	54.18	53.19
M41 (been drunk last 30 days)	67.13	70.02	75.58	71.81
M44 (cannabis last 30 days)	69.51	71.65	92.42	94.31
M46 (age of first sexual intercourse)	58.16	66.62	88.00	91.23
M58 (bullied past 2 months)	82.06	84.07	73.43	74.65
M59 (bullied others past 2 months)	63.34	63.84	60.56	60.62

Notes: I. Only individual level variables, II. Individual and class level variables, III. All types of variables, IV. The most easily measurable variables.

In the case of SVM (Table 2) we can see the increase in the average accuracy after the addition of class level variables. In contrast, after the addition of school level variables for most of the used output variables there can be seen a decrease in the average accuracy. However, in case of variables M44 and M46, there were relatively large increases in accuracy. But in case of these variables there were used the smallest samples of data. When using the fourth set of input variables, containing only the most easily measurable variables, the obtained values of average accuracy are comparable with the results of other sets of variables.

Table 3. Average accuracy after 10-fold cross-validation for Naïve Bayes Classifier algorithm for different combinations of input and output variables

Output variable	I.	II.	III.	IV.
M39 (smoked cigarettes last 30 days)	70.21	73.86	73.83	76.17
M40 (drunk alcohol last 30 days)	61.44	61.37	61.84	59.58
M41 (been drunk last 30 days)	67.88	71.10	71.40	75.32
M44 (cannabis last 30 days)	68.79	63.08	75.38	69.28
M46 (age of first sexual intercourse)	72.39	63.05	67.83	62.01
M58 (bullied past 2 months)	84.19	86.82	86.48	84.17
M59 (bullied others past 2 months)	63.27	64.42	63.16	63.69

Notes: I. Only individual level variables, II. Individual and class level variables, III. All types of variables, IV. The most easily measurable variables.

In case of NBC (Table3) can be seen a greater decrease in the average accuracy for variable M46, even after the addition of class level variables; although it is possible to talk about an increase of accuracy in the case of other variables. There is no significant change in the average accuracy in most of the variables after the addition of school level variables, with the exception of the mentioned variables M44 and M46. In case of NBC the Achieved accuracy for the fourth set of input variables is also comparable with the results of other sets of variables.

Table 4. Average accuracy after 10-fold cross-validation for J48 machine learning algorithm for different combinations of input and output variables

Output variable	I.	II.	III.	IV.
M39 (smoked cigarettes last 30 days)	73.86	77.30	76.77	76.28
M40 (drunk alcohol last 30 days)	62.02	62.38	62.97	62.30
M41 (been drunk last 30 days)	68.94	71.64	75.70	78.36
M44 (cannabis last 30 days)	63.08	75.33	84.12	84.25
M46 (age of first sexual intercourse)	62.28	72.76	78.54	80.65
M58 (bullied past 2 months)	85.59	86.94	86.62	85.11
M59 (bullied others past 2 months)	62.95	65.43	64.30	65.03

Notes: I. Only individual level variables, II. Individual and class level variables, III. All types of variables, IV. The most easily measurable variables.

In the case of J48 machine learning algorithm (Table 4) after the addition of class level variables, there can be seen an increase in the accuracy for all variables. The results obtained for the third and fourth set of variables are similar with the results obtained by SVM a NBC.

There are some differences between the results obtained for compared machine learning methods but these differences are not significant. It is interesting that for most models there was found significantly fewer false positive errors than false negatives (the positive class indicating risky behavior). This tendency was mostly prominent for the use of NBS, although similar results were obtainable for SVM with appropriately selected penalty parameters for each class.

4   Conclusions

The results of realized experiments confirm the suitability of the using of KDD methods to develop models for the identification of the school-aged children with a high probability of risky behavior on the basis of easily measurable variables. The achieved accuracies of models are for most forms of risk behavior sufficiently high for their practical use as screening tools in the prevention programs. Relatively high accuracies of the classification models were achieved even when using the input variables that are part of school records and they don't need be separately measured. However, as it's evident from the results, the achieved average accuracies are highly dependent on the input variables and in several cases the additional variables don't lead to the higher accuracies. Based on these findings, as well as on the some additional experiments conducted with other input variables, we recommend a systematic verification of the application possibilities of attribute selection methods. Differences among compared machine learning methods are not significant. Within the frame of following research activities, we should also look on the possibility of the identifying classes and schools with a high probability of children risky behavior.

Acknowledgement. The work presented in this paper was supported by the Slovak Research and Development Agency under the contract No. VMSP-P-0048-09 (30%); the Slovak Grant Agency of Ministry of Education and Academy of Science of the Slovak Republic under grant No. 1/0042/10 (40%) and project implementation: Development of the Center of Information and Communication Technologies for Knowledge Systems (ITMS project code: 26220120030) (30%) supported by the Research & Development Operational Program funded by the ERDF.

References

1. Li, J., Fu, A.W.-c., Fahey, P.: Efficient discovery of risk patterns in medical data. Artificial intelligence in Medicine 45, 77–89 (2009)
2. Sibbritt, D., Gibberd, R.: The Effective Use of a Summary Table and Decision Tree Methodology to Analyze Very Large Healthcare Datasets. Health Care Management Science 7, 163–171 (2004)
3. Expert Health Data Programming, http://www.ehdp.com/links/index.htm
4. Holmes, J.H., Durbin, D.R., Winston, F.K.: Discovery of predictive models in an injury surveillance database: an application of data mining in clinical research. In: Proc. AMIA Symp., pp. 359–363 (2000)
5. Orlygsdottir, B.: Using knowledge discovery to identify potentially useful patterns of health promotion behavior of 10–12 year old Icelandic children. The University of Iowa (2008)
6. Flouris, A.D., Duffy, J.: Applications of Artificial Intelligence Systems in the Analysis of Epidemiological Data. European Journal of Epidemiology 21, 167–170 (2006)

7. Poynton, M.R., McDaniel, A.M.: Classification of smoking cessation status with a back-propagation neural network. Journal of Biomedical Informatics 39, 680–686 (2006)

8. Lemon, S., Roy, J., Clark, M., Friedmann, P., Rakowski, W.: Classification and regression tree analysis in public health: Methodological review and comparison with logistic regression. Annals of Behavioral Medicine 26, 172–181 (2003)

9. MacDowell, M., Somoza, E., Rothe, K., Fry, R., Brady, K., Bocklet, A.: Understanding birthing mode decision making using artificial neural networks. Medical Decision Making 21, 433–443 (2001)

10. Goodwin, L.K., Iannacchione, M.A., Hammond, W.E., Crockett, P., Maher, S., Schlitz, K.: Data Mining Methods Find Demographic Predictors of Preterm Birth. Nursing Research 50, 340–345 (2001)

11. Bertsimas, D., Bjarnadóttir, M.V., Kane, M.A., Kryder, J.C., Pandey, R., Vempala, S., Wang, G.: Algorithmic Prediction of Health-Care Costs. Operations Research 56, 1382–1392 (2008)

12. Yu, W., Liu, T., Valdez, R., Gwinn, M., Khoury, M.: Application of support vector machine modeling for prediction of common diseases: the case of diabetes and pre-diabetes. BMC Medical Informatics and Decision Making 10, 16 (2010)

13. Health Behaviour in School-Aged Children, http://www.hbsc.org/index.html

14. Vapnik, V.: The nature of statistical learning theory. Springer-Verlag New York, Inc. (1995)

15. Abe, S.: Support Vector Machines for Pattern Classification (Advances in Pattern Recognition). Springer-Verlag New York, Inc. (2005)

16. Chang, C.-C., Lin, C.-J.: LIBSVM: A library for support vector machines. ACM Trans. Intell. Syst. Technol. 2, 1–27 (2011)

17. Paralic, J., Furdik, K., Tutoky, G., Bednar, P., Sarnovsky, M., Butka, P., Babic, F.: Dolovanie znalostí z textov. Equilibria, s.r.o. (2010)

18. Quinlan, J.R.: C4.5: programs for machine learning. Morgan Kaufmann Publishers Inc. (1993)

MedReminder – An Interactive Multimedia Medical Application for the IPTV Environment

Jože Guna[1], Rok Kovač[1], Emilija Stojmenova[2], and Matevž Pogačnik[1]

[1] Faculty of Electrical Engineering, University of Ljubljana, Slovenia
[2] Iskratel, Kranj, Slovenia
joze.guna@fe.uni-lj.si, rok.kovac@ltfe.org,
stojmenova@iskratel.si,
matevz.pogacnik@fe.uni-lj.si

Abstract. We present the MedReminder, an interactive multimedia medical application, integrated into an existing IPTV service framework. The MedReminder application is implemented within XBMC multimedia platform and is integrated alongside interactive TV live and on demand multimedia services, providing easy to use and intuitive user experience. It is a client-server based application connecting different target user roles: doctors as medicine prescribers, patients as medicine consumers and patient caregivers. It allows for a centralized collection of medicine related reminder information. Consequently, the system provides user notifications on TV screen and through other communication channels, such as SMS messages, e-mail and telephone calls, which are used in case the consumption of prescribed medicine has not been confirmed. Several use case scenarios are discussed including the possibility of dynamic medicine prescriptions, based on doctor's remote readings of patient's medical parameters (e.g. blood pressure, body weight, temperature etc.), using the integrated personal health system.

Keywords: telemedicine, medicine reminder, IPTV, personal health systems.

1 Introduction and Motivation

Medical care and health oriented services represent one of the key strategic areas in modern societies, essentially ensuring a greater quality of life. As the percentage of elderly population is increasing medical related costs are significantly increasing. To alleviate this situation, telemedicine stands out as a possible solution. In its essence, telemedicine [1, 2] and related e-health oriented services provide the delivery and exchange of health-care information across distances by means of telecommunications and information technologies. Using these, both the improvement of quality of life and the significant reduction of costs, can be achieved. When comparing the costs of clinical care compared to telemedicine oriented approaches, a cost reduction in the range of hundreds up to several thousands of times is possible [3], which provides an important motivation towards utilization of telemedicine and related services.

A. Holzinger and K.-M. Simonic (Eds.): USAB 2011, LNCS 7058, pp. 635–644, 2011.

To critically appraise the effects of telemedicine, several comprehensive reviews [4 and 5] were conducted. Both studies conclude that telemedicine is effective. Beside the significant reduction of costs, other benefits can be identified, such as therapeutic effects, increased efficiencies in the health services, as well as travel time savings, increased user satisfaction and technical usability. Although the study results show that telemedicine is promising and good for patients, some critique has been expressed as well. Mainly a lack of detailed knowledge and understanding of the effects of telemedicine and higher quality evidence to inform policy decisions on how best to use telemedicine in health care is still lacking, suggesting further studies.

With recent advances in ICT and especially multimedia and human-computer interaction (HCI) technologies, their impact toward telemedicine and e-health oriented services is ever increasing [6, 7]. Multimedia technologies are enabling more comprehensive and intuitive uptake of information, suitable for all target user groups. User interaction, usability and information presentation are therefore as important as the content of the service itself. Personal computers and smart phones can in this regard be, in a way, intimidating for the elderly, which are the main target user group. On the other hand, the classical television interface and related services are not [8]. Telemedicine and related services are also recognized as an important part of the comprehensive service set of the modern digital television and IPTV systems [9].

A comprehensive study of previous exposure to technology and its acceptance with aspects of usability and accessibility focusing on the elderly has been conducted in [10]. The authors also provide usability metrics and insights gained when confronting the elderly people with technology in general.

Medicine reminder systems [11] represent a small but important part of a wide range of telemedicine services. They essentially provide medicine schedule and usage related information and are suitable for all target user groups. As shown by a study in [12], non-attendance at outpatient clinics and medication non-adherence lead to significant time wasting and inefficient use of resources. Forgetfulness has been identified as one of the key reasons for this behavior. Electronic reminders are an efficient and also acceptable solution to this problem, according to [13]. Reminder systems can further be improved by integrating personal health systems (PHS) [14], which allows for home collection and monitoring of various additional patients' medical parameters. Thus, greater therapeutic efficiency and significant cost reductions can be achieved.

With this in mind, we present the MedReminder, an interactive multimedia medical application, integrated into an existing IPTV service framework. The MedReminder application allows for a centralized collection and admission of medicine related reminders on the TV screen using an intuitive and simple user interface.

The rest of the paper is organized as follows: related work is presented in section 2; a detailed description of the proposed MedReminder application, including functionalities, use case scenarios and architecture is described in section 3; and finally discussion, key conclusion and references for future work are drawn in section 4 respectively.

2   State of the Art

The field of telemedicine and related services has received a lot of research attention due to its importance and benefits. Medical reminders are among the most effective methods of persuading individuals to perform healthy behavior such as taking their medication and performing exercises. These reminders often represent a task interruption for users who are engaged in work activities. However, as shown in [15], it is interesting that the degree of perceived politeness of such interruptions is positively correlated with predicted long-term adherence, but negatively correlated with short-term compliance. To this end we have chosen the television medium as the interface for relating medicine reminder information as the users will be more attentive and more favourably inclined to these interruptions.

In [16] researchers present the design and exploratory evaluation of a sensor-driven adaptive reminder system for home medical tasks. A mobile reminder delivery device and ambient sensors are used for determining opportune moments for reminder delivery. The results show that context-sensitive reminders might improve adherence levels, the manner of their representation is still very important. Similarly, an adaptive notification framework for optimal delivery and handling of multimedia requests and alerts in a nursing home is presented in [17]. Device selection, content adaptation and specific user delivery properties are considered. Study results show improved quality of life of elderly people as well as the efficiency of the medical staff.

A mobile health monitoring system for the elderly called iCare is presented in [18]. Wireless body sensors and smart phone based interface are used to monitor the wellbeing of the elderly. Besides monitoring features, a relatively simple regular medicine reminder is implemented as well, which implies at the importance of such reminders in general. A more complex smart phone based medicine in-take scheduler named Wedjat is described in [19]. Beside simple on time medicine reminders the system allows for user notification and avoidance of potential drug-drug or drug-food related interactions and schedule revisions in case a medicine dose was missed. Finally, a web based medicine e-Reminder is presented in [20]. The system is managed via a web based interface, where relevant medicine reminder information is entered by professional personnel. The reminders themselves are sent as voice or SMS messages and e-mails.

Relatively little research effort, however, has been afforded to integration of medicine based reminder systems and IPTV services. In this regard we present our own solution for delivering medicine reminders, which is especially designed for the IPTV environment. To further extend the functionality of the MedReminder system, it is also integrated with our PHS system [14]. The PHS allows for monitoring of blood pressure and body weight parameters and supports on-line medical interviews. Consequently, remote monitoring of patient's medical parameters and dynamic changes to the medicine schedule information are possible.

3   The MedReminder System

The MedReminder medical application is directly integrated into an existing IPTV environment. Various communication channels such as text, voice messages and e-mail are supported. From the user's point of view the application allows for viewing and setting of medicine intake related reminders.

The XBMC multimedia platform [21], as one of the possible platforms for the IP television set-top boxes, was used for front-end TV implementation. Integrated graphical user interface (GUI) allows the user to easily manage videos, photos, music and applications using a remote control. MedReminder application's user interface is designed in such a way that it is easy to use for the users already familiar with the usage of other television services.

The MedReminder application is automatically started after the XBMC platform initialization. Depending on the user type, application can operate in different modes. Advanced users may choose information from a database of existing medical drugs or enter new drug descriptions. Reminders can be set for an unlimited number of drugs. It is possible to select a notification interval, a number and dose of drugs or enter additional descriptions, as shown in Fig. 1. Choices of language, phone number and type of notification are possible. On the other hand, the basic user has no access to the MedReminder settings, as these are reserved for doctors, pharmacists or patient caregivers. It should be noted that the medical professional can access these settings irrespective of the user type.

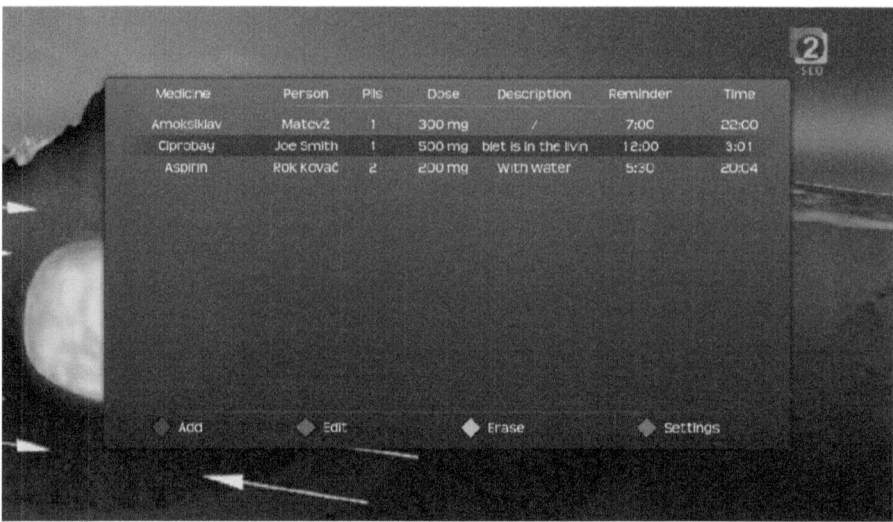

Fig. 1. A MedReminder parameter input screenshot

At the preset time a medicine reminder appears on the television screen overlaying the current picture. The patient can act upon the information provided and acknowledge the medicine usage, view additional instructions or start an emergency (video) call, to authorized medical personnel, as illustrated in Fig. 2. If no

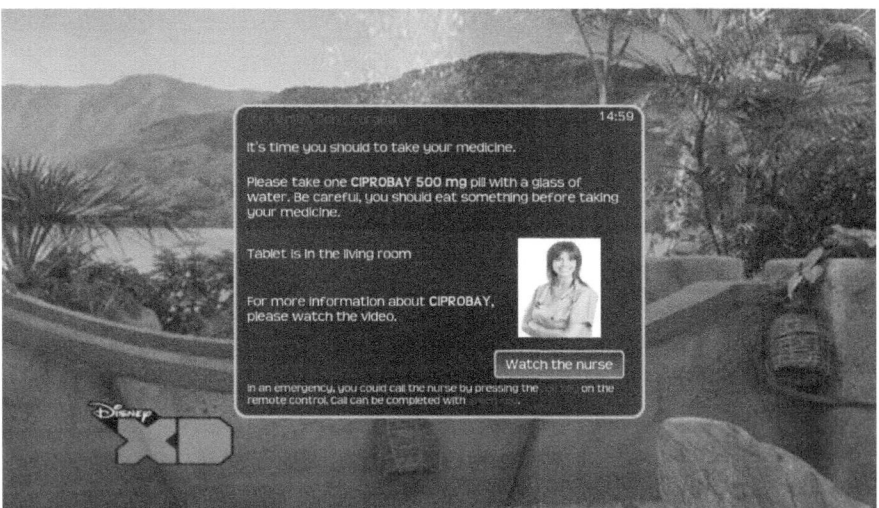

Fig. 2. A MedReminder notification window screenshot

acknowledgement is received within the preset time interval (set to 1-5 minutes), a back-end server triggered voice call, SMS message or e-mail notifications are sent.

3.1   Use Case Scenarios

To illustrate the usage possibilities, two typical use case scenarios for the proposed system were considered. Presented use cases are graphically illustrated in Fig. 3.

In the first scenario, a typical example of medicine reminders is presented. The patient visits a doctor and after personal examination, the doctor decides to prescribe drugs to the patient. The prescribed drugs are delivered to the patient through a pharmacist, who also inscribes appropriate medicine reminders using a dedicated web based user interface or standalone application. This information is inserted into the back-end database server. The MedReminder XBMC application periodically connects to the back-end database server and downloads all medicine reminders for selected users. At the appropriate time a notification appears on the television screen and the patient confirms (or not) the successful medicine usage by pressing OK button on the remote control. An application report is sent to the back-end database server and no other action is required by the patient.

In the second scenario, a patient uses his personal health system to conduct blood pressure measurements. This data is automatically sent to the back-end database server. The doctor, who has access to those remote PHS parameters, decides to change the drug dose. Medicine reminder related modifications made and stored in back-end database server. The updated information is then available to the MedReminder XBMC application. At the appropriate time notification appears on the television screen, but no successful confirmation by the patient is received. In this case the back-end server triggers the Call Server to make a voice call to the patient.

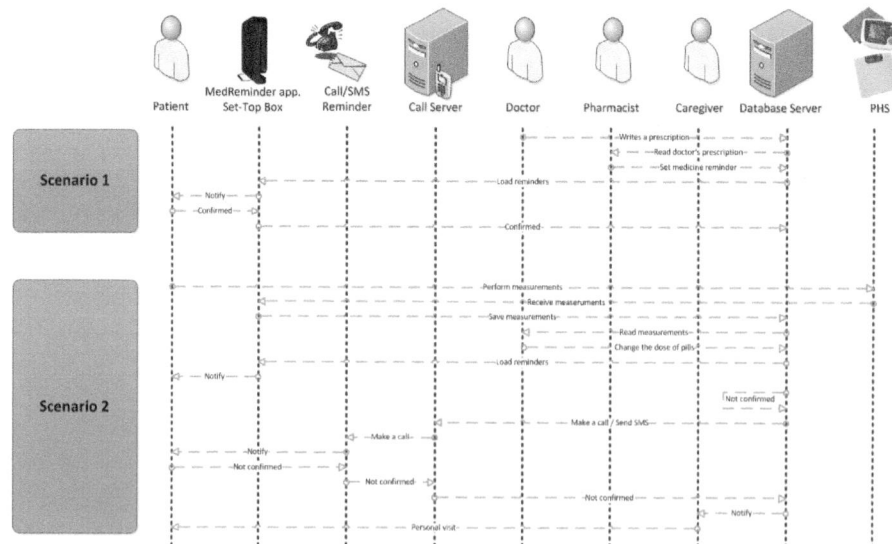

Fig. 3. Use case scenarios

Because still no response to the call is received, a notification is sent to the caregiver. Caregiver decides to visit the patient in person to examine his situation or state of health.

3.2   System Architecture Overview

Modular system architecture was designed to implement the described functionalities and use case scenarios. It is being implemented in phases.

The MedReminder system (Fig. 4) consists of the front-end graphical user application and back-end central server database and business logic. MedReminder XBMC application was implemented as a front-end application for the XBMC multimedia platform using the existing framework and additional Python scripts to develop the graphical user interface (GUI) and decision logic. Considering the graphical design it was very important that the original appearance and navigation was adopted thus making the application user-friendly for average users and especially for elderly people. Special attention was devoted to this aspect of implementation.

In the initialization phase, application connects to the back-end database server and downloads all medicine reminders for selected users. Connection is established through multiple protocol standards and data formats such as Internet Protocol suite (IP), Simple Object Access Protocol (SOAP) and Extensible Markup Language (XML). After the successful data transfer, the connection is closed. Any further checking is done at predefined intervals (preset to two hours). Access to the database server is possible also via a web based or standalone application, by which the patient's medicine reminders can be inserted, modified, deleted or cancelled by doctors, pharmacists or patient caregivers.

When a MedReminder notification appears on the television screen, the patient has a predefined time interval (a few minutes; set by medical professionals) to acknowledge a successful medicine administering. It is important that the MedReminder application and the back-end database server are synchronized. A network time protocol (NTP) is therefore used for time synchronization. When medicine administering is acknowledged, a report is sent to the back-end database server. In case no report from the MedReminder application is received, the back-end server assumes no user confirmation was given and consequently the medicine schedule was not properly adhered to. Described scenario could also happen in case of network related problems. In the latter scenario the back-end server contacts the Call Server, which triggers the dispatch of SMS text message or voice call reminders. Notifications can also be sent to the caregiver. Call Server constitutes a separate part of the network and is responsible for setting up calls and sending messages.

To further enhance the functionality, we connected MedReminder system to the personal health telemonitoring services, developed at the Faculty of Electrical Engineering [14]. Monitoring of blood pressure and body weight medical parameters are currently enabled and uploaded to the back-end database server. This enables the doctors to remotely monitor patient's medical parameters and dynamically change medicine doses and schedule, if necessary.

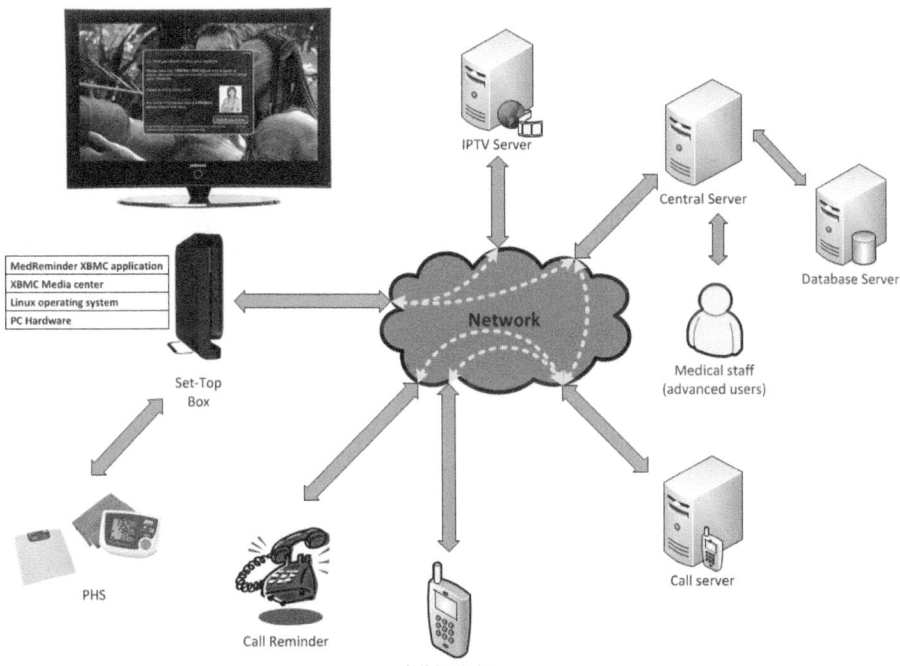

Fig. 4. MedReminder system architecture

4   Discussion and Conclusions

The presented reminder/PHS medical application was designed and implemented, based on evident need for such systems. As the average age of population in developed countries is increasing, the need for optimization of health care is becoming of high importance. Such systems, if designed appropriately, can bring a number of benefits to the society. On one hand, we can achieve significant cost reductions due to faster processing of patient's needs and medical measurements, which would normally require patient's visits to medical institutions. Related to the above are time savings of all actors: patients, doctors and patient caregivers, and to some extent indirect benefits to fuel consumption, traffic and consequently the environment. Proposed medical application can therefore be considered as green technology in this aspect.

On the other hand, such centralized data systems allow for smart gathering and analyzing of medical data, thus providing the possibility to identify the correlations between measured medical parameters, consumed medicines, medical disorders, etc. These kinds of analyses have undoubtedly been performed in the past for decades, but the access to useful medical information is much simplified in case of such centralized information system. Furthermore, such systems, if upgraded with data mining and reasoning algorithms, may potentially identify anomalies or problems based on measured medical parameters, prescribed medicines, etc. and alert medical personnel in real-time accordingly.

In addition to benefits of the described system, serious consideration needs to be given to privacy and security issues. Medical and health related information are one of the most sensitive, therefore sufficient security mechanisms need to be enforced in order to protect the information exchange and storage. Fortunately, current state of security mechanisms has reached a mature stage, and can be applied with reasonable investment.

The proposed medical application is still being enhanced and developed and therefore currently has some limitations as well. The most obvious limitation is when the TV set or the set-top box devices are turned off for any reason (user action, no power available, equipment malfunction, etc.). In this case the TV reminder cannot be delivered, however alternative communications channels have been foreseen for this case in form of SMS, telephone call or e-mail messages, delivered directly to the patients and/or their caregivers. As shown in [11] and [13], reminders are an effective and acceptable solution to reduce costs in general and to prevent time wasting and inefficient use of resources, according to [12]. Also, in combination with personal health systems the overall service to patients can be further improved [14]. Since the majority of users are not technical experts and some are even negatively disposed to new technologies and approaches, this can be considered as an important, non-technical limitation, as well. However, the proposed medical application has been carefully designed with usability and ease of use aspects in mind, to provide great user experience for all target user groups. For this reason well known non-computer like technologies, primarily the TV screen and secondary the mobile phone (SMS, call) were selected as interfaces between users and the system. Also, as shown in [10], previous exposure to technology can significantly improve its acceptance, especially with the elderly users.

To test our medical application and to gain insights in real-life usage, we plan to perform an extensive usability study. We will test the proposed two existing and additional scenarios using established usability methods, including System Usability Scale (SUS) and heuristic approaches. We will include users of different genders, technical backgrounds and ages, with an emphasis on the elderly. A short preliminary user evaluation study has indicated a positive acceptance of the proposed medical application. Therefore, we expect similar results in the detailed user evaluation study as well.

There are a number of ways how to improve such systems. Firstly, the inclusion of additional medical devices is foreseen to extend the number of measured medical parameters. Secondly, the inclusion of security standards, defined by the medical organizations is to be included in one of the future releases. In case such a system is used in real-life scenarios, the integration into existing medical information systems will be required. Regardless of the above, we must strive to keep the system modular and leave room for later inclusion of new functionalities. Most of all, we should keep it simple, intuitive and easy to use for all actors as this is one of the foremost important adoption factors for all interactive systems.

References

1. Wootton, R., et al.: Introduction to Telemedicine. The Royal Society of Medicine Press (1999)
2. Jorda, E.G.: Telemedicine: shortening distances. Clin. Transl. Oncol. 12, 650–651 (2010)
3. Wartena, F., Muskens, J., Schmitt, L.: Continua: The impact of a Personal Telehealth Ecosystem. In: Proceedings International Conference on eHealth, Telemedicine, and Social Medicine, eTELEMED, pp. 13–18 (2009)
4. Hailey, D., Ohinmaa, A., Roine, R.: Study quality and evidence of benefit in recent assessments of telemedicine. Journal of Telemedicine and Telecare 10, 318–324 (2004)
5. Ekeland, A., Bowes, A., Flottorp, S.: Effectiveness of telemedicine: A systematic review of reviews. International Journal of Medical Informatics 79, 736–771 (2010)
6. Duplaga, M., Zieliński, K.: Evolution of IT-Enhanced Healthcare: From Telemedicine to e-Health. Springer, London (2006)
7. Kim, J., Wang, Z., Cai, W., Feng, D.: Multimedia for Future Health: Smart Medical Home. Biomedical Information Technology. Elsevier Press, San Diego (2007)
8. Rodriguez, T., Fischer, K., Kingston, J.: Intelligent Services for the Elderly Over the TV. Journal of Intelligent Information Systems 25(2), 159–180 (2005)
9. ITU-T IPTV Focus Group Proceedings, http://www.itu.int/pub/T-PROC-IPTVFG-2008
10. Holzinger, A., Searle, G., Wernbacher, M.: The effect of previous exposure to technology on acceptance and its importance in usability and accessibility engineering. Univ. Access Inf. Soc. 10, 245–260 (2011)
11. Bennison, C.: Medication reminders. Occupational Therapy Now 8, 3–6 (2006)
12. Hogan, A.M., Mc Cormack, O., Traynor, O., Winter, D.C.: Potential impact of text message reminders on non-attendance at outpatient clinics. Ir. J. Med. Sci. 177, 355–358 (2008)

13. Sahm, L., MacCurtain, A., Hayden, J., Roche, C., Richards, H.L.: Electronic reminders to improve medication adherence—are they acceptable to the patient? Pharm. World Sci. 31, 627–629 (2009)
14. Pustišek, M., Zebec, L., Stojmenova, E., Kervina, D.: Bringing Health Telemonitoring into IPTV Based AMI Environment. In: SAME Workshop 2011 in conjuct with C&T 2011 Brisbane, Australia (2011)
15. Bickmore, T., Mauer, D., Crespo, F., Brown, T.: Persuasion, task interruption and health regimen adherence. In: de Kort, Y.A.W., IJsselsteijn, W.A., Midden, C., Eggen, B., Fogg, B.J. (eds.) PERSUASIVE 2007. LNCS, vol. 4744, pp. 1–11. Springer, Heidelberg (2007)
16. Kaushik, P., Intille, S.S., Larson, K.: Observations From a Case Study on User Adaptive Reminders for Medication Adherence. In: Pervasive Computing Technologies for Healthcare, pp. 250–253 (2008)
17. Betge-Brezetz, S., Dupont, M.P., Ghorbel, M., Kamga, G.B., Piekarec, S.: Adaptive Notification Framework for Smart Nursing Home. In: Engineering in Medicine and Biology Society, pp. 7244–7247 (2009)
18. Lv, Z., Xia, F., Wu, G., Yao, L., Chen, Z.: iCare: A Mobile Health Monitoring System for the Elderly. In: IEEE/ACM International Conference on Green Computing and Communications & 2010 IEEE/ACM International Conference on Cyber, Physical and Social Computing, pp. 699–705 (2010)
19. Zao, J.K., Wang, M.Y., Tsai, P., Liu, W.S.: Smart Phone Based Medicine In-take Scheduler, Reminder and Monitor. In: 2010 12th IEEE International Conference on e-Health Networking Applications and Services (Healthcom), pp. 162–168 (2010)
20. Cimerman, P., Borštnar, T., Rudel, D., Oberžan, D.: e-Reminder for Self-Health Care - Presentation of a Solution. Informatica Medica Slovenica 15(supl.), 51–52 (2010)
21. XBMC Wiki portal, http://wiki.xbmc.org

A Logical Approach to Web User Interface Adaptation

Jesia Zakraoui and Wolfgang Zagler

Institute "integrated study"
Vienna University of Technology, Austria
e9827053@student.tuwien.ac.at, zw@fortec.tuwien.ac.at

Abstract. This article presents a logical framework that allows the generation of Web user interfaces depending largely on user's needs and meaningful contextual information. In order to provide means for that, relevant parts of formally connected knowledge in user interaction processes are used to support a reasoning component, which is based on Answer Set Programming (ASP). This task is achieved through generation of visual aspects of user interfaces such as sizes of user interface elements, colours, relative position of the elements or navigation devices used. In Web environments, user interface adaptation is needed to tailor user interfaces to older people's needs and impairments while preserving their independence.

Keywords: Ontology, Answer Set Programming, Web accessibility, Usability, Context, User interaction.

1 Introduction

The ageing of the population is a phenomenon faced by many nations, such as Austria, where $17,5\%$ of the population are more than 65 years old in 2011 [1]. In many countries the ratio between the number of old and young people is constantly growing. This means that the number of old people will be a sizeable percentage of the whole population. We want these people to have good quality of life while keeping expenses as low as possible. In fact, studies on the acceptance of technologies for care [23], [9] show that older people tend to look for social networking as well as accepting new technological assistances. In this context, many factors are supposed to influence the older users' acceptance of software. The extent of previous exposure to technology and other factors are evaluated in [12] to provide short guidelines for software developers on how to design and develop software for the older population. The authors in this work emphasize that expectations, behavior, abilities, and limitations of prospective end users are considered of primary importance for the development of technology.

These considerations lead us to regard diversities of users, and particularly age related specificities, as a potential enrichment in Web user interface design. As a contribution, this paper suggests a logical framework to adaptive user interfaces (UI), as a possibility to automatically generate user interface characteristics.

A. Holzinger and K.-M. Simonic (Eds.): USAB 2011, LNCS 7058, pp. 645–656, 2011.

As a consequence, providing accessible and usable user interfaces to any Web information is crucial for e-Inclusion and e-Health of these people.

The design of such effective Web interfaces is difficult due to the variety of users' interests, perceptive capabilities or other meaningful factors. Unfortunately, because of the great diversity of users and their context of use, manually designing interfaces for each one of them is impractical and not scalable. One possible solution to this problem is to use a semi-automatic mechanisms to detect the type of user of the Web application and his/her contextual information related to the interaction process and then adapt its interaction mechanism. The usage of style sheets for providing personalized user interfaces is very beneficial in such environment where users' conditions and time constraints do not permit optimally to shift the interaction settings from one mode to another. In this paper, we show that Web interface characteristics can automatically be generated according to users' capabilities and to relevant contextual information using a decision mechanism based on Answer Set Programming [8]. Basically the generation of colours and their contrasts, sizes or position of the different components of the Web interface are considered.

This approach takes away a significant amount of overhead related to manual coding of style sheets in Web applications. The execution of rules consists of abstract user interfaces suggestions according to user profile and contextual information. In the light of these suggestions the style sheets can be generated and/or adapted on the fly. Similarly, relations between information entities in any information system such as eHealth systems may also be automated in this way. Consequently, our logical framwork could be usefully exploited towards the automation of usability metrics [11]. In particular, the authors in this work [11] investigate metrics-based benchmarks which are crucial for measuring different aspects of usability for older users; whether in passive or active interaction.

The rest of this document is organized as follows: the next Section gives the related work. Section 3 recalls Web accessibility and usability. Section 4 gives an overview of the integration of knowledge using formally connected Ontologies and Answer Set Programming. The results are explained in Section 5, followed by conclusions and future work in Section 6.

2   Related Work

Several approaches to automatic user interface generation can be found in the literature, some of them have been developed with a particular subset of motor-impaired user or only visual-impaired user or both such as [7], however without the consideration of any contextual information.

Other general approaches such as [10] have developed new design methodologies for creating interfaces that can be dynamically adapted by the end-user for their individual needs, however the user may not be able to adjust his/her settings due to disabilities, the user may not know what options exist or how she/he can set them. She/he may have no idea what the best setting is for her/him. A few other interfaces have been created, particularly in the Web domain, but most lack any such adaptation capabilities. Shuaib et al. introduced the concept Connecting Ontologies [20] with the help of SWRL [21] for providing universal Accessibility. However, due to lack of support for rules or for some concepts (e.g., transitive closure, negation as failure, cardinality constraints), some queries can not be represented concisely and some queries can not be represented at all. In this sense, the use of a rule mechanism such as Answer Set Programming provides a more expressive formalism to represent rules, concepts, constraints, and queries than the rule mechanism used in this approach.

In the healthcare sector, a number of adaptive user interfaces has been developed and integrated in many devices such as [24], which proposes a personalized smart phone to assist older people. The smart phone has been optimized to ease interaction of the device for senior citizens. In [19], the authors use a fuzzy expert system to decide which information is relevant for the user based on the user model. The goal is to provide the data that meet the user's current profile and location. They do not, however, follow a clear separation of layers in their adaptation framework. This makes support for different devices and output modalities more difficult.

Our logical framework derives the user interface characteristics according to the user profile, user's impairments profile and contextual profile. Therefore, the obvious candidates for interaction are the style sheets for use in browsers as well as for integration in some applications adressed to diversities of users.

3   Web Accessibility and Usability

Web accessibility corresponds to making the Web possible to any user by using some user agent, to understand and interact with a website, despite of disabilities, languages or technological constraints. The W3C/WAI [22] Working Group offers standards which are internationally accepted. They offer quantifiable rules such as using alt text for non textual content so that it can be changed into other forms people need like speech. Such rules are technically applied and, therefore, the website is accessible, however, sometimes alt text is not suitable so that the usability of the site is not suitable for anyone who relies only on alt text. Other kinds of experiences show that guidelines have not been successful in producing accessible and usable websites [18].

For older people, accessibility and usability of the Web is very important, and will become more important in the future. As the demographic balance changes, older people will need as much technological support as they can use to reach a certain level of independance. As the older population grows, the likelihood of impairments increases with age such as poor vision which is the most common impairment affecting older people. Many works have been done toward the investigation of new usability metrics for older people such as [12]. In [13] the author draws attention to the user interfaces, which should be easily accessible, but also useful, usable and enjoyable for all people.

On the other hand, many assistive tools have been developed to modify non-accessible Web interfaces and translate them into accessible components such as browsers built-in extensions. They aim at making easy for older users to view and navigate through Web content. Web Accessibility Toolbar [1] is an example. However, such solutions are mostly used by developers who want to check or correct certain aspects of Web applications. The variety of such tools is wide that users do not want spending their time learning about their activation or use.

In fact, Web accessibility and usability benefits also users with disabilities, mobile device users, and other individuals, since the needs and preferences that are essential to a user are a consequence of having a disability and/or it may be that the circumstances, devices, or other factors have led to a mismatch between them and the resources they wish to use. Web accessibility is likely to bring about new opportunities, but, at the same time, new challenges for access to Web services by old people, which can not be addressed through ad hoc assistive technology solutions. Instead, there is a need for more approaches. A promising approach is the semantic knowledge about users und his/her context of use. This could be very helpful in adapting the Web interfaces to their. Such semantic knowledge is not very useful if the semantic of different information items with each other and with other meaningful information components are not established. The following Section shows how it is possible to integrate different semantic components together and exploit them for deriving the most suitable Web interface characteristics.

4   Integrating Knowledge from Ontologies

In a previous work, we have modelled knowledge about the user, his/her impairment and his/her contextual information which are meaningful in the user interaction process in OWL-DL Ontologies [17] and formally connected them together. The connections are developed following a semi-automatic approach using Distributed Description Logics (DDL) [2]. DDL follow the ontology mapping [17] paradigm. It allows to connect multiple DL Knowledge bases with bridge rules [2], a new kind of axioms that represents the mapping. We have chosen DDL since it allows for inter-ontology subsumption [2], a notion that combines well with the vision of Semantic Web [14].

We built our instances for the User Profile Ontology UPO by first exporting user FOAF[2] profile from a social networking site like Twitter. We used http://semantictweet.com/, a FOAF generator for Twitter profiles, to get a FOAF profile of the user. We could use this approach with other social networking sites that produce FOAF data such as Facebook (Facebook FOAF generator not working at the moment). Since not all required details are available in resulting FOAF file, we use default reasoning, a feature of Answer Set Programming [8], assuming to know user's details and we add this information manually in the UPO. Only a restricted set of data is requested from UPO:

---

[1] http://www.wat-c.org/

[2] http://www.foaf-project.org/

```
observedU(User,Age,Gender,Ability,Imp,T):-
timestamp(T),defaultMS(User,MaritalStatus),
defaultAge(User,Age),defaultGender(User,Gender),
defaultAbility(User,Ability), defaultImp(User,Imp).
```

Information about the user's disabilities is requested from User Impairment Ontology UIO - if exists - otherwise, default reasoning allows us to assume it as follow:

```
observedI(Imp,Perception,Pmeasure,Capability,Cmeasure,T):-
timestamp(T),
defaultaffectsPerception(Imp,Perception),
defaultperceptionMeasure(Perception,Pmeasure),
defaultaffectsCapability(Perception,Capability),
defaultcapabilityMeasure(Capability,Cmeasure) .
```

Moreover, the user interface element could be influenced by additional contextual information observed at a given time T. Such information becomes significant and thus is represented in OWL-DL and used in the inference process. Contextual information can be related either to the user or to an element of the interface or to the environment, so that we can generally extract contextual information form the Context Ontology CO following the form bellow:

```
observedC(Context,Decibel,Intensity,Reso,Contrast,T):-
timestamp(T), location(Context),
defaultLight(L,Decibel),defaultNoise(N,Intensity),
defaultdevice(Device,Software,Reso,Size,Contrast,Volume).
```

The declarative nature of this approach allows to easily extend the amount of information extracted from the connected Ontologies to consider other contextual information, and correspondent new logic predicates can be included in the inference process.

5   Decision Mechanism

In order for the information presentation to be fully accessible and usable, it must be shaped based on users' characteristics and their contextual information. This can be achieved by a decision mechanism. The decision mechanism provides ways of adaptation decisions at either level of the user interaction. It comprises the default rules, which refer to static users' characteristics and the run-time rules, which refer to dynamic user characteristics and contextual information. Rules describe system behavior and are represented internaly as dl-rules/dl-programs [6]. Consequently, a set of these rules has been defined for providing the decision for the selection of appropriate user interaction styles. That most of the information consists actually of defaults and that the connected Ontologies contains incomplete knowledge motivated us to use a non-monotonic formalism to build a rule layer over them. We might want to express preferences (e.g. aggregate functions) as well as constraints (e.g. integrity constraints) while querying the knowledge stored in Ontologies to be able to discover new knowledge. Answer Set Programming provides an expressive language to express these knowledge and efficient solvers, like DLV-Hex [4] built over DLV [3] to reason about it, this motivated us to use ASP as such a non-monotonic formalism. Additionaly, the non-monotonicity is important to allow updates to the user interaction model.

Furthermore, such concept allow us to choose the most relevant answer sets in order to allow the user interface characteristics to change dynamically according to this knowledge. This could make improvements of user interaction for all impairments or the combinations of impairments of the users in a generic way instead of focusing only on the stereotypical disabilities. Our approach may be used in context of the user's personal information management systems as well as in mobile computing systems.

5.1   Answer Set Programming

Answer Set Programming (ASP) [8] has emerged as an important tool for declarative knowledge representation and reasoning. This approach is rooted in semantic notions and is based on methods to compute stable models [8]. ASP is one of the most prominent and successful semantics for *non-monotonic* logic programs. The specific treatment of default negation under ASP allows for the generation of multiple models for a single program, which in this respect can be seen as the encoding of a problem specification. With ASP, one can encode a problem as a set of rules and the solutions are found by the stable models (Answer sets) of these rules.

An Answer Set Program consists of rules of the form *head :- body* that can contain variables. The head can be a disjunction or empty and the body is a conjunction or empty. A *term* is either a constant or a variable. An *atom* is defined as $p(t_1, ...t_k)$ where k is called the arity of p and $t_1, ...t_k$ are terms. A *literal* is an atom p or a negated atom $\neg p$, also strong negation (also often referred to as classical negation). A rule without head literal is an *integrity (strong) constraint*. A rule with exactly one head literal is a *normal rule*. If the body of the rule variable-free is empty then this rule is a *fact*. A *negation as failure literal* (or NAF-literal) is a literal l or a default-negated literal *not l*. Negation as failure is an extension to classical negation, it represents default negation in a program, and infers negation of a fact if it is not provable in a program. Thus, *not l* evaluates to true if it cannot be proven that l is true. This is relevant in our work since we don't have complete information about the user interaction process and we must assume some defaults reasoning until we confirm the reasoner with a new knowledge.

In order to solve a problem in ASP, a logic program should be constructed so that its answer sets correspond to the solutions of the problem. By adding new knowledge, not only new answer sets become possible, but old answer sets are defeated, so that the sets do not grow monotonically. ASP provides us this *non-monotonicity*. An important feature of ASP is that the body of a rule can also contain negation, which is handled as negation as failure, thus allowing methods from non-monotonic reasoning, since additional information might lead to retraction of a previously made inference [5].

In order to compute these answer sets, there exist ASP solvers or engines such as DLV [3], a highly efficient reasoner for ASP which extends the core language with various sophisticated features such as aggregates or weak constraints [15].

5.2   Default Reasoning

In default reasoning one can specify general knowledge for standard cases and modulary add exceptions. When one adds an exception to default, one can not conclude what one could before. In that default reasoning is told non-monotonic. Static user characteristics represented in the UPO have been selected to serve as the basis for the default reasoning. The selection of such meaningful characteristics was made so as to ensure that adequate knowledge exists for the system. Such characteristics have been selected also to serve as the basis for reasoning. These include: user's impairments, familiarity of the user with the Web etc. The dynamic user characteristics and other dynamic contextual information are responsable for the system inference to be triggered. The evaluation of such data can be based on results of specific data aggregation e.g. quality of navigation/user error rate, results of ad-hoc logic rules e.g. user idle time/user response time.

By default, a user interface (UI) element in the interface does not have to be adapted if the User Profile Ontology does not trace any anomaly in the way the user could interact with it. Such anomalies are to be specified in a declarative form, by using predicates. By default, UI style in the Web interface is favorite style, if it has generic usability characteristics like sufficient colour contrast, suitable font size etc. A favorite style is classified as usable or as unusable. The correspondent rules in our framework are as follows:

```
%The contrast ratio
%For large text it's 3:1 for AA and 5:1 for AAA.
%For small text it's 5:1 for AA and 7:1 for AAA.
fav(UI,FontSize,W,Font,Style,ColorBG,ColorFG) :-
hasContrast(Color,W),
W >= 3, vis(UI,W,ColorBG,ColorFG),
text_profile(UI,FontSize,Font,Style), FontSize >= 18,
timestamp(T1), not rem(UI,T1), n_bold(UI).

fav(UI,FontSize,W,Font,Style,ColorBG,ColorFG) :-
hasContrast(Color,W),
W >= 3, vis(UI,W,ColorBG,ColorFG),
text_profile(UI,FontSize,Font,Style), FontSize >= 14,
timestamp(T1), bold(Style), not rem(UI,T1).

fav(UI,FontSize,W,Font,Style,ColorBG,ColorFG) :-
hasContrast(Color,W),
```

```
W >= 5,vis(UI,W,ColorBG,ColorFG),
text_profile(UI,FontSize,Font,Style), FontSize < 18,
timestamp(T1),not rem(UI,T1), n_bold(UI).
```

Contrast ratios can range from 1 to 21 (commonly written 1:1 to 21:1). For the purpose of Success Criteria 1.4.3 and 1.4.6 [22], contrast is measured with respect to the specified background over which the text is rendered in normal usage. If no background colour is specified, then white is assumed. Black and white create the highest contrast possible. Using 3:1 contrast ratio or higher for the default presentation is required to conform the AA level. Large text has wider character strokes and is easier to read at lower contrast. The contrast requirement for larger text is, therefore, lower. The correspondent rules in our framework are as follows:

```
vis(UI,W1,C2,C1) :- uicomponent(UI),
color(C1),color(C2), hasContrastW(C1,W1),
hasContrastW(C2,W2), defaultFG(UI,C1),
defaultBG(UI,C2),
C1 != C2, W1>=5, W2=1.

vis(UI,W1,C2,C1) :- uicomponent(UI),
color(C1),color(C2), hasContrastB(C1,W1),
hasContrastB(C2,W2), defaultFG(UI,C1),
defaultBG(UI,C2),
C1 != C2, W1>=5, W2=1.


%If no background color is specified, then white is assumed.
defaultBG(UI,C) :- uicomponent(UI),color(C),white(C),
#count{P: colorBG(UI,P)} = 0.
defaultBG(UI,C) :- uicomponent(UI),color(C), colorBG(UI,C).


%If no foreground color is specified, then black is assumed.
defaultFG(UI,C) :- uicomponent(UI),color(C),black(C),
#count{P: colorFG(UI,P)} = 0.
defaultFG(UI,C) :- uicomponent(UI),color(C), colorFG(UI,C).
```

We apply a default rule of the following form, where not is to be intended as *negation as failure*. A style is classified as usable or unusable. A UI style is usable according to general usability measures if it is considered as favorite style or a followed suggestion from a previous inference step. The following correspondent rules in our framework indicate that, by default, all UI elements are usable. This holds unless unusability of a UI element is inferred by the inference process:

```
usable(UI,FontSize,W,Font,Style,ColorBG,ColorFG) :-
not n_usable(UI), fav(UI,FontSize,W,Font,Style,ColorBG,ColorFG).

usable(UI,"-",W,Usa,Sig,ColorBG,ColorFG) :-
not n_usable(UI), foll(UI,W,Usa,Sig,ColorBG,ColorFG).
```

When a UI element is inferred to be unusable, the default mechanism allows us to detect an exception to default by applying following rule:

```
n_usable(UI) :- unusable(UI).
```

The predicate *unusable(UI)* can be derived in following cases:

(i) UI has no modality
(ii) UI text element has no legibility measure
(iii) non textual content has no alternative text
(iv) UI has been discared by the user with a frequency N greater than a given minimum *Min*.
(v) UI has been removed by the user at a time T and is not a favorite style.

The correspondent rules in the our framework are as follows:

```
unusable(UI) :- uicomponent(UI), not n_modality(UI).
unusable(UI) :- text(UI), not n_hasLegibility(UI).
unusable(UI) :- uicomponent(UI), not n_altText(UI), not text(UI).
unusable(UI) :- disc(UI,N), N > min.
unusable(UI) :- rem(UI,T),timestamp(T1),
text_profile(UI,FontSize,Font,Style),vis(UI,W,ColorBG,ColorFG),
not fav(UI,FontSize,W,Font,Style,ColorBG,ColorFG), T1 > T.
```

In addition, a consistency constraint of following form is added to assure that a UI style cannot be considered both usable und unusable at the same time:

```
:- usable(UI,FontSize,W,Font,Style,ColorBG,ColorFG), n_usable(UI).
```

5.3   Generic Accessibility Rules

A generic accessibility rule is extendable to cover various scenarios. When an adaptation is needed, the default mechanism detects an exception to default. This might happen in cases such as:

(i) UI has a lack of usability
(ii) UI is explicitly said to require an adaptation, eventually according to some contextual details different from those in default case

The correspondent logic rules are listed below:

```
% UI suggestions determined by usability criteria
suggests(UI,W,Usa,Sig,ColorBG,ColorFG):-
unusable(UI),foll(UI,W,Usa,Sig,ColorBG,ColorFG).

% generic adaptation
suggests(UI,W,Font,Style,ColorBG,ColorFG) :-
observedC(Context,Decibel,Intensity,Reso,Contrast,T),
observedU(User,Age,Gender,Ability,Imp,T),
observedI(Imp,Perception,Pmeasure,Capability,Cmeasure,T),
size2reso(D,UI),
usable(UI,FontSize,W,Font,Style,ColorBG,ColorFG).
```

6   Results and Discussion

Preliminary evaluations show that the combination of an ASP-based reasoning component and a connected knowledge base is a good solution for creating an integrated information system in general. Preliminary scenarios on a few instances showed that answer sets computed by the DLV-Hex [4] solver provide a significant set of user interface styles. These details can also be easily analysed by interface designer, thus supporting them in deriving hints for improving the interface final design.

For example, for an aged user suffering from yellow-blue color blindness and low visual acuity and using a device with a small screen. Suggestions are generated including size increase for all text elements on the Web interface and maximum colour contrast of all UI elements. We assume, additionally that colour contrast sensitivity decreases with age, therefore, by adding following weak constraint [16] we obtain the most promising answer sets.

```
:~ suggests(UI,ColorContrast,Font,Style,ColorBG,ColorFG),
   observedU(User,Age,Gender,Ability,Imp,T),
   Age > 65.[ColorContrast:1]
```

Using weak constraints the answer sets are resulting in a cost ordering, from the cheapest answer sets to expensive ones. Here, the costs were comprised of the facts that weight the importance of a property, such as the colour contrast as given in the scenario.

Since the actual generated model is verbose and difficult to read, therefore, we need to do some post-parsing operations to get a better overview of the generated model and pass it to *gnuplot* [3] for visualization.

6.1   Answer Sets

Figure 1 shows some of the suggestions of text sizes and colours contrasts of UI elements according to screen resolution and user impairments, generated by the DLV-Hex solver. These suggestions can be stored for reuse until there are some further changes in the participating Ontologies. These suggestions could be processed for adapting the *Cascading Style Sheet CSS* of websites.

For example, there is a range of recommended text sizes for the user's low visual acuity. The highest suggested *TextSize_20*, this could be mapped to the HTML tag *h1*, the next *TextSize_14* to *h2* and so on. Since the used device has small screen, no *RadioButtons* or *ComboBoxes* have been recommended, instead there are the elements *ListBox_1* and *TabbedPane_1* which seem to be suitable for this case, however the recommended colour contrast shows that the later has better usability for our case.

---

[3] http://gnuplot.info/

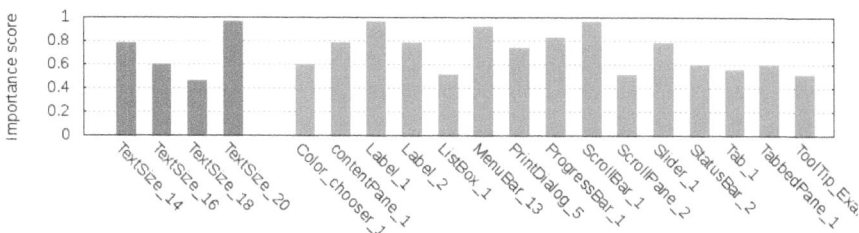

Fig. 1. UI suggestions according to yellow-blue color blindness with low visual accuracy and a mobile device

7   Conclusion and Future work

We have presented a logical framework for integrating relevant parts of semantic knowledge in user interaction process using Semantic Web technologies, Answer Set Programming and DLV-Hex as a solver. This approach allowed us by the use of constraints to limit and to prioritize the set of fired answer sets. We have achieved thereby an efficient problem reduction, since this approach scales the size of the answer sets and the run time.

It should be noted, that although the users' characteristics are uniformly static, they are not all assumed to remain unchanged. In fact, it is foreseen that future work will include a methode to detect and record changes in these characteristics over time, thus causing different adaptations to be effected in the Web interface. Furthermore, we plan to automatically detect the user's intention.

References

1. http://www.euromonitor.com/austria/country-factfile
2. Borgida, A., Serafini, L.: Distributed Description Logics: Assimilating Information from Peer Sources. In: Spaccapietra, S., March, S., Aberer, K. (eds.) Journal on Data Semantics I. LNCS, vol. 2800, pp. 153–184. Springer, Heidelberg (2003)
3. DLV, http://www.dbai.tuwien.ac.at/proj/dlv/ (last accessed on 2011-04-10)
4. DLV-HEX, http://www.kr.tuwien.ac.at/research/systems/dlvhex/
5. Eiter, T.: Answer Set Programming for the Semantic Web. In: Dahl, V., Niemelä, I. (eds.) ICLP 2007. LNCS, vol. 4670, pp. 23–26. Springer, Heidelberg (2007)
6. Eiter, T., Ianni, G., Schindlauer, R., Tompits, H.: dlvhex: A tool for semantic-web reasoning under the answer-set semantics. In: Proceedings of International Workshop on Applications of Logic Programming in the Semantic Web and Semantic Web Services, pp. 33–39 (2006)
7. Gajos, K.Z., Wobbrock, J.O., Weld, D.S.: Automatically generating user interfaces adapted to users' motor and vision capabilities. In: Proceedings of the 20th Annual ACM Symposium on User Interface Software and Technology, UIST 2007, pp. 231–240. ACM (2007)
8. Gelfond, M., Lifschitz, V.: The stable model semantics for logic programming. In: ICLP/SLP, pp. 1070–1080 (1988)

9. Giuliani, M.V., Scopelliti, M., Fornara, F.: Elderly people at home: technological help in everyday activities, pp. 365–370 (2005)

10. Gregor, P., Newell, A.F.: Designing for dynamic diversity interfaces for older people. In: Proceedings of 5th ACM/SIGAPH Conf. on Assistive Technologies, pp. 151–156. ACM Press (2002)

11. Holzinger, A., Searle, G., Kleinberger, T., Seffah, A., Javahery, H.: Investigating Usability Metrics for the Design and Development of Applications for the Elderly. In: Miesenberger, K., Klaus, J., Zagler, W.L., Karshmer, A.I. (eds.) ICCHP 2008. LNCS, vol. 5105, pp. 98–105. Springer, Heidelberg (2008)

12. Holzinger, A., Searle, G., Wernbacher, M.: The effect of previous exposure to technology on acceptance and its importance in usability and accessibility engineering. In: Universal Access in the Information Society, pp. 245–260 (2011)

13. Holzinger, A., Ziefle, M., Röcker, C.: Human-Computer Interaction and Usability Engineering for Elderly (HCI4AGING): Introduction to the Special Thematic Session. In: Miesenberger, K., Klaus, J., Zagler, W., Karshmer, A. (eds.) ICCHP 2010, Part II. LNCS, vol. 6180, pp. 556–559. Springer, Heidelberg (2010)

14. Lee, B.: Weaving the Web. The origial design and ultimate destiny of the Wold Wide Web by its inventor. Harper, San Fransisco (1999)

15. Leone, N., Pfeifer, G., Faber, W., Eiter, T., Gottlob, G., Perri, S., Scarcello, F.: The dlv system for knowledge representation and reasoning. ACM Trans. Comput. Logic 7, 499–562 (2006)

16. Leone, N., Pfeifer, G., Faber, W., Eiter, T., Gottlob, G., Perri, S., Scarcello, F.: The DLV System for Knowledge Representation and Reasoning. ACM Transactions on Computational Logic 7(3), 499–562 (2006)

17. mcbride, B.: The resource description framework (RDF) and its vocabulary description language RDFS. In: Staab, S., Studer, R. (eds.) Handbook on Ontologies, pp. 51–66 (2004)

18. Milne, S., Dickinson, A., Carmichael, A., Sloan, D., Eisma, R., Gregor, P.: Are guidelines enough?: an introduction to designing web sites accessible to older people. IBM Syst. J. 44, 557–571 (2005)

19. Portmann, E., Andrushevich, A., Kistler, R., Klapproth, A.: Prometheus – fuzzy information retrieval for semantic homes and environments. In: Proc. for the 3rd Int. Conference on Human System Interaction, pp. 757–762 (2010)

20. Karim, S., Latif, K., Tjoa, A.M.: Providing Universal Accessibility Using Connecting Ontologies: A Holistic Approach. In: Stephanidis, C. (ed.) HCI 2007, Part III. LNCS, vol. 4556, pp. 637–646. Springer, Heidelberg (2007)

21. SWRL, http://www.w3.org/Submission/SWRL/ (last accessed on 2011-04-09)

22. WAI (2007), http://www.w3.org/WAI/ (last accessed on 2011-03-10)

23. Wilkowska, W., Ziefle, M.: Which Factors Form Older Adults' Acceptance of Mobile Information and Communication Technologies? In: Holzinger, A., Miesenberger, K. (eds.) USAB 2009. LNCS, vol. 5889, pp. 81–101. Springer, Heidelberg (2009)

24. Zao, J.K., Fan, S.-C., Wen, M.-H., Hsu, C.-T., Hung, C.-H., Hsu, S.-H., Chuang, M.-C.: Activity-oriented design of health pal: a smart phone for elders' healthcare support. EURASIP J. Wirel. Commun. Netw. 2008, 27:1–27:10 (2008)

Exploring Training Issues in Healthcare: Towards Identifying Barriers to Increase Electronic Medical Records Adoption by Healthcare Professionals

A. Aktta Patel and A. Ant Ozok

Department of Human-centered Computing,University of Maryland Baltimore County,
1000 Hilltop Circle, Baltimore Maryland, United States of America
{Akttal,ozok}@umbc.edu

Abstract. Many healthcare organizations in the U.S are working on the implementation of Electronic Medical Record (EMR) Systems. This literature review identifies technology training related factors that hinder adoption of technologies by clinical and non-clinical staff during implementation. We present the important concepts as defined by the literature within EMR context and the importance of analyzing training barriers and the role of Human-centered computing (HCC) in healthcare. We conclude that there is a need to create specific HCC focused training guidelines to effectively train end users in the healthcare domain. Major concepts of these guidelines can include consistency in training, providing feedback, reducing cognitive load and recognizing user diversity which includes understanding the user profiles and tasks required for those users functioning in a time-pressured environment such as healthcare.

Keywords: Electronic Medical Records (EMR), Training, Technology, Human-centered computing (HCC) and Healthcare.

1 Introduction

This review is an introductory study to analyze the literature that exists on training related factors concerning technology adoption among care givers [1]. We focused on the technology training factors that may limit technology adoption and training related barriers that exist to learning new technology as it pertains to healthcare professionals going through a transition from paper to paperless when incorporating Electronic Medical Records (EMR). The identification of factors that promote adoption of electronic medical records in the healthcare environment can help future trainers, educators, implementers, and organizational management teams to be successful and effective in the implementation of new technologies in the healthcare domain as they relate to patient care and safety.

1.1 Technology Training

Technology training provided in this domain can be seen as considerably different from training provided in other industries not directly affecting patient care. Even

A. Holzinger and K.-M. Simonic (Eds.): USAB 2011, LNCS 7058, pp. 657–671, 2011.

though there are many similarities between healthcare and other safety critical industries such as nuclear energy, aviation, mining and some others, there are distinct differences as well. Aviation industry has influenced healthcare towards adopting practices such as checklists, simulator based training and management training [2].

There are indications that both healthcare and aviation uses highly skilled and trained professionals who have to work as a team and achieve common goals, and depend on technology that may affect safety of everyone involved. Some fundamental differences are that medicine is lengthier than aviation and medical training requires more hands-on learning whereas aviation relies on simulated training [3]. Another difference is that patients are more complex than airplanes and the information that is needed to care for patients is complex and changes continuously. In aviation, air traffic control highly influences the overall flight operations, but in healthcare there is no single influence on patient's health operations. These basic differences are the reason why training provided in healthcare is or should be different from training provided in other time sensitive, safety critical industries [3].

This literature review will address some of the fundamental questions regarding EMR, including what they are and how they differ from Electronic Health records (EHR) and paper-based records. Researchers need to truly understand what EMRs are in order to gain a deeper understanding of how the implementation of such technology affects end users such as physicians and nurses from a training perspective. Better technology training for healthcare givers can improve the quality of service in healthcare and also result in significant financial and other patient-related gains. This understanding can also help end users (care givers) prepare for challenges in learning new technology applications in the healthcare domain including EMR.

This literature review aims at answering some fundamental questions in technology use within the healthcare domain. It is very clear that the use of technology is very much related to its design. However, in our study we do not focus on design issues. Rather, we aim at determining the training related factors relating to technology that play a significant role in adoption of technologies.

The significant goals of our literature review include answering the following questions:

- What is the difference between an EMR and EHR?
- What training related barriers hinder EMR adoption?
- Do users in general prefer EMR over Paper based records?

2   Role of Human-Centered Computing *Training* in Healthcare

Human Centered Computing (HCC) can play a critical role in design, implementation and training of computing systems in various disciplines, including health care, to support people's activities. HCC aims to integrate social and cognitive sciences with computer science (e.g. Human-computer Interaction, HCI) in an effort to design and deliver intuitive computing systems with a human focus [4]. Human-centered systems should be adaptive, responding to requests in a contextually sensitive manner. They should also be reactive, responding reasonably and unprompted to events in the environment, and end users should be empowered to modify and extend the behavior of the systems using natural interaction modes [5]. End user empowerment involves training and educating users to manipulate and accentuate the behavior of the systems. In order to include the characteristic of empowerment in a human-computer system, on top of the design issues, proper training and education to the end users may be required

2.1 Patient Care, Technology and Training

Technology is an ever increasing adjunct in the healthcare domain assisting care givers in providing better, more efficient and safe patient care. In particular, a user's technologic proficiency is an under-recognized act of caring; whereby, the caregiver can utilize the technologies features to fully understand the patient's healthcare needs in an effort to provide better, more comprehensive care. Many times the use of technology and caring are thought to be mutually exclusive. This belief prevents healthcare professionals from using technology to its fullest potential. When new applications are implemented, technology use is viewed as another task or hurdle demoting the patient to an object necessary in completing the task [6]. Due to these erroneous beliefs held by both healthcare givers as well as patients; a new updated definition of patient care must be established. The perspective "to fully care in this increasingly sophisticated world, nurses generally recognize that technologic proficiency is a desirable attribute and not a substitute for caring but an important variation of caring" [6] helps nurses view the technology they encounter in their workplaces as a tool to know patients as human beings, and not just another task to be completed [6]. It is easy to take the tasks out of context and just focus on completing the tasks. However, in critical environments such as healthcare, it is very important to remember the goal is not to just complete the tasks required within the system but to ultimately provide better patient care and this should be addressed during training.

2.2 Value of Healthcare Training Research

Ford, Menachemi and Phillips [7] provide the perspective on how healthcare professionals relate to the increasing use of technology in their work place. Healthcare has many professions and there is a wide range of complex information needs, which vary from task to task within a group.

There are about fifty physician specialties, each with unique software needs, not to mention the software needs of other clinical groups such as nurses, dieticians, medical assistants and front office staff [8]. Each discipline may have several different task scenarios in a day, with each scenario requiring a different interface design. In order to provide scenario-based training effectively, it is important to conduct research in the areas of training and implementation methods along with system design as they pertain to user adoption rates.

There is no denying that wide system adoption and successful systems primarily require good designs complying with well-established usability and user satisfaction rules. This study aims at understanding user training related issues in the technology context and makes an assumption that user training occurs on systems with at least acceptable levels of usability.

3 Review of Literature

A literature review was conducted to learn about the existing barriers to learning technology in systems with no major usability problems. We expected and found many articles about designing and developing EMR and their value to the organization and if they increase patient safety. Our scope was to identify the literature regarding barriers to learning and adopting EMR and if proper training can assist with some of those barriers. This section presents the manner in which relevant articles were identified.

3.1 Inclusion and Exclusion Criteria

Most of the papers generated in the survey were between the years 1994 and 2010. Articles published in the English language were used. Although cultural differences could contribute to conflicting data with regards to training factors that increase EMR adoption; studies from foreign authors, countries, and healthcare systems were included since this paper is more of an exploration of the current literature. Unless otherwise noted, our results reflect adoption in United States-based and situated institutions. If the article discussed what made EMR implementations successful, it was selected. Articles that focused on the design and development of the EMR application with structural, database and programming foci were not selected. The search resulted in 81 relevant articles which were summarized to help extract factors which are barriers to EMR adoption by healthcare professionals.

3.2 Search Methods

The literature was searched using several different databases: PubMed, Associations of Computer Machinery (ACM), Institute for Electrical and Electronics Engineers (IEEE) and The Journal of the American Medical Informatics Association (JAMIA).

Most search terms were chosen due to their relation to the research goals in Chapter 1. The keywords used in different combinations included: *electronic medical record, electronic health record, EMR, EHR, adoption, training, barriers, learning, technology, healthcare, physicians, nurses, clinicians, clinical staff, software applications*. The titles, abstracts and manuscripts were examined before being included in the review. Duplicate articles were excluded.

4 Literature Findings

With the implementation of technology in healthcare, there has been an ever increasing number of terms and concepts. Some of the important terms and concepts found in the literature are first presented in this section. The evolution and significance of EMR are presented along with the differences between EMR and EHR, and user issues involving technology use apart from design are presented based on the literature survey.

4.1 What Is an Electronic Medical Record (EMR)?

Electronic Medical Records (EMR) are computerized medical records created in a care delivery organization (CDO) such as a hospital. According to the National Alliance of Health Information Technology (NAHIT) [9], an EMR is described as "an electronic record of health-related information on an individual that can be created, gathered, managed and consulted by authorized clinicians and staff within one's healthcare organization. According to HIMSS Analytics [8], "the EMR is the legal record created in hospitals and ambulatory environments that is the source of data for the Electronic Health Record (EHR)".

4.2 Evolution of EMR

In the 1960s, a physician named Lawrence L. Weed first had the idea of computerized electronic medical records (EMR). Weed described the EMR as a system to automate and organize patient information in such a way as to enhance its utilization and lead to improved patient care [10]. The work towards building an EMR started as the PROMIS project at the University of Vermont in 1967. These efforts led to the development of problem oriented medical record (POMR). In 1970, the POMR was used at the Medical Center Hospital of Vermont for the first time [11]. During the 1970s and 1980s, several electronic medical record systems were developed and further refined by various academic and research institutions. Several EMR that were developed included Harvard's COSTAR and Technicon and Duke's 'The Medical Record' and HELP system. Indiana's Reganstrief record was one of the earliest combined in-patient and outpatient systems.

Since the 1960's when EMR were first introduced, significant technological advances have been made. The availability of mass storage was once an issue, but is no longer a significant problem anymore. Starting with a 7-MB-per-freezer-size-disk drive, we now have enterprise storage systems that provide large amounts of storage for less than one dollar per gigabyte. Advances in storage are accompanied by advances in file structures, database design, and database maintenance utilities, greatly simplifying and accelerating data access and maintenance [12].

The human-machine interface has also improved with the evolution of the mouse as a pointing device and the emergence of touch screens. We have also seen the development of the graphical user interface, which has facilitated user multitasking. A significant area of technological improvement has been in the acquisition, processing, transmission, and presentation (display) of graphical images [12].

4.3 What Is the Significance of EMR?

There are a number of studies that suggest EMR can lead to a significant cost savings over a period of time. From a financial standpoint, a study conducted by Wang *et al.* [13], found the estimated money saved by an organization per provider to be approximately $86,400. From a patient safety standpoint, a study conducted by Hollingworth *et al.* [14] found that using EMR for prescribing does not disrupt clinical workflow, and enhances patient safety and quality of care. Also, EMR have the potential to improve communication between a patient's multiple health-care givers, eliminate needless medical testing, decrease medical errors and decrease paperwork and improve legibility [12].

4.4 How Are EMR Used?

Electronic medical records (EMR) have the potential to advance quality of care; but studies have shown mixed results. A study by Zhao *et al.* [15] linked two data sources: a statewide survey of physician's adoption and use of EMR and claims data reflecting quality of care as indicated by physicians' performance on widely used quality measures. They found that the percentage of physicians reporting adoption of EMR doubled between 2000 and 2005. In this cross-sectional study, the authors found no association between duration of using an EMR system and the performance with respect to quality of care. The physicians did not use clinical decision support tools, but they claimed clinical decision support may improve the quality of EMR usage. They indicated that future studies should examine the relationship between the extent to which physicians use key EMR functions and their performance on quality measures over time.

4.5 What Are the User Profiles of EMR, and What Is Their Technology Usage?

Any clinical or non-clinical staff that may access a patient's paper chart will need to access the electronic chart once an EMR system is implemented. User profiles range from physicians, residents/fellows, nurses, medical students to medical assistants and front desk triage.

An investigation by Anderson *et al.* [16] studied the knowledge and use of information technology by Kentucky physicians. In particular, the study assessed the willingness to employ technology in the care of patients, as well as trying to identify some of the factors that influence attitudes concerning EMR implementation. They hypothesized that physicians who voluntarily listed their email address with the Kentucky Board of Medical Licensure (KBML) are more likely to use e-mail and therefore EMR and other aspects of information technology (IT) in their medical practice. Of the 9,375 licensed physicians, 6,328 physicians recorded an e-mail address on their application. Additionally, physicians from both cohorts (listing or not listing an email) were contacted by fax, telephone or email which gained an additional 29% response rate from both groups. The results of this study concluded that a majority of Kentucky physicians (68%) express some knowledge of information technology. Not surprisingly, physicians who are younger and a part of a large healthcare organization have more experience with information technology and are more likely to use it.

In the United States, the National Ambulatory Medical Care Survey (NAMCS) found that approximately 40% of office-based physicians used electronic medical records in 2008 which was a 19% increase from 2007. Surprisingly, Only 4.4% of physicians reported having a "fully functional" EMR system, which consists of the functionalities of the "basic system" but also has the ability to retrieve, store and follow up on a patient's medical history, order sets, and send prescriptions electronically. The NAMCS data was generated by a mail survey which was sent out to 2000 physicians as well as in-person interviews with an additional 3,200 physicians. In Canada, only 25% of physicians have adopted electronic medical record (EMR) systems [17].

Information presented in this section helps us better understand the current technology knowledge of EMR users. Currently, some users are exposed to EMR and are using it in their practices; however there are a number of users in the United States and abroad who have not converted to electronic records and there is still an opportunity to provide proper training for when they convert to electronic records.

4.6   What Is an Electronic Health Record (EHR)?

Electronic health records are reliant on EMR being in place, and EMR will never reach their full potential without interoperable EHRs in place. The EHR represents the ability to easily share medical information among stakeholders allowing patient information to be accessible throughout the various modalities of care engaged by an individual. Stakeholders are composed of patients, healthcare givers, employers and payers/insurers, including the government [8].

4.7   What Is the Difference between EMR and EHR?

EMR is a legal record of the care delivery organization (CDO) whereas an EHR is a subset of information from various CDO's at which patients have had encounters. EMR is owned by the CDO, whereas EHR is owned by the patient or stakeholder. EMR systems are sold by vendors and are installed in hospitals and clinics to maintain the patient's data in an electronic form. This data from various CDOs combined can help create EHRs that can be maintained by the patient or stakeholder. Many patients have access to some medical test result information through the EMR patient portal in a limited capacity; an EHR provides interactive patient access as well as the ability for the patient to append information. EHR is connected to the National Health Information Network but an EMR is only connected to the local health Information network within the organization. EMR contains patient data for one CDO only; EHR contains patient information from multiple CDOs.

4.8   Do Users Prefer EMR over Paper Records?

A survey conducted in 2007 asked the general population if they had a preference between paper and electronic medical records and concluded that U.S. adults favored providers and insurance carriers that use electronic medical records. Almost 75% of Americans said that they believe in the benefits of electronic records, such as better care in emergencies and reduction in medical errors, which outweigh the potential privacy risks [18]. Paper based records have been the standard due to the low cost as well as ease of data entry; however, they require a significant amount of storage. In the United States, most states require physical records be held for a minimum of seven years. The costs of media storage, such as paper and film, per unit of information differ dramatically from that of electronic storage media. When paper records are stored in different locations, collating them to a single location for review by a healthcare provider can be time consuming and complicated.

U. S. Congress has included incentives such as up to 44,000 dollars a year for up to six years for EMR adoption and penalties of decreased Medicare and Medicaid reimbursements to doctors who continue to use paper based records and fail to use EMR by 2015 as a part of the American Recovery and Reinvestment Act of 2009 (AARA) [19]. We can conclude to a great extent that the majority of healthcare givers believe in the benefits of EMR and are willing to use it.

4.9   How Are Organizations Affected by the Move to EMR?

EMR implementation is a lengthy process and a course of action that requires time and attention [20]. There are many changes in the transition from the medium used (paper charting vs. electronic charting) to the processes in which data is collected, roles of users, and the sheer amount of information that is collected. Healthcare organizations need to comply with AARA guidelines of capturing accurate and sufficient information in the EMR in order to receive the government funding [19]. Due to strict guidelines and changes in workflows, processes and design, users undergo psychological stress [21]. Change in the environment due to EMR creates stress, uncertainty and role confusion (e.g., a physician might say "my nurse usually documents the diagnosis, is it my responsibility now?"). Despite the fact that EMR systems are well structured and the programs are well supported, factors such as the computer aptitude of physicians and complexity in graphical user interfaces are not being considered as hindrances to adoption. The organizations provide coaching to healthcare professionals, but time constraints hinder physicians from taking full advantage of this support. Also, lack of user acceptance and staff attitudes have been cited as factors that may hinder EMR implementation from a training perspective [22].

4.10   Why Is there Is Need for Success in EMR Implementation?

Physicians and nurses together make up the largest group of end users that interact with the EMR system; and therefore, these users will be the largest group impacted if their organization decides to implement such a technology. It is hypothesized that an EMR system that is implemented and utilized properly can enhance patient care workflow and improve the quality of care provided to patients [23]. There is little research conducted on end user understanding of their new role and related task as well as the ability of the end user to accomplish these new tasks within the confines of the new EMR system.

Many questions still remain as to the best way to train and educate end users prior to, during, and after the implementation for optimal results for both healthcare givers and receivers alike. Making EMR implementation efficient and successful is of paramount importance to providing better, safe patient care. One cannot deny the role of compliant designs in increasing adoption of any medium, and EMR in that regard is surely no different. However, there is an opportunity to investigate factors that can improve the training and delivery process to reduce barriers to adoption and increase acceptance by healthcare professionals; this contribution to the literature may prepare healthcare organizations in planning for future EMR implementations.

4.11   What Are the Barriers to EMR Adoption from Technology Training Perspectives?

An ethnography study conducted by Ventres *et al.* [24] studied the effects of EMR on physician-patient encounters. The objectives of this study were to identify the factors that influence the manner by which physicians use EMR. This study identified 14 factors that influence how EMR are used and perceived in medical practice. The 14 factors were categorized into 4 themes: **spatial** – effect of the physical presence and location of EMR on interactions between physicians; **relational** - perceptions of physicians and patients about EMR and how those perceptions affect its use; **structural issues** -institutional and technological forces that influence how physicians perceive their use of EMR; and **educational** issues of developing physician proficiency with and improving patients' understanding about EMR use.

They found that the introduction of EMR into the clinic influences multiple cognitive and social dimensions. Of the 4 domains classified in this research study, one of them was education. There is an opportunity to expand upon this domain and create guidelines to improve the learnability of EMR to further influence cognitive and social dimensions. A similar study conducted by Ludwick and Doucette [25] assessed the relevance and impact of risk and insulating factors of information technology adoption in the context of primary care. The interviews they conducted showed that physicians struggle to get appropriate training and technical support for their systems. The authors concluded that in adapting technology, factors such as physician computer aptitude and complexity of GUIs are not considered as hindrances. Despite medical associations providing valuable coaching to clinical staff on system procurement, time sensitive environments preclude the staff from taking advantage of the tools provided. Creating guidelines to provide appropriate training has the potential to provide the physicians with necessary skills to perform the tasks electronically.

Two other studies, conducted by Granlien & Hertzum *et al.* [26], presented barriers that prevent adoption of EMR by healthcare systems. These barriers are related to knowledge, approval, design and implementation. Lack of time and resources are identified as an important barrier. Some of the barriers mentioned include poor usability, lack of time, lack of knowledge, poor information delivery and insufficient training provided.

One study by Patterson *et al* in 2003 [1] focused specifically on human factors to identify barriers to the effective use of health information systems and identified an array of barriers, one of which was the limited and insufficient training provided to the clinical staff.

4.12   Technology Acceptance

Understanding why people accept or do not accept technological innovation remains one of the most challenging and complex issues. Technology Acceptance Model (TAM) was proposed by Davis in 1989 [27] as a measure that could explain system use. According to Davis, reasons for acceptance can depend on perceived ease of use (PEU) and perceived usefulness (PU). A study conducted by Liu and Ma [28], focused on the technology acceptance model (TAM) and proposes new detriments, perceived system performance (PSP) and Behavioral Intention (BI)for examination and tested on EMR applications.

They concluded that Perceived system performance has a direct positive impact on the perceived ease of use of a system and finally perceived system performance has a direct positive impact on the user's behavioral intention to use a system. Understanding these variables and their influence may assist trainers understand users better and provide efficient training.

4.13 Interface Barriers

In a panel presentation, Jiajie Zhang [29] focused on the interface barriers of EMR and the things that were wrong with today's EMR. In order for EMR to succeed, it is imperative that users are able to easily and accurately retrieve, seek, gather, encode, transform, organize and manipulate important information to accomplish desired tasks. EMR is developed to aid user activities, not to generate secondary tasks that demand extra cognitive resources. It is crucial for users to directly interact with the task domains, not the interfaces mediating the system. The human mind is very limited in its bandwidth of information processing, capacity of working memory and attention, speed of mental operations and other cognitive functions. It usually cannot allocate the cognitive resources to processes that are not essential to the task. A good system should have an interface that is transparent to users such that the users can directly and completely engage in the primary desired task. Unfortunately, the current EMR is far from meeting such requirements of direct interaction. Human centered principles have not been systematically applied in the design of current EMR. In order for EMR to perform the functions that it promised and to be universally accepted by healthcare professionals, human factors principles should be applied to the design of EMR at the earliest possible stage.

Vimla L. Patel [29] recognized that the current way of designing and training EMR is by using the "paper chart" metaphor. Dr. Patel argues that there is a problem using the "paper chart" metaphor for designing and training EMR. The problems that exist in paper charts have also been transferred to designing EMR, when using this metaphor. It is proposed that a medical chart should be a scientific problem solving manuscript which should accurately represent decisions made by the user in a form of clinical investigation and rather than borrowing the paper chart metaphor which does not currently reflect a protocol for sound clinical investigation. This suggests that creating HCI-based guidelines is important for development of future EMR design as well as trainings guidelines.

Some cognitive issues with the EMR include cognitive overload, disorientation, blind acceptance of information and recommendations [29]. In conjunction with EMR design methods complying with the rules of usability, user-centered design and other human factors principles, providing better training to reduce cognitive overload and disorientation could reduce these barriers to adoption.

A literature review study by Boonstra and Broekhuis [30] indicated an array of barriers to the acceptance of electronic medical records by physicians. Their review included twenty-two articles and identified eight categories of barriers with a total of 31 sub categories. The review concluded that some physicians have insufficient technical knowledge to deal with EMR, a problem that may be generalized to the support staff as well.

Pizziferri *et al.* [31] carried out a time and motion study on physicians' time utilization before and after implementing an EMR system and found that most physicians were able to avoid "sacrificing time with patients or overall clinic time, but they do spend more time on documentation outside of clinic sessions". Given the technical problems noted earlier, such as physicians' lack of computer skills and the complexity of EMR systems, an EMR system's ease of use is a key element in the efficiency and acceptance of such systems.

Only a few researchers have considered the possibility of interaction problems between doctors and patients when using EMR. In a research study by Shachak [32], 92% of physicians felt EMR use did disturb communication with their patients. Physicians have to turn to the computer to complete electronic forms during the patient visit and this can be time consuming especially when they have basic computer training. In the research by Ludwick *et al.* [25], some physicians reported that EMR are hard to use because hunting for menu items and identifying actions with the correct buttons disrupts their time with the patients. Shachak *et al.* [32] mentioned using EMR increases the average screen gaze time of physicians from 25% to 55% of the consultancy session, inevitably resulting in less eye-contact and less conversation with the patient. Consequently, physicians have to spend more time per patient. Further, as some EMR are patient-accessible, they might even distort the clinical encounter with more interference and distractions from the patient [33]. Thus, the traditional doctor-patient relationship has been changed by the EMR. However, whether this is really a problem for physicians and patients requires further empirical research since this issue has so far been largely neglected by researchers. Proper training must be provided to prepare physicians and alleviate some of the disruptions that affect the doctor-patient relationship.

A study by Holzinger *et al.* [34] explored factors that influence older user's acceptance to technology and found that Previous Exposure to Technology (PET) goes hand in hand with the acceptance of technology. Some of the other factors were expectations, behavior, abilities, and limitations of the user. Since users in the healthcare environment have limited time, understanding a user's PET may be extremely useful when providing training.

5 Conclusion

Although difficult to scientifically prove, proper training and education techniques may increase acceptance of technology and adoption of EMR. Our study is a preliminary review to understand what types of technology training related barriers have been discovered when implementing healthcare technology. Based on the findings here we plan on conducting more extensive literature reviews along with empirical studies in determining the factors that play the most critical roles in training the clinical and non-clinical staff on EMR, as this was found to be largely missing in the literature.

We discovered that there is little research conducted on the applicability of human factors principles in designing and delivering EMRs to end users as well as properly training users for EMRs. A study conducted by Jiajie Zhang *et al*, developed a methodology called human-centered distributed information design (HCDID), which incorporated distribution cognition theory with the need for multiple levels of analysis in system design [21].

The authors decided to apply this methodology to EMR systems "because HCC is almost nonexistent in EMR systems" and also EMR can be improved dramatically with human centered design. When an organization adopts a new technology, it can be challenging and cumbersome to all users [35]. Certain human-factors processes such as task analysis and user analysis need to be conducted to understand the tasks that need to be completed by the users. Then training guidelines can be created based on the results of the analysis. Task analysis is the process of identifying system functions that have to be performed, procedures and actions that have to be carried out to achieve task goals, information to be processed, and communication needs that are consistent with the technology.

This way only the information that is necessary for the end users to perform required duties are included in the training guidelines (primary information). Information that is not critical to perform required duties (secondary or tertiary information) could require extra cognitive bandwidth, and could be presented either if there is demand, or could be learned by the users at their own time. Some questions we would like to raise and answer in the future include:

1. Along with system and interface design, if ineffective training is one of the barriers to adoption of EMR in healthcare organizations,

    a. What is the current most used training methodology? (Training using "paper chart" metaphor? Training based on existing end-user mental models or training based on hypothetical conceptual models?)

    b. If users in high impact environment and training time are limited, how can we design training to deliver important concepts without causing cognitive overload?

2. What human factors principles can be applied to training EMR to foster adoption?

    a. In the context of task and user analysis, would it be ideal to conduct a clinic or setting specific to healthcare technology needs analysis?

    b. What is the general perceived ease of use (PEU) and perceived usefulness (PU) of current EMR systems and what is the Previous exposure to technology (PET) level among EMR users?

    c. What changes should be made in the training and delivery domain to increase PEU and PU?

3. Finally, how do usability design of EMR systems and training of EMR fit in? Should design and training be developed concurrently, and should in some cases designs of EMR be adjusted for the purposes related to training?

6 Future Research

There is not a sufficient amount research conducted regarding effective training principles and guidelines for applications in the healthcare domain. The use of conceptual frameworks in this area of study is limited. There were no articles found that addressed usability as it pertains to training and delivery, that specifically incorporated technology adoption, electronic medical records and care givers.

With an eye towards usability design, next we would like to answer the questions above to attempt developing a set of human factors-based electronic medical records training guidelines for users in the healthcare domain.

Acknowledgments. Special thanks to Sedona Learning Solutions for their support and sponsorship. Sedona is committed to excellence in healthcare IT training. Along with providing learner-focused education, Sedona's goal is to help learners use their new knowledge and skills on the job, thus improving accuracy, efficiency and quality of care in healthcare.

References

1. Patterson, E.S., Nguyen, A.D., Halloran, J.M., Asch, S.M.: Human factors barriers to the effective use of ten HIV clinical reminders. J. Am. Med. Inform. Assoc. 11-1, 50–59 (2004)
2. Anderson, J.: What are the Challenges for Health Care in Learning from Other Industries? Beyond Traditional Patient Safety Tools and Techniques 28-1, 4–5 (2010)
3. Thomas, E.J., Helmreich, R.L.: Will airline safety models work in medicine? In: Sutcliffe, K.M., Rosenthal, M.M. (eds.) Medical Error, pp. 217–234. Jossey-Bass, San Francisco (2002)
4. Jaimes, A., Sebe, N., Gatica-Perez, D.: Human-centered computing: a multimedia perspective. In: Proceedings of the 14th Annual ACM Interaction Conference on Multimedia, Santa Barbara, CA, USA (2006)
5. Gajos, K., Fox, H., Shrobe, H.: End user empowerment in human centered pervasive computing. In: Proceedings of Pervasive, pp. 1–7 (2002)
6. Locsin, R.C.: Technological competency as caring in nursing: A model for practice. Sigma Theta Tau International, Indianapolis (2005)
7. Ford, E.W., Menachemi, N., Phillips, M.T.: Predicting the adoption of electronic health records by physicians: When will health care be paperless? J. Am. Med. Inform. Assoc. 13-1, 106–112 (2006)
8. EHR Usability Task Force, Defining and Testing EMR Usability: Principles and Proposed Methods of EMR Usability Evaluation and Rating. In: Healthcare Information Management Systems Society (2009)
9. Ebadollahi, S., Chang, S.-F., Syeda-mahmood, T., Coden, A.R., Amir, A., Tanenblatt, M.A.: Concept-Based Electronic Health Records: Opportunities and Challenges. In: Multimedia, pp. 997–1006 (2006)
10. Weed, L.L.: Medical records that guide and teach (Part I). NEJM 278-11(11), 593–599 (1968)
11. Matsumura, Y., Kuwata, S., Kusuoka, H., et al.: Dynamic viewer of medical events in electronic medical record. Medinfo 10, 648–652 (2001)

12. Stephen, V., Cantrill, M.D.: FACEP.: Computers in Patient Care: The Promise and the Challenge. ACM Queue 8-8, 20–27 (2010)
13. Wang, S.J., et al.: A Cost-Benefit Analysis of Electronic Medical Records in Primary Care. J of Medicine 114, 397–402 (2003)
14. Hollingworth, W., Devine, E.B., Hansen, R.N., Lawless, N.M., Comstock, B.A., Wilson-Norton, J.A., et al.: The impact of e-prescribing on prescriber and staff time in ambulatory care clinics: a time-motion study. The Journal of the American Medical Informatics Association 14-6, 722–730 (2007)
15. Zhou, L., Soran, C.S., Jenter, C.A.: The relationship between electronic health record use and quality of care over time. J. Am. Med. Inform. Assoc. 16, 457–464 (2009)
16. Anderson, D.M., Asher, L.M., Wilson, E.A.: Physician computer skills: a prerequisite to the future in healthcare services. J. Kentucky Medical Association 105-2, 67–71 (2009)
17. Davis, K., Doty, M.M., Shea, K., Stremiks, K.: Health information technology and physician perceptions of quality of care and satisfaction. Health Policy 90 (2009)
18. Swartz.: Americans prefer electronic health record. The Information Management Journal 4-8 (2007)
19. U.S. Department of Health and Human Services Centers for Medicare & Medicaid Services 42 CFR Parts 412, 413, 422 et al. Medicare and Medicaid Programs; Electronic Health Record Incentive Program; Final Rule
20. Karnas, J., Robies, J.: Implementing the electronic medical record: Big bang or phased rollout? Creative Nursing 2, 13–14 (2007)
21. Zhang, J., Patel, V.L., Johnson, K.A.: Panel Presentation. In: IEEE Intelligent Systems (2002)
22. Ash, J.S., Bates, D.W.: Factors and forces affecting EHR adoption: Report of a 2004 ACMI discussion. Journal of the American Medical Informatics Association 12-1, 8–12 (2005)
23. Deese, D., Stein, M.: The ultimate health care IT consumers: How nurses transform patient data into a powerful narrative of improved care. Nursing Economics 22-6, 336–341 (2004)
24. Ventres, W., Kooienga, S., Vuckovic, N., Marlin, R., Nygren, P., et al.: Physicians, patients, and the electronic health record: An ethnographic analysis. Ann. Fam. Med. 4, 124–131 (2006)
25. Ludwick, D., Manca, D., Doucette, J.: Primary care physicians' experiences with electronic medical records. Implementation experience in community, urban, hospital, and academic family medicine. Can Fam Physician 56-40 (2010)
26. Granlien, M.S., Hertzum, M.: Implementing new ways of working: interventions and their effect on the use of an electronic medication record. In: Proceedings of the ACM 2009 International Conference on Supporting Group Work, Sanibel Island, Florida, USA. ACM (2009)
27. Davis, D.F.: Perceived usefulness, perceived ease of use and user acceptance of information technology. MIS Quarterly 13(3), 319–340 (1989)
28. Liu, L., Ma, Q.: Perceived system performance: a test of an extended technology acceptance model. ACM SIGMIS Database 37, 2–3 (2006)
29. Cimino, J.J., Teich, J.M., Patel, V.L., Zhang, J.: What is wrong with EMR? Panel proposal for AMIA 1999 (1999)
30. Boonstra, A., Broekhuis, M.: Barriers to the acceptance of electronic medical records by physicians from systematic review to taxonomy and interventions. BMC Health Serv. Res. 10-231 (2010)

31. Pizziferri, L., Kittler, A.F., Volk, L.A., Honour, M.M., Gupta, S., Wang, S., Wang, T., Lippincott, M., Li, Q., Bates, D.W.: Primary Care Physician Time Utilization Before and After Implementation of an Electronic Health Record: A time-motion Study. Journal of Biomedical Informatics 38-3, 176–188 (2005)

32. Shachak, A., Hadas-Dayagi, M., Ziv, A., Reis, S.: Primary Care Physicians' Use of an Electronic Medical Record System: A Cognitive Task Analysis. Journal of General Internal Medicine 24-3, 341–348 (2009)

33. Earnest, M.A., Ross, S.E., Wittevrongel, L., et al.: Use of a Patient-Accessible Electronic Medical Record in a Practice for Congestive Heart Failure: Patient and Physician Experiences. Journal of the American Medical Informatics Association 11-5, 410–417 (2004)

34. Holzinger, A., Searle, G., Wernbacher, M.: The effect of previous exposure to technology on acceptance and its importance in usability and accessibility engineering. Universal Access in the Information Society 10-3, 245–260 (2011)

35. Schoolfield, M., Orduna, A.: Understanding staff nurse responses to change: Utilization of a grief-change framework to facilitate innovation. Clinical Nurse Specialist 8, 57–62 (1994)

Requirements of Indoor Navigation System from Blind Users

Mei Miao, Martin Spindler, and Gerhard Weber

Department of Computer Science, University of Technology Dresden
Noethnitzer Str. 46, 01187 Dresden, Germany
{Mei.Miao,Martin.Spindler,Gerhard.Weber}@tu-dresden.de

Abstract. Most blind people navigate within buildings with help only from other people. One of the reasons is that there isn't enough information about the buildings available to them. To address this problem, we are working on a project named MOBILITY. One of the goals is that an application should be developed, which helps blind people navigating themselves in public buildings independently. This application is multimodal and can be installed on mobile phones. Auditory and tactile output can be used for the navigation in buildings. A thorough user requirements analysis of this application has been carried out with blind users. In this paper we report on the results of the user requirements analysis.

Keywords: Blind users, user requirements analysis, indoor navigation system.

1 Motivation

1.1 Mobility and Disability

Disabilities mostly lead to less mobility. Particularly, blind people and wheelchair users are at a disadvantage. There are sometimes digital plans for public buildings available. Information like path structure and space are offered on such plans. However, most of them are prepared just for sighted people, but not accessible for blind people. Therefore, it is especially difficult for blind people to get some information about an unknown building in advance. This makes the navigation in buildings for blind people more difficult. The most often used method to get information about an unknown building in advance is to ask friends.

Some blind people also use tactile maps, but there are very few tactile maps available. As tactile maps are usually produced by sighted people, they are often incomprehensible for blind people. Therefore, many blind people do not like working with tactile maps. Another disadvantage of tactile maps is that there are often obstacles for blind people such as billboards and they can't be mapped. Many blind people do not go to an unknown building without accompaniment. For the orientation in buildings, they usually have to stop passersby and ask for help.

A. Holzinger and K.-M. Simonic (Eds.): USAB 2011, LNCS 7058, pp. 673–679, 2011.

1.2   The Project MOBILITY

To address these problems, a project named MOBILITY has been started in 2011. One of the goals within this project is that a multimodal application should be developed, which will help people with disabilities, especially blind people. So they can orient and navigate in public buildings independently. A sighted person creates content and annotation into digital plans of public buildings like airports and train stations. This information of digital plans will be offered both for mobile phones and for the web. Furthermore, additional information for example how does a drinks machine work, will also be integrated. This information will be then converted automatically in an accessible format for the users.

1.3   User Centered Design

Since the 90s, the User-Centred Design (UCD) [1] has had increased attention, particularly in the area of human-computer interaction. UCD is applied to develop this application within this project. Within a UCD the needs and wants of future users guide the development. UCD is characterized by two main features: firstly, the users are actively involved from the start of the development. Secondly, the development process is iterative. User requirements analysis is the first milestone of UCD [2]. To identify the needs from blind users on this application, a thorough user requirements analysis has been carried out with blind users. We identified the requirements and classified them into two groups: the requirements of functionality and usability of the application and of route description. In this paper we report on the results from the user requirements analysis.

2   Related Work

Several navigation systems are developed based on GPS (Global Positioning System) for visually impaired people, like *Trekker*[1], *LoadStone*[2], and *Wayfinder Access*[3]. They talk to you about what is around you, your position, and the street name and so on. Therefore, blind people can move outdoors on their own with these assistive technologies.

However, navigation systems for indoors have not been developed as much as for the outdoors, because GPS is not available in buildings. It requires other location methods like WiFi access points, RFID tags and so on. The TANIA system[4] [4] aims to provide blind, visually impaired, and deaf-blind people to navigate on their own, both indoors and outdoors. For the indoor navigation they used a step-based tracking method, and for outdoors GPS signals. One problem with a step-based tracking method is the inaccuracy due to the varied step lengths or changing floors.

---

[1]   Trekker: http://www.atkratter.com/index.html
[2]   Loadstone: http://www.loadstone-gps.com/
[3]   Wayfinder Access: http://www.dvlop.nl/saveWayfinder/main/home.php
[4]   TANIA system: http://www.blindnavigationinternational.org/projects_en.htm

Most of the developments are just based on developers' Ideas. Users' real wants and needs will often not be thorough analyzed.

3   Procedure of the User Requirements Analysis

In this section, we briefly describe our procedure of the user requirements analysis which was based on [1-3]. The user requirements analysis consist of the following 6 steps: (1) Extensive literature research, (2) Creation of user profile, (3) Analysis of the environment, (4) Interview of mobility coach and mobility coaching, (5) Requirements gathering from blind users, (6) Confirmation of requirements derived from steps 1 to 4 with blind users.

(1) Extensive literature research
In the first step, we did an extensive literature research in respect of indoor/outdoor navigation, navigation systems, and route description for blind people. Some possible requirements are derived from this step.

(2) Creation of user profile
We designed a questionnaire to figure out blind users characteristics, like remaining visual acuity, experience with pedestrian navigation systems, mobile phone, and Internet, etc. 6 blind users (2 female and 4 male) were asked to fill in the Questionnaire. Half of them are congenitally blind and the other half are adventitiously blind. From the questionnaires we created a general user profile for blind users. After that, we derived possible requirements from the user profile.

(3) Analysis of the environment
In this step, we analyzed 2 typical public buildings. They were one airport and one train station. We also derived possible requirements which were depending on the environment of use.

(4) Interview of mobility coach and mobility coaching
We interviewed a mobility coach for blind people. We got useful advice concerning the orientation and perception of blind people. One of our developers was blindfolded and then navigated in a train station and an unknown building to get a sense of what the blind people experienced. Some possible requirements could be derived again.

(5) Requirements gathering from blind users
In this step, we conducted structured interviews [6] with the 6 blind users. We asked the blind users, which functionalities they want to have and how they want to have the functionalities.

(6) Confirmation of requirements derived from steps 1 to 4 with blind users
As mentioned, we derived requirements from 4 aspects: literature research (in step 1), user profile (in step 2), environment (in step 3), and interview of mobility coach (in step 4). In order to verify if these requirements are really important for blind users, they will be confirmed by the 6 blind users.

4   User Requirements of the Application

After conducting the 5 steps, we identified a set of requirements from blind users on the application. In this section we describe the main results. The total requirements are classified in two categories: *requirements of functionalities and usability* of the application and *requirements of route description*. Requirements of functionalities and usability mean which functionalities do blind users want to have and how do they want to have them. Route description is a very important part of a navigation system. It is essential that blind users understand the route descriptions so that they arrive at the destination effectively and efficiently. Helpful information for sighted people is not necessarily helpful for blind people. For example, "Turn to the right after a big plant." this is almost meaningless for blind people, because they cannot see where the big plant is. Therefore, it is necessary to figure out which information helps them to orient in public buildings.

4.1   Requirements of Functionalities and Usability

According to the results of user profile in step 2, most of the blind users are not familiar with pedestrian navigation systems. This indicates a need for ease of learning. For example, the design of menu navigation and the key mapping should be learned and memorized as easy as possible.

Furthermore, the blind users have taken the following main functionalities for important of a pedestrian navigation system:

4.1.1   PC Version of the Application
As expected, blind users want to have the application on a mobile phone while on the move as well as on a computer at home. The PC version does not have to have the same functionalities like the mobile phone version. But the same functionalities of both versions should be represented in similar interfaces. Using PC version blind users can get more information about buildings and plan the routes in advance.

4.1.2   Input Destination/Stopover
This function is one of the main functions of navigation system. One new thing is that blind users would like to input their destination/stopover, both on mobile phones and on the computer. For planning a route, they can do it on a computer in advance. The Route should then be transmitted to the mobile phone. On mobile phones, most of the blind users prefer speech input, but only if the speech recognition works well.

They also want to use virtual keyboard, standard typewriter keyboard (QWERTY/ QWERTZ keyboard) and standard mobile phone keyboard. All of the destination/interim destination inputted should be saved for the further use.

— *"Where am I" function*

Users can get Information about the current position.

– *"What is next to me" function*

The immediate Point of Interests (POI) will be announced along the route. They should be categorized and the user can select the categories which are interesting for them.

– *"What is around me" function*

With this function users will get information about what there are after they have defined a certain direction and a certain distance. How to define the directions should be investigated further.

– *Overview of the buildings*

Auditory information about the overview of buildings should be supported. This information comprises the structure, the primary and secondary goals of the buildings.

– *Feedback of input and actions*

Feedback of input and actions should be presented in tactile or speech form.

– *Warning of obstacles*

The Warning should occur early enough. Emergency stop should not be used too much.

– *Warning of poor signals*

Tactile and auditory information should be provided for poor signals, as well as when the signal is back again. The last route description should be repeated following the absence of the signal.

– *Warning of being off track*

Tactile and auditory information for a warning of being off track.

– *Pause, repeat and stop function for route descriptions*

Blind users should have control over the route descriptions.

– *Create and annotate POIs*

For the further use, blind users can add POIs which are interesting for them in the database.

– *Transfer of configuration to other mobile phones*

If users change their mobile phones, they do not need to configure it once more, but just transfer the configuration to a new one.

4.2   Requirements of Route Descriptions

A route description describes how you can move from your start point to your destination. As mentioned above in everyday life, blind people have to face many problems with route descriptions of sighted people. We begin this section with the general requirements of route description, followed by detailed requirements of the route description representation.

4.3   General Requirements of Route Description

— Personalization of the route description

Route descriptions should be personalized. Depending on how well blind users know the building, how they orient in a building and which information is interesting for them, they should have the possibility of adapting the route description to their own preference flexibly. For example, because of a guide dog, a blind user may prefer a lift instead of stairs. Another example is that a blind user can select the categories of the POIs which will be outputted.

— A short but meaningful overview of the route

Blind users considered that before starting, an overview of the route can be helpful. The overview begins with information about the current location, and then a summary about the total route. It should comprise information about the main areas and the floors on the route.

— Description of functional waypoints

Functional waypoints mean an object that the users have to use, such as doors, stairs/staircase, and lifts etc. It is very helpful for blind users to know how to use them. For example, for a lift it is important to know if there is a speech output and where the buttons are.

— Integration of helpful environmental pattern

Environmental pattern for blind people means tactile, auditory and olfactory information from the environment. As an example, "In front of the stairs there is a doormat."

4.4   Detailed Requirements of the Route Description Representation

— Description of direction changes

"left/right/forward/back" was accepted by all of the blind users and none of them want "north/south/west/east" for indoor. In contrast to our assumption, most of the blind users can not deal with the "clock hand" system (e.g.: 3 o'clock means turn right). The degree system excepting "90°/180°" was also rejected.

— Description of Distance

For describing distance the unit meter is suitable, but not for the number of steps. None of the blind users find the number of steps helpful.

− Estimation of effort

Most of the blind users find an estimation of effort with reference to time as unnecessary, but half of the blind users would like to get information about distance.

− Information about the current position after changing of floor and area

In order to help the blind users to build a correct mental map, it is necessary to tell them where they are after the changing of floor and area.

5   Conclusion and Future Work

To ensure a successful outcome, a thorough user requirements analysis is the first step. It is essential that the requirements should be gathered directly from future users, but not just from literature research, experiences or other ways. In our case, an interview with a mobility coach, who teaches orientation and perception of environmental cues to blind people, is a domain expert to get more information about the navigation of blind people.

We described in this paper the results of user requirements analysis with blind users on an indoor navigation application. In our project, the user requirements in respect of functionality, usability, and route description will guide the development of design concepts of the application. Subsequently the design concepts will be evaluated by blind users.

Acknowledgments. This work has been funded by the Federal Ministry of Education and Research (BMBF). We want to thank the participants and collaborators for spending their time on the user requirements analysis.

References

1. ISO 9241-210: Ergonomics of human-system interaction. Part 210: Human-centred design for interactive systems (2010)
2. Mayhew, D.: The Usability Engineering Lifecycle – A practitioner's handbook for user interface design. Morgan Kaufmann, San Francisco (1999)
3. Miao, M.: Usability-Methoden für multimodale Anwendungen mit blinden Benutzern. Thesis. University of Technology Dresden. Dresden. Department of Computer Science (in progress)
4. Hub, A.: Precise Indoor and Outdoor Navigation for the Blind and Visually Impaired Using Augmented Maps and the TANIA System. In: Proceedings of the 9th International Conference on Low Vision, Vision 2008, Montreal, Quebec, Canada (2008)
5. Völkel, T., Kühn, R., Weber, G.: Mobility Impaired Pedestrians Are Not Cars: Requirements for the Annotation of Geographical Data. In: Miesenberger, K., Klaus, J., Zagler, W.L., Karshmer, A.I. (eds.) ICCHP 2008. LNCS, vol. 5105, pp. 1085–1092. Springer, Heidelberg (2008)
6. Maguire, M., Bevan, N.: User requirements analysis – A review of supporting methods. In: Proceedings of IFIP 17th World Computer Congress, Montreal, Canada, pp. 133–148 (2002)

Empirical Study on the Relevance of Factors Influencing Readability of Instruction Manuals for Elderly

Claudia M. Nick[1], Alexander Mertens[1], Stefan Krüger[2], and Christopher M. Schlick[1]

[1] Chair and Institute of Industrial Engineering and Ergonomics of RWTH Aachen University,
Germany
{c.nick,a.mertens,c.schlick}@iaw.rwth-aachen.de
[2] Medical Clinic I, Medical Faculty, RWTH Aachen, Germany
{stkrueger}@ukaachen.de

Abstract. Demographic Change leads to an increase of elderly users relying on supportive systems, such as "E-Health Assistants". Acceptance and ease of use of those systems are highly dependent on an age-appropriate design. Especially readability of instructions should be taken into account in this respect, since users find themselves confronted with the manual as soon as questions concerning the system arise. There has only been little research on the relevance of different factors influencing readability of manuals for elderly. The objective of this research was to evaluate the relevance of temporal iconicity, linguistic factors (foreign words, signal words, active/passive voice), and layout factors (visual emphasis of keywords, visual structuring through sequences) in the context of written instructions. An empirical survey was designed in which 45 elderly participated voluntarily. 4x3 instructions were presented to the subjects. The task was to execute those instructions accordingly as correct and quickly as possible.

Keywords: readability, 50+, temporal iconicity, linguistic factors, layout factors.

1   Introduction

Heterogeneity among the elderly population must be identified as one of the main characteristics of this age group. Different biographies, educational standards and diseases make it very difficult to speak of "the" group of elderly. Still, it is commonly agreed on that with growing age, cognitive and physiological capacity changes occur. These changes often alter self-reliance. New technologies challenge these changes and offer the opportunity of an autonomous lifestyle. Thus, a special demand is given to the design of manual instructions. A technology may offer the most convenient solution, but if the target group does not comprehend accordingly a benefit will not occur. Wirtz, Jakobs and Ziefle (2009) have identified 20 types of usability problems and assigned them to 5 categories [1]. These categories are coherence, feedback, layout, structural and linguistic factors. This study analyzes 3 of these categories: layout, structure and linguistic factors.

A. Holzinger and K.-M. Simonic (Eds.): USAB 2011, LNCS 7058, pp. 681–689, 2011.
© Springer-Verlag Berlin Heidelberg 2011

2   Structural Factors

The problem occurring with structural design concerns the overall design of content. For this study the aspect of temporal iconicity was evaluated.

2.1   Temporal Iconicity

As proven by Smith et al. a non-chronological text structure lowers comprehension relative to a text which is structured according the chronological order of its content [2]. The latter describing temporal iconicity. Enkvist defined temporal iconicity as given"…whenever the linear relations in a text stand for temporal (…) relations between the referents in the world described by that text [3]. A famous example for temporal iconicity can be found in Haspelmath (2003), where he exemplified iconicity with the famous dictum "Veni, vidi, vici" (He came, he saw, he conquered) [4]. Contrary, "Prior to his victory, he came and saw", would be an non iconic expression.

Until now, there are diverging results and interpretations on the relevance of temporal iconicity. Whilst Van Horen et al. clearly say that "the results (…) suggest that temporal iconicity of instructions is not helpful" [5], Maxim and Bryan investigated that "sentences in which the order of mention was the same as the order of occurrence were significantly easier to understand than sentences where the order of mention was not the order of occurrence" [6].

Regarding the fact that with increasing age short-term memory capacities decrease [7], and non iconic sentences place a high cognitive load on the reader, since the reader has to store information in his memory, in order to reconstruct the sequence of occurrence, elderly should highly benefit from temporal iconicity in texts. Thus temporal iconicity must be a central design factor if cognitive change in age is considered within text comprehension. As a result this factor was given priority during the test phase of this study.

3   Linguistic Factors

The analyzed linguistic factors during testing were the use of foreign- and signal words as well as the use of passive voice.

3.1   Foreign Words

A survey carried out by Jakobs et al. investigated interfering factors of instruction manuals [8]. 45,8% of participants stated that the manual was incomprehensible. The reason for this being technical expressions, acronyms or other unknown items and terms. Similarly, *ETSI 2006 user education guidance and guidelines* discusses the use of inappropriate language [9].

An important aspect of textual comprehension is the awareness level of used terms: It is obvious that terms, rarely occurring, are less familiar and thus demand a higher effort in terms of decoding, than commonly used terms [10]. Terms possessing a low level of awareness among the reader are referred to as foreign words. This includes foreign language expressions and technical terms as well native language terms which are less common. Ownby stated that "…complexity of vocabulary is the most consistent aspect of text that differentiates text … whose overall ratings indicate that they are easier or more difficult to read" [11]. Ziefle and Bay also suggest that foreign words, acronyms and technical terms are to be avoided [12].

Thus, only terms with a high level of awareness are to be used [13], or if unavoidable, adequate descriptions are to be delivered to the reader [8].

3.2   Signal Words

Signal words do not provide new content but rather point out certain aspects of semantic content or text structure e.g. *eventually, at last, in order to* [14]. They facilitate comprehension of certain textual structures and help to establish a correct, coherent and representative structure of the text [15]. Hence, as signal words reduce cognitive load [16], especially the elderly should benefit from their use [5].

3.3   Passive Voice

A central aspect of designing technologies is the fulfillment of user expectations and desires. Especially elderly expect target group oriented addressing e.g. "direct addressing of the user" [8]. It was shown by Obler et al that the use of passive phrasing increases difficulties in text comprehension [17]. This was also shown by Ownby in a more recent study [11].

4   Layout Factors

In consideration of layout aspects, the visual emphasizing of various elements as well as the overall structuring through sequencing of text were analyzed. Other ergonomic aspects such as contrast of color, typeface, font size etc. were not evaluated in this study, as there has already been sufficient research on those factors.

4.1   Visual Signaling

Signals reducing the cognitive load for understanding a text may not only be given through certain use of words. Signals may also be given acoustically or visually. The acoustic emphasis on single words [18], finds its counterpart in the style and design of words e.g. font style, underlining, certain positioning [14]. Independent from the type of signaling, elderly generally benefit from elements capturing their attention [13].

4.2   Visual Structuring

Changes in spatial layout can have significant consequences on accuracy and speed of comprehension [19]. Cohen stated that age differences are less evident if the transported information is well structured [20]. This finding is consistent with the results of the survey done by Jakobs et al. (2008). Asked the question "what irritates you most about instruction manuals?" 39.6% of the subjects criticized irritating structure and imprecise step by step instructions [8].

A well structured text allows the reader to easily switch between the written instructions and a technical device [21]. Segmentations mark the spots, where the user may take a break from reading the manual, in order to execute the given instruction. Further, they enable easy navigation through the text, thus reducing the probability of repeating or skipping an instructional step [5].

5   Empirical Study

In order to gain an understanding of the process, the study design and dependent and independent variables are explained. Further, the group of subjects is outlined.

5.1   Study Design

The test carried out was a reaction test. A reaction test asks the subjects to execute written instructions presented to them. Their reaction, measured in time needed to complete the task and the amount of errors made during the execution, allows to draw conclusions regarding the general textual comprehension [10]. In this study, the subjects were asked to execute instructions presented on a 10 inch tablet pc with touch screen. In order to minimize quantifiable effects created by age related change in the subject´s visual reception, font size 18 was chosen for the entire text [13]. It was also decided to use a sans-serif typeface [22]. Further, the screen was positioned according to the anthropometric position of the subject. There were three different types of instructions in four different modes each. These four versions consist of the combination of the two independent variables (Table 1):

- Iconic vs. non-iconic formulation
- Other supportive layout and linguistic factors incorporated vs. other supportive layout and linguistic factors not incorporated

Among the instructions the following types were differentiated:

1.) The type "place pills" (P) asked the subjects to arrange pills of different colors in a pill box according to a particular order described in the instruction.
2.) Instructions of the type "make appointment" (N) asked the subject to navigate through the environment of the tablet pc and make an appointment for a certain service e.g. a cleaning lady, on a certain day and time.
3.) "Body coordination" (M) demanded the coordination of movement, e.g. right hand to chin and left hand above head.

Table 1. Overview of combinations tested

Version	Independent Variable 1	Independent Variable 2
A	temporally iconic	textual structuring through sequences, active voice, visual signaling of keywords, no foreign words, use of signal words
B	temporally iconic	no textual structuring, passive voice, no visual signaling of keywords, use of foreign words, no signal words
C	temporally non-iconic	textual structuring through sequences, active voice, visual signaling of keywords, no foreign words, use of signal words
D	temporally non-iconic	no textual structuring, passive voice, no visual signaling of keywords, use of foreign words, no signal words

These instructions were given to the subjects in varying sequences. The construction of sequences was done according to the Williams design. The Williams design is a special case of the cross-over and Latin square designs. A Latin square, in which every treatment is represented once, and once only, in each column and in each row, yields uniform cross-over designs. Such a cross-over design is said to be balanced with respect to first-order carry-over effects [23]. Distinctive for this design is that each variation occurs only once during each sequence and at a different position in each sequence.

Thus, every subject participated in four test sequences. Each of those four test sequences consisted of three instructions with each instruction type (P,N,M) occurring only once in each sequence and no formulation version (A, B, C, D) occurring twice in each sequence. Additionally, the order of versions in each sequence varied. This reduced positioning effects for later analysis. There was also a 30 min. break between each sequence in order to reduce learning effects. Dependent variables are, as previously mentioned, execution time required (t) and error rate (F).

5.2 Subjects

45 subjects were tested. Eight of those participated in the pretest. The other 37 took part in the actual data collection. Of those 37, one was excluded due to the fact, that he was not a native speaker, so difficulties in text comprehension could not be clearly associated with the factors evaluated. 24 subjects were male, 12 female. The age group of 61 years to 70 years was represented by 47,2% of the subjects, while 33,3% were between 71 and 80 years, 11,1% were aged between 50 and 60 years. 8,3% were between age 81 and 90 years.

5.3 Results

During the analysis ANOVAs were created for reaction time and amount of mistakes of all instructions. Here, time (p = 0,03) and mistake evaluation (p=0,00) lead to significant differences during the application of temporal iconicity. Hence, iconic formulations seem to be more comprehensive than non iconic formulations. The average mistake for instructions of the category A and B was $\varnothing F = 0,5$ (SD 0,84), while instructions of category C and D were at $\varnothing F = 1,78$ (SD 1,86). The time average for instructions of category A and B was at $\varnothing t = 90,57$ s (SD 43,78), C and D resulted in $\varnothing t = 106,34$ s (SD 60,75). A Bonferroni test showed no significant differences for time and error results in between the two iconic/ non iconic versions respectively though.

Table 2. Means of time (t) and error (F) rates

	Instructiontype „make appointment" (N)		Instructiontype „body coordination" (M)		Instructiontype „place pills" (P)	
	$\varnothing F$	$\varnothing t$	$\varnothing F$	$\varnothing t$	$\varnothing F$	$\varnothing t$
Version A	0,639	112,5	0,167	70,61	0,722	74,31
Version B	0,472	123,61	0,333	83,28	0,667	79,14
Version C	1,431	128,61	0,472	89,92	3,111	82,39
Version D	1,583	133,5	0,722	102,03	3,347	101,6

Looking at the means for each instruction type (Table 2), it stands out that both instructions of category P and M, show lower error rates in version B than instructions formulated in version A. M received in version A 8,25% more mistakes than instructions of type B. Instructions of group P received even 35,38% more mistakes in variation A.

However, subjects took approximately 6,5% more time in version B of group M. The difference between version A and B was at 9,88% in time for instructions of group P, inclining towards A. Correlation coefficients between time and error rates were computed in order to detect traces of time-accuracy trade-offs, but the results showed no sign thereof.

The calculated means for time and error rate include all results from all tested subjects. Considering the great intra-individual performance differences between the subjects, a more differentiated look on the results might be necessary in order to determine which formulation type obtained the best results. Therefore, for each subject was determined in which formulation type the best and worst outputs were produced (Table 3). This was done for all instruction categories. Afterwards results were compared again.

This comparison of worst and best output showed that formulation type D is always joined with the highest amount of worst results – both for time and for error rates in all instruction categories. Thus in formulation type D 36.11% of the subjects performed worst time-wise in the category P, even 41.67% in categories N and M. Instructions in type D lead to 22.22% of the worst results error-wise in category N and up to 42.86% in category P.

In contrast most of the best results were joined with formulation type A. The only exception is the finding for best time results in category M. There 38.89% of the best performances were achieved in connection with formulation type B. All the other "best performance" outcomes, up to 44.44%, were linked to formulation type A.

Table 3. Results for best/ worst analysis. Percentage of best /worst results time-/error-wise achieved under certain formulations

	Instructiontype „make appointment" (N)		Instructiontype „body coordination" (M)		Instructiontype „place pills" (P)	
	%	formulation	%	formualtion	%	formulation
Best (time)	44.44	A	38.89	B	44.44	A
Best (error)	5.56	A	25	A	22.22	A
Worst (time)	41.67	D	41.67	D	36.11	D
Worst (error)	22.22	D	36.11	D	42.86	D

At last, influencing factors were calculated in a multivariate data analysis. It turned out that regarding the error rate the type of formulation and frequency of computer use were always influencing factors (Table 4).

Table 4. Multivariate Analysis of factors influencing time and error rate

Instruction-type	Source	Typ III SS	Med.square	F-statistics	Pr>F
N	Formulation	5.88002021	1.96000674	2.78	0.0437 *
N	Appear-Ord	2.00502021	0.66834007	0.95	0.4196
N	Sex	0.55072282	0.55072282	0.78	0.3785
N	Comp-Use	6.80869707	2.26956569	3.22	0.0249*
M	Formulation	232.3524306	77.4508102	39.44	<.0001 *
M	Appear-Ord	15.6024306	5.2008102	2.65	0.0515
M	Comp-Use	40.9727722	13.6575907	6.96	0.0002 *
P	Formulation	34.53805923	11.51268641	9.21	<.0001 *
P	Appear-Ord	18.17694812	6.05898271	4.85	0.0031 *
P	Age	7.39775670	2.46591890	1.97	0.1213
P	Comp-Use	11.63821919	3.87940640	3.10	0.0289*

So it can be said that besides the way of formulation, a strong effect roots back to the general use of computer systems. The analysis of a questionnaire completed prior to the test, states that 21,6% of the subjects never used a computer before. 45,9% operate a computer on a daily basis, 21,6 % use it 2-3 times a week. 10,8% rarely use a computer. The difference in time and error results, between those who have never used a computer and those who have some level of experience with a computer system, is highly significant ($p_t = 0,00$; $p_F = 0,00$). The mean for mistakes made by computer users was at $\varnothing F = 0,97$ (SD 1,41) mistakes per instruction, while the group that never used a computer system was at $\varnothing F = 1,84$ (SD 1,99) mistakes per instruction. The means for time were $\varnothing t = 113,32$ s (SD 70,14) for the non users and $\varnothing t = 94,87$ s (SD 48,05) for the experienced.

5.4   Conclusion

The study results imply that temporal iconicity plays a key role in the design of instructions. Instructions that were temporally iconic were executed faster and at a smaller error rate than instructions that were non iconic. A detailed evaluation of the other factors relevance was not possible within the frame of this study but looking at the differences regarding time and error rate between the non iconic versions C and D, instructions that respect other supporting factors as active voice, text structure, signal wording and avoidance of foreign words, perform better with regard to the evaluated variables.

An explanation why most results for instruction category M were best performed in formulation type B, might be, that some of the subjects were confused by the layout structure of the instructions provided in version A. Just as inappropriate accentuation slows language processing [18], a text structure that does not appeal to the reader might rather hinder than support textual understanding [24]. 11,1% of the study participants stated in a questionnaire that was conducted right after the experiment, that they found the structural layout not helpful.

As for the reason why computer use seems to play such a significant role in the overall results, it can only be assumed, that since the entire instructions were presented on a tablet pc, those with a certain amount of experience in computer use benefited from their know-how with a more confident and less anxious approach which ultimately resulted in higher performance levels.

The study focused on an age group above 50 years. However, ergonomic design of instruction manuals has an independent positive effect on comprehension of instructions and thus results in an increased impression of control on the user side – independent of age.

Acknowledgments. We would like to thank everyone who participated in this study, as well as the Clinical Trial Center Aachen , who was a great support. This research is funded by the German Federal Ministry of Education and Research BMBF (01FG10004) and the body responsible for the project is DLR.

References

[1] Wirtz, S., Jakobs, E.M., Ziefle, M.: Age-specific usability issues of software interfaces. In: Proceedings of the IEA 2009 – 17th World Congress on Ergonomics, Bejing (2009)

[2] Smith, S.W., Rebok, G.W., Smith, W.R., Hall, S.E., Alvin, M.: Adult age differences in the use of story structure in delayed free recall. Experimental Aging Research 9(3), 191–195 (1983)

[3] Enkvist, N.E.: Experiential iconicism in text strategy. Text 1(1), 97–111 (1981)

[4] Haspelmath, M.: Against Iconicity and Markedness (2003),
http://email.eva.mpg.de/~haspelmt/IconicityMarkedness.pdf

[5] Van Horen, F., Jansen, C., Noordman, L., Maes, A.: Manuals for the elderly: Text characteristics that help or hinder older users. In: Hayhoe, G.F., Grady, H.M. (eds.) Connecting people with technology – Issues in professional communication, pp. 43–53. Baywood Publishing Company, Inc., New York (2009)

[6] Maxim, J., Bryan, K.: Language of the elderly: A clinical perspective. Whurr Publishers, Ltd., London (1994)

[7] McDaniel, M.A., Einstein, G.O., Jacoby, L.L.: New considerations in aging and memory: The glass may be half full. In: Craik, F.I., Salthouse, T.A. (eds.) The Handbook of Aging and Cognition, pp. 251–310. Psychology Press, New York (2008)

[8] Jakobs, E.M., Lehnen, K., Ziefle, M.: Alter und Technik – Studie zu Technikkonzepten, Techniknutzung und Technikbewertung älterer Menschen. Apprimus Verlag, Aachen (2008)

[9] Stephanidis, C.: The Universal Access Handbook. CRC Press, New York (2009)

[10] Amstad, T.: Wie verständlich sind unsere Zeitungen? Abhandlung zur Erlangung der Doktorwürde der Philosophischen Fakultät I der Universität Zürich. Studenten-Schreib-Service, Zürich (1978)

[11] Ownby, R.L.: Influence of Vocabulary and Sentence Complexity and Passive Voice on the Readability of Consumer-Oriented Mental Health Information on the Internet. In: AMIA 2005 Symposium Proceedings, pp. 585–588 (2005)

[12] Ziefle, M., Bay, S.: How older adults meet complexity: aging effects on the usability of different mobile phones. Behaviour & Information Technology 24(5), 375–389 (2005)

[13] Fisk, A.D., Rogers, W.A., Charness, N., Czaja, S.J., Sharit, J.: Designing for older adults – Principles and Creative Human Factors Approaches. CRC Press, New York (2004)

[14] Meyer, B.J.F.: The organization of prose and its effects on memory. North Holland Pub. Co., Amsterdam (1975)

[15] Lorch Jr., R.F., Lorch, E.P.: Effects of organizational signals on free recall of expository-text. Journal of Educational Psychology 88, 38–48 (1996)

[16] Meyer, B.J.F., Marsiske, M., Willis, S.L.: Text processing variables predict the readability of everyday documents read by older adults. Read Res. Q 28(3), 235–248 (1993)

[17] Obler, L.K., Nicholas, M., Albert, M.L., Woodward, S.: On comprehension across the adult lifespan. Cortex 21, 273–280 (1985)

[18] Cohen, G., Faulkner, D.: Does "Elderspeak" work? The effect of intonation and stress on comprehension and recall of spoken discourse in old age. Language & Communication 6, 91–98 (1986)

[19] Detweiler, M.C., Ellis, R.D.: The Effects of Display Layout on Keeping Track of Visual-Spatial Information. In: Rogers, W.A., Fisk, A.D., Walker, N. (eds.) Aging and Skilled Performance, pp. 157–184. Lawrence Erlbaum Associates, Inc. Publishers, Mahwah (1996)

[20] Cohen, G.: Speech comprehension in the elderly. British Journal of Audiology 21, 221–226 (1987)

[21] Steehouder, M., Karreman: De verwerking van stapsgewijze instructies. Tijdschrift voor Taalbeheersing 22, 218–237 (2000)

[22] Hartley, J.: Designing instructional text for older readers: A literature review. British Journal of Educational Technology 25, 172–188 (1994)

[23] Wang, B.S., Wang, L.X.J., Gong, L.K.: The Construction of a Williams Design and Randomization Cross-Over Clinical Trials Using SAS. Journal of Statistical Software 29 (2009)

[24] Kauffman, D.F., Kiewra, K.A.: What makes a matrix so effective? An empirical test of the relative benefits of signaling, extraction, and localization. Instructional Science 38(6), 679–705 (2010)

Dispedia.de – A Linked Information System for Rare Diseases

Romy Elze[1], Tom-Michael Hesse[2], and Michael Martin[1]

[1] University of Leipzig, Institut for Computer Science,
Department of Business Information Systems
[2] Institute for Applied Informatics (InfAI) e.V.
{lastname}@informatik.uni-leipzig.de, tommichael.hesse@googlemail.com
http://bis.informatik.uni-leipzig.de

Abstract. The challenge of developing information systems for rare diseases is in harmonizing social care conditions and health care conditions with the focus on personalization and patient autonomy. Knowledge about the most rare diseases is limited, which is the result of poorly funded research and the existence of only a few specialized experts. Furthermore, the treatment and care of the affected patients is very complex, cost-intensive, time critical, and involved stakeholders are very heterogeneous. The information needed by the patient depends on his or her personal situation and constitution. To support the information logistics between patients of rare diseases and (all) other stakeholders (e.g. physicians, therapists, and researchers), we developed an information system with Linked Open Data technologies in order to create a platform and tool independent solution addressing the heterogeneity of the stakeholders. To engineer system and data model requirements of our approach we analyzed the rare disease *Amyotrophic Lateral Sclerosis* (ALS), which have wide-spreaded characteristics. The resulting formal knowledge representation was encoded in OWL, which allows, for instance, a modular development of complex areas and also the re-usage of existing knowledge bases.

1 Introduction

The field of research about rare diseases is extremely complex, because of multifaceted disease progressions, the existence of many stakeholders from different sectors (i.e. social care, health care, therapists, and aid suppliers) and the high costs incurred by treatment and care. A disease is defined as rare if less than one of 2000 people are diseased by it [2]. Consequently, the available qualitative knowledge about it is limited to a few experts [4]. The complex treatment and care is carried out by a variety of actors who do not always have the special expertise [5]. One example of a rare disease is Amyotrophic Lateral Sclerosis (ALS)[1].

---

[1] Definition:https://uts.nlm.nih.gov///metathesaurus.html#C0002736;0;1;
CUI;2011AA;EXACT_MATCH;*;

A. Holzinger and K.-M. Simonic (Eds.): USAB 2011, LNCS 7058, pp. 691–701, 2011.
© Springer-Verlag Berlin Heidelberg 2011

It is a degenerative disease of the nervous system [12]. The clinical manifestations include progressive weakness, atrophy, dysphagia, and further problems that limit the quality of life and the self-determination of the concerned people. Diseases such as ALS, which follows the definition of a rare disease, are characterized by very different courses and prognoses [9]. There is neither a fixed time frame in which a patient is in a certain state of health nor does a certain state of health follow specific existing conditions. A general provision of information in advance like in disease-management-programs [10] is not possible. Since there is normally no cure for rare diseases, the care of these patients focuses on improving living conditions and maintenance of self-determination. During the course of the disease, a constant flow of new information on the patient's respective state of health is required in order to notify stakeholders about new treatment methods or aids [13]. The demand for information about the disease is very high but individually different and influenced by many factors. The WWW contains a big set of (semi-)structured information about varying diseases which are currently difficult to filter by the particular patient needs[2]. Due to the lack of quantitative and qualitative information, patients can be confused easily [16]. Furthermore, information for patients with rare diseases requires qualified and sensitive intermediation. Hence, there is a need to select and aggregate information that is relevant for a particular disease or health condition.

To address these requirements, our approach aims to handle the health state and the patient's characteristics on the one hand and the expert knowledge, which has to be adapted to the patient's requirements, on the other hand. Therefore, the aspect of information logistics for ALS patients was analysed. This analysis resulted in a knowledge model which is presented in section 2. To create a basis for a holistic information system, which can also be reused for other rare diseases, we decided to develop a domain ontology [6], the Dispedia Ontology. The formalization of that ontology including the conceptual model of diseases, patients, proposals as well as its structure and functions is presented in section 3. In order to formalize our approach, we used the Resource Description Framework (RDF) [11] and the Web Ontology Language (OWL) [18] as representation languages. With respect to reusing and extending the Dispedia Ontology in a decentralized web of information, we furthermore followed the principles of Linked Open Data (LOD) [1]. To publish that ontology in a dereferenceable manner, we used OntoWiki [7] as an application framework sketched in section 4. We conclude our approach in section 5 and provide a short outlook on future research and development.

2   Analysis of a Rare Disease

To identify the deficits in information, communication, and coordination in the management of rare diseases, we analyzed the disease Amyotrophic Lateral Sclerosis (ALS). Initially, 19 medical records of patients and their families from books and web sites were analyzed. To structure the knowledge from this analysis, we

---

[2] http://www.patientslikeme.com/

extracted the most important keywords and their relations as a Concept Map [3]. Using this method, the knowledge about each case was graphically structured, semantically annotated, and summarized as a knowledge model or rather a concept model. Included in this analysis were 41 expert interviews with 20 patients respectively members, eight doctors, seven social consultants, two aid advisers, two health insurance representatives, one speech therapist, and a dietician were considered in this way. To develop a domain specific knowledge scheme, each concept model was consolidated into a complete model and iteratively revised by experts[3], such as computer scientists, physicians, and further stakeholders acting in other research areas. The revised holistic presentation is called Disease Concept Model and a cut-out is shown in Figure 1.

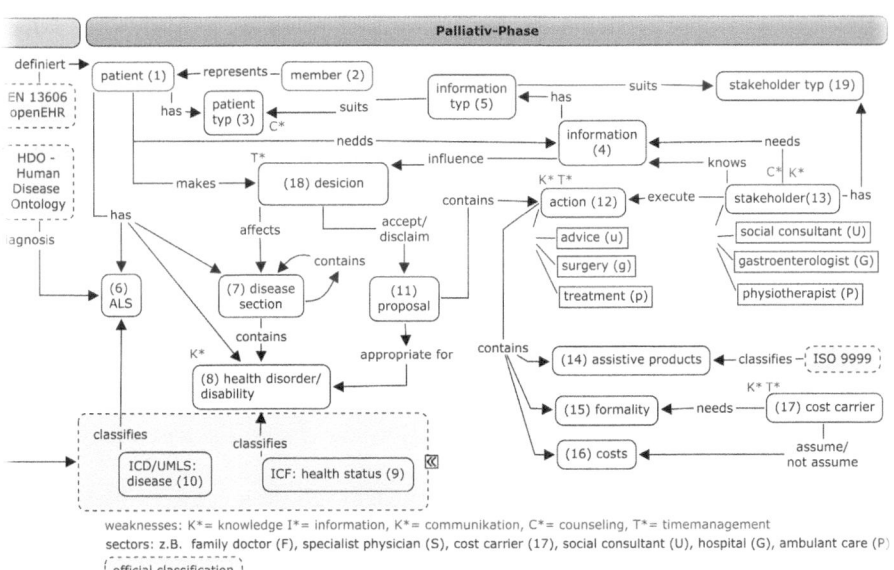

Fig. 1. Disease Concept Model

On the Basis of the depicted conceptualization, we were able to engineer the requirements, such as important concepts and relations of the desired information system. For instance, the patient (1) as the central role has a health state (8), which describes the disorders and disabilities including the environmental facts such as profession or living situation. For this patient's needs, there is a proposal (11) that could improve the patient's situation. The proposal contains actions (12). Actions are executed by stakeholders (13). The stakeholders have special knowledge that could be captured as information. The information (4) can be selected in information types (5), which are suitable for special patient

---

[3] University of Leipzig: `http://bis.informatik.uni-leipzig.de/`; Charité Campus Virchow-Klinikum Neurological Clinic: `http://www.als-charite.de/`; German Society for Muscle Diseases e.V.: `http://www.dgm.org/`

types (3) or stakeholder types (19). With this information (5), the patient (1) is able to make the decision (18) to either accept or disclaim the proposal. For instance, a patient (1) of a specific type (3) has severe swallowing disorders (8) and he needs information (5) about supplemental tube feeding (11) that prolongs the patients life. It is on the patient to decide whether the feeding tube will improve his quality of life and thus whether he should accept this proposal.

For the provision of such a patient-specific information system, the Disease Concept Model shows which software development sections are to be developed. One must create a knowledge base about the patient, which provides information about the patient, an expert knowledge base to deliver proposals to the patient, and the information allocations that provide the adapted information with the special type to the patient with the relevant parameters. Medical classifications and standards play a significant role in this environment, and the Disease Concept Model shows which concepts must be created to apply them. In this case, for instance, the International Classification of Disease (ICD [20]), the Electronic Health Record (openEHR [8]) and the International Classification of Functioning, Disability and Health (ICF [19]) are relevant. Most medical classifications and ontologies are available in the description language OWL (Web Ontology Language). The above-mentioned aspects establish our further proceedings, in which we develop a domain-specific ontology in the formal description language RDF/OWL.

3   Formalization and Knowledge Representation

To provide a flexible and extensible solution on the one hand, which is also standardized and easy to use on the other, we developed the Dispedia Ontology hold under the domain Dispedia[4].

The name Dispedia is derived from the goal of this designed knowledge base to make disease-specific information available and usable for humans and machines. As section 2 indicates, the concepts and instances were modeled in RDF/OWL. The Dispedia Ontology includes the vocabulary or scheme (Core Ontology), the expert knowledge base (Proposal Ontology), the knowledge base about the patient (Case Ontology), the allocation of proposal information for patient parameters and the concepts to interlink additional classifications (cf. Figure 2).

1. The **Core Ontology** is the Dispedia vocabulary and it implements all relevant concepts to model the linked information system for rare diseases. The Core Ontology provides a total of 25 classes with 72 object properties and 52 data properties coded by 744 triples. More specifically, the Core Ontology provides classes and properties to model two aspects of information, information *about* patients and information *for* them. An overview of this vocabulary is shown in Figure 3. This scheme defines the allocation classes and object properties which enable the connection and respectively the *Allocation* of the *Case* and *Proposal* knowledge. The vocabulary is available via http://www.dispedia.de/.

---

[4] http://www.dispedia.de/

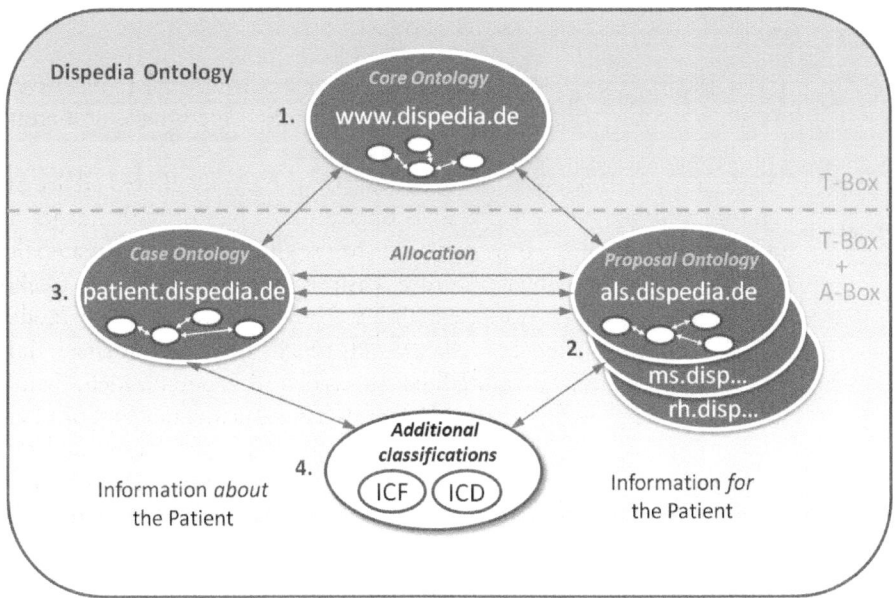

Fig. 2. Architectural overview about the Dispedia Ontology

2. The **Proposal Ontology** includes concepts and relations, which contain disease specific information *for* the patient. Therefore, the relevant concepts of the Core Ontology should be imported to the Proposal Ontology and instantiated. These instances are expert proposals of certain stakeholders, which are adapted to the different patient types. The Proposal Ontology for ALS is specified in `http://als.dispedia.de/`. In the future other Proposal Ontologies for other diseases, such as multiple sclerosis `http://ms.dispedia.de/` or rheumatism `http://rh.dispedia.de/`, may be integrated as well.

3. The **Case Ontology** is the part of the knowledge base, that includes the information *about* the patient. It is defined at `http://patient.dispedia.de/`. This Case Ontology imports the relevant concepts of the Core Ontology and *additional classifications* to standardize the patients parameters. To deliver information from the Proposal Ontology according to the Case Ontology both sides use the *Allocation*.

4. **Additional classifications** like the International Classification for Diseases (*ICD*) [14] or the International Classification of Functioning, Disability and Health (*ICF*) [19] can be linked to the Case and Proposal Ontology providing extra vocabularies e.g. for the description of health conditions.

Each ontology should import the Core Ontology to be able to use the comprehensive semantics provided by it. This allows standardization and integration of knowledge to be combined with the flexibility for heterogeneous points of view by different stakeholders. The structure and functions of the Dispedia Ontology should be presented as follows.

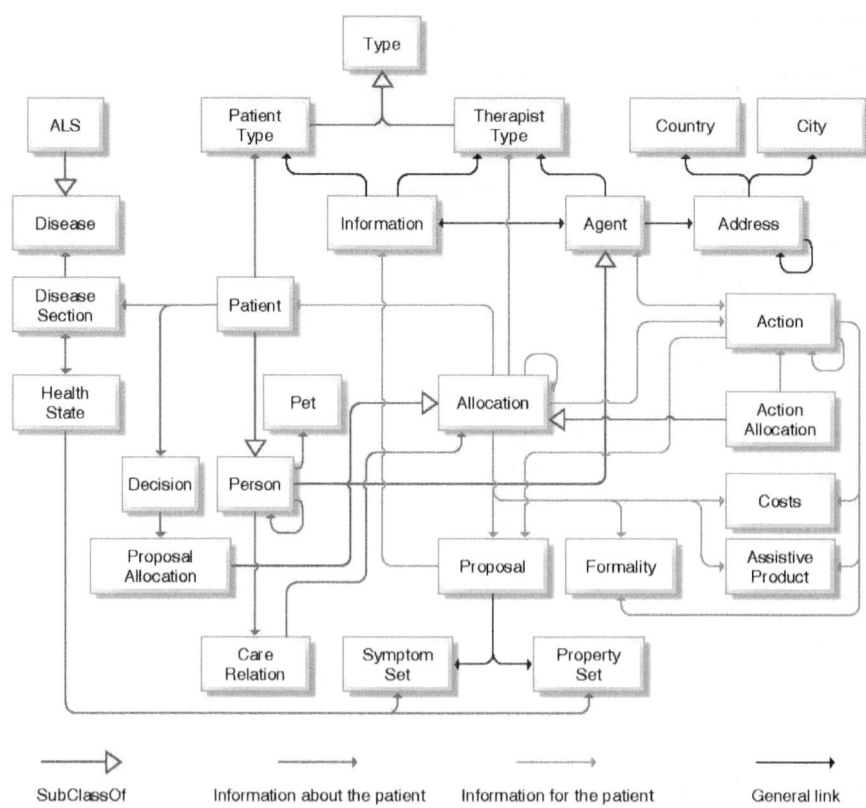

Fig. 3. Vokabulary of the Dispedia Ontology

The central class is the *Patient*, which is a subclass of `foaf:Person`[5]. Knowledge about the patient is stored in *Disease Sections* structuring the phases in which the disease advances. *Health States* are divided into *Symptom Sets*, which are sets of occurring symptoms, and *Property Sets*, which are additional disabilities that the patient has. Moreover, descriptions about the patient can be added by using relations to tag friends and relatives. Personal attributes, such us the living situation or care requirements,can be added as well.

Representing knowledge for the patient is done by linking the patient to a set of *Proposal Allocations* and *Decisions* modelling treatment options and the patients particular attitude towards them. Clusters of *Information*, which are defined by the patient's condition (e.g. experienced or sensitive) as *Patient Type* can be provided as well. The *Proposals* represent a generalized treatment option (e.g. a PEG tube) and are linked to the individual patient by an allocation as mentioned above. It can consist of one or more *Actions*, which can also be allocated to the involved stakeholders in *Action Allocations*. Actions indicate

---

[5] `http://xmlns.com/foaf/0.1/Person`

necessary procedures with *Formalities* as the used formal artefacts, *Costs* to represent financial aspects or necessary *Assistive Products* for the patient.

In the Proposal Ontology, these concepts can be instantiated to represent the stakeholder-dependent knowledge. We will use Joe Public as an example for a patient who suffers from severe dysphagia. For dysphagia this severe, the proposal of installing a PEG tube can be described by a physician as an expert knowledge fact in the Proposal Ontology. It includes numerous actions concerning the procedure performing surgery to place the tube. Figure 4 illustrates some of the RDF instances needed for this representation.

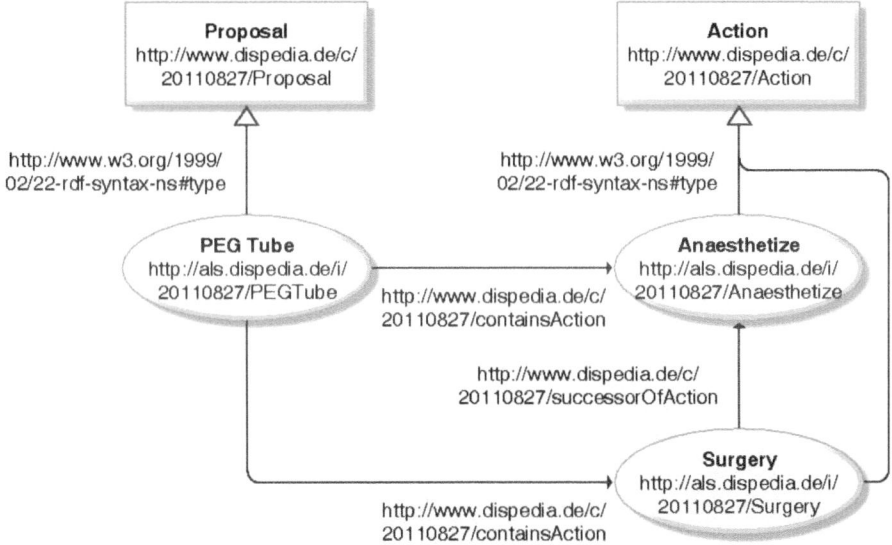

Fig. 4. The proposal for a PEG tube as RDF representation

The acquired information is linked to the individual patient's case in the Case Ontology by instances of the allocation concepts for proposals and actions. Therefore, the patient's case is represented by the patient knowledge instances consisting of the instantiated concepts of Patient, Health State, etc. The generalized information about a procedure stored in the Proposal Ontology can be adapted to the individual needs of a patient and the specific personal situation. Regarding the case of Joe Public, the anaesthesiologist would store his protocol of the pre-operation discussion here as an information instance. In addition, the corresponding ALS physician can choose to estimate the life expectancy when using the PEG tube and share this information with Joe if desired. Finally, the surgeon can create the information about the surgery procedure and link it to the appropriate patient type "experienced". Because Joe is marked as an experienced type of patient, this information will be shown to him. The RDF resources structuring this information are depicted in Figure 5.

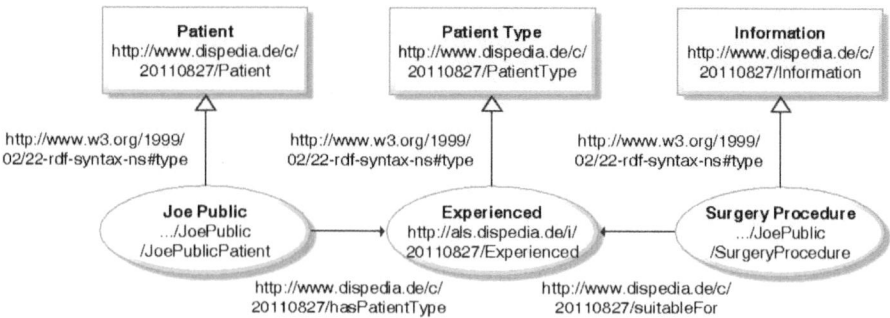

Fig. 5. The surgery procedure information for Joe Public

4   Deployment and Application

By utilizing this formalization and knowledge representation, our system provides the needed flexibility in structuring and linking the knowledge of physicians, speech and occupational therapists, neurologists, counselors and many
more. Especially for the ALS disease this approach supports the management
of these different points of view regarding the implications of an underlying disease with a broad variety of symptoms and treatment options. The focus is on
tailoring the given information towards the needs of the involved stakeholders
with the patient as the first priority.

In order to improve the collaborative knowledge acquisition and publication
of qualitative and quantitative information about diseases like ALS, we decided
to use a content management system that follows the WIKI principles. Furthermore, because of the required re-usability of encoded conceptual information of
the Dispedia Ontology on the one hand and because of required re-usage of existing knowledge bases in the Linked Open Data Web, we decided to use a semantic
wiki system. In addition to conventional wiki systems, it is possible to add and
manage structured semantically annotated information instead of textual elements. One particular wiki system that follows the semantic wiki approach is
OntoWiki which offers the following set of general functionalities.

- *Exploration Interfaces:* OntoWiki supports ontology exploration in multiple
  ways. Each RDF resource, which is represented as an HTML page for humans, can be (full-text) searched, explored in faceted browsing, or queried
  with content and use-case specific browsing interfaces. The last listed interfaces can be developed with OntoWiki's integrated extension system.
- *Authoring of Semantic Content:* Content is represented as a resource description following the RDF data model in OntoWiki. These RDF resource
  descriptions can be managed in OntoWiki with (a) an RDFauthor [17] (to
  manually add, update, and delete resources), (b) with a versioning component (to keep track of all changes), and (c) with EvoPat [15], which supports
  ontology evolution and refinement tasks.

– *Access Interfaces:* In addition to human-targeted exploration interfaces, OntoWiki supports the re-usage of RDF data by offering interfaces such as the SPARQL-endpoint and the Linked-Data-endpoint. Unlike the Linked-Data-endpoint, which is used to publish data according to the LOD principles, OntoWiki also contains a data gathering component, which is used to consume information from the Linked Data Web. By using that component, linked resources in the Dispedia Ontology can be resolved and the referenced RDF can be received after requesting the remote Linked-Data-endpoint.

We deployed OntoWiki with an underlying Virtuoso RDF Store on `http://www.dispedia.de/` for the purpose of storing and publishing all conceptual RDF resources of the Dispedia ontology in a dereferencable manner (the web domain is part of every RDF resource URI). To publish the two A-Box Ontologies (Patient and ALS-Proposal) we deployed them in a similar manner on `http://patients.dispedia.de/` and `http://als.dispedia.de/`. To improve the usability of the OntoWiki GUI interfaces for humans, we developed a form extension for OntoWiki and created a set of Dispedia specific form definitions. By using this extension, users are able to access and maintain RDF resources without having any knowledge of the underlying architecture itself. Figure 6 shows one of the predefined templates for adding and editing patient information nested in OntoWiki.

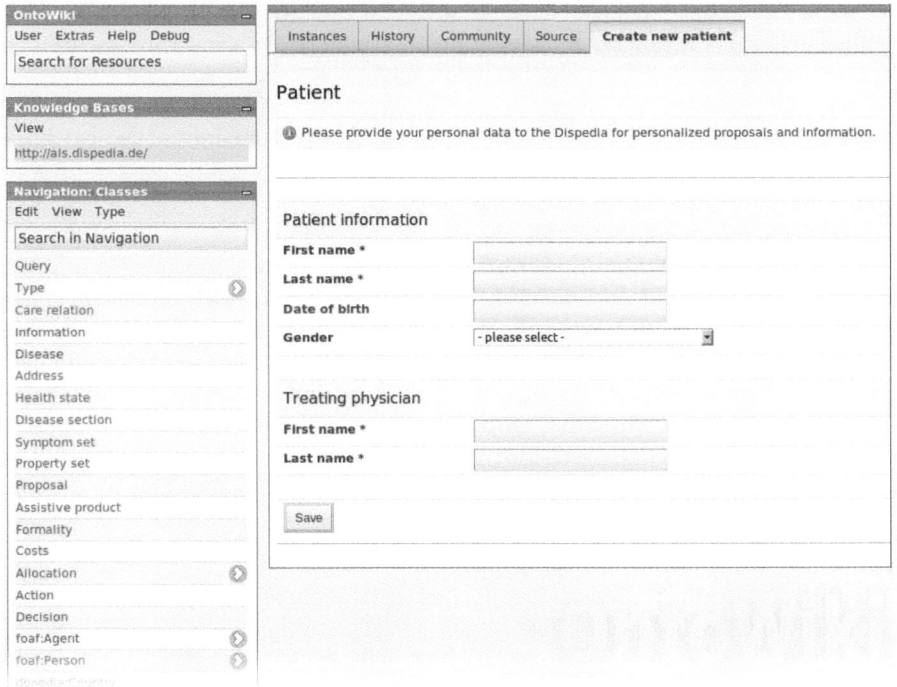

Fig. 6. Screenshot of a patient formular nested in OntoWiki

5   Conclusion and Future Work

Our work focused on improving the information logistics in the existing health system regarding ALS. The actual state of our approach, which was evaluated by using select patients with ALS and the course of the disease in their specific cases, combines the following different advantages:

1. Different information providers can operate on the same standard using the structure given by the Architecture concepts and their relations.
2. The ontological model of the system is extendible by interlinking and flexible with regards to accommodating new concepts.
3. General aspects of the health care processes for the disease can be represented and linked to their implications for the individual stakeholder.
4. Existing knowledge bases like the ICD and ICF can be connected and re-used.
5. Existing technologies like the OntoWiki can be used with low effort to make the information accessible to patients and other stakeholders.

To improve our existing approach, we will evaluate our system setup (ontology, architecture, and applications) in real environments. Furthermore, we will integrate existing ontologies like ICD and ICF in more depth in order to support better results while interlinking resources on the conceptual and individual level with further knowledge bases in the linked data web. In the existing development state, we focus on functionalities supporting knowledge acquisition in order to allow the approach of Dispedia itself to evolve. Therfore, it was and is still very important to create the Dispedia-specific forms and workflows to abstract the underlying RDF model for users. In a later state, if the amount of patient information is increased, technologies such as OWL reasoning can be used to improve the conceptual parts of Dispedia Ontologies.

The general architecture will also be improved in the future (cf. Figure 3). Similar to the possibility of interlinking further proposal Ontologies in addition to the actual existing ALS Ontology, we will pursue the idea of decentralizing data in the web also for patients. We have currently only designed one patient knowledge base, which could be outdated when the idea of the WebID for people has been established. When using RDF and OWL as a representation for the different parts of Dispedia, Dispedia can easily be interlinked with multiple decentralized knowledge bases for individual patients.

References

1. Bizer, C., Heath, T., Berners-Lee, T.: Linked data - the story so far. Int. J. Semantic Web Inf. Syst. 5(3), 1–22 (2009)
2. BMBF. Rare diseases (2010), http://www.bmbf.de/en/1109.php
3. Cañas, A.J., Carff, R., Hill, G., Carvalho, M., Arguedas, M., Eskridge, T.C., Lott, J., Carvajal, R.: Concept Maps: Integrating Knowledge and Information Visualization. In: Tergan, S.-O., Keller, T. (eds.) Knowledge and Information Visualization. LNCS, vol. 3426, pp. 205–219. Springer, Heidelberg (2005)

4. Eidt, D., et al.: Maßnahmen zur Verbesserung der gesundheitlichen Situation von Menschen mit Seltenen Erkrankungen in Deutschland, Berlin (2009)
5. Gastl, R., Ludolph, A.C.: Amyotrophe Lateralsklerose. Der Nervenarzt 78, 1449–1459 (2007)
6. Gmez-Prez, A., Benjamins, R.: Overview of knowledge sharing and reuse components: Ontologies and problem-solving methods. In: 16th International Joint Conference on Artificial Intelligence (IJCAI 1999) Workshop KRR5: Ontologies and Problem-Solving Methods: Lesson Learned and Future Trends, Stockholm, Sweden, vol. 18 (1999); IJCAI and the Scandinavian AI Societies. CEUR Workshop Proceedings
7. Heino, N., Dietzold, S., Martin, M., Auer, S.: Developing Semantic Web Applications with the Ontowiki Framework. In: Pellegrini, T., Auer, S., Tochtermann, K., Schaffert, S. (eds.) Networked Knowledge - Networked Media. SCI, vol. 221, pp. 61–77. Springer, Heidelberg (2009)
8. Kalra, D., Beale, T., Heard, S.: The openehr foundation. Stud Health Technol. Inform. 115, 153–173 (2005); Kalra, D., Beale, T., Heard, S.: Netherlands Studies in health technology and informatics. Stud. Health Technol. Inform. 115, 153–173 (2005)
9. Kempf, K.U.: Analyse des Phänotyps von an familiärer amyothropher Lateralsklerose erkrankter Familien ohne Mutation der Superoxid-1-dismutase: Eine Untersuchung zur Vorbereitung von Kopplungsanalysen, Ulm (2006)
10. Kuschel, F.: Die medizinische Versorgung erwachsener Patienten mit Muskelerkrankungen, Berlin (2006)
11. Manola, F., Miller, E.: Rdf primer (2004), http://www.w3.org/TR/rdf-primer/
12. Mitchell, J.D., Borasio, G.D.: Amyotrophic lateral sclerosis. The Lancet 369(9578), 2031 (2007)
13. Musca, G., Cuccurullo, O.: Chronic Heart Failure management program. BMC Geriatrics 10, 1 (2010)
14. Möller, M., Ernst, P., Sintek, M., Biedert, R., Dengel, A., Sonntag, D.: Representing the international classification of diseases version 10 in owl. In: Proc. of KEOD, Spain (2010)
15. Rieß, C., Heino, N., Tramp, S., Auer, S.: EvoPat – Pattern-Based Evolution and Refactoring of RDF Knowledge Bases. In: Patel-Schneider, P.F., Pan, Y., Hitzler, P., Mika, P., Zhang, L., Pan, J.Z., Horrocks, I., Glimm, B. (eds.) ISWC 2010, Part I. LNCS, vol. 6496, pp. 647–662. Springer, Heidelberg (2010), http://svn.aksw.org/papers/2010/ISWC_Evolution/public.pdf
16. Taruscio, D., Seyoum, I.M.: Tackling the problem of rare diseases in public health: the Italian approach. Community Genet. 6, 123–124 (2003)
17. Tramp, S., Heino, N., Auer, S., Frischmuth, P.: RDFauthor: Employing RDFa for Collaborative Knowledge Engineering. In: Cimiano, P., Pinto, H.S. (eds.) EKAW 2010. LNCS, vol. 6317, pp. 90–104. Springer, Heidelberg (2010), http://svn.aksw.org/papers//2010/EKAW_RDFauthor/public.pdf
18. W3C. OWL Web Ontology Language Overview, W3C Recommendation. Online (February 2004), http://www.w3.org/TR/owl-features/
19. WHO. Icf the international classification of functioning, disability and health (2002)
20. WHO. International classification of diseases (icd) (2006)

How Medical Expertise Influences the Understanding of Symptom Intensities – A Fuzzy Approach

Franziska Bocklisch[1], Maria Stephan[1], Barbara Wulfken[1],
Steffen F. Bocklisch[2], and Josef F. Krems[1]

Chemnitz University of Technology,
[1] Cognitive and Engineering Psychology
[2] Systems Theory, 09107 Chemnitz, Germany
franziska.bocklisch@psychologie.tu-chemnitz.de

Abstract. This paper examines the role of imprecision in the interpretation of verbal symptom intensities (e.g., *high* fever) depending on the level of medical expertise. In a contrastive study we compare *low*, *medium* and *high* level experts (medical students vs. physicians with $M = 5.3$ vs. $M = 24.9$ years of experience) concerning their interpretation of symptom intensities. For obtaining and modeling of empirical data a fuzzy approach was used. The resulting fuzzy membership functions (MF) reflect the meanings of the verbal symptom intensities. The two main findings are: (1) with increasing expertise the precision of the MF increase such that *low* level experts have very vague concepts compared to *high* level experts and (2) the precision depends on the symptom (e.g., intensities of *fever* are more precise than *pain* intensities).

Keywords: level of medical expertise, imprecision, fuzzy approach.

1 Introduction

Physicians have to process a huge amount of information. For instance, they deal with the patient's state of health, disease history, diseases, symptoms and their intensities. A variety of studies (see [1] and [2] for reviews) consistently showed the influence of knowledge and knowledge organization on medical decisions. Feltovich and colleagues [1] postulated that novices have rather imprecise clinical expectations compared to medical experts. Expert's knowledge base is assumed to be dense and precise. Boegl and colleagues [3] as well as Seising [4] emphasized that vagueness can be found during the whole process of medical reasoning. Fuzzy MFs are generally considered appropriate for the description of vagueness. Wallsten et al. [5] pointed out that people prefer to use words for communication. The objective of this paper is to explore the imprecision of linguistic terms (LT) such as verbal symptom intensities (e.g., *high* fever) depending on the level of medical expertise (*low* vs. *medium* vs. *high*). We assume that the higher the expertise the more precise the meanings of the LTs are. We use a fuzzy approach [6, 7] to measure and model the LTs. The resulting fuzzy MFs reflect the imprecision of the LTs meanings. Discriminatory power values (*dp*) that based on the MF overlap [6] serve as a measure of distinctiveness of MF.

A. Holzinger and K.-M. Simonic (Eds.): USAB 2011, LNCS 7058, pp. 703–706, 2011.

2   Method

Participants. Ninety-eight participants (35 males) took part in the study. Seventy-one were medical students with completed preliminary medical examination but no remarkable practical experiences (*low* expertise). Thirteen were physicians with *medium* practical expertise ranging between one and twelve years ($M=5.3$ years, $SD=3.7$ years) and fourteen physicians with *high* expertise ranging from sixteen to thirty-two years ($M=23.9$ years, $SD=5.2$ years). The physicians (*medium* and *high* expertise groups) had different areas of specialisation: two were general practitioners, six anaesthetists, two ophthalmologists, one surgeon, five dermatologists, two gynaecologists, five internists, one orthopaedist, one paediatrician, one psychiatrist, and one was urologist. All participants were Germans studying or working in different regions of Germany.

Material and Procedure. The survey instrument was an online questionnaire. It consisted of four descriptions of general medical cases describing symptom pattern that pointed to meningitis and common cold as disease causes. The cases were characterized concerning patient's sex, age, body weight and disease symptoms (e.g., body temperature, pain, blood pressure, CRP-value) and the observed symptom intensities (e.g., *slight* fever, *immense* pain). The main task was to state a diagnosis. A variety of different dependent variables were measured (e.g., confidence in diagnosis, difficulty, diagnostic relevance of symptoms). Here, we only report the results of the translation of the verbal symptom intensities for *slight* and *high* fever as well as *strong* and *immense* pain.

Translation Procedure and Fuzzy Analysis. The verbal symptom intensities were translated using the two-step translation procedure outlined in [7, 8]. In the first step participants estimated three numerical values: (1) the "typical value" that best represented the given symptom intensity, (2) the "minimal value", and (3) "maximal value" that correspond to the given verbal expression. In the second step this data was used to model parametric fuzzy MFs of the potential type. For a detailed description of the translation procedure, the function type and modelling please see [6].

3   Results and Discussion

3.1   Descriptive Statistics

Table 1 presents the descriptive statistics for the empirical estimates of the typical values that correspond to the presented symptom intensities depending on the level of expertise. The minimal and maximal estimates were used for the modelling of the MFs. Body temperatures (fever estimates) are given in °C and pain estimates are based on the pain scale ranging from 0 (no pain) to 10 (extreme pain). Results show that means and standard deviations are almost equal between levels of expertise. The differences between the verbal intensities (approximately 1°C for body temperature or 1 unit on the pain scale) are also very small.

Table 1. Descriptive statistics for the estimates (typical values)

Symptom intensity	Level of Expertise					
	low		medium		high	
	M	SD	M	SD	M	SD
Slight Fever	38.12	0.38	38.23	0.33	38.06	0.46
High Fever	39.69	0.55	39.68	0.42	39.38	0.23
Strong Pain	6.96	1.20	7.08	0.76	7.43	0.85
Immense Pain	8.48	1.00	8.42	0.90	8.77	0.93

3.2 Fuzzy Analysis

Figure 1 shows the MFs for the verbal symptom intensities for fever and pain. The membership represents the value of truth that an object belongs to a specific class. (e.g., the numerical temperature 38 °C belongs to the class *slight* fever).

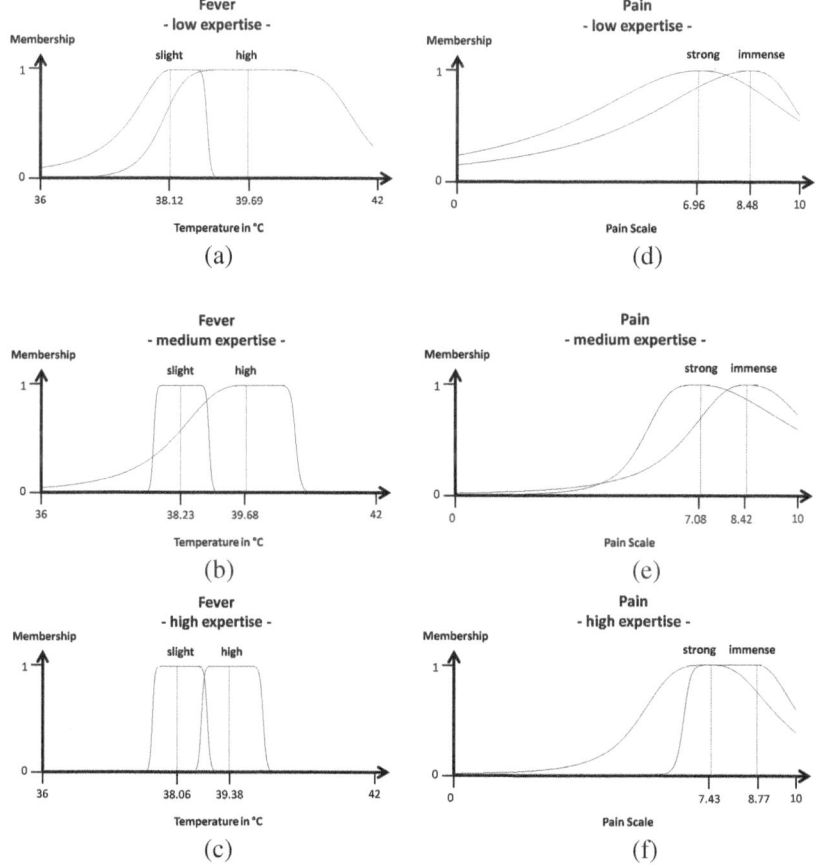

Fig. 1. Membership functions of the verbal symptom intensities (fever and pain)

Figure 1 (a) shows the MFs for *slight* and *high* fever for low level experts. Obviously, the MFs are very broad in shape and overlap very much. This is also evident for pain (see 2 (d)). Medium level experts (2 (b) and (e)) show narrower MFs and high level experts (2 (c) and (f)) the most precise ones. Both symptoms show this pattern of result but it is clearer for fever than for pain. The dp [6] is standardized taking values from 0 (MFs are identical) to 1 (no overlap at all). Therefore, small dp values (< 0.7) represent large overlaps of MFs and high similarity in LT's meanings. Low and medium level experts show smaller dps (low: $dp_{fever} = 0.62$ and $dp_{pain} = 0.16$; medium: $dp_{fever} = 0.58$ and $dp_{pain} = 0.18$) than high level experts ($dp_{fever} = 0.89$ and $dp_{pain} = 0.23$). The MFs of high level experts (slight vs. high fever) are the most distinct ones.

3.3   Discussion

Results show that (1) the vagueness of symptom intensities decreases with increasing medical expertise, (2) the precision of LTs meanings depends on the symptom (intensities of *fever* are more precise than *pain* intensities). These findings are consistent with former results reported in [1] and [8]. They show that medical expertise and the imprecision of medical concepts are related, at least, for some concepts such as verbal symptom intensities. The results have implications for the understanding of medical reasoning processes, for the representation of knowledge in medical decision support systems as well as training and acquisition of medical competence.

References

1. Feltovich, P.J., Johnson, P.E., Moller, J.H., Swanson, D.B.: LCS: the role and development of medical knowledge in diagnostic expertise. In: Clancey, W.J., Shortliffe, E.H. (eds.) Readings in Medical Artificial Intelligence: The First Decade, pp. 275–319 (1984)
2. Patel, V.L., Glaser, R., Arocha, J.F.: Cognition and expertise: aquisition of medical competence. Clinical and Investigative Medicine 23(4), 256–260 (2000)
3. Boegl, K., Adlassnig, K.-P., Hayashi, Y., Rothenfluh, T.E., Leitich, H.: Knowledge acquisition in the fuzzy knowledge representation framework of a medical consultation system. Artificial Intelligence in Medicine 30, 1–26 (2004)
4. Seising, R.: From vagueness in medical thought to the foundations of fuzzy reasoning in medical diagnosis. Artificial Intelligence in Medicine 38, 237–256 (2006)
5. Wallsten, T.S., Budescu, D.V., Zwick, R., Kemp, S.M.: Preferences and reasons for communicating probabilistic information in numerical or verbal terms. Bulletin of the Psychonomic Society 31, 135–138 (1993)
6. Bocklisch, F., Bocklisch, S.F., Krems, J.F.: Sometimes, often and always: Exploring the vague meanings of frequency expressions. Behavior Research Methods (2011), doi:10.3758/s13428-011-0130-8
7. Bocklisch, F., Bocklisch, S.F., Krems, J.F.: How to Translate Words into Numbers? A Fuzzy Approach for the Numerical Translation of Verbal Probabilities. In: Hüllermeier, E., Kruse, R., Hoffmann, F. (eds.) IPMU 2010. LNCS, vol. 6178, pp. 614–623. Springer, Heidelberg (2010)
8. Murphy, G.L., Wright, J.C.: Changes in conceptual structure with expertise: differences between real-world experts and novices. Journal of Experimental Psychology: Learning, Memory and Cognition 10(1), 144–155 (1984)

Older Adults' Perception of Costs and Benefits of Web-Based and Mobile PHR Technologies: A Focus Group Approach

Oliver Sack[1], Richard Pak[2], and Martina Ziefle[1]

[1] Human Technology Centre (Humtec),
RWTH Aachen University, Theaterplatz 14
52062 Aachen, Germany
{sack,ziefle}@humtec.rwth-aachen.de
[2] Richard Pak
Department of Psychology, Clemson University, Clemson, SC, 29634, USA
richpak@clemson.edu

Abstract. The goal of the study was to explore older adults perceived benefits and costs of relatively new personal health records (PHR) technologies: web-based PHRs versus mobile PHRs. Twenty-six older adults (ages 63-79 years) participated in a focus group. The results showed a significantly different cost-benefit relation between the PHR technologies. The results showed that older adults perceived more benefits than costs with web-based PHRs but more balanced costs and benefits with mobile PHRs. These results suggest that the adoption of e-health may be hindered by this lack of perceived benefits relative to costs.

Keywords: e-health, personal health records, older people, perceived costs and benefits, focus group.

1 Introduction

So-called "e-health" tools such as personal health records (PHR) enable patients to manage and share their health information [1]. Due to PHR, health consumers can be more proactive in the management of their health; more so for older adults and with chronic illness. Although older adults may have more difficulty using new technologies [2], it is not accurate that they are resistant to technology adoption. For older adults' adoption of new communication technologies (e.g. mobile phones) the absence of benefits is more influential to the adoption of email and cell phones compared to the perceived costs. Older adult's choices are based on a cost-benefit analysis, before deciding to make an investment [3].

There is currently no study, which has examined the cost-benefit-relationship between different technologies in a PHR context. Our goal was to use focus groups to explore how older adults perceive the benefits and costs of web-based PHRs compared to mobile PHRs.

A. Holzinger and K.-M. Simonic (Eds.): USAB 2011, LNCS 7058, pp. 707–710, 2011.
© Springer-Verlag Berlin Heidelberg 2011

2   Method

2.1   Participants

Twenty-six old participants (14 female and 12 male) took part in focus groups. They ranged in age from 63 to 79 years (M=71, SD=4.9). The participants had extensive computer experience. Although most of the focus group participants were aware of web-based health information tracking using PHRs, the majority were unaware that such information was also available on mobile phones.

2.2   Procedure and Material

In seven focus group sessions participants discussed two ways of accessing and maintaining personal health information: using a web-based system (Google Health website) and a mobile-based system (Google Health as iOS-based application (app) on a mobile device that access a Google Health profile).

After an introduction (e.g. "personal health records".) participants were given demonstrations of the Google Health website and the mobile app. Both systems were shown on a projector. Additionally the mobile system was demonstrated individually to each participant on a mobile phone. After each system demonstration the moderator led a discussion of costs and benefits of each system. Order of system presentation was counterbalanced.

Each system demonstration showed typical PHR usage scenarios based on earlier research [4]. In the discussion of motivational factors, the moderator specifically asked for benefits of using the technology (e.g. "Why might you use the Google Health website?"), followed by expected drawbacks of using the technology (e.g. "Why might you not use the Google Health website?"). Finally, participants were asked to discuss ideas and suggestions about what they would like to add to a hypothetical, ideal technology (a "magic box") to better fit to their needs. Each session was audio-recorded.

2.3   Data Analysis

Transcriptions were analyzed with top-down enforcement of categories. Two independent coders reached an inter-rater reliability of 86% on a sample of the data.

We used a previously developed coding scheme [3] and used the responses of the participants to develop sub-categories of the coding scheme. Comments were coded along two dimensions: (A) the communication technology, which consisted of two levels "web-based PHR" and "mobile PHR" and (B) motivational factor as a consideration for using this method on two levels "benefit" and "cost". Benefit was defined as an advantage or positive statement about using a method (e.g. keep "everything in one place"). Cost was defined as a disadvantage, or negative statement (e.g. "privacy issue"). The subcategories were mutually exclusive and were created from a portion of data. Additionally, we coded "desired features", which were mentioned during the group discussion. Desired features were defined as a missing aspect which would give a benefit e.g. "magic mouse to track out vital parameter" or a negatively stated comment about a benefit e.g. "for me it is not useful".

For the statistical analysis we used the Fisher's exact test of a 2x2 table. The level of significance was set at 5%.

3   Results

3.1   Effects of Communication Technology (Web-Based PHR vs. Mobile PHR) on Cost-benefit Relationship

Perceived costs and benefits for the two communication technologies (web-based PHR vs. mobile PHR) were quantitatively contrasted. In 7 group sessions we gathered 342 comments. Of those, 150 comments were about the web-based application, while 192 comments were about the mobile phone application. The website averaged 5.8 entries per person and cellphone averaged 7.4. Participants, on average, made 12% more statements for the cellphone application than for the website.

The benefits category accounted for 60% of all the comments in comparison to 40% of comments about costs. For the web-based PHR, 66% of comments were about benefits and 34% were about costs. For mobile PHR 55% of comments were about of benefits in comparison to 45% of comments regarding costs.

Fisher exact test showed that the cost-benefit relation within the web-based PHR (benefits: 66%, costs: 34%) is significantly different from the cost-benefit relation within the mobile PHR application (benefits: 55%, costs: 45%) (Fisher's exact test, $p<.05$). Participants mentioned proportionally more benefits than costs for the web-based PHR in comparison to the more balanced cost-benefit-relationship of the mobile PHR.

3.2   Qualitative Analysis of Desired Features

Another technique to understand barriers to technology adoption is to ask what features are missing from existing systems. To that end, we asked our focus group participants to imagine a non-existent technology ("magic box"). Participants imagined what features an ideal technology would have without regard for any technological limitations. Desired features, which were mentioned in each technology, were "medication interaction warnings" and "diagnosis and prognosis". An example which addressed web-based PHR were a `magic computer mouse to track continuous vital parameters". Mentioned desired features for the mobile PHR were "voice commands", "print possibility" or "security password for medicals e.g. in EMS-situations".

4   Discussion

The present study supports the assumption of recent research [3] that older adults tended to associate using a relatively new technology in a PHR context primarily with its benefits. Twenty-six participants mentioned predominantly more benefits than costs for the website. In contrast, the cost-benefit relationship for the cellphone was balanced. This difference between the two systems suggests that our older adults, because of the maturity of web-based tools, are more able to see the benefits versus the costs. However, our highly experienced older participants may have more issues perceiving the unique benefits of mobile health applications compared to the costs. These results suggest that the adoption of e-health may be hindered by this lack of perceived benefits relative to costs.

With the view on the qualitative analysis of the subcategories, we can conclude that our sample of older participants are aware of general PHR related benefits and additionally of the unique characteristics of a communication technology. Whether this finding generalizes to most older adults is a topic for future research.

Further research may compare different age-groups. Although young people do not have as many health issues, they tend to be more familiar with mobile applications. Therefore the cost-benefit relations of both technologies may not differ between age groups. Additionally future research may approach to investigate different cultural effects. The participants in the study were all U.S. citizens.. They might be more familiar with the technologies than other cultures where technology adoption tends to be slower. Furthermore data from this study could be used to help better communicate benefits of this technology to older adults.

Acknowledgement. We thank the older adults, which participated in the study. Additionally we want to thank Margaux Price and Jeremy Mendel for their comments. This research was supported by a Google Research Award to Richard Pak.

References

1. WebMD, http://www.webmd.com/phr
2. Czaja, S.J., Sharit, J.: Age differences in attitudes toward computers. Journal of Gerontology 53B(5), 329–340 (1998)
3. Melenhorst, A.S., Rogers, W.A., Caylor, E.C.: The use of communication technologies by older adults: exploring the benefits from the user's perspective. In: Proceedings of the Human Factors and Ergonomics Society 45th Annual Meeting. Human Factors and Ergonomics Society, Santa Monica (2001)
4. Price, M.M., Pak, R., Müller, H., Stronge, A.: Enhancing the adoption of personal health records by older adults: A qualitative analysis of older user's health information needs and strategies. Poster presented at the biannual Cognitive Aging Conference, Atlanta, G (2010)

Biomedical Informatics: Defining the Science and Its Role in Health Professional Education

Edward H. Shortliffe

AMIA, Bethesda, MD, USA
shortliffe@amia.org

Abstract. There is a growing appreciation that information technology is no longer an option but a necessity in the management of clinical and health information. This imperative has increasingly led to questions regarding the field of biomedical informatics (BMI) and its relationship to health information technology. Emerging in the 1960s from an academic base, with an emphasis on research and education, some 50 years later we see large numbers of applied informatics practitioners as well as both basic and applied researchers in the discipline. The information technology that has emerged from the research environment is now changing the practice of medicine, its financing, and our ability to monitor both health care and the preservation of health in the populace. The scholarly base of the fields still requires nurturing, but its concepts and practical applications are no longer esoteric and require study and incorporation into the knowledge base of all 21st century health professionals.

Keywords: biomedical informatics, health information technology, education, health professionals.

1 Introduction

Medical students, residents, physicians, nurses, and other health professionals today are increasingly savvy about technology. It is a rare young physician who lacks a smart phone, tablet computer, laptop, or desktop computer—some have all of these. Yet this increased computer literacy and routine use of electronic tools does not mean that modern health professionals have a conceptual understanding of the issues that confront those who are attempting to design, implement, or use health information technology to manage patients, conduct clinical research, or promote human health. Physicians use pharmacologic agents in the treatment of patients, practicing applied pharmacology, but we require that they first understand the *science* of molecular pharmacology—topics such as toxicity, drug tolerance, structure-activity relationships, antibiotic resistance, and even modern drug design. By analogy, in the increasingly wired world, where patient data are captured, shared, accessed, and analyzed electronically, there is another science that our health professionals must understand in order to be adequately prepared for the realities of practice: *biomedical informatics*.

A. Holzinger and K.-M. Simonic (Eds.): USAB 2011, LNCS 7058, pp. 711–714, 2011.
© Springer-Verlag Berlin Heidelberg 2011

2   The Scientific Discipline

According to AMIA[1], biomedical informatics (BMI) is defined as "the interdisciplinary field that studies and pursues the effective uses of biomedical data, information,
and knowledge for scientific inquiry, problem solving, and decision making, motivated by efforts to improve human health" [1]. It has a theoretical and methodological base and is closely tied to computer science, communications, and information
science. Extremely broad in its applications scope, ranging from molecules and cells
to individual patients and populations, the field is also closely tied to the behavioral
and social sciences, with major research and educational activities related to cognition, ethics, economics, and organizational theory. Graduate students who are formally trained in BMI are highly multidisciplinary in their perspectives, learning about
computing and communications, basic life sciences, clinical care, epidemiology, decision science, cognitive science, management science, and even some biomedical engineering (notably in the areas of imaging and smart devices). One view of the field
and its terminology is summarized in Figure 1, which outlines the relationship between the basic discipline and its broad areas of application. Note that in this view
bioinformatics is an application domain of BMI and not another name for the field as
a whole. Many people also use the term *health informatics* to refer to applied research and practice in clinical and public health informatics.

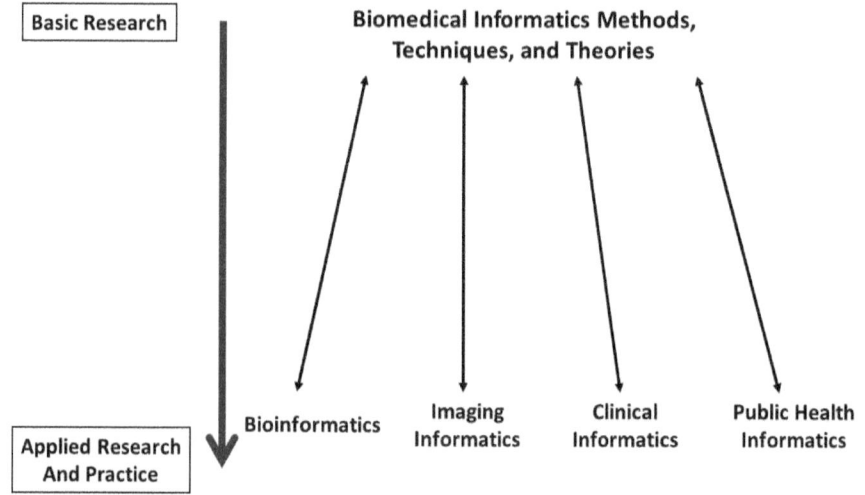

Fig. 1. Biomedical informatics in perspective. Basic work is motivated by needs identified in
one or more of the applied spheres.

---

[1] Formed in 1988 as the American Medical Informatics Association, this professional society is
now known simply as AMIA, thereby deemphasizing the outdated term "medical
informatics".

Many BMI trainees also have health professional training and view informatics as highly relevant to their area of clinical interest and practice. Others come from technical computing backgrounds or other non-health disciplines, learning about the methods of BMI and the cultural and logistical issues involved in their implementation in busy healthcare settings.

Major introductory textbooks are available in the field [2], [3], as are more focused books and peer reviewed journals that capture both the underlying science and its applications [4], [5], [6], [7]. There are professional societies for biomedical informatics in many countries and all regions of the world, with a federation of these organizations, IMIA [8], which holds international scientific meetings biannually that complement the regional- and country-based meetings that occur throughout the world.

There has been explosive growth in the BMI field as reflected in the number of new academic programs at medical schools and health science universities, the increasing numbers of applicants for both graduate degree programs and shorter-term certificate training opportunities, and the growing investments in both research and applied health information technology by many governments.

3   Relationship to Health Information Technology

Early research on electronic health records (EHRs) began in the 1960s, when the power of database technology was being recognized and there were demands to apply the methods in socially useful settings. Those who have watched the evolution of the BMI field can attest to the slow but steady progress that was subsequently made, with the eventual introduction of the first companies that built and sold EHRs for use in hospitals, clinics, and private offices. The penetration of such technologies into routine practice was slow until recently. Progress has been facilitated not only by research but also by the remarkable advancement in computing technology along almost every dimension: cost, power, size, portability, reliability, familiarity.

Thus the health information technology (HIT)[2] of today is a product of decades of research, most of which has been funded by government entities, foundations, and healthcare institutions rather than by the companies themselves. Today there are rich opportunities for synergistic interactions between the research and academic communities in BMI and the more applied development and implementation of systems that is occurring in hospitals and practices. Many HIT workers were trained initially in BMI settings, and the research being pursued by BMI faculty and students is increasingly driven by feedback and insights gleaned by those who are working in HIT settings and can identify clearly the limitations of technologies and capabilities that are currently available.

---

[2] Outside North America, HIT is often referred to as HICT (health information and communications technology). In the US, communications technology is generally viewed as simply one of many information technologies, so the simpler HIT has been used.

4   Implications for Health Professional Education

Given the central role of informatics notions in clinical practice, plus the inevitability of increasing use of, and dependence on, health information technology, many observers have argued that the discipline ought to be taught to all health professionals, including physicians in training, from the preclinical years through graduate medical education and beyond [9]. The Association of American Medical Colleges first called for inclusion of informatics in the medical curriculum in the General Professional Education of the Physician report in 1984 [10], so this is not a new concept. I have argued elsewhere that we are failing to prepare future physicians adequately if we leave BMI and its applications out of the medical curriculum [11], so I will not repeat all those points here. But it is clearly time for health professional schools to embrace BMI as part of the scientific and practical base of what practitioners need to know in order to deliver care and manage disease prevention in the modern world. We have for too long viewed computing and informatics concepts as foreign to the "medical model" that dominates what we teach in medical schools and other health professional training programs.

References

1. Biomedical informatics core competencies,
   http://www.amia.org/biomedical-informatics-core-competencies
   (accessed September 25, 2011)
2. Coeira, E.: Guide to Health Informatics, 2nd edn. Oxford University Press, USA (2003)
3. Shortliffe, E.H., Cimino, J.J. (eds.): Biomedical Informatics: Computer Applications in Health Care and Biomedicine, 3rd edn. Springer, New York (2006)
4. Journal of the American Medical Informatics Association (BMJ Group),
   http://www.jamia.org (accessed September 25, 2011)
5. Journal of Biomedical Informatics (Elsevier),
   http://www.elsevier.com/locate/yjbin (accessed September 25, 2011)
6. International Journal of Medical Informatics (Elsevier),
   http://ees.elsevier.com/ijmi/ (accessed September 25, 2011)
7. Methods of Information in Medicine (Schattauer),
   http://www.schattauer.de/de/magazine/uebersicht/
   zeitschriften-a-z/methods.html (accessed September 25, 2011)
8. International Medical Informatics Association (IMIA), http://www.imia.org (accessed September 25, 2011)
9. Stead, W.W., Searle, J.R., Fessler, H.E., Smith, J.W., Shortliffe, E.H.: Biomedical informatics: Changing what physicians need to know and how they learn. Acad. Med. 86, 429–434 (2011)
10. Association of American Medical Colleges. Physicians for the Twenty-first Century. Report of the Project Panel on the General Professional Education of the Physician and College Preparation for Medicine. J. Med. Educ. 59(11) (part 2), 1-208 (1984)
11. Shortliffe, E.H.: Biomedical informatics in the education of physicians. J. Amer. Med. Assoc. 304(11), 1227–1228 (2010)

Author Index